GARTNER AND HIATT'S

Atlas and Text of

Histology

EIGHTH EDITION

GARTNER AND HIATT'S

Atlas and Text of

Histology

EIGHTH EDITION

Leslie P. Gartner, PhD

Professor of Anatomy (Retired)
Department of Biomedical Sciences
Baltimore College of Dental Surgery
Dental School
University of Maryland
Baltimore, Maryland

Lisa M. J. Lee, PhD

Associate Professor
Department of Cell and Developmental Biology
University of Colorado School of Medicine
Aurora, Colorado

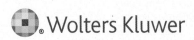

Philadelphia • Baltimore • New York • London
Buenos Aires • Hong Kong • Sydney • Tokyo

Acquisitions Editor: Crystal Taylor
Development Editors: Andrea Vosburgh and Kelly Horvath
Editorial Coordinator: Sean Hanrahan
Editorial Assistant: Parisa Saranj
Marketing Manager: Phyllis Hitner
Production Project Manager: Bridgett Dougherty
Design Coordinator: Stephen Druding
Manufacturing Coordinator: Margie Orzech
Prepress Vendor: S4Carlisle Publishing Services

Eighth edition

9 8 7 6 5 4 3 2 1

Printed in Mexico

Translations:
Chinese (Taiwan): Ho-Chi Book Publishing Company
Chinese (Mainland China): Liaoning Education Press/CITIC
Chinese (Simplified Chinese): CITIC/Chemical Industry Press
French: Wolters Kluwer France
Greek: Parissianos
Indonesian: Binarupa Publisher
Italian: Masson Italia; EdiSES
Japanese: Igaku-Shoin; Medical Sciences International (MEDSI)

Korean: E Public, Co., Ltd
Portuguese: Editora Guanabara Koogan
Russian: Logosphera
Spanish: Editorial Medica Panamericana; Gestora de Derechos Autorales; Libermed Verlag
Turkish: Gunes Bookshops
Vietnamese: Hanoi Medical University

Library of Congress Cataloging-in-Publication Data
Names: Gartner, Leslie P., 1943- author. | Lee, Lisa M. J., author.
Title: Gartner and Hiatt's atlas and text of histology / Leslie P. Gartner, Lisa M.J. Lee.
Other titles: Color atlas and text of histology | Atlas and text of histology
Description: Eighth edition. | Philadelphia: Wolters Kluwer Health, [2023] | Preceded by Color atlas and text of histology / Leslie P. Gartner. Seventh edition. [2018].
Identifiers: LCCN 2021037960 | ISBN 9781975164256 (paperback)
Subjects: MESH: Histology | Atlas
Classification: LCC QM557 | NLM QS 517 | DDC 611/.0180222—dc23
LC record available at https://lccn.loc.gov/2021037960

shop.lww.com

QUADM0322

To my wife Roseann, my daughter Jen, and in loving memory of my parents
–LPG

To my best friend and husband, Suraj Pradhan.

–LMJL

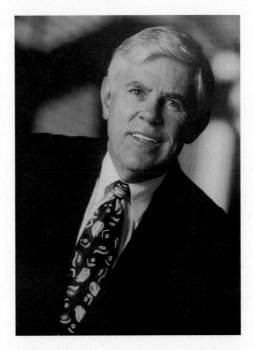

We wish to dedicate the eighth edition of *Gartner and Hiatt's Atlas and Text of Histology* in memory of Dr. James L. Hiatt (1934–2021).

–LPG and LMJL

Reviewers

Faculty

Erin M. Brannick, DVM, MS, ACVP

Associate Professor and Veterinary Anatomic Pathologist
University of Delaware
Newark, Delaware

Rebecca Grandy Brown, MPAS, PA-C

Assistant Coordinator for Physician Assistant Studies
Le Moyne College
Syracuse, New York

Eduard I. Dedkov, MD, PhD

Associate Professor
Cooper Medical School
Rowan University
Camden, New Jersey

Abimbola Farinde, PhD, Pharm D

Professor
Columbia Southern University
Phoenix, Arizona

Kiran Matthews, MD

Director, Anatomical Donor Program
CUNY School of Medicine
City University of New York
New York, New York

Students

Kathryn Hughes, MD

Rush Medical College
Chicago, Illinois

Christine M. Ly

State University of New York
Upstate Medical University
Syracuse, New York

Ramona Mittal

St. George's University
True Blue, Grenada

Preface

Unlike most prefaces, this preface to the eighth edition of *Gartner and Hiatt's Atlas and Text of Histology* is presented in two parts because I, as the senior author, wish to announce how pleased I am to be able to present my new coauthor, Dr. Lisa M. J. Lee, who was kind enough to accept my invitation to join me in this revision of the previous edition. Dr. Lee is a distinguished faculty member of the Department of Cell and Developmental Biology at the University of Colorado School of Medicine, who has taught histology, as well as additional aspects of the anatomical sciences for a number of years. Her many contributions to the current edition are invaluable, and I thank her for all of her hard work in making the eighth edition far better than its predecessors.

Leslie P. Gartner

Dr. Lee and I are very pleased to be able to present the eighth edition of our *Gartner and Hiatt's Atlas and Text of Histology*, an atlas that has been in continuous use since its first publication as a black-and-white atlas in 1987. The success of that atlas prompted us to revise it considerably, retake all of the images in full color, change its name, and publish it in 1990 under the title *Color Atlas of Histology, 3rd edition*. In the past 32 years, the Atlas has undergone many changes. We added color paintings, published a corresponding set of Kodachrome slides, and added histophysiology to the text. The advent of high-resolution digital photography allowed us to reshoot all of the photomicrographs for the fourth edition, and we created a digital resource that accompanied this text. The eighth edition includes the following resources online: over 300 additional photomicrographs with more than 900 interactive fill-in-the-blank questions organized in a fashion to facilitate the student's learning and preparation for practical examinations; approximately 100 USMLE Step 1 style multiple-choice questions based on photomicrographs; and nearly 50 new identification questions based on images featured in the "Tissues That Resemble Each Other" appendix.

We are grateful to the many faculty members throughout the world who have assigned our Atlas to their students whether in its original English or in its translated form that now counts twelve languages. We have received many compliments and constructive suggestions not only from faculty members but also from students, and we tried to incorporate those ideas into each new edition. One suggestion that we have resisted, however, was to change the order of the chapters. There were several faculty members who suggested a number of varied sequences and they all made sense to us and would have been very easy for us to adopt any one of the suggested chapter orders. However, we feel partial to and very comfortable with the classical sequence that we adopted so many years ago; it is just as valid and logical an arrangement as all the others that were suggested and, in the final analysis, instructors can simply tell their students to use the chapters of the Atlas in a different sequence without harming the coherence of the material.

Major changes have been introduced in this eighth edition. We have rewritten the introductory matter to each chapter, added new photomicrographs to the textual material, and we have added new tables for many of the chapters. Each chapter is revised to apply many of the cognitive theory of multimedia learning. It is our hope that these evidence-based pedagogical approaches applied in this edition will enhance learner experience and outcome. We have also enlarged what was the Appendix in the previous edition and is now Chapter 1, which describes and illustrates many of the common stains used in the preparation of histologic specimens. Probably the most exciting change that we have introduced in this edition is the addition of USMLE Step 1 type questions in every chapter, except Chapter 1 (answers to the questions appear on pp. 592–593, in Appendix B). Another feature of this edition is the enlarged chapter, titled "Tissues That Resemble Each Other" (now, Appendix A) where we present tissues that are easily confused with other—similar appearing—structures and describe how to differentiate them from one another.

As in the previous editions, most of the photomicrographs of this Atlas are of tissues stained with hematoxylin and eosin. All indicated magnifications in light and electron micrographs are original magnifications. Many of the sections were prepared from plastic-embedded specimens, as noted. Most of the exquisite electron micrographs included in this Atlas were kindly provided by our colleagues throughout the world as identified in the legends.

This Atlas has been written with the student in mind, and thus the material is complete but not esoteric. We wish to help the student learn and enjoy histology, not be overwhelmed by it. Furthermore, this Atlas is designed not only for use in the laboratory but also as preparation for both didactic and practical examinations. Although we have attempted to be accurate and complete, we know that errors and omissions may have escaped our attention. Therefore, we welcome criticisms, suggestions, and comments that could help improve this Atlas; please address them to LPG21136@yahoo.com.

Leslie P. Gartner
Lisa M. J. Lee

Acknowledgments

We would like to thank Todd Smith for the rendering of the outstanding full-color plates and thumbnail figures, Jerry Gadd for his paintings of blood cells, and our many colleagues who provided us with electron micrographs. We are especially thankful to Dr. Stephen W. Carmichael of the Mayo Medical School for his suggestions concerning the suprarenal medulla, Dr. Cheng Hwee Ming of the University of Malaya Medical School for his comments on the distal tubule of the kidney, and Dr. Matthijs Valstar of the Stichting Het Nederlands Kanker Instituut - Antoni van Leeuwenhoek Ziekenhuis for his two photomicrographs of his newly discovered tubarial salivary glands. Additionally, we are grateful to our good friends at Wolters Kluwer, including our most wonderful senior acquisitions editor, Crystal Taylor, who has been instrumental in launching not only this but several previous editions of this book; Andrea Vosburgh, our development editor who also worked on the seventh edition of this Atlas; Kelly Horvath, the best, kindest, and most efficient freelance editor one can wish for; Sean Hanrahan, editorial coordinator who kept the project going in a timely fashion, making sure that we adhered to all the deadlines; Parisa Saranj, editorial assistant; and Jen Clements, art designer.

Finally, we wish to thank our families for encouraging us during the preparation of this work. Their support always makes the labor an achievement.

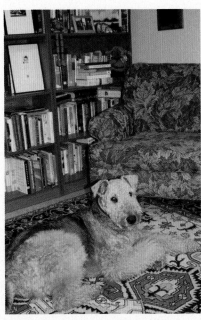

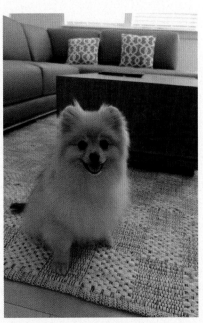

Although it has been stated that writing is a lonely profession, I have been very fortunate in having the company of my faithful Airedale Terrier, Skye, who, as is evident in the accompanying photograph, kept me company as I was sitting at my computer. It is with a sad heart that I have to add that my sweet Skye died between the completion of the manuscript and the publication of the Atlas.

–LPG

I share Dr. Gartner's love of canine family members. Like him, I have been very fortunate to have the company of my loving and playful Pomeranian, Phoebe, while working on this text during the particularly challenging period of global pandemic and unrest.

–LMJL

Contents

INTRODUCTION TO HISTOLOGIC TECHNIQUES

The modern scope of histology is the study of cells, tissues, and organs of the body by magnification techniques involving various types of microscopy. The only available technique up to the mid-20th century was the use of optical microscopy that used natural and, later, electrically produced light as the illumination source. But, in the 1950s, transmission electron microscopy (TEM) that used electrons as a light source was invented. Somewhat later, scanning electron microscopy (SEM) was developed, as well as other forms of illumination that permitted visualization of structures and even of functions of cells, organs, and organ systems. Because an *Atlas and Text of Histology* presents images procured mostly by light microscopy, TEM, and SEM, only these techniques are described.

Light Microscopy

The light microscopic study of cells, tissues, and organs requires that the material to be examined be sectioned thinly enough to permit light or electrons to penetrate it and that the light be sufficient to be collected by the lenses of the microscope and to reach the retina of the examiner. Moreover, the tissue must maintain its natural, living characteristics; otherwise, the viewer will have a distorted image of the tissue. Over the years, numerous procedures were developed and refined to ensure a close resemblance between the image under the microscope and the properties of the tissue during its living state. These procedures include fixation, dehydration, clearing, embedding, sectioning, mounting, staining, and the affixing of a coverslip over the tissue section.

- **Fixation** is the use of chemicals that inhibit tissue necrolysis and prevent alteration of its normal morphology. For light microscopy, the fixative of choice is neutral buffered formalin, although many other fixatives are commonly used.

- **Dehydration** and **clearing** are accomplished using an increasing concentration of ethanol (from 50% to 100%) followed by a clearing agent such as xylene to make the tissue transparent and miscible with an embedding material.

- **Embedding** is the process that permeates the tissue with an agent, such as **paraffin** or a **plastic polymer**, to make it firm enough to be sliced into sections (**sectioning**) thin enough to be transparent to visible light. Tissues embedded in paraffin are usually sectioned 5 to 10 μm in thickness, whereas those embedded in plastic are sectioned much thinner (0.1 μm or less). Many other embedding media and sectioning techniques are also available.

- Sections obtained from paraffin or plastic blocks are **mounted** on glass slides coated with an adhesive material, such as albumin, to ensure that the sections adhere to the glass slides.

- **Staining** of the sections is necessary because the optical densities of the various tissue elements are so similar that they are indistinguishable from one another without being treated with various dyes. Because many of the stains used are water miscible (i.e., capable of being mixed with water without becoming separated), the sections must be deparaffinized and rehydrated before they can be stained.

- The stained sections are once again dehydrated and are made permanent by placing and affixing a **coverslip** over the tissue section.

Terminology of Staining for Light Microscopy

Commonly, when staining histologic sections, a **principal stain** is used in conjunction with a **counterstain**, a contrasting color that stains those components of the tissue that are not stained well with the principal stain. Usually, the stains are either **acidic (anionic)** or **basic (cationic)** and are attracted to those components of the cell or tissue that are basic or acidic, respectively. Therefore, the acidic components of the cell, such as nucleic acids, attract the basic stains and are said to be **basophilic**. Those components of the cell whose pH is greater than pH 7, such as many cytoplasmic proteins, attract acidic stains and are said to be **acidophilic**.

Common Stains Used in Histology

Although a great number of histologic and histopathologic stains have been developed, only the most commonly used stains are listed in this chapter (Figs. 1-1 to 1-14).

Transmission Electron Microscopy

Transmission electron microscopes, unlike light microscopes, use electron beams as their light source. Because electrons have a negative charge, it is possible to use electromagnets to focus and spread the electron beams in a manner analogous to the use of glass lenses in compound light microscopy. Because the resolving power of a microscope is indirectly dependent on the wavelength of the light source, the much shorter wavelength of electrons provides TEM a 1,000-fold greater resolving power than that of a light microscope (0.2 nm vs. 200 nm).

The basic processing techniques for TEM are the same as for light microscopy; however, the tissue samples must be much smaller—no larger than 1 mm^3—because the fixatives and the heavy metal stains do not penetrate as well as those of light microscopy. Additionally, the tissues must be embedded in a much harder embedding material, namely epoxy resins (e.g., epon and araldite), and the sections must be much thinner, usually between 25 and 100 nm so that the electrons are not absorbed by the embedding material. The sections, procured by glass or diamond knives, are placed on perforated copper disks.

The electron microscope generates a high-energy electron beam within an evacuated chamber, and the beam is spread and then focused on the specimen by electromagnets; additional electromagnets focus the electrons onto a fluorescent plate. As the electrons interact with the tissue stained with heavy metal, they lose some of their kinetic energy. As they hit the fluorescent plate, their kinetic energy is converted into points of light. The more kinetic energy the electron lost in its interaction with the heavy metal–stained tissue, the less light is produced as the electron impinges on the fluorescent plate; therefore, the image on the fluorescent screen is due to the various intensities of light produced by the interaction of the electrons with the fluorescent plate. The image may be captured by replacing the fluorescent screen with an electron-sensitive film that captures a photographic record of the image or by a charge-coupled sensor that captures a digital record of the image.

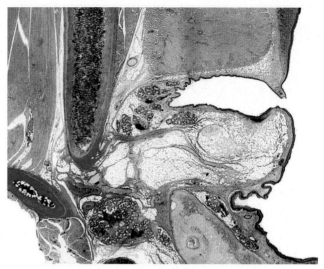

FIGURE 1-1. Hematoxylin and eosin.

Hematoxylin, in conjunction with the counterstain eosin, is one of the most commonly used stains in histologic and histopathologic preparations. Hematoxylin is a basic stain that dyes nuclei, nucleoli, and ribosomes blue to purple in color. Eosin stains basic components of the cell, including myofilaments of muscle, pink to light red in color. Red blood cells stain orange to bright red in color. Additionally, extracellular matrix proteins, such as collagen, are also stained pink to light red.

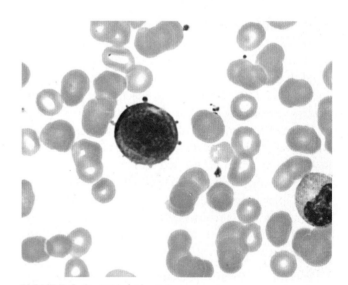

FIGURE 1-2. Wright's stain.

Wright's stain and the related Giemsa's stain are designed specifically for staining blood cells. It stains erythrocytes salmon pink; nuclei of leukocytes and granules of platelets stain dark blue to purple, whereas the specific granules of eosinophils stain salmon pink and those of basophils stain dark blue to black. The cytoplasm of lymphocytes and monocytes stain light blue.

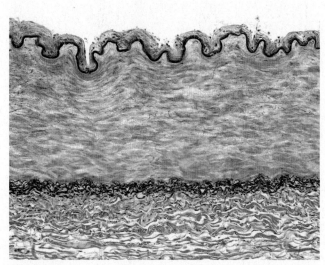

FIGURE 1-3. Weigert's method for elastic fibers and elastic van Gieson's stain.

Weigert's method and van Gieson's stain for elastic fibers are both commonly used to stain elastic fibers. They both dye elastic fibers dark blue to black. Because nuclei also stain dark gray to black, the fibroblasts present among the elastic fibers are very difficult to see.

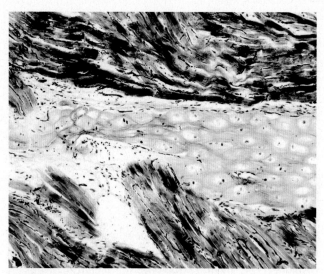

FIGURE 1-5. Iron hematoxylin.

Iron ammonium sulfate is a mordant (used to ensure strong adherence of the hematoxylin to the tissue), permitting very good visualization of cell membranes and membrane complexes, such as terminal bars, cross-striations of skeletal and cardiac muscle, and intercalated disks of cardiac muscle.

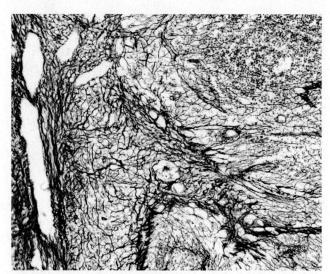

FIGURE 1-4. Silver stain.

Silver stain uses silver salts in solution, which precipitate out as silver metal on the surfaces of type III collagen fibers (reticular fibers), staining them black. Some cells, such as diffuse neuroendocrine (DNES) cells, also stain with silver stains and are called argentaffin or argyrophilic cells. Their granules stain brown to black with silver stains.

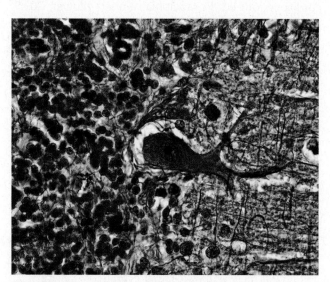

FIGURE 1-6. Bielchowsky's silver stain.

Bielchowsky's stain uses silver salts to permeate the tissue and then the silver is reduced so that it stains dendrites and axons black. The surrounding tissues are golden brown-yellow with a tinge of red in the cytoplasm and black nucleoli.

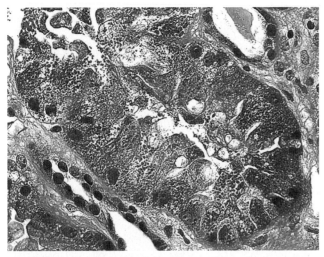

FIGURE 1-7. Masson trichrome.

As the name implies, this stain produces three colors and is used to differentiate collagen of connective tissues from muscle and other cell types. Depending on the variant used, collagen is stained blue or green, muscle cells red, cytoplasm of nonmuscle cells pink to light red, and nuclei stain black. (Reprinted with permission from Mills SE, et al., eds. *Sternberg's Diagnostic Surgical Pathology*, 6th ed. Philadelphia: Wolters Kluwer, 2015. p. 1893, Figure 41-22.)

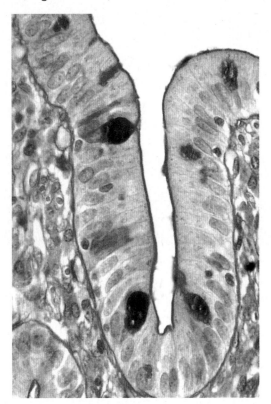

FIGURE 1-8. Periodic acid–Schiff reaction (PAS).

PAS reaction stains glycogens, glycoproteins, mucins, and glycolipids. Thus, basement membranes stain pinkish red, whereas mucins of goblet cells and mucous salivary glands stain a deep red to magenta. (Reprinted with permission from Mills SE, ed. *Histology for Pathologists*, 5th ed. Philadelphia: Wolters Kluwer, 2020. p. 619, Figure 23-8.)

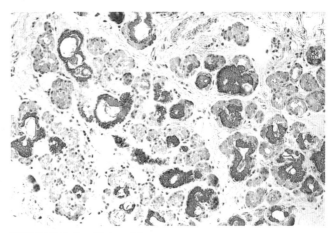

FIGURE 1-9. Alcian blue.

Alcian blue is specific for staining mucins, glycoproteins, and the matrix of cartilage blue in color, whereas the cytoplasm stains a light pink and nuclei stain red. (Reprinted with permission from Mills SE, ed. *Histology for Pathologists*, 5th ed. Philadelphia: Wolters Kluwer, 2020. p. 408, Figure 14-24.)

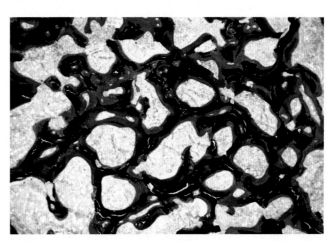

FIGURE 1-10. Von Kossa stain.

Von Kossa stain uses silver salts that become reduced to demonstrate calcification and calcified tissues, which stain black. (Reprinted with permission from Strayer DS, et al., eds. *Rubin's Pathology: Mechanisms of Human Disease*, 8th ed. Philadelphia: Wolters Kluwer, 2020. p. 1359, Figure 30-26.)

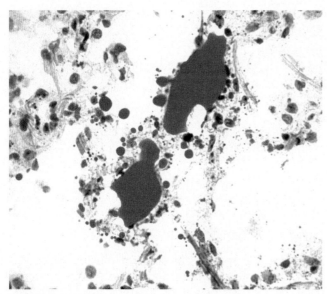

FIGURE 1-11. Sudan red.

Sudan red is used to stain lipids, phospholipids, lipoproteins, and triglycerides, all of which stain an intense red with this dye. (Reprinted with permission from Strayer DS, et al., eds. *Rubin's Pathology: Mechanisms of Human Disease*, 8th ed. Philadelphia: Wolters Kluwer, 2020. p. 336, Figure 7-24B.)

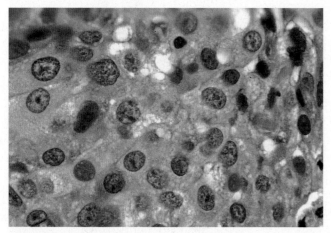

FIGURE 1-12. Mucicarmine stain.

As its name implies, mucicarmine is used to localize mucin, which stains a deep red color. The cytoplasm appears light, salmon pink; nuclei are stained bluish-black; and connective tissue is stained yellowish orange. (Reprinted with permission from Strayer DS, et al., eds. *Rubin's Pathology: Mechanisms of Human Disease*, 8th ed. Philadelphia: Wolters Kluwer, 2020. p. 757, Figure 18-85D.)

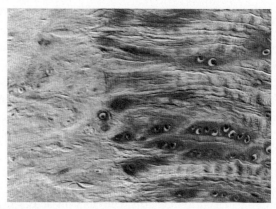

FIGURE 1-13. Safranin-O.

Safranin-O is used to localize granules of mast cells, cartilage matrix, and mucin of goblet cells, all of which stain orange to red. Nuclei appear dark blue to black. (Reprinted with permission from Mills SE, ed. *Histology for Pathologists*, 5th ed. Philadelphia: Wolters Kluwer, 2020. p. 120, Figure 5-18C.)

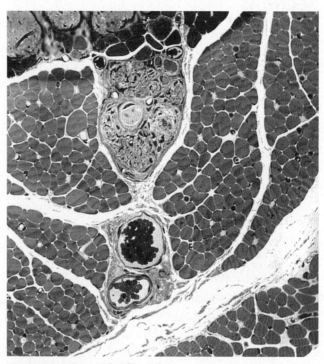

FIGURE 1-14. Toluidine Blue.

Toluidine blue is a metachromatic stain in that it changes color with specific substances, such as the granules of mast cells and cartilage matrix, both of which stain reddish purple. It acts as a normochromatic stain in that acidic components of the cell, such as ribosomes and nuclei, stain blue. Toluidine blue is especially useful in staining thin, plastic-embedded tissue sections. (Reprinted with permission from Mills SE, ed. *Histology for Pathologists*, 5th ed. Philadelphia: Wolters Kluwer, 2020. p. 176, Figure 7-12.)

Scanning Electron Microscopy

Instead of capturing images of ultrathin sections, SEM provides a three-dimensional image of the surface of a solid object that was coated with an exceptionally thin layer of metal (such as gold or palladium). An electron beam is directed at the specimen in an evacuated chamber, and the electrons that are not absorbed by the specimen but are reflected back (backscatter electrons), as well as those electrons that are dislodged from the heavy metal coat of the specimen (secondary electrons), are captured by electron detectors. The electron detectors are coupled to a computer that collates and interprets the image thus gained and displays it on a monitor and that can also capture the image on a photographic film or capture it digitally.

Interpreting Microscopic Sections

An image produced by a light or by a transmission electron microscope, is, in effect, a two-dimensional (2D) section procured from a three-dimensional (3D) object. The task of the viewer is to reconcile the 2D image with the actual structure of the 3D object. This is a difficult task that takes time and perseverance on the part of the student. The following three images—sections from three familiar objects: a hardboiled egg without its shell (Fig. 1-15), a lemon (Fig. 1-16), and a coiled garden hose (Fig. 1-17)—permit the student to understand how these 2D images may be compiled mentally to provide the correct 3D structure.

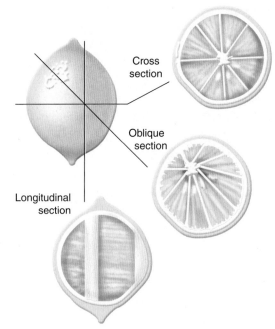

FIGURE 1-16. Lemon in cross, oblique, and longitudinal sections.

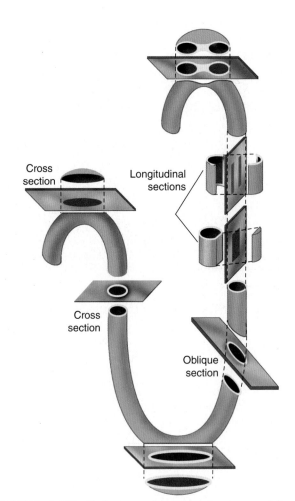

FIGURE 1-17. Coiled garden hose in cross, oblique, and longitudinal sections.

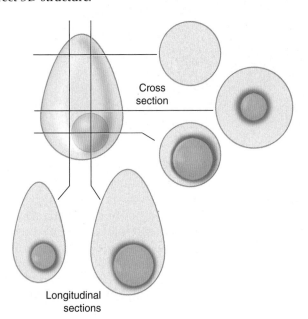

FIGURE 1-15. Hardboiled egg without its shell in cross and longitudinal sections.

CELL BIOLOGY

Cells not only constitute the basic units of the human body but also function in executing all activities the body requires for survival. Although there are more than 200 different cell types, most cells possess common features that permit them to perform their varied responsibilities. The living component of the cell is known as the **protoplasm**, and the nonliving components are known as **inclusions**. The cell is bounded by a **plasmalemma** (**cell membrane, plasma membrane**) and houses the nucleus, which is enclosed by the **nuclear envelope** (Fig. 2-1). The portion of the protoplasm located between the plasmalemma and the nuclear envelope is the **cytoplasm**, whereas the portion of the protoplasm confined by the nuclear envelope is the **nucleoplasm**. The cell possesses distinct metabolically active structures, the **organelles**, many of which are composed of membranes similar to but not identical with the plasmalemma.

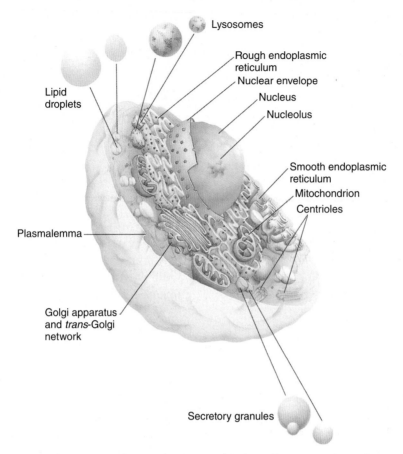

FIGURE 2-1. Schematic illustration of the cell and its organelles.

Plasmalemma

The semipermeable **plasmalemma** is a phospholipid bilayer that provides a selective, structural barrier between the cell and the outside world. The functions of **plasma membrane** include the following:

- cell–cell recognition;
- exocytosis and endocytosis;
- as receptor sites, such as **G proteins** (Table 2-1), for signaling molecules; and
- as initiators and controllers of the secondary messenger system.

Table 2-1	Functions and Examples of Heterotrimeric G Proteins	
Type	**Function**	**Examples**
G_s	Activates adenylate cyclase, leading to the formation of cAMP thus activating protein kinases	Binding of epinephrine to β-adrenergic receptors increases cAMP levels in the cytosol
G_i	Inhibits adenylate cyclase, preventing the formation of cAMP, thereby protein kinases are not activated	Binding of epinephrine to α_2-adrenergic receptors decreases cAMP levels in cytosol
G_q	Activates phospholipase C, leading to formation of inositol trisphosphate and diacylglycerol, permitting the entry of calcium into the cell that activates protein kinase C	Binding of antigen to membrane-bound IgE causes the release of histamine (and other preformed agents) by mast cells
G_o	Opens K^+ channels, allowing potassium to enter the cell and closes Ca^{2+} channels, thereby calcium movement in or out of the cell is inhibited	Inducing contraction of smooth muscle
G_{olf}	Activates adenylate cyclase in olfactory neurons, which open cAMP-gated sodium channels	Binding of odorant to G protein–linked receptors initiates generation of nerve impulse
G_t	Activates cGMP phosphodiesterase in rod cell membranes, leading to hydrolysis of cGMP resulting in the hyperpolarization of the rod cell plasmalemma	Photon activation of rhodopsin causing rod cells to fire
$G_{12/13}$	Activates Rho family of GTPases, which control the formation of actin and the regulation of the cytoskeleton	Facilitating cellular migration

cAMP, cyclic adenosine monophosphate; cGMP, cyclic guanosine monophosphate; IgE, immunoglobulin E.

The plasmalemma bilayer consists of an inner and an outer leaflet of phospholipids; the **inner leaflet** is in contact with the cytoplasm, and the **outer leaflet** faces the extracellular space. **Phospholipids** are amphipathic molecules with a polar head and two short fatty acid nonpolar tails. The polar, hydrophilic heads face the membrane surfaces; the nonpolar, hydrophobic tails of each leaflet project into the internal aspect of the membrane, facing each other, and form noncovalent bonds that hold the two leaflets together. Cholesterol, peripheral proteins, and integral proteins are embedded in the phospholipid membrane.

Materials may enter (**endocytosis**) or leave (**exocytosis**) the cell through the plasmalemma by several means. They may enter via:

- **pinocytosis** (nonspecific uptake of molecules in an aqueous solution),
- **receptor-mediated endocytosis** (specific uptake of substances, such as low-density lipoproteins), or
- **phagocytosis** (uptake of particulate matter).

Cytoplasm

The major component of the cytoplasm is a fluid, the **cytosol**, in which the cell's organelles, cytoskeleton, and inclusions are suspended. The cytosol is composed mostly of water in which various organic and inorganic substances are either dissolved or suspended.

Mitochondria

Mitochondria are composed of a smooth outer and folded inner membrane separated from each other by the **intermembrane space**. The folded inner membrane, rich in the phospholipid **cardiolipin**, forms flat, shelf-like structures known as **cristae** (that are tubular in steroid-manufacturing cells) and encloses a viscous fluid-filled space known as the **matrix space** (Fig. 2-2). Almost all mitochondria are derived from the ovum; spermatozoa contribute only a very limited amount of mitochondria to the offspring.

Mitochondria **generate ATP** (adenosine triphosphate) utilizing a chemiosmotic coupling mechanism that employs a specific sequence of enzyme complexes and proton translocator systems (**electron transport chain** and the ATP-synthase containing **elementary particles**) embedded in their cristae; they **generate** heat in **brown fat** instead of producing ATP, and they assist in the **synthesis** of certain **lipids** and **proteins** (Fig. 2-3; also see Fig. 2-1).

Mitochondria possess the enzymes of the **tricarboxylic acid** (TCA) **cycle (Kreb's cycle)**, **mitochondrial DNA (mtDNA)**, and matrix granules in their matrix space. The

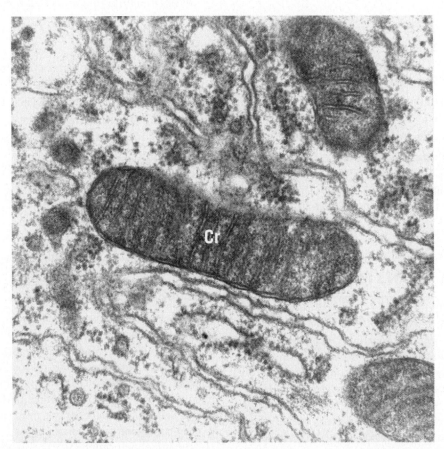

FIGURE 2-2. Transmission electron micrograph of several mitochondria. Note that their outer membranes are smooth, whereas their inner membranes are folded to form cristae (Cr). ×39,700.

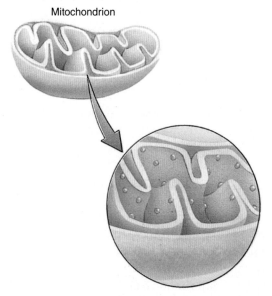
Mitochondrion

FIGURE 2-3. Mitochondria synthesize adenosphine triphospahte (ATP) and lipids; elementary particles couple oxidation to phosphorylation.

mtDNA possesses only a small number of genes; most of the genes required for the functioning and reproduction of mitochondria are located in the chromosomes of the nucleus. Mitochondria increase in number by undergoing binary fission.

Ribosomes

Ribosomes are small, bipartite, nonmembranous macromolecular assemblies that exist as individual particles that do not coalesce with each other until protein synthesis begins (Fig. 2-4 and Fig. 2-5; also see Fig. 2-1). The two subunits are of unequal size and constitution: the large subunit is 60S and the small subunit 40S (Table 2-2). Each subunit is composed of proteins and rRNA, and, together, they function as an interactive "workbench" that not only provides a surface upon which protein synthesis occurs but also acts as a catalyst that facilitates the synthesis of proteins.

Endoplasmic Reticulum

The **endoplasmic reticulum (ER)**, tortuous, membrane-enclosed spaces shaped into tubules, sacs, and flattened compartments, occupies much of the intracellular space (Fig. 2-5; also see Figs. 2-1 and 2-4). Members of **ER-shaping protein families** form the framework responsible for the specific configurations of the ER. The two types are smooth and rough.

- **Smooth endoplasmic reticulum (SER)** functions in the synthesis of **cholesterols** and **lipids**, as well as in the **detoxification** of certain drugs and toxins (e.g., barbiturates and alcohol). Additionally, in striated muscle cells, this organelle is specialized to sequester and release calcium ions and thus regulate muscle contraction and relaxation (Fig. 2-6).
- **Rough endoplasmic reticulum (RER)**, whose cytoplasmic surface possesses receptor molecules for ribosomes and signal recognition particles (SRPs; known as **ribophorins** and **docking protein**, respectively), is continuous with the **outer nuclear membrane**. The RER functions in the **synthesis** and **modification of proteins** that are to be **packaged**, as well as in the synthesis of membrane lipids and proteins.

Golgi Apparatus

The **Golgi apparatus (complex)** is composed of a specifically oriented cluster of vesicles, tubules, and flattened membrane-bounded cisternae. Each Golgi complex has a convex entry face, known as the *cis* face closer to the nucleus, a concave exit face, known as the *trans* face oriented toward the cell membrane; between the *cis* face and the *trans* face are several intermediate cisternae known as the **medial face** (Figs. 2-7 and 2-8; also see Figs. 2-1 and 2-5).

CLINICAL CONSIDERATIONS 2-1

Leber Hereditary Optic Neuropathy

Leber hereditary optic neuropathy (LHON), one of the inherited mitochondrial diseases, is caused by mutations in mtDNA and transmitted mostly to male offspring, but females can also be affected. It is characterized by loss of vision due to the deterioration of axons and cell bodies of the ganglion cells of the retina. Usually, the vision begins to deteriorate at an early age in one eye followed by vision decline in the other eye within 2 months. Currently, no effective treatment exists, although the administration of estrogen has shown considerable improvement in some patients. Additionally, clinical trials are underway to attempt the reversal of LHON using mitochondrial gene therapy as well as by administering cardiolipin-stabilizing agents that protect mitochondria from the toxic effects of oxygen-containing free radicals formed during oxidative metabolism of mitochondria.

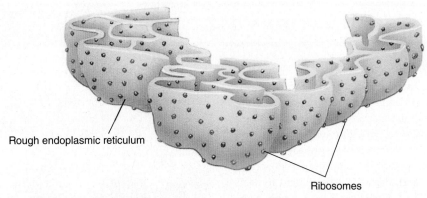

Rough endoplasmic reticulum

Ribosomes

FIGURE 2-4. Ribosomes.

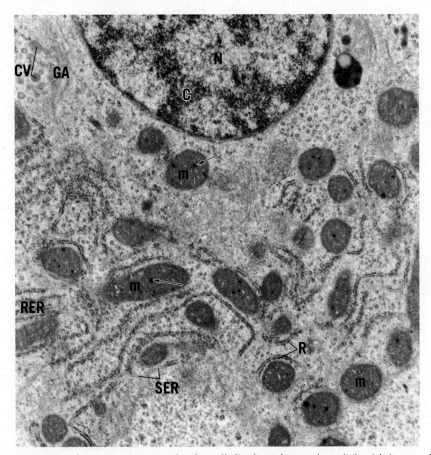

FIGURE 2-5. This transmission electron micrograph of a cell displays the nucleus (N) with its condensed chromatin (c) as well as many cytoplasmic organelles. Note that the mitochondria (m) have electron-dense matrix granules (*arrows*) scattered in the matrix of the intercristal spaces. The perinuclear area presents the Golgi apparatus (GA), which is actively packaging material in condensing vesicles (CV). The rough endoplasmic reticulum (RER) is obvious because of the presence of its ribosomes (R), whereas the smooth endoplasmic reticulum (SER) is less obvious. × 10,300.

Table 2-2	Ribosome Composition		
Subunit	Size	Number of Proteins	Types of rRNA
Large	60S	49	5S
			5.8S
			28S
Small	40S	33	18S

rRNA, ribosomal ribonucleic acid; S, Svedberg unit.

Membrane Trafficking

Substances such as **secretory products** may leave the cell by one of two means:

• **Constitutive secretion**, using non–clathrin-coated vesicles, is the **default pathway** that does not require an extracellular signal for release; thus, the secretory product (e.g., procollagen) leaves the cell in a continuous fashion.

CLINICAL CONSIDERATIONS 2-2

Hydropic Swelling

When cells that become injured, by coming into contact with toxins, are placed in areas of low or high temperature or low-oxygen concentration, or are being exposed to various inimical conditions, their cytoplasm swells and takes on a pale appearance. This characteristic is usually reversible and is called hydropic swelling. Usually, the nuclei occupy their normal position and their organelle content remains unaltered, but here the organelles are located farther away from each other and the cisternae of their ER are dilated.

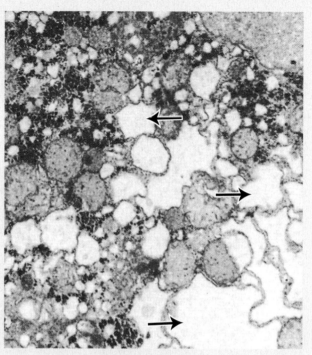

An electron micrograph of a liver with hydropic swelling shows enlarged cisternae (*arrows*) of the endoplasmic reticulum that causes the liver cells to be swollen. (Reprinted with permission from Strayer DS, et al., eds. *Rubin's Pathology: Mechanisms of Human Disease*, 8th ed. Philadelphia: Wolters Kluwer, 2020. Figure 1-2B.)

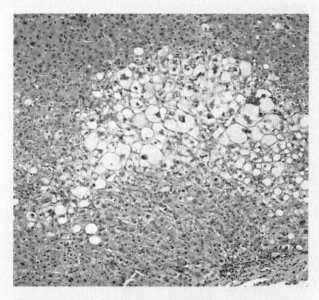

This light photomicrograph of a liver of a patient with toxic hepatic injury shows hydropic swelling. Note that the affected cells are enlarged with accumulations of fluid, but the nuclei of most cells appear to be at their normal location. The cells at the periphery seem to be healthy. (Reprinted with permission from Strayer DS, et al., eds. *Rubin's Pathology: Mechanisms of Human Disease*, 8th ed. Philadelphia: Wolters Kluwer, 2020. p. 3, Figure 1-1.)

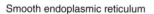
Smooth endoplasmic reticulum

FIGURE 2-6. Smooth endoplasmic reticulum.

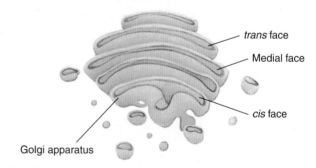
trans face
Medial face
cis face
Golgi apparatus

FIGURE 2-7. Golgi apparatus.

- **Regulated secretion** requires the presence of clathrin-coated storage vesicles whose contents (e.g., pancreatic enzymes) are released only after the initiation of an extracellular signaling process.

The fluidity of the plasmalemma is an important factor in the processes of membrane function, including **membrane trafficking**, a process that conserves the membrane as it is transferred through the various cellular

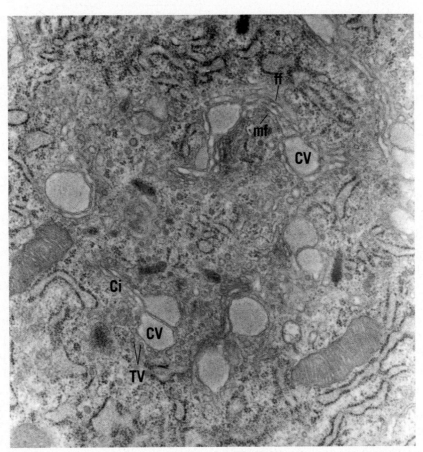

FIGURE 2-8. The extensive Golgi apparatus of this secretory cell presents several flattened membrane-bound **cisternae** (Ci), stacked one on top of the other. The convex face (*cis* face) (ff) receives **transfer vesicles** (TV) derived from the rough endoplasmic reticulum. The concave, ***trans*-Golgi network** (mf) releases **condensing vesicles** (CV), which house the secretory product. (Reprinted with permission from Gartner LP, et al. A fine-structural analysis of mouse molar odontoblast maturation. *Acta Anat (Basel)* 1979;103(1):16–33. Copyright © 1979 Karger Publishers, Basel, Switzerland.) ×18,500.

CLINICAL CONSIDERATIONS 2-3

Hereditary Hemochromatosis

Excessive iron storage in hereditary hemochromatosis, if left untreated, can be a lethal disorder. The individual absorbs too much iron, which accumulates in the parenchymal cells of vital organs such as the liver, pancreas, and heart. Because it may affect organs in different sequence, the symptoms vary and diagnosis may be difficult. Testing the blood levels for high concentration of ferritin and transferrin can provide definitive diagnosis, which can be confirmed by genetic testing. As this is a hereditary disorder, the close relatives of the positive individual should also undergo genetic testing.

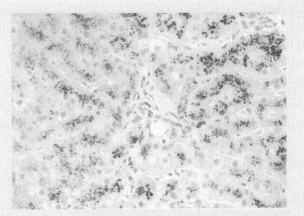

In the case of the liver displayed in this photomicrograph of a Prussian blue–stained specimen, the lysosomes of hepatocytes are congested by large accumulations of iron (appearing as small, granular deposits). (Reprinted with permission from Strayer DS, et al., eds. *Rubin's Pathology: Mechanisms of Human Disease,* 8th ed. Philadelphia: Wolters Kluwer, 2020. Figure 1-4F.)

compartments during endocytosis and exocytosis (see Fig. 2-1, Fig. 2-9, and Fig. 2-10). The degree of fluidity is influenced

- directly by temperature and the degree of unsaturation of the fatty acyl tails of the membrane phospholipids and

- indirectly by the amount of cholesterol present in the membrane.

Ions and other hydrophilic molecules are incapable of passing through the lipid bilayer; however, small nonpolar molecules, such as oxygen and carbon dioxide, as well as uncharged polar molecules, such as water and glycerol, all diffuse rapidly across the lipid bilayer, although special water transporter channels, known as **aquaporins**, specialize in facilitating the very rapid movement of water molecules in and out of the cell. Specialized multipass integral proteins, collectively known as **membrane transport proteins**, function in the transfer of substances such as ions and hydrophilic molecules across the plasmalemma. The two types of such proteins are ion channels and carrier proteins. Transport across the cell membrane may be

- **passive** down an ionic or concentration gradient (**simple diffusion**);

- **facilitated diffusion** via ion channel or carrier proteins (no energy required); or

- **active**, only via carrier proteins; these require the expenditure of energy because the transport is usually against an energy gradient.

Ion channel proteins possess an aqueous pore and may be **ungated** or **gated**. Ungated ion channels are always open, whereas gated ion channels require the presence of a stimulus (alteration in voltage, mechanical stimulus, presence of a ligand, G protein, neurotransmitter substance, etc.) that opens the gate. **Ligands** and **neurotransmitter substances** are types of signaling molecules. **Signaling molecules** are either hydrophobic (lipid soluble) or hydrophilic and function in cell-to-cell communication.

- **Hydrophobic signaling molecules** diffuse through the cell membrane to activate **intracellular messenger systems** by binding to receptor molecules located either in the cytoplasm or in the nucleus.

- **Hydrophilic signaling molecules** initiate a specific sequence of responses by binding to **receptors** (integral proteins) embedded in the cell membrane.

Carrier proteins, unlike ion channels, can permit the passage of molecules with or without the expenditure of energy. If the material is to be transported against a concentration gradient, then carrier proteins can utilize ATP-driven methods or sodium ion concentration differentials to achieve the desired movement. Unlike ion

channels, the materials to be transported bind to the carrier protein. The materials may be transported

- individually (**uniport**) or

- in concert with another molecule (**coupled transport**), and the two substances may travel

- in the same direction (**symport**) or

- in opposite directions (**antiport**).

Role of Golgi Apparatus in Protein Modification and Packaging

The Golgi complex not only **packages** but also **modifies** macromolecules synthesized on the surface of the RER. Newly synthesized proteins pass from the region of the RER, known as the **transitional endoplasmic reticulum**, to the **vesicular-tubular cluster (VTC)** by **transfer vesicles** whose membrane is covered by the **protein coatomer II (COPII)** and are, therefore, also known as **coatomer II–coated vesicles**. From the VTC, the proteins are delivered to the *cis*-Golgi network, probably via **coatomer I–coated vesicles (COPI-coated vesicles)**. The proteins continue to travel to the *cis*-, medial-, and *trans* faces of the Golgi apparatus (most probably) by COPI-coated vesicles (or, according to some authors, via cisternal maturation). Lysosomal oligosaccharides are phosphorylated in the VTC and/or in the *cis* face; mannose groups are removed, and galactose and sialic acid (**terminal glycosylation**) are added in the medial face; whereas selected amino acid residues are phosphorylated and sulfated in the *trans* face.

Sorting and the final **packaging** of the macromolecules are the responsibility of the *trans*-**Golgi network (TGN)**. Mannose 6-phosphate receptors in the TGN recognize and package enzymes destined for lysosomes. These **lysosomal enzymes** leave the TGN in clathrin-coated vesicles. **Regulated secretory proteins** are separated and are also packaged in clathrin-coated vesicles. **Membrane proteins** and proteins destined for constitutive (unregulated) transport are packaged in non–clathrin-coated vesicles (Fig. 2-10).

It should be noted that material can travel through the Golgi complex in an **anterograde fashion**, as just described, as well as in a **retrograde fashion**, which occurs in situations such as when escaped proteins that are residents of the RER or a particular Golgi face have to be returned to their compartments of origin in COPI-coated vesicles.

Protein Synthesis

Protein synthesis requires the code-bearing messenger RNA (mRNA), amino acid-carrying tRNAs, and ribosomes (Figs. 2-11 through 2-14). Proteins that will not be packaged are synthesized on **ribosomes** in the cytosol, whereas **noncytosolic proteins** (secretory, lysosomal, and membrane proteins) are synthesized on ribosomes on the **rough endoplasmic reticulum**. The complex of mRNA and ribosomes is referred to as a **polysome**.

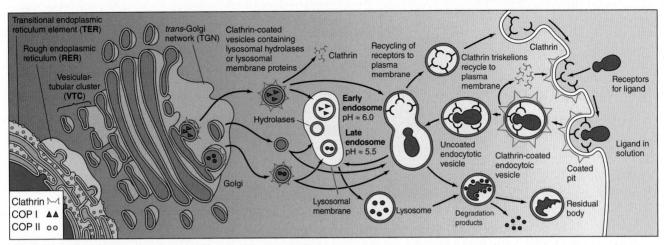

FIGURE 2-9. Schematic diagram of membrane trafficking.

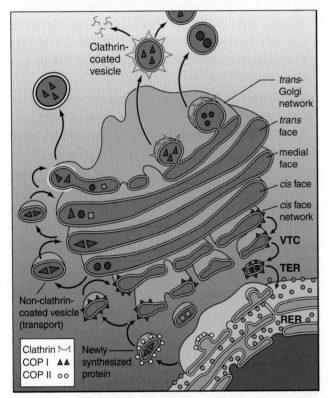

FIGURE 2-10. Schematic diagram of the modification and packaging of the newly formed protein that is to be packaged for exocytosis. RER, rough endoplasmic reticulum; TER, transitional endoplasmic reticulum element; VTC, vesicular-tubular cluster.

The code for the amino acid sequence of proteins and the site for its synthesis is housed in the chromosomes of the nucleus, where the DNA code is transcribed into mRNA. As the mRNA leaves the nucleus and enters the cytoplasm, it associates with the small subunit of a ribosome. The small subunit has a binding site for mRNA as well as three binding sites (A, P, and E) for tRNAs.

1. Once the initiation process is completed, the **start codon** (AUG for the amino acid methionine) is recognized, and the **initiator tRNA** (bearing methionine) is attached to the **P site** (peptidyl-tRNA-binding site), the large subunit of the ribosome, which has corresponding A, P, and E sites, becomes attached to the small subunit, and protein synthesis can begin (Fig. 2-11).

2. The next codon is recognized by the proper acylated tRNA, which then binds to the **A site** (aminoacyl-tRNA-binding site). Methionine is uncoupled from the initiator tRNA (at the P site) and a **peptide bond** is formed between the two amino acids (forming a **dipeptide**) so that the tRNA at the P site loses its amino acid and the tRNA at the A site now has two amino acids attached to it (Fig. 2-12). The formation of this peptide bond is catalyzed by **peptidyl transferase**, an enzyme that belongs to the large ribosomal subunit.

3. As the peptide bond is formed, the large subunit shifts in relation to the small subunit and the attached tRNAs wobble just enough to cause them to move a little bit, so that the initiator tRNA (the one that lost its amino acid at the P site) moves to the **E site** (exit site), and the tRNA that has two amino acids attached to it moves from the A site to the P site. Thus, the A site becomes empty (Fig. 2-13).

4. As this shifting occurs, the small ribosomal subunit moves the space of a single codon along the mRNA, so that the two ribosomal subunits are once again aligned with each other and the A site is located above the next codon on the mRNA strand (see Fig. 2-13).

5. As a new tRNA with its associated amino acid occupies the A site (assuming that its anticodon matches the newly exposed codon of the mRNA), the initiator RNA drops off the E site, leaving the ribosome. The dipeptide is uncoupled from the tRNA at the P site, and a peptide bond is formed between the dipeptide and the new amino acid, forming a tripeptide.

6. The empty tRNA again moves to the E site to fall off the ribosome, as the tRNA bearing the tripeptide moves from the A site to the P site. In this fashion, the peptide chain is elongated to form the coded protein (see Fig. 2-13).

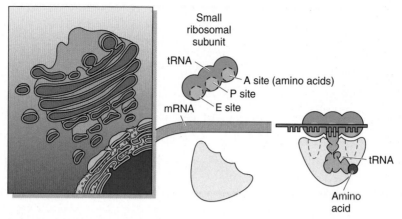

FIGURE 2-11. Protein synthesis step 1: ribosome assembly.

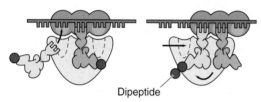

FIGURE 2-12. Protein synthesis step 2: peptide bond formation.

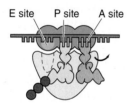

FIGURE 2-13. Protein synthesis steps 3 to 5: movement of tRNA and tripeptide formation.

If a protein is to be inserted into the plasmalemma, is destined for lysosomes, or is to be packaged for export out of the cell, it follows the procedures depicted by the **signal hypothesis**. The synthesis of the protein begins in the cytosol, on the ribosomes, but the first 20 to 30 amino acid sequence forms the signal peptide, which is recognized by cytosol-resident proteins, known as **signal recognition particles (SRPs)**.

1. SRP binds to the signal protein, inhibits the continuation of protein synthesis, and the entire polysome proceeds to the RER (Fig. 2-14).

2. A **signal recognition particle receptor**, a transmembrane protein located in the membrane of the RER, recognizes and properly positions the polysome.

3. The docking of the polysome results in the movement of the SRP–ribosome complex to the **protein translocator**, a pore-forming complex, which creates a pore in the RER membrane.

4. The large subunit of the ribosome binds to and forms a tight seal with the protein translocator, aligning the pore in the ribosome with the pore formed by the protein translocator.

5. The SRP and its receptor leave the polysome, permitting protein synthesis to resume, and the forming protein chain can enter the RER cisterna through the aqueous channel that was created by the protein translocator.

6. During this process, the enzyme **signal peptidase**, located in the RER cisterna, cleaves signal peptide from the growing polypeptide chain and protein synthesis continues.

7. Once protein synthesis is complete, the two ribosomal subunits fall off the RER, the pore in the RER membrane closes, and the ribosomal subunits return to the cytosol (Fig. 2-15).

8. The newly synthesized protein is modified in the RER by glycosylation as well as by the formation of disulfide bonds, which transforms the linear protein into a globular form (Fig. 2-16).

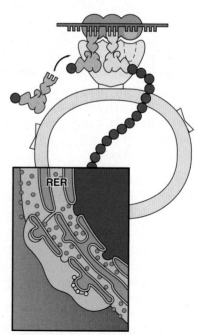

FIGURE 2-14. Polysome docking. RER, rough endoplasmic reticulum.

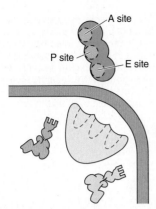

FIGURE 2-15. Ribosomal subunits return to cytosol once protein synthesis is complete.

Endosomes

Endosomes are intermediate compartments within the cell, utilized in the destruction of endocytosed, phagocytosed, or autophagocytosed materials as well as in the formation of lysosomes. Endosomes possess **proton pumps** in their membranes, which pump H$^+$ into the endosome, thus acidifying the interior of this compartment.

The process of endocytosing specific ligands can be accelerated when receptors, designed to recognize these ligands, are assembled on the cell membrane. Receptors permit the endocytosis of a much greater concentration of ligands than would be possible without receptors. This process is referred to as **receptor-mediated endocytosis** and involves the formation of a **clathrin-coated endocytic vesicle**, which, once within the cell, sheds its clathrin coat and fuses with an **early endosome** (Fig. 2-17).

- **Early endosomes** are located at the periphery of the cell and contain receptor–ligand complexes. Their acidic contents (pH 6) are responsible for the uncoupling of receptors from ligands. The receptors are usually carried into a system of tubular vesicles, the **recycling endosomes**, from which the receptors are returned to the plasmalemma, whereas the ligands are translocated to late endosomes located deeper in the cytoplasm.

- **Late endosomes** have an even more acidic content (pH 5.5). Many investigators have suggested that early endosomes mature into late endosomes by the fusion of vesicles with one another as well as with late endosomes that have been formed earlier.

Lysosomes

Lysosomes are formed by the utilization of **late endosomes** as an intermediary compartment. Both lysosomal membranes and lysosomal enzymes are packaged in the TGN and are delivered in separate **clathrin-coated vesicles** to late endosomes, forming **endolysosomes**, which then mature to become **lysosomes** (see Fig. 2-9 and Fig. 2-17).

These membrane-bound vesicles, whose proton pumps are responsible for their very acidic interior (pH 5.0), contain various **hydrolytic enzymes** that function in **intracellular digestion**.

- These enzymes degrade certain macromolecules as well as phagocytosed particulate matter (**phagolysosomes**) and autophagocytosed material (**autophagolysosomes**).

- Frequently, the indigestible remnants of lysosomal degradation remain in the cell, enclosed in vesicles referred to as **residual bodies** or **lipofuscin**.

- The lysosomal membrane maintains its integrity possibly because the luminal aspects of the membrane proteins are glycosylated to a much greater extent than those of other membranes, thus preventing the degradation of the membrane.

Peroxisomes

Peroxisomes are membrane-bounded organelles housing **oxidative enzymes** such as **urate oxidase**, D-**amino acid oxidase**, and **catalase**. These organelles function in the

- formation of free radicals (e.g., superoxides), which destroy various substances;

- protection of the cell by degrading hydrogen peroxide by catalase; and

- **detoxification** of certain toxins and elongation of some fatty acids during **lipid synthesis**.

CLINICAL CONSIDERATIONS 2-4

Lysosomal Storage Diseases

Certain individuals suffer from lysosomal storage diseases, which involve a hereditary deficiency in the ability of their lysosomes to degrade the contents of their endolysosomes. One of the best-characterized examples of these diseases is **Tay-Sachs disease** that occurs mostly in children whose parents are descendants of Northeast European Jews. Because the lysosomes of these children are unable to catabolize GM2 gangliosides, owing to hexosaminidase deficiency, their neurons accumulate massive amounts of this ganglioside in endolysosomes of ever-increasing diameters. As the endolysosomes increase in size, they obstruct neuronal function, and the child dies by the third year of life.

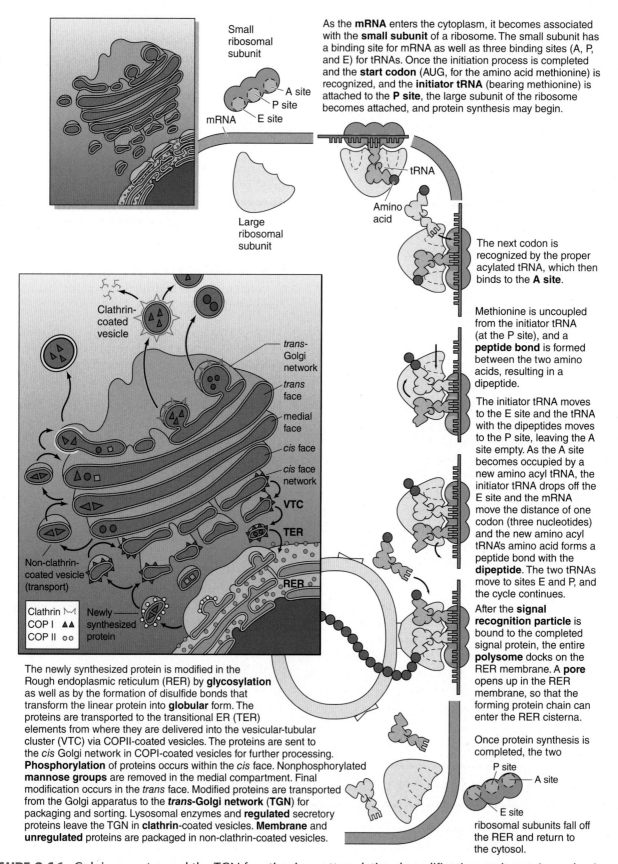

Small ribosomal subunit

A site
P site
E site

mRNA

Large ribosomal subunit

As the **mRNA** enters the cytoplasm, it becomes associated with the **small subunit** of a ribosome. The small subunit has a binding site for mRNA as well as three binding sites (A, P, and E) for tRNAs. Once the initiation process is completed and the **start codon** (AUG, for the amino acid methionine) is recognized, and the **initiator tRNA** (bearing methionine) is attached to the **P site**, the large subunit of the ribosome becomes attached, and protein synthesis may begin.

tRNA

Amino acid

The next codon is recognized by the proper acylated tRNA, which then binds to the **A site**.

Methionine is uncoupled from the initiator tRNA (at the P site), and a **peptide bond** is formed between the two amino acids, resulting in a dipeptide.

The initiator tRNA moves to the E site and the tRNA with the dipeptides moves to the P site, leaving the A site empty. As the A site becomes occupied by a new amino acyl tRNA, the initiator tRNA drops off the E site and the mRNA move the distance of one codon (three nucleotides) and the new amino acyl tRNA's amino acid forms a peptide bond with the **dipeptide**. The two tRNAs move to sites E and P, and the cycle continues.

After the **signal recognition particle** is bound to the completed signal protein, the entire **polysome** docks on the RER membrane. A **pore** opens up in the RER membrane, so that the forming protein chain can enter the RER cisterna.

Once protein synthesis is completed, the two

P site
A site
E site

ribosomal subunits fall off the RER and return to the cytosol.

Clathrin-coated vesicle

trans-Golgi network

trans face

medial face

cis face

cis face network

VTC

TER

RER

Non-clathrin-coated vesicle (transport)

Clathrin
COP I
COP II

Newly synthesized protein

The newly synthesized protein is modified in the Rough endoplasmic reticulum (RER) by **glycosylation** as well as by the formation of disulfide bonds that transform the linear protein into **globular** form. The proteins are transported to the transitional ER (TER) elements from where they are delivered into the vesicular-tubular cluster (VTC) via COPII-coated vesicles. The proteins are sent to the *cis* Golgi network in COPI-coated vesicles for further processing. **Phosphorylation** of proteins occurs within the *cis* face. Nonphosphorylated **mannose groups** are removed in the medial compartment. Final modification occurs in the *trans* face. Modified proteins are transported from the Golgi apparatus to the ***trans*-Golgi network** (TGN) for packaging and sorting. Lysosomal enzymes and **regulated** secretory proteins leave the TGN in **clathrin**-coated vesicles. **Membrane** and **unregulated** proteins are packaged in non-clathrin-coated vesicles.

FIGURE 2-16. Golgi apparatus and the TGN function in posttranslational modification and protein packaging.

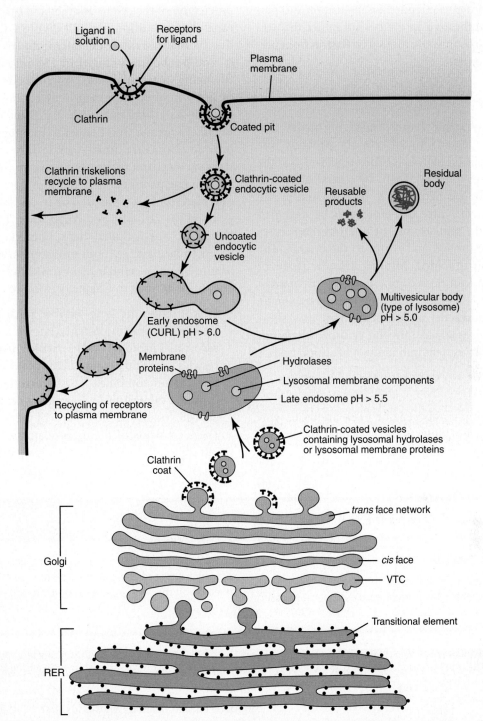

FIGURE 2-17. Receptor-mediated endocytosis of a ligand (e.g., low-density lipoprotein) and the lysosomal degradative pathway. Clathrin triskelions quickly recycle back to the cell membrane. The receptors and ligands then uncouple in the early endosome (compartment for uncoupling of receptors and ligands [CURL]), which is followed by recycling of receptors back to the cell membrane. The late endosome is the primary intermediate in the formation of lysosomes (e.g., multivesicular bodies). Material that is phagocytosed or organelles that undergo autophagy do not use the early endosomal pathway. RER, rough endoplasmic reticulum; VTC, vesicular-tubular cluster. (Reprinted with permission from Gartner LP. *BRS Cell Biology and Histology*, 8th ed. Philadelphia: Wolters Kluwer, 2019. Figure 1-12.)

Most of the proteins intended for inclusions into peroxisomes are synthesized in the cytosol rather than on the RER. All peroxisomes are formed by **fission** from pre-existing peroxisomes.

Proteasomes

Proteasomes are small, barrel-shaped organelles that function in the degradation of cytosolic proteins. The process of cytosolic proteolysis is highly regulated, and the candidate protein must be tagged by several **ubiquitin** molecules before it is permitted to be destroyed by the proteasome system. Once the protein to be degraded begins to enter the proteasome, the ubiquitin molecules detach from the protein and return to the cytosol. The protein becomes unfolded, forming a linear chain of amino acids that can be accommodated by the narrow lumen of the proteasome. Within the lumen, enzymatic degradation reduces the amino acid chain into short peptides that are released into the cytosol, where enzymes further cleave them into individual amino acids.

Cytoskeleton

The **cytoskeleton** is composed of a filamentous array of proteins that act not only as the structural framework of the cell but also to **transport** material within it from one region of the cell to another and provide it with the capability of **motion** and cell division. Components of the cytoskeleton include **microtubules** (consisting of α- and β-tubulins arranged in 13 protofilaments); **thin filaments** (**actin filaments**, **microfilaments**, composed of actin monomers arranged in a double helix); and **intermediate filaments** with the diameter between the microtubules and thin filaments. Intermediate filaments provide a structural framework to the cell and assist in resisting mechanical stresses placed on cells (Table 2-3). Thin filaments function in the movement of cells from one place to another as well as in the movement of regions of the cell with respect to itself. **Thick filaments** (**myosin**), not included here, interact with thin filaments to facilitate cell movement either along a surface or movement of cellular regions with respect to the cell. They are described in Chapter 7, Muscle.

- **Microtubules** are long, hollow, polar structures that are associated with proteins, known as **microtubule-associated proteins** (**MAPs**), which permit organelles, vesicles, and other components of the cytoskeleton to bind to microtubules. Most microtubules originate from **the microtubule-organizing center** (MTOC) of the cell, located in the vicinity of the Golgi apparatus. These elements of the cytoskeleton are pathways for intracellular translocation of organelles and vesicles;

CLINICAL CONSIDERATIONS 2-5

Zellweger Disease

Zellweger disease is an inherited autosomal-recessive disorder that interferes with normal peroxisomal biogenesis.

Characteristics include renal cysts, hepatomegaly, jaundice, hypotonia of the muscular system, and cerebral demyelination resulting in psychomotor retardation.

Table 2-3	Major Intermediate Filaments	
Type	**Location**	**Function**
Keratin	Epithelial cells / Cells of hair and nails	Support; tension bearing; withstands stretching; associated with desmosomes, hemidesmosomes, and tonofilaments; immunologic marker for epithelial tumors
Vimentin	Mesenchymal cells, chondroblasts, fibroblasts, endothelial cells	Structural support, forms cage-like structure around nucleus; immunologic marker for mesenchymal cell tumors
Desmin and vimentin	Muscle: skeletal, smooth, cardiac	Link myofibrils to myofilaments; desmin is an immunologic marker for tumors arising in muscle
GFAP and vimentin	Astrocytes, oligodendrocytes, Schwann cells, and neurons	Support; GFAP is an immunologic marker for glial tumors
Neurofilaments	Neurons	Support of axons and dendrites; immunologic marker for neurologic tumors
Lamins A, B, and C	Line nuclear envelopes of all cells	Organize and assemble nuclear envelope; maintain organization of nuclear chromatin

GFAP, glial fibrillary acidic protein.

CLINICAL CONSIDERATIONS 2-6

Giant Axonal Neuropathy

Giant axonal neuropathy (GAN) is a recessive hereditary condition resulting in the presence of very large, poorly functioning axons. This condition is recognizable even in very young children because of their ambulatory problems. As the child ages, other symptoms become evident, such as lack of muscle strength and neuromuscular coordination, followed by poor reflexes and ataxia. Later in life, intellectual function declines, as well as eyesight and hearing. Few patients with GAN live into their early 30s. Interestingly, most patients with GAN have very tightly curled hair.

during cell division, chromosomes are moved into their proper locations. Two important MAPs, **kinesin** and **dynein**, are motor proteins that facilitate anterograde and retrograde intracellular vesicular and organelle movement, respectively. The **axonemes** of cilia and flagella, as well as a framework of centrioles, are formed mostly of microtubules.

- **Thin filaments** are polar structures, 7 nm in diameter that, similar to microtubules, are able to vary their length via the intermediary of **actin-binding proteins**. Thin filaments function in the movement of nonmuscle cells, in the attachment of cells to the extracellular matrix, epithelial folding during embryogenesis, and structural maintenance of some microvilli. In muscle cells, they interact with myosin to affect the contraction of muscle cells.

- **Intermediate filaments** are 8 to 10 nm in diameter and have structural supportive functions in the cytoplasm as well as in the nucleus. The molecular building blocks of intermediate filaments are diverse and tissue specific; thus, they can be useful markers of tissue origin in metastatic tumors.

Inclusions

Cytoplasmic **inclusions**, such as **lipids**, **glycogen**, **secretory granules**, and **pigments**, are also consistent constituents of the cytoplasm. Many of these inclusions are transitory in nature, although some pigments (e.g., **lipofuscin**) are permanent residents of certain cells.

Nucleus

The **nucleus** is enclosed by the **nuclear envelope**, composed of an **inner** and an **outer nuclear membrane** with an intervening **perinuclear cistern** (Fig. 2-18; also see Fig. 2-5). The inner nuclear membrane is supported by a complex of four types of nuclear intermediate filaments (lamins A, B_1, B_2, and C), collectively known as **nuclear lamins**. The outer nuclear membrane is studded with **ribosomes** and is continuous, in places, with the **rough endoplasmic reticulum**. In areas the inner and outer nuclear membranes fuse with each other, forming circular perforations in the nuclear envelope, known as **nuclear pores**. These perforations of the nuclear envelope are guarded by the assembly of a large number of proteins,

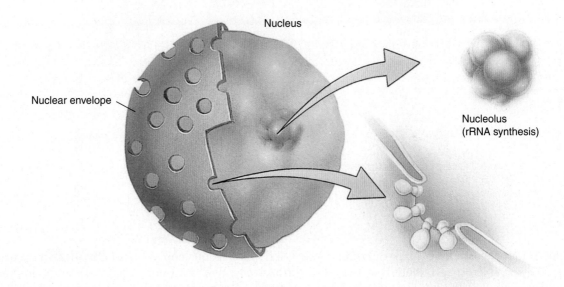

Nucleus

Nuclear envelope

Nucleolus
(rRNA synthesis)

Nuclear pore complex

FIGURE 2-18. Nucleus and the nuclear pore complex.

nucleoporins, which, together with the perforations, are known as **nuclear pore complexes**. They provide passive as well as regulated passageways for the movement of materials in and out of the nucleus. Substances that are less than 9 to 11 nm in diameter can usually enter and leave the nucleus passively. Molecules larger than 9 to 11 nm in diameter require transporter proteins known as **exportins** and **importins** that can identify specific polypeptide signals indicating "permission" to traverse the nuclear pore.

The bulk of the nucleus is composed of a viscous fluid that houses **chromosomes** and nuclear particles such as interchromatin and perichromatin granules. The nucleus is the location of **DNA, mRNA and tRNA synthesis**.

Nucleolus

The **nucleolus**, present in cells only during the interphase (cells that are not in the process of cell division), is located within the nucleus but is not surrounded by a membrane. Some cells have only a single nucleolus, whereas other cells have multiple nucleoli. Nucleoli are assembled around the regions of chromosomes that house the genes for rRNA, known as the **nucleolar organizing regions** (NORs) of the chromosomes. Additional genes of the NOR include those that code for SRPs and the enzyme RNA polymerase I, necessary for rRNA synthesis.

The nucleolus is also the site of assembly of ribosomal proteins and rRNA into the small and large subunits of **ribosomes** (Fig. 2-19). The two types of ribosomal subunits leave the nucleus and enter the cytosol separately.

Chromatin and Chromosomes

The double helix DNA and its associated histone and nonhistone proteins that are suspended in the nucleus are referred to as **chromatin**. Most of the chromatin is partially wound, making it unavailable for translation; this inactive chromatin, referred to as **heterochromatin**, presents under the light microscope as basophilic clumps of material at the periphery of the nucleus. Approximately 10% of chromatin is completely unwound, is available for transcription, and is known as **euchromatin**. It is invisible with the light microscope, thus appearing as pale-staining areas within the nucleus, but with high-resolution transmission electron microscopy

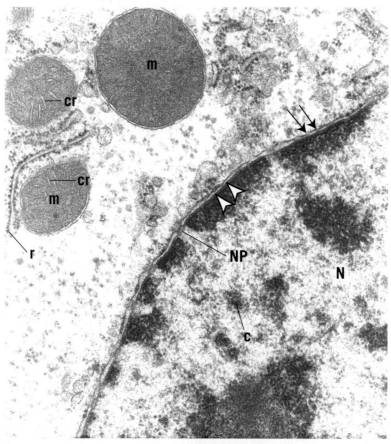

FIGURE 2-19. The **nucleus** (N) of this mouse liver cell displays its nucleoplasm and **chromatin** (c) to advantage in this electron micrograph. Note that the inner (*arrowheads*) and the outer (*double arrow*) membranes of the nuclear envelope fuse in areas to form **nuclear pores** (NP). The rough endoplasmic reticulum is richly endowed by **ribosomes** (r). Note the presence of **mitochondria** (m) whose double membrane and cristae (cr) are quite evident. ×22,100.

(TEM), it resembles a string of pearls, 10 nm in width. DNA, the string, instead of piercing each histone complex, the pearl, wraps twice around the pearl and continues on to do the same for each consecutive pearl. Each "pearl" is comprised of four pairs of histone proteins, the **nucleosome** (H_2A, H_2B, H_3, and H_4). The DNA string between adjacent nucleosomes is known as the **link DNA** (2.5 nm in width). An additional histone, H_1, is responsible for folding the 10-nm wide nucleosome sequence into 30-nm filaments that constitute the heterochromatin. Because euchromatins are the DNA regions available for transcription, the amount of euchromatin versus heterochromatin in the nucleus can be an indicator of cellular activity: A mostly euchromatic nucleus may indicate that the cell has high transcription activity, and coupled with punctate or duplicate nucleoli, may indicate high translation activity as well. A mostly heterochromatic nucleus may indicate that the cell has low transcription activity.

Chromosomes are formed from tightly wrapped and precisely arranged 30-nm nucleosome sequences that are formed in preparation for **mitosis** or **meiosis**. Each species has a precise **genome** consisting of an explicit number of chromosomes. The human genome is composed of 23 pairs of chromosomes, including a single pair of sex chromosomes and 22 pairs of autosomes. The genetic sex of an individual is determined by the sex chromosomes, with XX representing a female and XY male.

Cell Cycle

The **cell cycle** is the sequence of processes that occurs in a cell from the end of one cell division to the next. The cell cycle is governed by the cell cycle control system that not only

---

CLINICAL CONSIDERATIONS 2-7

Cancer

Recent studies have suggested that most **cancers** arise not from mutations in individual genes but from the formation of aneuploidy (abnormal number of chromosomes). In fact, within the same tumor, the chromosomal configurations of individual cells vary greatly and the DNA content of the cells may be 50% to 200% of the normal somatic cell. Interestingly, in the apparently chaotic reshuffling and recombination of chromosomes in cancer cells, there appears to be an order, as in Burkitt lymphoma, in which chromosomes 3, 13, and 17 usually displayed translocations and chromosomes 7 and 20 were usually missing segments.

CLINICAL CONSIDERATIONS 2-8

Genital Herpes Infection

One of the most common sexually transmitted diseases, **herpes simplex virus** (**HSV-2, genital herpes**) is the infection of the cervix (although **HSV-1**, usually associated with cold sores on the lips and, occasionally, the eyes, can also be a causative factor). Usually, HSV infection displays the presence of painful blisters that discharge a clear fluid, form a scab within a week or so, and disappear. During this episode, the genital area in females is painful and urination may be accompanied by a burning feeling. However, if the affected region is the cervix or the vagina, the pain may be much less severe. When the blisters break, the fluid within them is filled with HSV and the individual is infectious. Subsequent to the outbreak of the blistering, the virus retreats along nerve fibers into the ganglion and remains there until the next episode. HSV infections cannot be cured, but the severity of the pain and the duration of the episode can be lessened by antiviral agents.

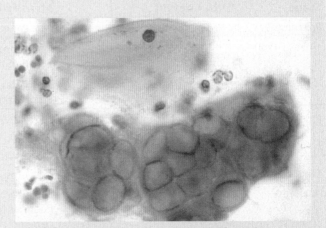

Note the healthy epithelial cell with its pink cytoplasm on top with a single healthy-appearing nucleus. The infected epithelial cells, below, possess multiple nuclei with a "ground-glass" appearance and with peripherally located chromatin. (Reprinted with permission from Rubin R, et al., eds. *Rubin's Pathology: Clinicopathologic Foundations of Medicine*, 5th ed. Philadelphia: Wolters Kluwer Health/Lippincott Williams & Wilkins, 2008. Figure 30-2.)

ensures the occurrence of the correct sequence of events in a timely fashion but also monitors and controls them.

Mitosis

The cell cycle is subdivided into four phases, G_1, S, G_2, and M.

- During the presynthetic phase, G_1, the cell increases its size and organelle content.
- During the **S phase**, DNA (plus histone and other chromosome-associated protein) synthesis and centriole replication occur.
- During G_2, ATP accumulates, centriole replication completes, and tubulin accumulates for spindle formation. G_1, S, and G_2 are also referred to as **interphase**.
- M represents **mitosis**, which is subdivided into prophase, prometaphase, metaphase, anaphase, and telophase (Table 2-4 and Fig. 2-20). The result is the division of the cell and its genetic material into two identical daughter cells.

The sequence of events in the cell cycle is controlled by a number of trigger proteins, known as **cyclin-dependent kinases** and **cyclins**.

There are three types of cell populations in the adult body based on their cell cycle: static, stable, and renewing. The static population of cells, such as neurons and cardiac muscle cells, do not usually divide, and any loss in this cell population is more or less permanent. Stable cell populations such as hepatocytes in the liver typically do not divide but can when stimulated to do so. The renewing cell population includes most epithelial cells that form lining membranes or glands in the body, which requires regular cell divisions to replace the cells that are shed continuously from the surface.

Meiosis

Although the somatic cells in the body divide by mitosis, germ cells (spermatocytes and oocytes) divide by meiosis, which has two division processes: meiosis I and meiosis II.

In meiosis I, the homologous chromosomes align side-by-side along the equator during metaphase I, which are then separated into two daughter cells. As the chromosomes in these daughter cells are no longer paired, the products of meiosis I are haploid cells containing only one copy of the genome. During meiosis II, the chromatids of the haploid chromosomes are separated. Thus, the final products of meiosis are four haploid daughter cells (Fig. 2-21).

In the beginning of meiosis, the germ cell is diploid (two sets of chromosomes), but each chromosome comprises two copies of the DNA (and its histones), referred to as chromatids; therefore, the germ cell has four total copies of DNA, which is denoted as 4CDNA (Fig. 2-21). After meiosis I, the paired chromosomes separate, resulting in haploid (one set of chromosomes) daughter cells, but because the chromosomes are still composed of two chromatids, they are denoted as 2CDNA. At meiosis II, the chromatids separate into new daughter cells; therefore, the sperm and the ovum are each haploid and have only one copy of the DNA (1CDNA). Fertilization

Table 2-4	Stages of Mitosis	
Stage	**DNA Content**	**Identifying Characteristics**
Prophase	DNA content doubles in the S phase of interphase (4n); also centrioles replicate.	Nuclear envelope begins to disappear, and the nucleolus disappears.
		Chromosomes have been replicated, and each chromosome is composed of two sister chromatids attached to each other at centromere.
		Centrioles migrate to opposite poles where they act as microtubule-organizing centers and give rise to spindle fibers and astral rays.
Prometaphase	DNA complement is 4n.	Nuclear envelope disappears.
		Kinetochores, additional microtubule-organizing centers, develop at centromeres, and kinetochore microtubules form.
Metaphase	DNA complement is 4n.	Chromosomes align at the equatorial plate of the mitotic spindle.
Anaphase	DNA complement is 4n.	Sister chromatids separate at the centromere and each chromatid migrates to an opposite pole of the cell along the microtubule, a process known as karyokinesis.
		In late anaphase, a cleavage furrow begins to form.
Telophase	Each new daughter cell contains a single complement of DNA (2n).	Deepening of the cleavage furrow restricts the continuity between the two developing daughter cells forming the mid-body. The two daughter cells separate from each other, a process known as cytokinesis.
		Nuclear envelope reforms, nucleoli reappear, chromosomes disperse forming a new interphase nucleus in each daughter cell.

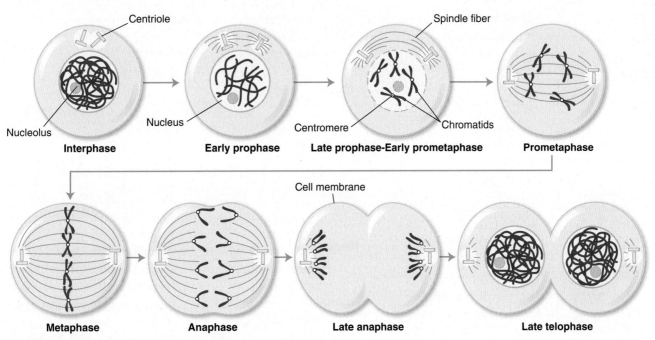

FIGURE 2-20. Schematic diagram of the stages of mitosis.

reconstitutes the diploid number of chromosomes in the resulting zygote.

Necrosis and Apoptosis

Both necrosis and apoptosis refer to cellular death, but they differ in the manner in which the cells die.

- **Necrosis** is a caspase-independent, *unregulated process*, in which cells die as a result of trauma. The plasmalemma of a necrotic cell becomes breached and the cytoplasm and nucleus are disgorged into the extracellular space, eliciting an inflammatory reaction that will eliminate the dead cell and its component parts. Necrosis is detrimental to the organism; indeed, unchecked widespread necrosis is very serious and may be fatal.

- **Apoptosis** is a genetically programmed cell death, a *regulated process* that ensures a specific, organized, methodical elimination of cells to balance a cell population, as in hemopoiesis or the preservation of the lining of mucosal surfaces, or during embryonic development. Therefore, apoptosis is advantageous to the organism. Apoptosis may be initiated by **caspases** or repressed by the presence of certain factors, known as **inhibitors of apoptosis**, which, by binding to caspases, prevent them from inducing apoptosis. The two pathways of apoptosis are extrinsic and intrinsic. The **extrinsic pathway** relies on cytokines released by a signaling cell, which activates the target cell to undergo apoptosis. The **intrinsic pathway**, instead of relying on external sources, relies on intracellular signals that cause the cell to enter apoptosis.

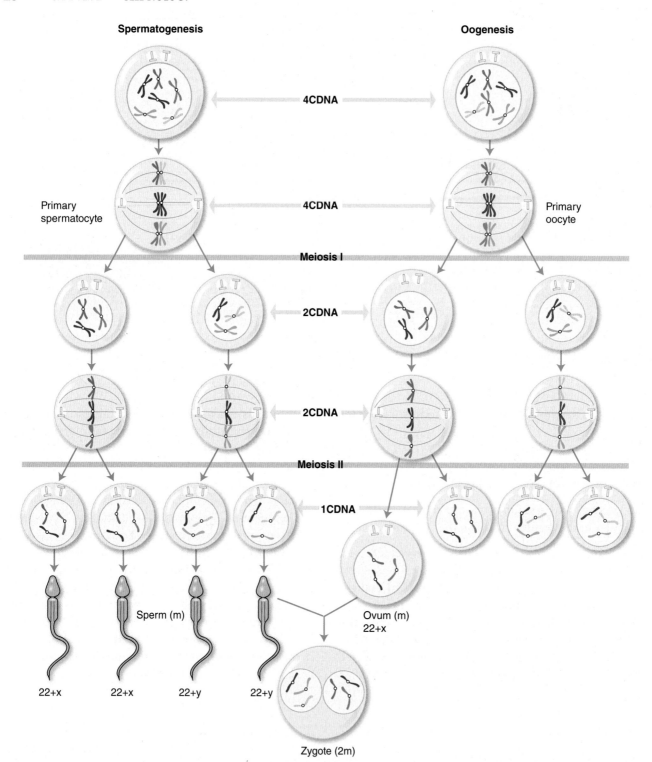

FIGURE 2-21. Schematic diagram of meiosis displays that in males (left), spermatogenesis gives rise to four haploid spermatozoa, whereas in females (right), oogenesis gives rise to a single haploid ovum and three polar bodies. Penetration of the ovum by a spermatozoon reconstitutes the number of chromosomes, forming a diploid zygote.

PLATE 2-1A   Typical Cell

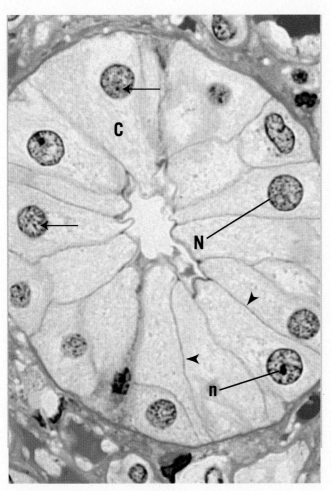

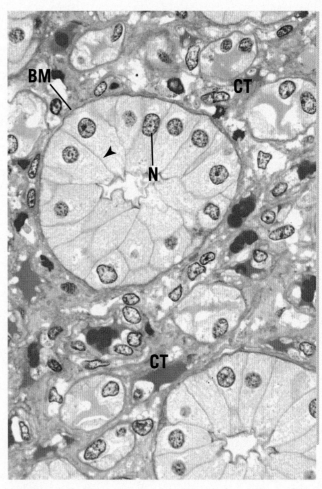

FIGURE 2-1-1. Cells. Monkey. Plastic section. ×1,323.

The typical cell is a membrane-bound structure that consists of a **nucleus** (N) and **cytoplasm** (C). Although the cell membrane is too thin to be visualized with the light microscope, the outline of the cell approximates the cell membrane (*arrowheads*). Observe that the outline of these particular cells more or less approximates a rectangle in shape. Viewed in three dimensions, these cells are said to be columnar in shape, with a centrally placed nucleus. The **nucleolus** (n) is evident, as are the heterochromatin granules (*arrows*) that are dispersed around the periphery as well as throughout the nucleoplasm. The pale or nonstaining areas in the nucleus likely contain euchromatin.

FIGURE 2-1-2. Cells. Monkey. Plastic section. ×540.

Cells may possess tall, thin morphologies, such as those of a collecting duct of the kidney. Their **nuclei** (N) are located basally, and their lateral cell membranes (*arrowheads*) are outlined. Because these cells are epithelially derived, they are separated from **connective tissue elements** (CT) by a **basal membrane** (BM).

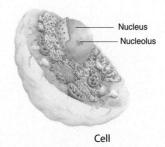

Nucleus
Nucleolus

Cell

KEY					
BM	basal membrane	**CT**	connective tissue	**n**	nucleolus
C	cytoplasm	**N**	nucleus		

PLATE 2-1B   Typical Cell

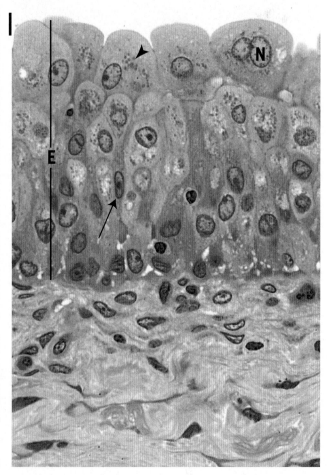

FIGURE 2-1-3. Cells. Monkey. Plastic section. ×540.

Cells come in a variety of sizes and shapes. Note that the **epithelium** (E) that lines the **lumen** of the bladder is composed of numerous layers. The surface-most layer consists of large, dome-shaped cells, some occasionally displaying two **nuclei** (N). The granules evident in the cytoplasm (*arrowhead*) are glycogen deposits. Cells deeper in the epithelium are elongated and narrow, and their nuclei (*arrow*) are located in their widest region.

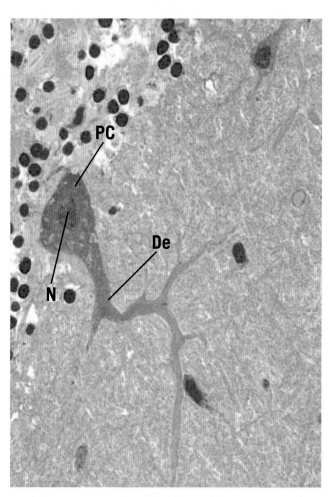

FIGURE 2-1-4. Cells. Monkey. Plastic section. ×540.

Some cells possess a rather unusual morphology, as exemplified by the **Purkinje cell** (PC) of the cerebellum. Note that the **nucleus** (N) of the cell is housed in its widest portion, known as the soma (perikaryon). The cell possesses several cytoplasmic extensions, **dendrites** (De), and axons. This nerve cell integrates the numerous digits of information that it receives from other nerve cells that synapse on it.

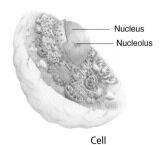

Nucleus
Nucleolus

Cell

KEY					
De	dendrite	**N**	nucleus	**PC**	Purkinje cell
E	epithelium				

PLATE 2-2A Cell Organelles and Inclusions

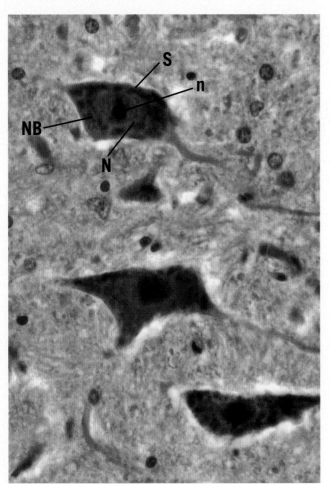

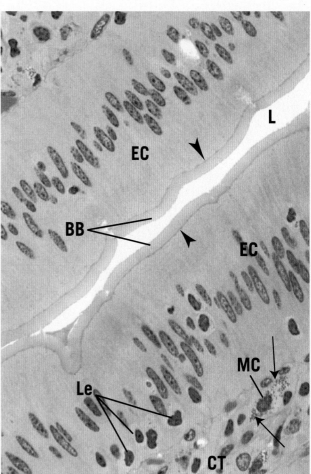

FIGURE 2-2-1. Nucleus and Nissl bodies. Spinal cord. Human. Paraffin section. ×540.

The motoneurons of the spinal cord are multipolar neurons because they possess numerous processes arising from an enlarged **soma** (S), which houses the **nucleus** (N) and various organelles. Observe that the nucleus displays a large, densely staining **nucleolus** (n). The cytoplasm also presents a series of densely staining structures known as **Nissl bodies** (NB), which have been demonstrated by electron microscopy to be rough endoplasmic reticulum. The staining intensity is due to the presence of ribonucleic acid of the ribosomes studding the surface of the rough endoplasmic reticulum. The motor neuron's high transcriptional and translational activities can be inferred from the large, euchromatic nuclei, distinct nucleoli, and abundant RER.

FIGURE 2-2-2. Mucosa of the duodenum. Mast cell in the connective tissue. Monkey. Plastic section. ×540.

The **connective tissue** (CT) subjacent to the epithelial lining of the small intestines is richly endowed with **mast cells** (MC). The granules (*arrows*) of mast cells are distributed throughout their cytoplasm and are released along the entire periphery of the cell. These small granules contain histamine and heparin as well as additional substances. Note that the **epithelial cells** (EC) are tall and columnar in morphology and that **leukocytes** (Le) are migrating, via intercellular spaces, into the **lumen** (L) of the intestines. *Arrowheads* point to terminal bars, junctions between ECs. The **brush border** (BB) has been demonstrated by electron microscopy to be microvilli.

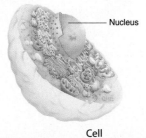

Nucleus

Cell

KEY							
BB	brush border	**Le**	leukocyte			**NB**	Nissl body
CT	connective tissue	**MC**	mast cell			**S**	soma
EC	epithelial cell	**N**	nucleus				
L	lumen	**n**	nucleolus				

PLATE 2-2B   Cell Organelles and Inclusions

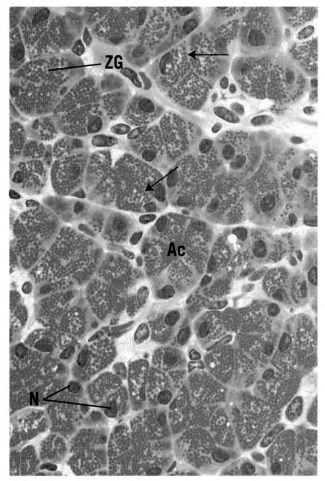

FIGURE 2-2-3. Zymogen granules. Pancreas. Monkey. Plastic section. ×540.

The exocrine portion of the pancreas produces enzymes necessary for the proper digestion of ingested food materials. These enzymes are stored by the pancreatic cells as **zymogen granules** (ZG) until their release is affected by hormonal activity. Note that the parenchymal cells are arranged in clusters known as **acini** (Ac), with a central lumen into which the secretory product is released. Observe that the zymogen granules are stored in the apical region of the cell, away from the basally located **nucleus** (N). *Arrows* indicate the lateral cell membranes of adjacent cells of an acinus.

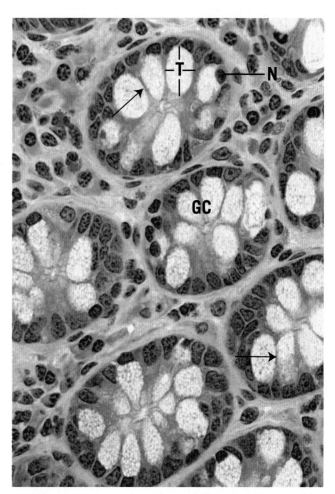

FIGURE 2-2-4. Mucous secretory products. Goblet cells. Large intestines. Monkey. Plastic section. ×540.

The glands of the large intestine house **goblet cells** (GC), which manufacture a large amount of mucous material that acts as a lubricant for the movement of the compacted residue of digestion. Each goblet cell possesses an expanded apical portion, the **theca** (T), which contains the secretory product of the cell. The base of the cell is compressed and houses the **nucleus** (N) as well as the organelles necessary for the synthesis of the mucinogen—namely, the rough endoplasmic reticulum and the Golgi apparatus. *Arrows* indicate the lateral cell membranes of contiguous goblet cells.

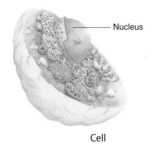

Nucleus

Cell

KEY					
Ac	acinus	**N**	nucleus	**ZG**	zymogen granule
GC	goblet cell	**T**	theca		

PLATE 2-3A Cell Surface Modifications

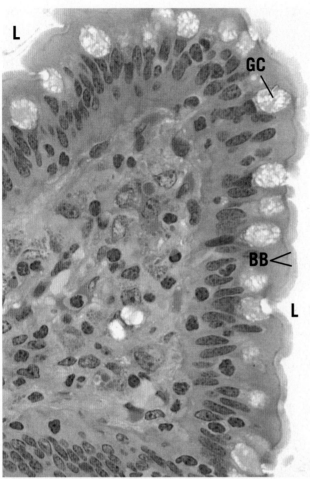

L

GC

BB

L

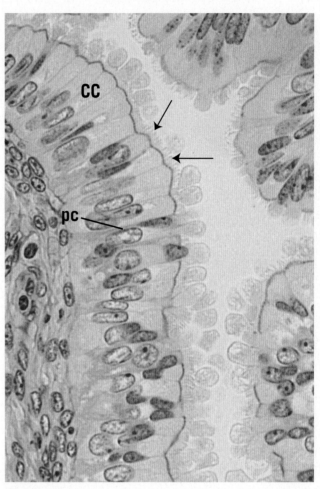

CC

pc

CC

FIGURE 2-3-1. Brush border. Small intestines. Monkey. Plastic section. ×540.

The cells lining the **lumen** (L) of the small intestine are columnar cells, among which are numerous mucus-producing **goblet cells** (GC). The function of the columnar cells is to absorb digested food material along their free, apical surface. To increase their free surface area, the cells possess a **brush border** (BB), which has been demonstrated by electron microscopy to be microvilli—short, narrow, finger-like extensions of plasmalemma-covered cytoplasm. Each microvillus bears a glycocalyx cell coat, which also contains digestive enzymes. The core of the microvillus contains longitudinally arranged actin filaments as well as additional associated proteins.

FIGURE 2-3-2. Cilia. Oviduct. Monkey. Plastic section. ×540.

The lining of the oviduct is composed of two types of epithelial cells: bleb-bearing **peg cells** (pc), which probably produce nutritional factors necessary for the survival of the gametes, and pale **ciliated cells** (CC). Cilia (*arrows*) are long, motile, finger-like extensions of the apical cell membrane and cytoplasm that transport material along the cell surface. The core of the cilium, as shown by electron microscopy, contains the axoneme, composed of microtubules arranged in a specific configuration of nine doublets surrounding a central pair of individual microtubules.

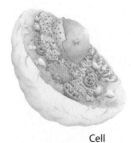

Cell

KEY					
BB	brush border	**GC**	goblet cell	**pc**	peg cell
CC	ciliated cell	**L**	lumen		

PLATE 2-3B   Cell Surface Modifications

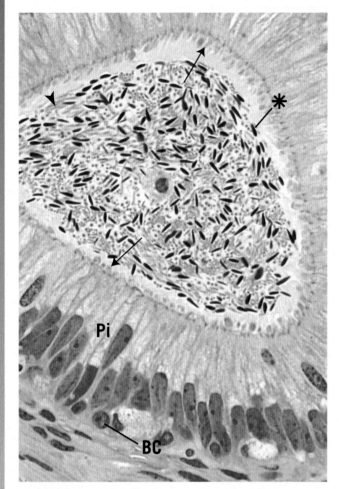

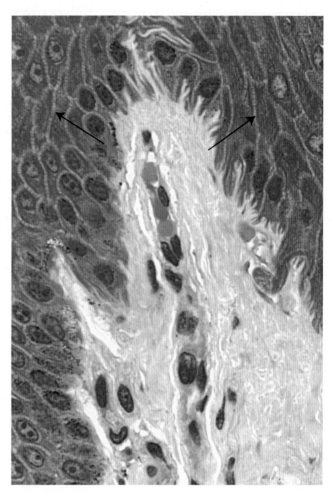

FIGURE 2-3-3. Stereocilia. Epididymis. Monkey. Plastic section. ×540.

The lining of the epididymis is composed of tall, columnar **principal cells** (Pi) and short **basal cells** (BC). The principal cells bear long stereocilia (*arrows*) that protrude into the lumen. It was believed that stereocilia were long, nonmotile, cilia-like structures. However, studies using the electron microscope have shown that stereocilia are actually long microvilli that branch as well as clump with each other. The function, if any, of stereocilia within the epididymis is not known. The lumen is occupied by numerous spermatozoa, whose dark heads (*asterisks*) and pale flagella (*arrowhead*) are clearly discernible. Flagella are very long, cilia-like structures used by the cell for propulsion.

FIGURE 2-3-4. Intercellular bridges. Skin. Monkey. Plastic section. ×540.

The epidermis of thick skin is composed of several cell layers, one of which is the stratum spinosum shown in this photomicrograph. The cells of this layer possess short, stubby, finger-like extensions that interdigitate with those of contiguous cells. Before the advent of electron microscopy, these intercellular bridges (*arrows*) were believed to represent cytoplasmic continuities between neighboring cells; however, it is now known that these processes merely serve as regions of desmosome formation so that the cells may adhere to each other.

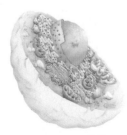

Cell

KEY			
BC	basal cell	**Pi**	principal cell

PLATE 2-4A   Mitosis, Light and Electron Microscopy

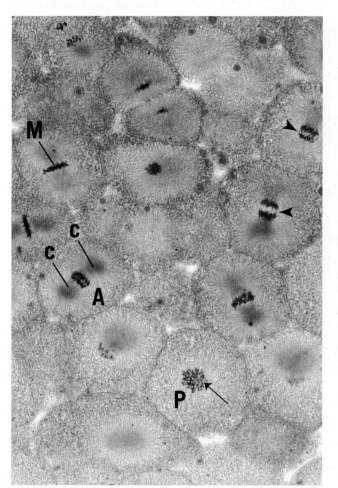

FIGURE 2-4-1. Mitosis. Whitefish blastula. Paraffin section. ×270.

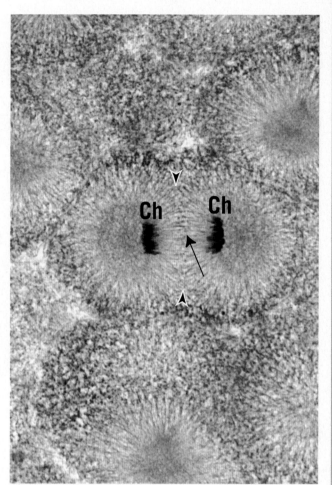

FIGURE 2-4-2. Mitosis. Whitefish blastula. Paraffin section. ×540.

This photomicrograph of whitefish blastula shows different stages of mitosis. The first mitotic stage, **prophase** (P), displays the short, threadlike chromosomes (*arrow*) in the center of the cell. The nuclear membrane is only partially present. During **metaphase** (M), the chromosomes line up at the equatorial plane of the cell. The chromosomes begin to migrate toward the opposite poles of the cell in early **anaphase** (A) and proceed farther apart as anaphase progresses (*arrowheads*). Note the dense regions, **centrioles** (c), toward which the chromosomes migrate.

During the early telophase stage of mitotic division, the **chromosomes** (Ch) have reached the opposite poles of the cell. The cell membrane constricts to separate the cell into the two new daughter cells, forming a cleavage furrow (*arrowheads*). The spindle apparatus is visible as parallel, horizontal lines (*arrow*) that eventually form the mid-body. As telophase progresses, the two new daughter cells will uncoil their chromosomes and the nuclear membrane and nucleoli will become reestablished.

KEY					
A	anaphase	Ch	chromosome	P	prophase
c	centriole	M	metaphase		

PLATE 2-4B Mitosis, Light and Electron Microscopy

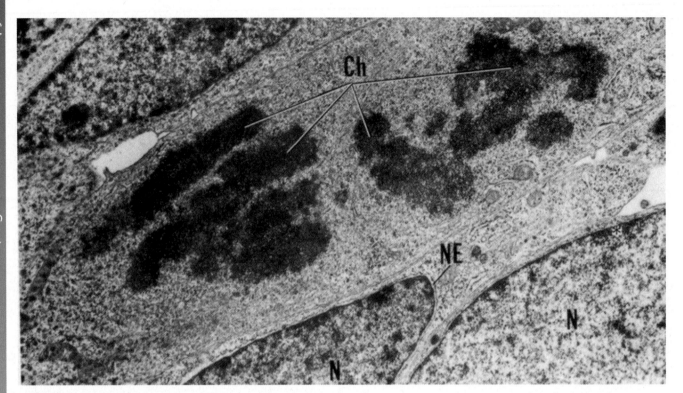

FIGURE 2-4-3. Mitosis. Mouse. Electron microscopy. ×9,423.

Neonatal tissue is characterized by mitotic activity, in which numerous cells are in the process of proliferation. Observe that the interphase **nucleus** (N) possesses a typical **nuclear envelope** (NE), perinuclear chromatin, nucleolus, and nuclear pores. A cell that is undergoing the mitotic phase of the cell cycle loses its nuclear envelope and nucleolus, whereas its **chromosomes** (Ch) are quite visible. These chromosomes are no longer lined up at the equatorial plate but are migrating to opposite poles, indicating that this cell is in the early- to mid-anaphase stage of mitosis. Observe the presence of cytoplasmic organelles such as mitochondria, rough endoplasmic reticulum, and Golgi apparatus.

KEY					
Ch	chromosome	**N**	nucleus	**NE**	nuclear envelope

PLATE 2-5   Typical Cell, Electron Microscopy

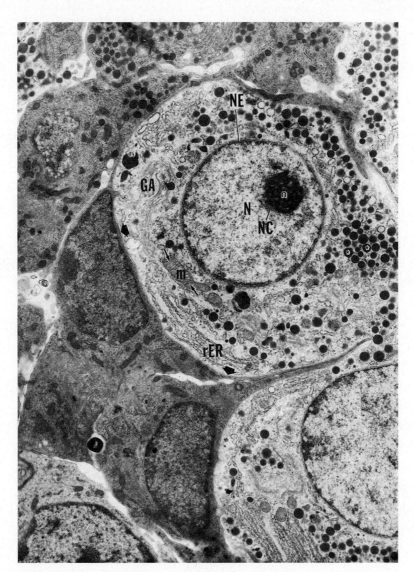

FIGURE 2-5-1. Typical cell. Pituitary. Rat. Electron microscopy. ×8,936.

The cytoplasm of this gonadotroph is limited by a cell membrane (*arrowheads*) **Mitochondria** (m) are not numerous but are easily recognizable because their cristae (*arrows*) are arranged in a characteristic fashion. This cell possesses a well-developed **Golgi apparatus** (GA), positioned near the **nucleus** (N). Note the presence of **rough endoplasmic reticulum**, as well as secretory products (*asterisks*), which are transitory inclusions.

The nucleus is bounded by the typical **nuclear envelope** (NE). The peripheral chromatin and chromatin islands are clearly evident, as is the **nucleolus-associated chromatin** (NC). The **nucleolus** (n) presents a spongelike appearance composed of electron-lucent and electron-dense materials, suspended free in the nucleoplasm. (Reprinted by permission from Springer: Stokreef JC, et al. A possible phagocytic role for folliculo-stellate cells of anterior pituitary following estrogen withdrawal from primed male rats. *Cell Tissue Res* 1986;243(2):255–261. Copyright © 1986 Springer Nature.)

Chapter Review Questions

2-1. Abnormal peroxisomal biogenesis is a characteristic of which of the following conditions?

   A. Sarcomas

   B. Tay-Sachs disease

   C. Adenomas

   D. Zellweger disease

   E. Marfan syndrome

2-2. Proteins that are to be degraded by proteasomes require the attachment of which of the following molecules?

   A. Ubiquitin

   B. Acetyl coenzyme A

   C. Adenosine triphosphate

   D. Guanosine triphosphate

   E. Regulatory particle

2-3. One of the characteristics of Leber hereditary optic neuropathy is that:

   A. it is transmitted from the father to the offspring

   B. it is a mitochondrial disorder

   C. it is a peroxisomal disorder

   D. usually only one eye is affected

   E. it is transmitted only to female offspring

2-4. Giant axonal neuropathy is a condition characterized by the presence of excess:

   A. microtubules

   B. thin filaments

   C. intermediate filaments

   D. early endosomes

   E. late endosomes

2-5. Which of the following nucleotides is characteristic of DNA only?

   A. Adenine

   B. Uracil

   C. Cytosine

   D. Thymine

   E. Guanine

EPITHELIUM AND GLANDS

Epithelial Tissue

Cells and extracellular matrix (ECM), which surrounds the cells and is composed of fibers and ground substance, constitute a tissue. The combination of particular cells surrounded by various types and proportions of ECM components determines the unique tissue morphology, which in turn dictates the function of that tissue. Four general tissue types comprise the human body: epithelial, connective, nervous, and muscle tissues. In this chapter, the histologic and functional characteristics of epithelial tissues and their derivatives, glands, will be explored.

Epithelial Tissue Characteristics

Epithelial tissues (epithelia) derive from all three embryonic germ layers (e.g., epithelium of the skin derives from ectoderm, those of the digestive and respiratory epithelia derive from endoderm, whereas vascular and much of the urogenital lining epithelia derive from mesoderm). Epithelial tissue is composed of abundant and tightly packed cells, with little to a negligible amount of ECM (Fig. 3-1).

Epithelia either form membranes or sheets that cover or line the external and internal surfaces of the body (such as the skin, respiratory tract, and body cavities), or form secretory elements known as glands (such as sweat glands, pancreas, and thyroid glands). Almost always, epithelia are separated from underlying or surrounding connective tissues by a thin, noncellular layer, the **basement membrane (basal membrane)** (see Fig. 3-1). Transmission electron microscopic images of the basement membrane demonstrate that it is usually composed of two regions, the **basal lamina** derived from epithelial cells and the **lamina reticularis** derived from the connective tissue (Fig. 3-2).

Epithelial tissues are avascular, and their cells receive nutrients via diffusion from blood vessels in the adjacent connective tissues. The lack of a vascular supply of their own limits the thickness of epithelial tissues. They form an interface between two different environments, whether it be between air and connective tissue or between a fluid and connective tissue. Epithelial tissue can regulate the transfer of materials between the two environments.

The cells of the epithelial tissues have polarity, meaning different sides of their cell surfaces are frequently specialized. Their free, apical surface may hold abundant **receptors** or **transporters**, or form **microvilli (brush border, striated border)**, **cilia**, or **stereocilia**. The lateral cell membranes are specialized to maintain various types of intercellular junctions with the neighboring cells, including **zonulae occludentes**, **zonulae adherentes**, **maculae**

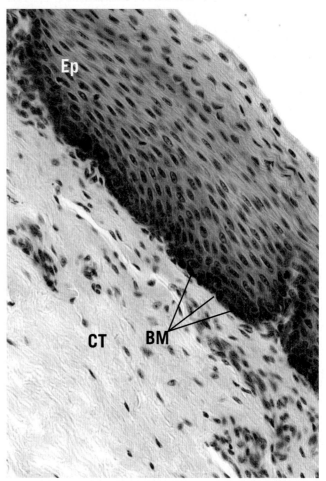

FIGURE 3-1. Epithelial tissue (Ep) separated from the underlying connective tissue (CT) by the basement membrane (BM).

adherentes, and **gap junctions**. The basal cell membrane forms **hemidesmosomes**, maintaining the cell's attachment to the basement membrane (Fig. 3-3).

Epithelial tissues have various functions that include

- protection from mechanical abrasion, chemical penetration, and bacterial invasion;
- reduction of friction;
- absorption of nutrients as a result of its polarized cells that are capable of performing vectorial functions;
- secretion;
- excretion of waste products;
- synthesis of various proteins, enzymes, mucins, hormones, and a myriad of other substances;
- receiving sensory signals from the external (or internal) milieu;
- **forming glands** whose function is **secreting** enzymes, hormones, lubricants, or other products; and
- movement of material along the epithelial sheet (such as mucus along the respiratory tract) by the assistance of cilia.

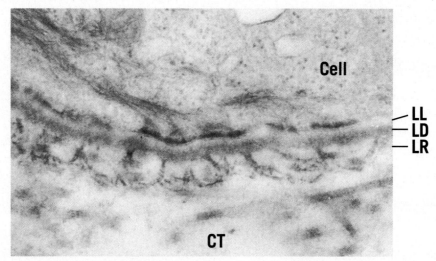

FIGURE 3-2. Viewed with the light microscope, the narrow acellular structure interposed between epithelium and the underlying connective tissue is known as the basement membrane. The same structure, when viewed with the electron microscope, has been resolved to have three components, **lamina lucida** (LL), **lamina densa** (LD; both manufactured by epithelial cells), and **lamina reticularis** (LR; manufactured by cells of connective tissue). The two epithelially derived components are collectively known as the basal lamina. Recently, some investigators have questioned the presence of the lamina lucida, and some suggest that it is an artifact of fixation. Additionally, some authors have stopped using the term basement membrane and substituted the term basal lamina for both light and electron microscopic descriptions. In this text, we continue to use basement membrane for light microscopic and basal lamina for electron microscopic descriptions. Moreover, certain cells, such as muscle cells and Schwann cells, invest themselves with an acellular material that resembles a basal lamina, which will be referred to as an external lamina. (Reprinted with permission from Strayer DS, et al., eds. *Rubin's Pathology: Mechanisms of Human Disease*, 8th ed. Philadelphia: Wolters Kluwer, 2020. Figure 28-7B.)

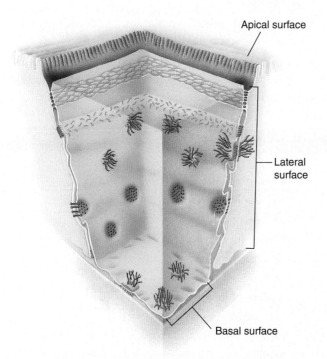

FIGURE 3-3. Epithelial cells have polarity with distinct apical, lateral, and basal surfaces, each specialized for interacting with the external environment, tightly attaching to the neighboring cells, and to the basement membrane, respectively.

Epithelial Tissue Classification

Epithelial tissues are classified according to two observational criteria. First is the shape of the most superficial cell layer as observed when sectioned perpendicular to the exposed surface epithelium. Therefore, the epithelium may be **squamous** (flat), **cuboidal**, or **columnar** in shape (Fig. 3-4). The second criterion is the number of cell layers composing the epithelium; thus, the epithelium is considered to be **simple** (a single layer of cells) or **stratified** (two or more layers of cells) (Table 3-1). In a simple epithelium, because it is composed of a single layer of epithelial cells, all of the cells contact the basement membrane and, in most cases, reach the free surface. There is a special type of simple epithelium all of whose cells contact the basement membrane, but some of the cells are taller than their neighbors making this epithelium *appear* to be stratified, and is consequently referred to as **pseudostratified epithelium** (whose taller cells may or may not possess cilia or stereocilia) (see Fig. 3-4).

There is a stratified type of epithelium that does not conform to this classification formula, namely the epithelium that lines various components of the urinary tract. Known as **transitional epithelium**, it is comprised of multiple layers of mostly cuboidal cells; however, the cells of the surface-most layer are dome-shaped. Depending on the level of organ distension, the number of

Cell shape:

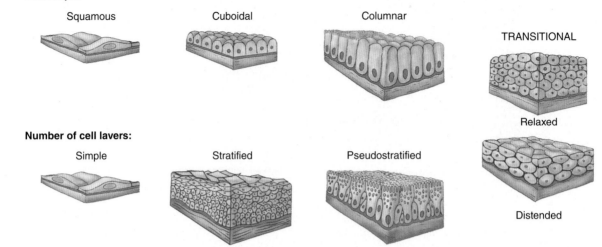

Squamous   Cuboidal   Columnar

TRANSITIONAL

Relaxed

Number of cell layers:

Simple   Stratified   Pseudostratified

Distended

FIGURE 3-4. Epithelial tissue classification criteria based on the epithelial cell morphology and the number of cell layers. Transitional epithelium is a unique tissue that changes in apical cell shape and number of cell layers depending on the level of distention. There are three types of stratified squamous epithelium, depending on the amount of frictional forces attendant on its free surface. If the forces are minimal, then the epithelium is said to be **nonkeratinized stratified squamous** (as in the esophagus); greater frictional forces demand better protection of the underlying cells and those epithelia are said to be **stratified squamous parakeratinized** (as in regions of the oral cavity); and epithelia where the frictional forces are considerable have a thicker layer of keratinized cells on the surface and are known as **stratified squamous keratinized** (as in skin, especially on the soles of the feet and on the palms of the hand) (Fig. 3-5). Keratinization refers to the amount of keratin present in the dead cells on the free surface of the epithelium.

cell layers and the shape of the surface cells can change, which prompted the name, transitional.

The epithelial tissue types are listed in Table 3-1.

Some epithelia in the body have unique names based on their function and location:

- Simple squamous epithelium that forms the serous membrane of the body cavities is referred to as **mesothelium**.

- Simple squamous epithelium that lines the blood, lymphatic vessels, and heart chambers is referred to as **endothelium**.

- Transitional epithelium that lines much of the urinary tract is called **urothelium**.

- Ciliated pseudostratified columnar epithelium that lines much of the upper respiratory tract is referred to as **respiratory epithelium**.

Table 3-1	Epithelial Tissue Types		
Number of Cell Layers	**Apical Cell Shape**	**Surface Specialization**	**Examples**
Simple	Squamous	–	Vascular lining, serous membranes, lung alveoli
	Cuboidal	–	Kidney tubules, small exocrine ducts
	Columnar	Ciliated	Uterine tube lining
		Nonciliated	Lining of small and large intestines
Stratified	Squamous	Keratinized	Skin
		Parakeratinized	Regions of the oral cavity
		Nonkeratinized	Esophagus, vagina
	Cuboidal	–	Large ducts
	Columnar	Ciliated	Some portions of the respiratory tract
		Nonciliated	Larger ducts, conjunctiva
Pseudostratified	Columnar	Ciliated	Upper respiratory tract
		Nonciliated	Epididymis, vas deferens
Transitional			Ureters, urinary bladder

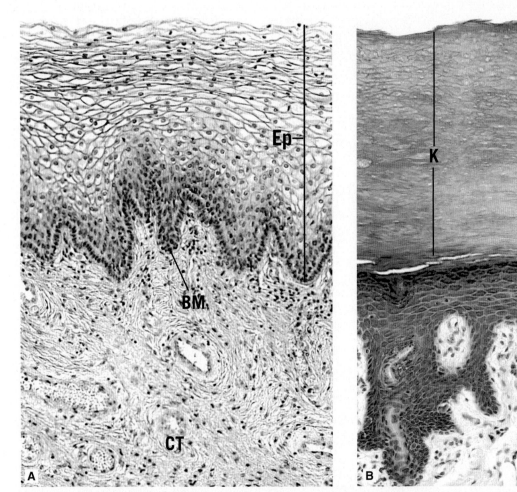

FIGURE 3-5. Nonkeratinized (A) vs. keratinized (B) stratified squamous epithelia. The stratified squamous epithelial tissues (Ep) in both micrographs are separated from the connective tissue (CT) by an inconspicuous basement membrane (BM). In keratinized stratified squamous epithelium (B), the keratin (K) layer on top of the living layer of epithelial cells provides an added protection from frictional forces.

Epithelial Cell Membrane Specializations

Epithelial cells may present specializations along their various surfaces. These surfaces are **apical** (microvilli, stereocilia, cilia, and flagella), **lateral or basolateral** (junctional complexes, zonula occludens, zonula adherens, macula adherens, and gap junctions), and **basal** (hemidesmosomes and basal lamina).

Apical Surface Modifications

Apical or surface membrane of epithelial cells may have specialized projections (Fig. 3-6).

Microvilli are closely spaced, finger-like extensions of the cell membrane that are employed to increase the surface area of those cells that function in absorption and secretion. Dense clusters of microvilli are evident in light micrographs as a **striated** or **brush border**. The core of each microvillus possesses a cluster of 25 or so microfilaments (actin filaments).

Cilia are elongated (7- to 10-μm long and 0.2 μm in diameter), motile, cellular projections that move material

along the apical cell surface. At the base of the axoneme is the **basal body** that resembles a centriole in that it is composed of nine microtubule triplets. The core of the cilium contains an **axoneme**, which is composed of nine pairs of peripherally located microtubule **doublets**, surrounding two single, centrally placed microtubule **singlets**. Each doublet is composed of a complete microtubule, **microtubule A**, consisting of 13 protofilaments and a **microtubule B**, composed of only 10 protofilaments. Microtubule A shares three of its protofilaments with microtubule B. The two singlets are surrounded by a **central sheet**, composed of an elastic material, and each doublet is attached to the central sheet by a **radial spoke**, also composed of an elastic material. Moreover, **nexin bridges**, again composed of an elastic material, bind adjacent doublets to each other. Microtubules of the doublets possess **dynein arms** with *ATPase activity*, which functions in energizing ciliary motion. These dynein arms form two rows and are located along the entire length of the A subunit resembling a centipede, and they project toward the B subunit of the adjacent doublet. The dynein arms hydrolyze ATP and utilize the

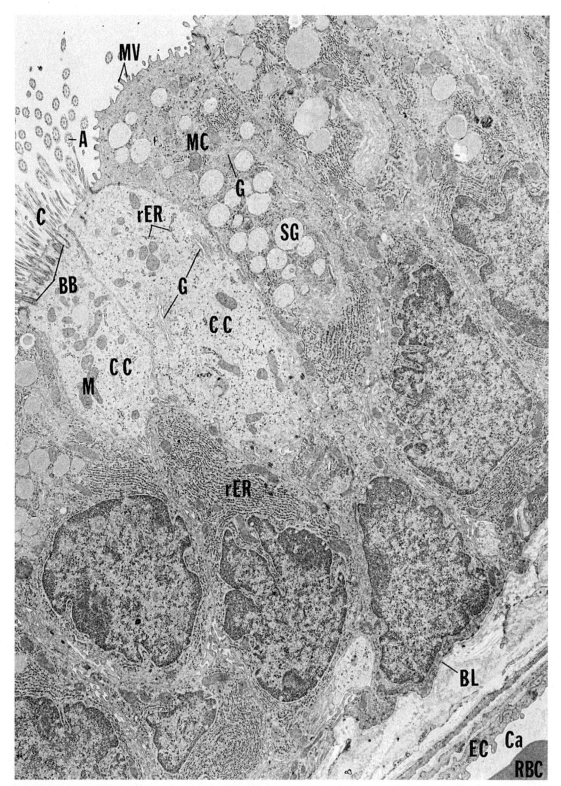

FIGURE 3-6. Pseudostratified ciliated columnar epithelium. Hamster trachea. Electron microscopy. ×6,480. The pseudostratified ciliated columnar epithelium of the trachea is composed of several types of cells, some of which are presented here. Because this is an oblique section through the epithelium, it is not readily evident here that all of these cells touch the basal lamina (BL). Note that the pale-staining ciliated cells (CC) display rough endoplasmic reticulum (rER), mitochondria (M), Golgi apparatus (G), and numerous cilia (C) interspersed with microvilli (MV). Each cilium, some of which are seen in cross section, displays its plasma membrane and its axoneme (A). The cilia are anchored in the terminal web via their basal bodies (BB). The second cell types to be noted are the mucous cells (MC), also known as goblet cells. The mucous cells are nonciliated but do present short, stubby microvilli (MV) on their apical surface. The lower right-hand corner of this electron micrograph presents a portion of a capillary (Ca) containing a red blood cell (RBC). Observe that the highly attenuated endothelial cell (EC) is outside of but very close to the basal lamina (BL) of the tracheal epithelium. (Courtesy of Dr. E. McDowell.) SG, secretory granules.

energy released to "climb" the adjacent B subunit, thus causing the cilium to bend thereby stretching the intricate group of elastic material of the axoneme. Once the dynein arms release their hold on the adjacent B subunit, the stretched elastic material returns to its resting length (without the requirement of energy consumption) and "snaps" the cilium back to its previous upright position. The whip-like motion of the cilium thus propels material on the surface of the cilium. In order to protect the cilium from bending too far, a somewhat rigid protein rod, composed of **tektin**, is nestled against each doublet, reinforcing it and reducing its flexibility.

Stereocilia are located in the epididymis, as well as in a few limited regions of the body. They were named cilia because of their length; however, electron micrography proved them to be elongated microvilli whose functions are, as yet, unknown. The core of these stereocilia is composed of actin filaments.

Basolateral Surface Modifications

The basolateral surface is really composed of a **lateral** and a **basal domain**. Each region has its own specialized adaptation and will be described as such. The lateral domain presents its specific junctional complexes, and the basal domain displays hemidesmosomes and the basal lamina.

Lateral Domain

Junctional complexes, which occupy only a minute region of the lateral cell surfaces, are visible with light microscopy as **terminal bars**, structures that encircle the entire cell. Terminal bars, as viewed by transmission electron microscopy, are composed of three components: **zonula occludens** (tight or occluding junction), **zonula adherens** (adhering junction), and **macula adherens** (**desmosome**, also adhering junction) (Fig. 3-7). The first two are located on the apical portion of the lateral membrane and are belt-like so that they encircle that very narrow adluminal region of the cell, whereas desmosomes do not; although in some epithelial cells, such as the endothelium, the tight junctions and adhering junctions are formed as ribbon-like configurations rather than belt-like and are known as fascia occludens and fascia adherens, respectively. Additionally, another type of junction, the **gap junction** (communicating junction), permits two cells to communicate with each other.

Zonulae occludentes are formed in such a fashion that the plasma membranes of the two adjoining cells are very close to each other and the transmembrane proteins of the two cells contact each other in the extracellular space. There are a number of transmembrane proteins that participate in the formation of the zonula occludens, **claudins**, **occludins**, **junctional adhesion molecules**, ZO-1, **ZO-2**, and **ZO-3 proteins**, among others. Although all

of these proteins are necessary to exclude material from traversing the paracellular route (the extracellular space between two cells), it is the claudins that form a physical barrier that cannot be penetrated. It is important to note that claudins do not require the presence of calcium ions to remain attached to their counterparts located in the adjacent cell membrane. Additionally, it should be noted here that some claudins possess aqueous channels that are designed to permit the movement of ions, water, and some very small molecules along the paracellular route. The proteins of the zonula occludens are preferentially adherent to the P-face (protoplasmic face) of the membrane and form characteristic ridges evident in freeze-fracture preparation, whereas the E-face (extracellular face) presents corresponding grooves. The zonulae occludentes are also responsible for preventing integral proteins of the cell from migrating from the apical surface to the basolateral surface and vice versa.

The plasma membranes of adjacent epithelial cells are farther apart in the region of the *zonula adherentes*. **Cell adhesion molecules** (CAMs) are the most significant components of adhering junctions of epithelial cells, and in the zonulae adherentes, they are calcium-dependent proteins, known as **E-cadherins**. The cytoplasmic moiety of the E-cadherins has binding sites for **catenins**, which, in turn, bind to **vinculin** and α-**actinin**, which are capable of forming bonds with the **thin filaments** of the cytoskeleton. In this fashion, in the presence of calcium in the extracellular space, the two epithelial cells adhere to each other and the adherence is reinforced by the cytoskeleton of the two cells. Moreover, the zonulae adherentes reinforce and stabilize the zonulae occludentes, which are just apically positioned, as well as distribute stresses across the epithelial sheet.

Maculae adherentes (**desmosomes**) resemble spot welding that holds the two cells together. As their name implies, they are not continuous structures as are the two zonulae but are discrete entities. Desmosomes require the presence of two cells, and they are composed of an outer and inner intracellular **attachment plaque** (**dense plaques**) in each cell. The outer attachment plaques are composed of **plakoglobins** and **plakophilins** that are attached to each other with the assistance of a family of proteins known as **desmoplakins**. The outer attachment plaques adhere to the cytoplasmic aspect of the two adjacent cell membranes as mirror images of each other. Intermediate filaments enter and leave the cytoplasmic aspect of the outer dense plaque resembling curved ends of hairpins, and these curved ends form the less dense inner attachment plaque. Embedded into the plaques are transmembrane, calcium-dependent cadherins, **desmogleins**, and **desmocollins**. The extracellular moieties of desmogleins and desmocollins of the adjoining cells contact each other in the extracellular space and, in the

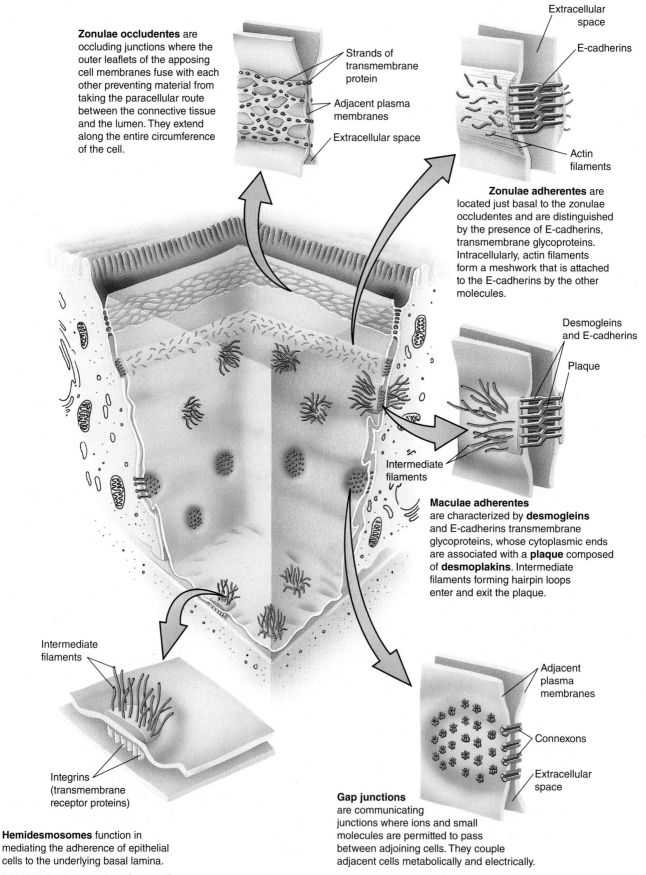

Zonulae occludentes are occluding junctions where the outer leaflets of the apposing cell membranes fuse with each other preventing material from taking the paracellular route between the connective tissue and the lumen. They extend along the entire circumference of the cell.

Strands of transmembrane protein

Adjacent plasma membranes

Extracellular space

Extracellular space

E-cadherins

Actin filaments

Zonulae adherentes are located just basal to the zonulae occludentes and are distinguished by the presence of E-cadherins, transmembrane glycoproteins. Intracellularly, actin filaments form a meshwork that is attached to the E-cadherins by the other molecules.

Desmogleins and E-cadherins

Plaque

Intermediate filaments

Maculae adherentes are characterized by **desmogleins** and E-cadherins transmembrane glycoproteins, whose cytoplasmic ends are associated with a **plaque** composed of **desmoplakins**. Intermediate filaments forming hairpin loops enter and exit the plaque.

Intermediate filaments

Integrins (transmembrane receptor proteins)

Hemidesmosomes function in mediating the adherence of epithelial cells to the underlying basal lamina.

Adjacent plasma membranes

Connexons

Extracellular space

Gap junctions are communicating junctions where ions and small molecules are permitted to pass between adjoining cells. They couple adjacent cells metabolically and electrically.

FIGURE 3-7. Junctional complex.

presence of calcium ions, attach the two cells to each other.

In the regions of **gap junctions** (communicating junctions, **nexus**), the two cell membranes are very close to each other, about 2 nm apart. Interposed within the cell membrane of each cell and meeting each other are **connexons**, composed of six subunits known as **connexins**; these multipass proteins form a cylindrical structure with a central pore. A connexon of one cell matches the connexon of the other cell and thus form an aqueous channel, about 2 nm in diameter, between the two cells that permit water, ions, and molecules smaller than 1 kD in size to traverse the channel and go from one cell to the next. Each cell has the ability to open or close the channel, and this regulation is calcium- and pH-dependent. In this fashion, a healthy cell can shut off communication with a cell that may be damaged. Each gap junction may be composed of several thousand connexons crowded together.

Basal Domain

The basal cell membrane of the cell is affixed to the basal lamina by adhering junctions known as **type I** or **type II hemidesmosomes**. Morphologically, they resemble half of a desmosome, but their biochemical composition and clinical significance demonstrate enough dissimilarity that hemidesmosomes are no longer viewed as being merely one-half of a desmosome. Type I hemidesmosomes are more intricate and are located in stratified squamous and pseudostratified epithelia, whereas type II hemidesmosomes are simpler and are located in simple cuboidal and simple columnar epithelia. Only the type I hemidesmosome will be described; it has an **intracellular plaque** composed mostly of **plectin, BP230 (plakin proteins)**, and **erbin. Tonofilaments** (intermediate filaments) terminate in the plaque by interacting with BP230 and plectin. Hemidesmosomes also possess dense clusters of transmembrane protein components known as $\alpha6\beta4$ **integrin molecules**, whose cytoplasmic moiety is embedded in the plaque and is attached to it by interacting with BP230 and erbin, thereby ensuring that the hemidesmosome is anchored to the cytoskeleton. The extracellular regions of the integrin molecules and the BP180 molecules contact laminin and type IV collagen of the basal lamina and bind to them if extracellular calcium is present. In this manner, hemidesmosomes assist in the anchoring of epithelial sheets to the adjacent basal lamina.

The **basement membrane**, interposed between epithelium and connective tissue, is composed of an epithelially derived component, the **basal lamina**, and a connective tissue–derived region, the **lamina reticularis**. The basal lamina is further subdivided into two regions, the **lamina lucida** and the **lamina densa**. Although some

investigators, using low-temperature, high-pressure freezing techniques of fixation, are beginning to question the existence of the lamina lucida, this *Text* will continue to adhere to the concept of a lamina lucida component of the basal lamina. The lamina lucida is that region of the basal lamina that houses the extracellular moieties of the transmembrane **laminin receptors**, namely, the **integrin** and **dystroglycan** molecules. The lamina lucida also houses the glycoproteins **laminin, entactin,** and **perlecan**. The lamina densa is composed of **type IV collagen**, coated by laminin, entactin, and perlecan on its epithelial surface, and **fibronectin** and perlecan on the lamina reticularis surface. Two other **collagen types, XV and XVIII**, are also present in the lamina densa. The lamina densa adheres to the **lamina reticularis**, the thickest region of the basement membrane. The lamina reticularis is composed mostly of **type III collagen**, proteoglycans, glycoproteins, as well as of **anchoring fibers (type VII collagen)** and **microfibrils (fibrillin)**. Type I and type III collagen fibers enter the lamina reticularis from its interface with the connective tissue to affix the two structures to each other. In this fashion, the epithelium and the connective tissue form firm bonds with each other. The basement membrane (and in certain areas where the lamina reticularis is absent and only the basal lamina is present) functions as structural supports for the epithelium, as molecular filters (e.g., in the renal glomerulus), in regulating the migration of certain cells across epithelial sheaths (e.g., preventing entry to fibroblasts but permitting access to lymphoid cells), in epithelial regeneration (e.g., in wound healing, where it forms a surface along which regenerating epithelial cells migrate), and in cell-to-cell interactions (e.g., formation of myoneural junctions).

Epithelial Cell Renewal

Epithelial cells usually undergo regular turnover because of their function and location. For example, cells of the epidermis that are sloughed from the surface originated approximately 28 days earlier by mitosis from cells of the basal layers. Other cells, such as those lining the small intestine, are replaced every few days. Still others continue to proliferate until adulthood is reached, at which time the mechanism is shut down. However, when large numbers of cells are lost, for example, because of injury, certain mechanisms trigger the proliferation of new cells to restore the cell population.

Glands

Most glands are formed during embryonic development by the downgrowth of the epithelial covering into the underlying connective tissue. There are two major classification of glands, exocrine and endocrine.

CLINICAL CONSIDERATIONS 3-1

Bullous Pemphigoid and Pemphigus Vulgaris

Bullous pemphigoid, a rare autoimmune disease, is caused by autoantibodies binding to some of the protein components of hemidesmosomes. Individuals afflicted with this disease exhibit skin blistering of the groin and axilla about the flexure areas and often in the oral cavity. Fortunately, it can be controlled by steroids and immunosuppressive drugs.

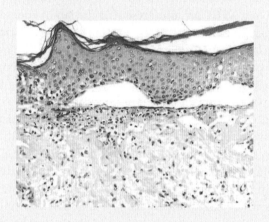

Bullous pemphigoid. Note that the epidermis is lifted from the dermis, a characteristic of bullous pemphigoid because the hemidesmosomes are attacked by the immune system thus separating the epidermis from the underlying dermis, which displays the presence of an inflammatory infiltrate of neutrophils, lymphocytes, and eosinophils. (Reprinted with permission from Mills SE, et al., eds. *Sternberg's Diagnostic Surgical Pathology*, 6th ed. Philadelphia: Wolters Kluwer, 2015. p. 18, Figure 1-28.)

Pemphigus vulgaris is an autoimmune disease, caused by autoantibodies binding to some of the components of desmosomes. This disease causes blistering and is usually found occurring in middle-aged individuals. Histologically, the blisters result from the separation of epithelial cells within the epidermis while the epidermal and dermal connection is preserved. It is a relatively dangerous disease because the blistering can easily lead to infections. Frequently, this disease also responds to steroid therapy.

CLINICAL CONSIDERATIONS 3-2

Cholera

Cholera toxins cause the release of tremendous volumes of fluid from the individual afflicted by that disease. The toxin attacks the zonulae occludentes by disturbing the proteins ZO-1 and ZO-2, thereby disrupting the zonula occludentes and permitting the paracellular movement of water and electrolytes. The patient has uncontrolled diarrhea and subsequent fluid and electrolyte loss. If the fluids and salts are not replaced in a timely manner, the patient dies.

- Glands that deliver their secretions onto the epithelial surface do so via ducts and are known as **exocrine glands**.

- Glands that do not maintain a connection to the outside (ductless) and whose secretions enter the vascular system for delivery are known as **endocrine glands** (see Chapter 11, Endocrine System).

The secretory cells of a gland, referred to as its **parenchyma**, are separated from surrounding connective tissue and vascular elements (collectively called the **stroma**) by a basement membrane.

- Exocrine glands are classified according to various parameters, for example, morphology of their secretory units, number of their ducts, types of secretory products that they manufacture, and the methods whereby secretory products are released from the secretory cells (Table 3-2).

- Generally, **acinar glands** are comprised of cuboidal to pyramidal cells that secrete watery proteinaceous fluids, whereas **tubular glands** are composed of columnar-shaped mucus-secreting cells. In **tubuloacinar glands**, both types of cells comprise the secretory units and often the serous cells can be observed as discrete hemispherical structures referred to as **serous demilunes** at the end of mucous tubes (Fig. 3-8). Recent investigations have suggested that serous demilunes are artifacts of fixation. These serous cells are believed to be located alongside their mucous counterparts but during fixation, as the mucus-producing cells swell, they force the serous cells to the periphery of the acinus.

- The classification of endocrine glands is much more complex, but, morphologically, their secretory units either are composed of **follicles** or are arranged in **cords** and clumps of cells.

CLINICAL CONSIDERATIONS 3-3

Psoriasis Vulgaris

Psoriasis affects approximately 2% of the population and may have a familial trait. It usually begins its course between 10 and 40 years of age, and it first appears as patches of dry skin that is raised and is reddish in color on the knees, scalp, elbows, back, or buttocks. It is believed to be an immune disorder that causes a higher than normal mitotic activity of the cells of the stratified squamous keratinized epithelium, the epidermis, of the skin. In most individuals, this condition has no symptoms other than the unsightly appearance of the skin. In some individuals, however, the condition is accompanied by pain and/or itching or both.

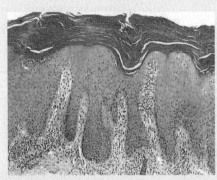

The normal keratinized stratified squamous epithelium of the skin of this patient is greatly modified. Note that the stratum spinosum layer is greatly thickened and the cells of the stratum corneum appear to possess nuclei. Higher magnification of that area, however (not shown), demonstrates that the nuclei belong to neutrophils that invaded the epithelium. Also, note the absence of the stratum granulosum and lucidum, which confirms that this specimen is not taken from regions of thick skin, such as the palm of the hand or the sole of the foot. The large number of nuclei present in the papillary layer of the dermis belongs to lymphocytic infiltrate. (Reprinted with permission from Mills SE, et al., eds. *Sternberg's Diagnostic Surgical Pathology*, 6th ed. Philadelphia: Wolters Kluwer, 2015. p. 7, Figure 1-5.)

CLINICAL CONSIDERATIONS 3-4

Tumor Formation

Of the four tissue types in the body, cells of the epithelial tissues on average turn over most frequently, which also puts the epithelial cells at most risk of incurring mutations that affect the cell cycle regulation. This also explains the fact that most tumors arise from epithelial origin. Under certain pathologic conditions, mechanisms that regulate cell proliferation becomes impaired; thus, epithelial proliferation gives rise to tumors that may be benign if they are localized or malignant if they wander from their original site and metastasize (seed) to another area of the body and continue to proliferate. Malignant tumors that arise from surface epithelium are termed carcinomas, whereas those developing from glandular epithelia are called adenocarcinomas.

Metaplasia

Epithelial cells are derived from certain germ cell layers, possess a definite morphology and location, and perform specific functions; however, under certain pathologic conditions, they may undergo **metaplasia**, transforming into another epithelial cell type. An example of such metaplasia occurs in the lining epithelium of the oral cavity of individuals who smoke or use chewing tobacco as well as in Barrett esophagus, where the long-term gastric reflux causes

the epithelium of the lower portion of the esophagus to resemble the cardiac stomach but with the presence of goblet cells rather than surface-lining cells.

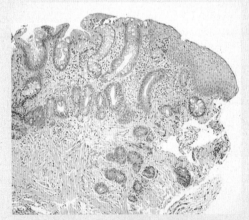

Metaplasia in a case of Barrett esophagus. Note that the normal esophageal epithelium, nonkeratinized stratified squamous, has been largely replaced by a simple columnar epithelium along with glands, resembling that of the cardiac stomach but rich in goblet cells. (Reprinted with permission from Montgomery EA, et al. *Biopsy Interpretation of the Gastrointestinal Tract Mucosa: Volume 2: Neoplastic*, 3rd ed. Philadelphia: Wolters Kluwer, 2018. Figure 1-179.)

Table 3-2	Exocrine Glandular Classification Criteria	
Cellular Composition	**Characteristics**	**Example**
Unicellular	Single isolated cell, either in covering or glandular epithelium, secreting specialized products	Goblet cell
Multicellular (more than one cell)	Collection of cells comprising a secretory unit in a gland	Salivary gland secretory acini
Type of secretion	**Characteristics**	**Example**
Serous	Watery, often proteinaceous fluid	Parotid salivary gland
Mucous	Viscous fluid containing highly glycosylated glycoproteins	Palatal salivary glands
Mixed	Both	Submandibular and sublingual salivary glands
Mode of secretion	**Characteristics**	**Example**
Merocrine	Secretory products are released via exocytosis.	Parotid salivary gland
Apocrine	Secretory products are collected within a cell and that portion of the cell is pinched off as the secretion.	Secretion of lipids by the lactating mammary gland may occur by the apocrine method of secretion.
Holocrine	Secretory products accumulate within the cell, and eventually, the cell dies and sheds as the secretion.	Sebaceous gland
Morphologic Classification		
Number of ducts	**Shape of secretory units**	**Examples**
Simple (single duct)	Acinar (oval to spherical)	Glands of Littre along the penile urethra
	Branched acinar (more than one acinus drain into a single duct)	Sebaceous glands
	Tubular (test tube-like)	Glands in the colon
	Branched tubular (more than one tubule drain into a short duct)	Glands in the stomach and small intestine
	Coiled tubular (long test tube coiled upon itself)	Sweat glands
Compound (more than one duct)	Acinar	Parotid glands
	Tubular	Duodenal (Brunner's) glands
	Tubuloacinar (mixture of acinus and tubule)	Submandibular and sublingual salivary glands

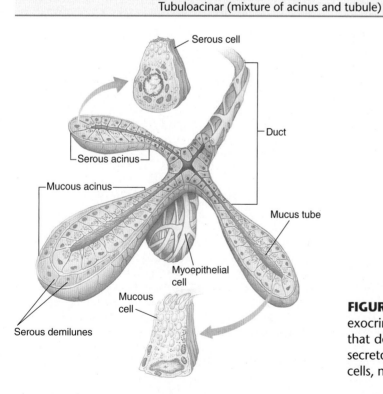

FIGURE 3-8. Schematic illustration of various forms of exocrine glands. Exocrine glands have ductal portions that deliver secretions to the surface or the lumen, and secretory portions that are composed of serous secreting cells, mucus-secreting goblet cells, or both types of cells.

PLATE 3-1A Simple Epithelia and Pseudostratified Epithelium

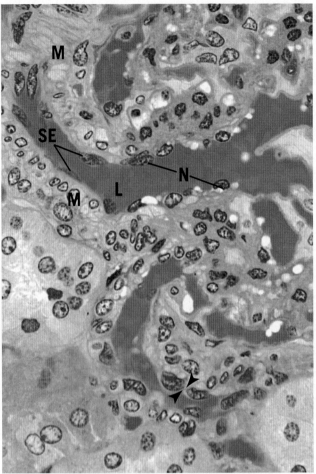

FIGURE 3-1-1. Simple squamous epithelium. Kidney. Monkey. Plastic section. ×540.

The lining of the **lumen** (L) of this small arteriole is composed of a simple **squamous epithelium** (SE) (known as the endothelium). The cytoplasm of these cells is highly attenuated and can only be approximated in this photomicrograph as a thin line (between the *arrowheads*). The boundaries of two contiguous epithelial cells cannot be determined with a light microscope. The **nuclei** (N) of the squamous epithelial cells bulge into the lumen, characteristic of this type of epithelium. Note that some of the nuclei appear more flattened than do others. This is because of the degree of agonal contraction of the **smooth muscle** (M) cells of the vessel wall.

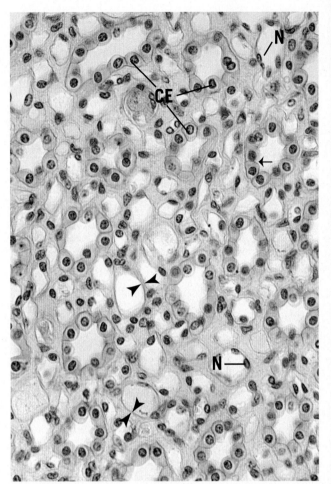

FIGURE 3-1-2. Simple squamous and simple cuboidal epithelia. x.s. Kidney. Paraffin section. ×270.

The medulla of the kidney provides an ideal representation of simple squamous and simple cuboidal epithelia. Simple squamous epithelium, as in the previous figure, is easily recognizable because of flattened but somewhat bulging **nuclei** (N). Note that the cytoplasm of these cells appears as thin, dark lines (between *arrowheads*); however, it must be stressed that the dark lines are composed of not only attenuated cells but also the surrounding basement membranes. The **simple cuboidal epithelium** (CE) is very obvious. The lateral cell membranes (*arrow*) are evident in some areas; even when they cannot be seen, the relationships of the round nuclei permit an imaginary approximation of the extent of each cell. Note that simple cuboidal cells, in section, appear more or less like small squares with centrally positioned nuclei.

SIMPLE

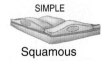

Squamous

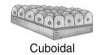

Cuboidal

KEY					
CE	simple cuboidal epithelium	M	smooth muscle	SE	simple squamous epithelium
		N	nucleus		

PLATE 3-1B   Simple Epithelia and Pseudostratified Epithelium

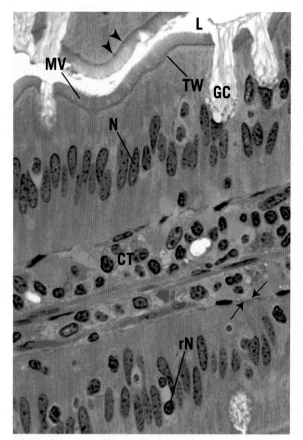

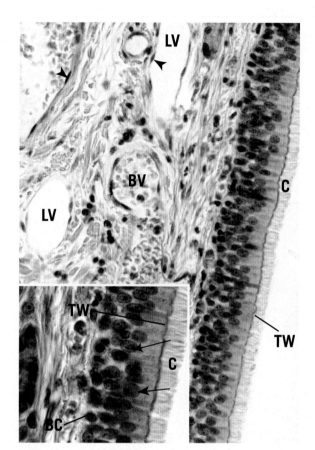

FIGURE 3-1-3. Simple columnar epithelium. Monkey. Plastic section. ×540.

FIGURE 3-1-4. Pseudostratified columnar epithelium with cilia. Paraffin section. ×270.

The simple columnar epithelium of the duodenum in this photomicrograph displays a very extensive **brush border** (MV) on the apical aspect of the cells. The **terminal web** (TW), where microvilli are anchored, appears as a dense line between the brush border and the apical cytoplasm. Distinct dots (*arrowheads*) are evident, which, although they appear to be part of the terminal web, are actually terminal bars, resolved by the electron microscope to be junctional complexes between contiguous cells. Note that the cells are tall and slender, and their **nuclei** (N), more or less oval in shape, are arranged rather uniformly at the same level in each cell. The basal aspects of these cells lie on a basement membrane (*arrows*), separating the epithelium from the **connective tissue** (CT). The **round nuclei** (rN) noted within the epithelium actually belong to leukocytes migrating into the **lumen** (L) of the duodenum. A few **goblet cells** (GC) are also evident.

The first impression conveyed by this epithelium from the nasal cavity is that it is stratified, being composed of at least four layers of cells; however, careful observation of the inset (×540) demonstrates that these are closely packed cells of varying heights and girth, each of which is in contact with the basement membrane. Here, unlike in the previous photomicrograph, the **nuclei** (N) are not uniformly arranged, and they occupy about three-fourths of the epithelial layer. The location and morphology of the nuclei indicate the cell type. The short **basal cells** (BC) display small, round to oval nuclei near the basement membrane. The tall, ciliated cells (*arrows*) possess large, oval nuclei. The **terminal web** (TW) supports tall, slender cilia (C), which propel mucus along the epithelial surface. The connective tissue is highly vascularized and presents good examples of simple squamous epithelia (*arrowheads*) that compose the endothelial lining of **blood** (BV) and **lymph vessels** (LV).

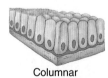

Columnar

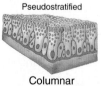

Pseudostratified

Columnar

KEY					
BC	basal cell	**GC**	goblet cell	**N**	nucleus
BV	blood vessel	**L**	lumen	**rN**	round nucleus
C	cilia	**LV**	lymph vessel	**TW**	terminal web
CT	connective tissue	**MV**	brush border		

PLATE 3-2   Stratified Epithelium and Transitional Epithelium

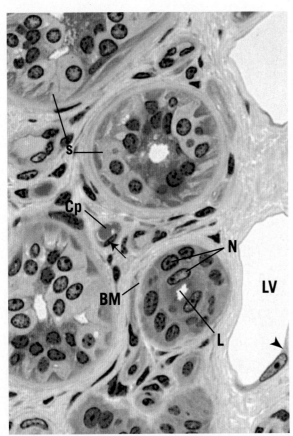

FIGURE 3-2-1. Stratified cuboidal epithelium. Monkey. Plastic section. ×540.

Stratified cuboidal epithelium is characterized by two or more layers of cuboid-shaped cells, as illustrated in this photomicrograph of a sweat gland duct. The **lumen** (L) of the duct is surrounded by cells whose cell boundaries are not readily evident, but the layering of the **nuclei** (N) demonstrates that this epithelium is truly stratified. The epithelium of the duct is surrounded by a **basement membrane** (BM). The other thick tubular profiles are tangential sections of the **secretory** (s) portions of the sweat gland, composed of simple cuboidal epithelium. Note the presence of a **capillary** (Cp), containing a single red blood cell, and the bulging nucleus (*arrow*) of the epithelial cell constituting the endothelial lining. The large empty space in the lower right-hand corner of this photomicrograph represents the lumen of a **lymph vessel** (LV) whose endothelial lining presents a flattened nucleus bulging into the lumen. Note that more cytoplasm is evident near the pole of the nucleus (*arrowhead*) than elsewhere.

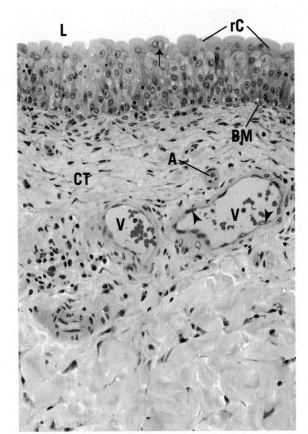

FIGURE 3-2-2. Transitional epithelium. Bladder. Monkey. Plastic section. ×132.

The urinary bladder, as most of the excretory portion of the urinary tract, is lined by a specialized type of stratified epithelium—the transitional epithelium. This particular specimen was taken from an empty, relaxed bladder, as indicated by the large, **round**, dome-**shaped** (rC) **cells**, some of which are occasionally binucleated (*arrow*), abutting the **lumen** (L). The epithelial cells lying on the **basement membrane** (BM) are quite small but increase in size as they migrate superficially and begin to acquire a pear shape. When the bladder is distended, the thickness of the epithelium decreases and the cells become flattened, more squamous-like. The connective tissue–epithelium interface is flat, with very little interdigitation between them. The **connective tissue** (CT) is very vascular immediately deep to the epithelium, as is evident from the sections of the **arterioles** (A) and **venules** (V) in this field. Observe the simple squamous endothelial linings of these vessels, characterized by their bulging nuclei (*arrowheads*).

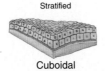

Stratified

Cuboidal

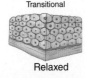

Transitional

Relaxed

KEY					
A	arteriole	**L**	lumen	**S**	secretory portion
BM	basement membrane	**LV**	lymph vessel	**V**	venule
Cp	capillary	**N**	nucleus		
CT	connective tissue	**rC**	round-shaped cell		

PLATE 3-3A   Epithelial Junctions, Electron Microscopy

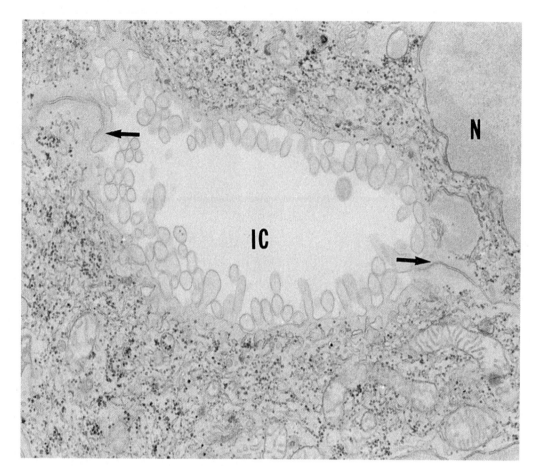

FIGURE 3-3-1. Epithelial junction. Human. Electron microscopy. ×27,815.

This electron micrograph represents a thin section of an intercellular canaliculus between clear cells of a human eccrine sweat gland stained with ferrocyanide-reduced osmium tetroxide. A tight junction (*arrows*) separates the lumen of the intercellular canaliculus (IC) from the basolateral intercellular space. Observe the nucleus (N). (From Briggman JV, et al. Structure of the tight junctions of the human eccrine sweat gland. *Am J Anat* 1981;162(4):357–368. Copyright © 1981 Wiley-Liss, Inc. Reprinted by permission of John Wiley & Sons, Inc.)

KEY

IC	intercellular canaliculus	**N**	nucleus

PLATE 3-3B Epithelial Junctions, Electron Microscopy

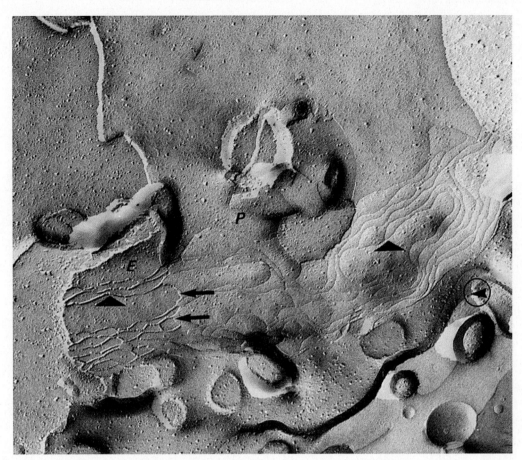

FIGURE 3-3-2. Epithelial junction. Zonula occludens. Human. Electron microscopy. ×83,700.

This is a freeze-fracture replica of an elaborate tight junction along an intercellular canaliculus between two clear cells. Note the smooth transition from a region of wavy, nonintersecting, densely packed junctional elements to an area of complex anastomoses. At the step fracture (*arrows*), it can be seen that the pattern of ridges on the E-face corresponds to that of the grooves on the P-face of the plasma membrane of the adjacent clear cell. In certain areas (*arrowheads*), several of the laterally disposed, densely packed junctional elements are separated from the luminal band. The direction of platinum shadowing is indicated by the *circled arrow*. (From Briggman JV, et al. Structure of the tight junctions of the human eccrine sweat gland. *Am J Anat* 1981;162(4):357–368. Copyright © 1981 Wiley-Liss, Inc. Reprinted by permission of John Wiley & Sons, Inc.)

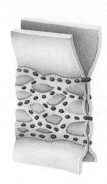

Zonulae occludentes

PLATE 3-4A Glands

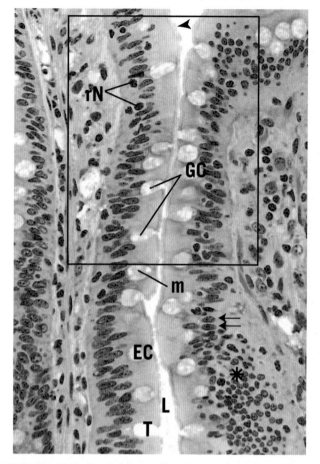

FIGURE 3-4-1. Goblet cells. Ileum. Monkey. Plastic section. ×270.

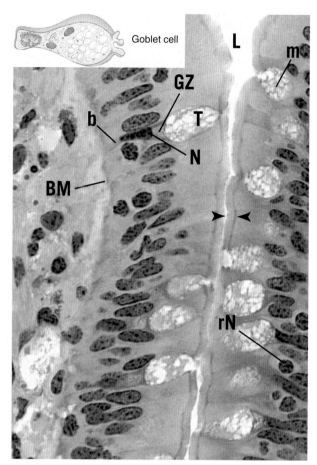

FIGURE 3-4-2. Goblet cells. Ileum. Monkey. Plastic section. ×540.

Goblet cells are unicellular exocrine glands that are found interspersed among simple columnar and pseudostratified columnar epithelia. This photomicrograph of an ileal villus displays numerous **goblet cells** (GC) located among the **simple columnar epithelial cells** (EC). The brush border (*arrowhead*) of the columnar cells is only scantly present on the goblet cells. The expanded apical region of the goblet cell is known as the **theca** (T) and is filled with **mucin** (m), which, when released into the lumen of the gut, coats and protects the intestinal lining. The lower right-hand corner of the simple columnar epithelium was sectioned somewhat obliquely through the nuclei of the epithelial cells, producing the appearance of a stratified epithelium (*asterisk*). Looking at the epithelium above the *double arrows*, however, it is clearly simple columnar. The occasional **round nuclei** (rN) are those of lymphocytes migrating through the epithelium into the **lumen** (L). Figure 3-4-2 is a higher magnification of the boxed area.

This photomicrograph is a higher magnification of the boxed area of the previous figure, demonstrating the light microscopic morphology of the goblet cell. The **mucinogen** (m) in the expanded **theca** (T) of the goblet cell has been partly precipitated and dissolved during the dehydration procedure. The **nucleus** (N) of the goblet cell is relatively dense owing to the condensed chromatin. Between the nucleus and the theca is the **Golgi zone** (GZ), where the protein product of the cell is modified and packaged into secretory granules for delivery. The **base** (b) of the goblet cell is slender, almost as if it were "squeezed in" between neighboring columnar epithelial cells, but it touches the **basement membrane** (BM). The terminal web and brush border of the goblet cell are greatly reduced but not completely absent (*arrowheads*). The **round nuclei** (rN) belong to leukocytes migrating through the epithelium into the **lumen** (L) of the ileum.

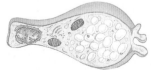

Goblet cell

KEY							
b	base	**GC**	goblet cell		**N**	nucleus
BM	basal membrane	**GZ**	Golgi zone		**rN**	round nucleus
EC	simple columnar epithelial cell	**L**	lumen		**T**	theca
		M	mucin			

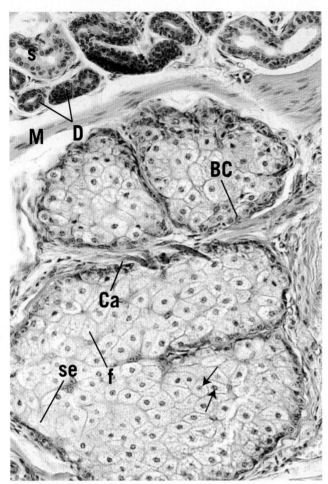

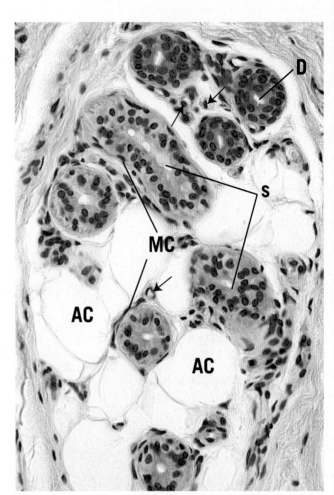

FIGURE 3-4-3. Sebaceous gland. Scalp. Paraffin section. ×132.

FIGURE 3-4-4. Eccrine sweat glands. Skin. Paraffin section. ×270.

Sebaceous glands are usually associated with hair follicles. They discharge their sebum into the follicle, although in certain areas of the body, they are present independent of hair follicles. These glands, surrounded by slender connective tissue **capsules** (Ca), are pear-shaped saccules with short ducts. Each saccule is filled with large, amorphous cells with nuclei in various states of degeneration (*arrows*). The periphery of the saccule is composed of small, cuboidal **basal cells** (BC), which act in a regenerative capacity. As the cells move away from the periphery of the saccule, they enlarge and increase their cytoplasmic **fat** (f) content. Near the duct, the entire cell degenerates and becomes the **secretion** (se). Therefore, sebaceous glands are classified as simple, branched, acinar glands with a holocrine mode of secretion. **Smooth muscle**s (M), arrector pili, are associated with sebaceous glands. Observe the **secretory** (s) and **duct** (D) portions of a sweat gland above the sebaceous gland.

Eccrine sweat glands are the most numerous glands in the body, and they are extensively distributed. The glands are simple, unbranched, coiled tubular, and producing a watery solution. The **secretory portion** (s) of the gland is composed of a simple cuboidal type of epithelium with two cell types, a lightly staining cell that makes up most of the secretory portion, and a darker staining cell that usually cannot be distinguished with the light microscope. Surrounding the secretory portion are **myoepithelial cells** (MC), which, with their numerous branching processes, encircle the secretory tubule and assist in expressing the fluid into the ducts. The **ducts** (D) of sweat glands are composed of a stratified cuboidal type of epithelium, whose cells are smaller than those of the secretory unit. In histologic sections, therefore, the ducts are always darker than the secretory units. The large, empty-looking spaces are **adipose** (fat) **cells** (AC). Note the numerous small blood vessels (*arrows*) in the vicinity of the sweat gland.

KEY					
AC	adipose cell	**D**	duct	**MC**	myoepithelial cell
BC	basal cell	**F**	fat	**S**	secretory
Ca	capsule	**M**	smooth muscle	**Se**	secretion

PLATE 3-4C   Glands

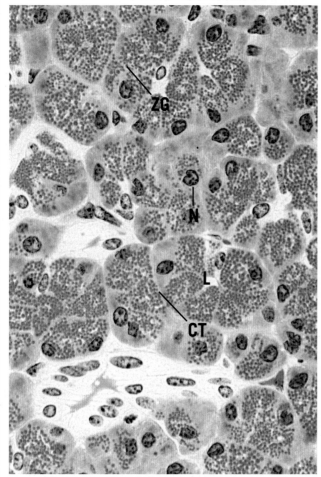

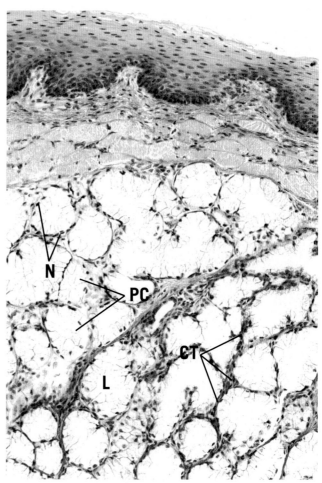

FIGURE 3-4-5. Compound acinar (alveolar) serous gland. Pancreas. Monkey. Plastic section. ×540.

This is a photomicrograph of the exocrine portion of the pancreas, a compound acinar (alveolar) serous gland. The duct system of this gland will be studied in Chapter 15 on the Digestive System. Only its secretory cells will be considered at this point. Each acinus, when sectioned well, presents a round appearance with a small central **lumen** (L), with the secretory cells arranged like a pie cut into pieces. The **connective tissue** (CT) investing each acinus is flimsy in the pancreas. The secretory cells are more or less trapezoid-shaped, with a round, basally situated **nucleus** (N). The cytoplasm contains numerous **zymogen granules** (ZG), which are the membrane-bound digestive enzymes packaged by the Golgi apparatus.

FIGURE 3-4-6. Compound tubular mucous glands. Soft palate. Paraffin section. ×132.

The compound tubular glands of the palate are purely mucous and secrete a thick, viscous fluid. The secretory tubules of this gland are circular in transverse section and are surrounded by fine **connective tissue** (CT) elements. The **lumina** (L) of the mucous tubules are clearly distinguishable, as are the trapezoid to columnar-shaped **parenchymal cells** (PC), which manufacture the viscous fluid. The **nuclei** (N) of the trapezoid-shaped cells are dark, dense structures that appear to be flattened against the basal cell membrane. The cytoplasm has an empty, frothy appearance, which stains a light grayish-blue with hematoxylin and eosin.

KEY					
CT	connective tissue	L	lumen	PC	parenchymal cell
D	duct	N	nucleus	ZG	zymogen granules

PLATE 3-4D Glands

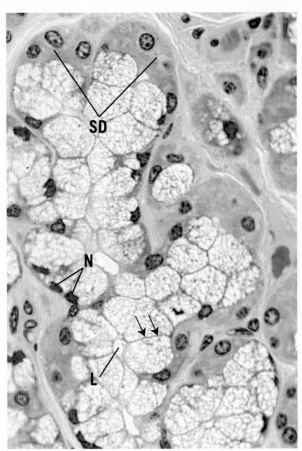

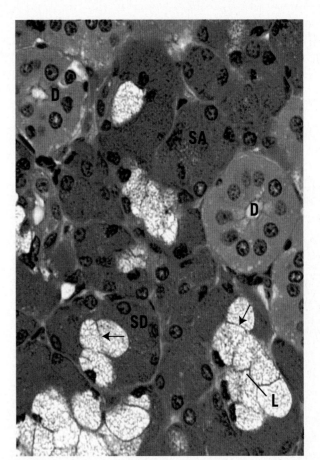

FIGURE 3-4-7. Compound tubuloacinar (alveolar) mixed gland. Sublingual gland. Monkey. Plastic section. ×540.

The sublingual gland is a mostly mucous, compound tubuloacinar gland that contains many mucous tubules and minor acini. These profiles of mucous tubules are well represented in this photomicrograph. Note the open **lumen** (L) bordered by several columnar to trapezoid-shaped cells whose lateral plasma membranes are evident (*double arrows*). The **nuclei** (N) of these mucous cells appear to be flattened against the basal plasma membrane and are easily distinguishable from the round nuclei of the cells of serous acini. The cytoplasm appears to possess numerous vacuole-like structures that impart a frothy appearance to the cell. The serous secretions of this gland are derived from the few serous cells that appear to cap the mucous units, known as **serous demilunes** (SD).

FIGURE 3-4-8. Compound tubuloacinar (alveolar) mixed gland. Submandibular gland. Monkey. Plastic section. ×540.

The submandibular gland is a compound tubuloacinar gland that produces a mixed secretion, as does the sublingual gland of the previous figure. However, this gland contains more **serous acini** (SA) and minor mucous tubules that are capped by **serous demilunes** (SD). Also, this gland possesses an extensive system of **ducts** (D). Note that the cytoplasm of the serous cells appears to be blue when stained with hematoxylin and eosin. Also note that the **lumina** of the acini are so small that they are not apparent, whereas those of mucous units (L) are obvious. Observe the difference in the cytoplasms of serous and mucus-secreting cells as well as the density of the nuclei of individual cells. Finally, note that the lateral cell membranes (*arrows*) of mucus-producing cells are clearly delineated, whereas those of the serous cells are very difficult to observe.

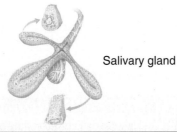

Salivary gland

KEY					
D	duct	**N**	nucleus	**SD**	serous demilunes
L	lumen	**SA**	serous acini		

Selected Review of Histologic Images

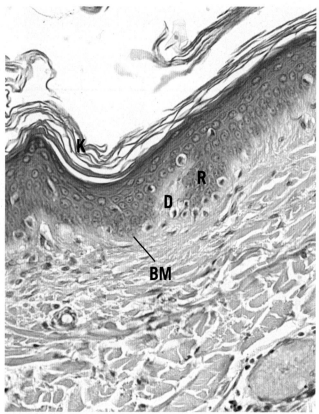

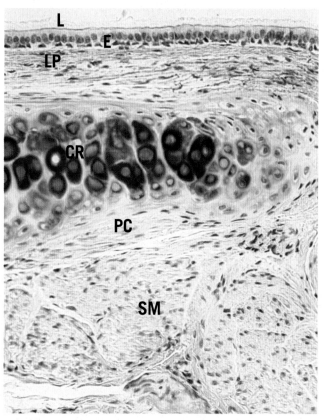

REVIEW FIGURE 3-1-1. Stratified squamous keratinized epithelium. Human glabrous skin. Paraffin section. ×270.

This photomicrograph of glabrous skin shows the **keratin** (K) sloughing off the free surface of the stratified squamous keratinized epithelium. Note that a **basement membrane** (BM) separates the epidermis from the dermis. Also observe the rete apparatus as evident from the presence of **epithelial ridges** (R) that interdigitate with **dermal ridges** (D) of the dermis.

REVIEW FIGURE 3-1-2. Trachea. l.s. Monkey. Paraffin section. ×270.

The **lumen** (L) of the trachea is lined by a **pseudostratified ciliated columnar epithelium** (E), which overlies the **lamina propria** (LP). The hyaline cartilage **C-ring** (CR) is the skeleton of the trachea, which maintains its patency. The dense irregular collagenous connective tissue **perichondrium** (PC) of the C-ring invests the entire hyaline cartilage. This section was taken from an area near the open ends of the C-ring, where the trachealis muscle, a **smooth muscle** (SM), fills in the gap.

KEY					
BM	basement membrane	**E**	pseudostratified ciliated	**LP**	lamina propria tissue
CR	C-ring		columnar epithelium	**PC**	perichondrium
D	dermal ridges	**K**	keratin	**R**	epithelial ridges
		L	lumen	**SM**	smooth muscle

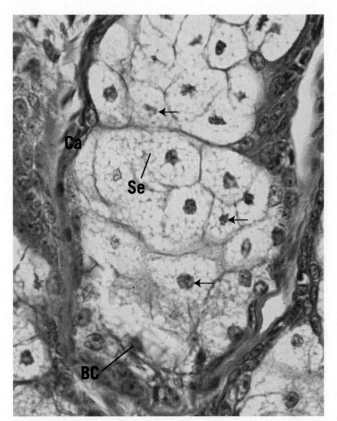

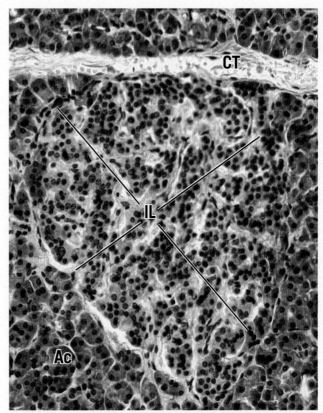

REVIEW FIGURE 3-1-3. Sebaceous gland. Human glabrous skin. Paraffin section. ×540.

This photomicrograph is a high magnification of a sebaceous gland displaying its **capsule** (Ca) as well as the regenerative **basal cells** (BC) that are responsible for the maintenance of the gland by providing new cells that replace the sebum-forming cells of the gland. **Sebum** (Se) collects in vesicles that fuse as the cell degenerates, and the entire dead cell is expressed as the secretory product of this holocrine gland. Observe that as the cell degenerates, its nucleus becomes more and more pyknotic (*arrows*).

REVIEW FIGURE 3-1-4. Pancreas including an islet of Langerhans. Human. Paraffin section. ×132.

This photomicrograph displays both the exocrine and the endocrine portions of the human pancreas where the **islets of Langerhans** (IL) constitute the endocrine portion. The **connective tissue** (CT) of the pancreas not only subdivides it into lobes and lobules but also conveys its vascular supply as well as the system of ducts that deliver the exocrine secretions of the acinar cells of the **serous acini** (Ac) and of the centroacinar cells and intercalated ducts into the duodenum. This particular duct is composed of a stratified cuboidal epithelium.

KEY					
Ac	serous acini	**Ca**	capsule	**IL**	islets of Langerhans
BC	basal cells	**CT**	connective tissue	**Se**	sebum

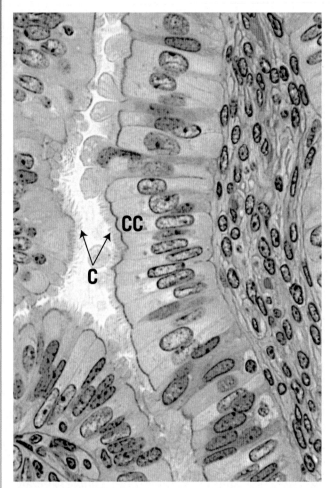

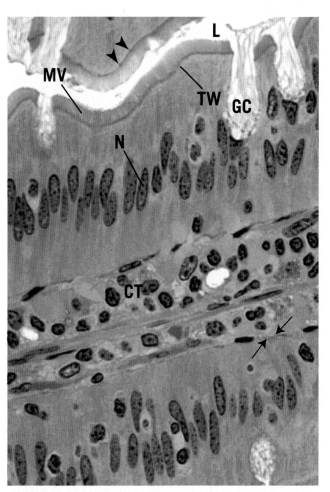

REVIEW FIGURE 3-1-5. Oviduct. x.s. Monkey. Plastic section. ×540.

This is the ciliated simple columnar epithelium lining the oviduct. Note the **cilia** (C) forming the apical specialization of the **ciliated cells** (CC). Transmission electron micrograph of the cilia would show the axonemes forming the core of each cilium, which, along with the function of dynein, allow the cilia to be motile. Although cilia tend to be longer and are larger in diameter than the microvilli forming the brush border, the two apical specializations can appear similar in light microscopy. However, upon closer inspection, the uniformity in length and staining pattern of the microvilli and the irregular length and shape of the cilia are apparent.

REVIEW FIGURE 3-1-6. Simple columnar epithelium. Monkey. Plastic section. ×540.

The simple columnar epithelium of the duodenum in this photomicrograph displays a very extensive **brush border** (MV) on the apical aspect of the cells. The **terminal web** (TW), where microvilli are anchored, appears as a dense line between the brush border and the apical cytoplasm. Distinct dots (*arrowheads*) are evident, which, although they appear to be part of the terminal web, are actually terminal bars, resolved by the electron microscope to be junctional complexes between contiguous cells. Note that the cells are tall and slender, and their **nuclei** (N), more or less oval in shape, are arranged rather uniformly at the same level in each cell. The basal aspects of these cells lie on a basement membrane (*arrows*), separating the epithelium from the **connective tissue** (CT). The round nuclei noted within the epithelium actually belong to leukocytes migrating into the **lumen** (L) of the duodenum. A few **goblet cells** (GC) are also evident.

KEY					
C	cilia	**GC**	goblet cells	**N**	nucleus
CC	ciliated cell	**L**	lumen	**TW**	terminal web
CT	connective tissue	**MV**	brush border		

Summary of Histologic Organization

I. EPITHELIUM

A. Types

1. Simple Squamous

Single layer of uniform flat cells.

2. Simple Cuboidal

Single layer of uniform cuboidal cells.

3. Simple Columnar

Single layer of uniform columnar cells.

4. Pseudostratified Columnar

Single layer of cells of varied shapes and heights. May or may not be ciliated.

5. Stratified Squamous

Several layers of cells whose superficial layers are flattened. These may be nonkeratinized, parakeratinized, or keratinized.

6. Stratified Cuboidal

Two or more layers of cells whose superficial layers are cuboidal in shape.

7. Stratified Columnar

Two or more layers of cells whose superficial layers are columnar in shape.

8. Transitional

Several layers of cells, characterized by large, dome-shaped cells at the free surface, which help maintain the integrity of the epithelium during distention of the various components of the urinary tract.

B. General Characteristics

1. Free Surface Modifications

Cells may possess **microvilli** (forming brush border, striated border), short finger-like projections that increase the surface area of the cell; **stereocilia** (long anastomosing microvilli), which are found almost exclusively in the epididymis; and **cilia**, which are long, motile projections of the cell with a 9 + 2 microtubular substructure (**axoneme**).

2. Lateral Surface Modifications

For the purposes of adhesion, the cell membranes form junctional complexes involving the lateral plasmalemma of contiguous cells. These junctions are known as **desmosomes** (maculae adherentes), **zonulae occludentes**, and **zonulae adherentes**. For the purpose of intercellular communication, the lateral cell membranes form **gap junctions** (nexus, septate junctions).

3. Basal Surface Modifications

The basal cell membrane that lies on the basement membrane forms **hemidesmosomes** to assist the cell to adhere to the underlying connective tissue.

4. Basement Membrane

The **basement (basal) membrane** of light microscopy is composed of an epithelially derived **basal lamina** (which has two parts, **lamina densa** and **lamina lucida**) and a **lamina reticularis** derived from connective tissue, which may be absent.

II. GLANDS

A. Exocrine Glands

Exocrine glands, which deliver secretions into a system of ducts to be conveyed onto an epithelial surface, may be **unicellular** (goblet cells) or **multicellular**.

Multicellular glands may be classified according to the number of their **ducts**. If there is one duct, the gland is **simple**; if there are more than one duct, the gland is **compound**. Moreover, the three-dimensional shape of the secretory units may be **tubular**, **acinar (alveolar)**, or a combination of the two, namely, **tubuloacinar (tubuloalveolar)**. Additional criteria include (1) the **type** of secretory product produced (**serous** [parotid, pancreas], **mucous** [palatal glands], and **mixed** [sublingual, submandibular], possessing serous and mucous acini and **serous demilunes**) and (2) the **mode of secretion** (**merocrine** [only the secretory product is released, as in the parotid gland], **apocrine** [the secretory product is accompanied by some of the apical cytoplasm, as perhaps in mammary glands], and **holocrine** [the entire cell becomes the secretory product, as in the sebaceous gland]). Large compound glands are subdivided by connective tissue septa into lobes and lobules, and the ducts that serve them are interlobar, intralobar, interlobular, and intralobular (striated, intercalated).

Myoepithelial (basket) cells are ectodermally derived myoid cells that share the basement lamina of the glandular parenchyma. These cells possess long processes that surround secretory acini and, by occasional contraction, assist in the delivery of the secretory product into the system of ducts.

B. Endocrine Glands

Endocrine glands are ductless glands that release their secretion into the bloodstream. These glands are described in Chapter 10.

Chapter Review Questions

3-1. A patient's esophageal biopsy reveals a well-organized simple columnar covering epithelium. What is this condition?

A. Adenocarcinoma

B. Bullous pemphigus

C. Carcinoma

D. Metaplasia

3-2. What type of epithelium should be expected from the normal esophageal lining?

A. Ciliated pseudostratified columnar epithelium

B. Nonkeratinized stratified squamous epithelium

C. Stratified cuboidal epithelium

D. Transitional epithelium

3-3. Which gland uses holocrine secretion?

A. Sebaceous gland

B. Sweat gland

C. Mammary gland

D. Parotid gland

3-4. A 38-year-old male patient suffers from frequent upper respiratory tract infection. Which epithelial cell specialization should be inspected for proper function?

A. Cilia

B. Stereocilia

C. Microvilli

D. Desmosome

3-5. If a high contrast dye in the intestine easily seeps into the underlying connective tissue, which protein should be suspected to be defective?

A. Claudin

B. E-cadherin

C. Integrin

D. Desmoplakin

E. Connexin

CONNECTIVE TISSUE

CHAPTER OUTLINE

The major structural constituents of the body are composed of connective tissues. Although seemingly diverse, they possess many shared qualities structurally and functionally; therefore, they are considered in a single category. Most connective tissues are derived from mesoderm, which forms the multipotential mesenchyme from which bone, cartilage, tendons, ligaments, capsules, blood and hematopoietic cells, and lymphoid cells develop. Functionally, connective tissues serve in support, defense, transport, storage, and repair, among other actions. Morphologically, connective tissues are composed mainly of **extracellular matrix** (ECM) and a relatively fewer number of **cells**. Recall that in epithelial tissues, cells are the major constituents with little to no amount of ECM.

Connective tissues are classified mostly based on their nonliving, ECM components rather than their cellular constituents. Although the precise ordering of the various subtypes differs from author to author, the following categories are generally accepted:

- Embryonic connective tissues
  - Mesenchymal
  - Mucous
- Adult connective tissues
  - Connective tissue proper
    - Loose (areolar)
    - Dense regular
    - Dense irregular
  - Specialized connective tissues
    - Reticular
    - Elastic
    - Adipose
      - Unilocular
      - Multilocular
    - Cartilage
    - Bone
    - Blood

Extracellular Matrix

The ECM of connective tissue proper is composed of **fibers, amorphous ground substance**, and **extracellular fluid (ECF; tissue** or **interstitial fluid)**.

Fibers

Three types of fibers are recognized histologically: collagen, reticular, and elastic.

Collagen Fibers

Collagen fibers are the most abundant of the fibers, forming about 20% to 25% of human protein content. They are nonelastic and usually occur as bundles of varied thicknesses. Their basic subunits are **tropocollagen molecules**, each of which is composed of three α chains wound around each other (Fig. 4-1). Interestingly, every third amino acid of the α chain is **glycine**, and a significant amount of **proline, hydroxyproline, lysine**, and **hydroxylysine** constitutes much of the tropocollagen subunit. Because glycine is a very small amino acid, the three α chains can form a tight helix as they wrap around each other. The hydrogen bonds of hydroxyproline residues of individual α chains hold the three chains together to maintain the stability of the tropocollagen molecule; hydroxylysine residues hold the tropocollagen molecules to each other to form collagen fibrils.

Currently, at least 35 different types of collagen proteins are known, each designated by a Roman numeral, depending on the amino acid composition of their α chains. The most common collagen proteins are type I (dermis, bone, capsules of organs, fibrocartilage, dentin, and cementum), type II (hyaline and elastic cartilages), type III (reticular fibers), type IV (lamina densa of the basal lamina), type V (placenta), and type VII (anchoring fibrils of the basal lamina). These 35 or so types of collagen proteins are grouped into four different classes: **fibril-forming, network-forming, fibril-associated**, and **transmembrane collagens (collagen-like proteins)** (Table 4-1). All collagen fibers composed of fibril-forming collagens display a **67-nm periodicity** as the result of the specific arrangement of the tropocollagen molecules (see Fig. 4-1). The non-fibril-forming collagen types, such as type IV collagen, which is present in basal laminae, do not exhibit this banding characteristic.

Synthesis of Fibril-Forming Collagens

Synthesis of fibril-forming collagen occurs on the rough endoplasmic reticulum (rER), where polysomes possess different mRNAs coding for the three α **chains (preprocollagens)**. Within the rER cisternae, specific proline and lysine residues are **hydroxylated**, and hydroxylysine residues are **glycosylated**. Each α chain possesses **propeptides (telopeptides)** located at both amino and carboxyl ends. These propeptides are responsible for the precise **alignment** of the α chains, resulting in the formation of the **triple-helical procollagen** molecule.

Coatomer-coated transfer vesicles convey the procollagen molecules to the **Golgi apparatus** for modification, mostly the addition of carbohydrate side chains. Subsequent to transfer to the *trans*-Golgi network, the **procollagen** molecule is exocytosed (via non-clathrin-coated vesicles), and the propeptides are cleaved by the enzyme **procollagen peptidase**, resulting in the formation of tropocollagen.

Tropocollagen molecules self-assemble in the ECM, forming fibrils with their characteristic 67-nm banding (see Fig. 4-1). Type IV collagen is composed of procollagen rather than tropocollagen subunits, hence the absence of periodicity and fibril formation in this type of collagen.

Reticular Fibers

Reticular fibers are thin, short, branching, fibers composed of type III collagen that possess a higher content of carbohydrate moieties than do the remaining collagen types. As a result, when stained with silver stain, the silver preferentially deposits on these fibers, giving them a brown to black appearance in the light microscope. Reticular fibers form delicate networks around smooth muscle cells, certain epithelial cells, adipocytes, nerve fibers, and blood vessels. They also constitute the structural framework of certain organs, such as the liver and the spleen.

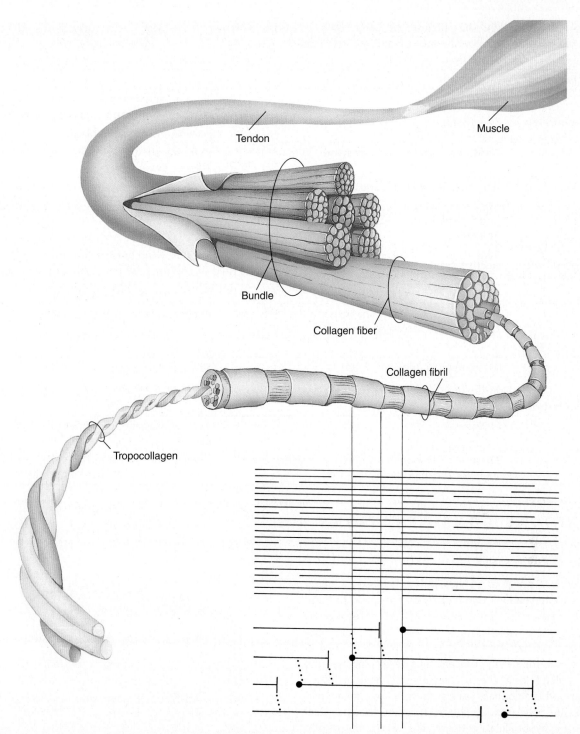

Tendon

Muscle

Bundle

Collagen fiber

Collagen fibril

Tropocollagen

FIGURE 4-1. Structural organization of typical collagen fibers. Each collagen fiber bundle is composed of smaller fibrils, which, in turn consist of aggregates of **tropocollagen molecules**. Tropocollagen molecules self-assemble in the extracellular environment in such a fashion that there is a gap between the tail of the one and the head of the succeeding molecule of a single row. As fibrils are formed, tails of tropocollagen molecules overlap the heads of tropocollagen molecules in adjacent rows. Additionally, the **gaps** and **overlaps** are arranged so that they are in register with those of neighboring (but not adjacent) rows of tropocollagen molecules. When stained with a heavy metal, such as osmium, the steam preferentially precipitates in the gap regions, resulting in the repeating **light** and **dark** banding of collagen.

Elastic Fibers

Elastic fibers, as their name implies, are highly elastic and may be stretched to about 150% of their resting length without breaking. They are composed of an amorphous protein, **elastin**, surrounded by a **microfibrillar** component, consisting of **fibrillin-5**, **fibrillin-1**, and the inelastic **type VIII collagen**. The fibrillin-1 molecules form a hollow, cylindrical configuration, and the soluble elastin

Table 4-1   Function and Location of the Most Common Collagen Types

Type	Function	Location
Fibril Forming		
I	Resists tension placed on it	Tendons and ligaments; dermis of skin, capsules of organs; bone; cementum; dentin
II	Resists tension placed on it	Hyaline and elastic cartilages
III	Constructs architectural framework	Liver; spleen; lymph nodes; smooth muscles; adipose tissue
V	Accompanies type I collagen	See type I; also placenta
VIII	May form a layer for the migration of endothelial cells and smooth muscle cells; limits the stretching ability of elastin	Endothelial basement membrane; corneal endothelium
XI	Type I and type II collagen form around it.	See type I and type II collagens
Network Forming		
IV	Affords support and acts as a filter	Lamina densa of the basal lamina
VII	Aids in attaching the lamina densa to the lamina reticularis of the basement membrane	Anchoring fibers of the basement membranes
Fibril Associated		
IX	Combines with type II collagen	See type II collagen
XII	Combines with type I collagen	See type I collagen
Transmembrane Collagens		
XVII	Unknown	Hemidesmosome (previous name: bullous pemphigoid antigen)
XVIII	Enzymatic cleavage transforms it into angiogenesis inhibitor and endostatin	Lamina reticularis of the basement membrane

CLINICAL CONSIDERATIONS 4-1

Keloid Formation

The body responds to wounds, including those caused by surgical intervention, by forming scars that repair the damage first with weak type III collagen that is later replaced by type I collagen, which is much stronger. Some individuals, especially African Americans, form an overabundance of collagen in the healing process, thus developing elevated scars called keloids. The collagen fibers in keloids are much larger and eosinophilic—said to have a "glassy" appearance—than the normal, fibrillar, collagen. Moreover, keloids are hypocellular, although they frequently display clusters of fibroblasts distributed among the large, glassy collagen fiber bundles.

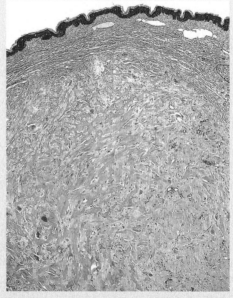

Keloid formation at the site of injury is evidenced by the excessively thick layer of the dermis whose large, eosinophilic, type I collagen fibers are clearly apparent. (Reprinted with permission from Mills SE, et al., eds. *Sternberg's Diagnostic Surgical Pathology*, 6th ed. Philadelphia: Wolters Kluwer, 2015. p. 30, Figure 1-54.)

CLINICAL CONSIDERATIONS 4-2

Scurvy

Scurvy, a condition characterized by bleeding gums and loose teeth among other symptoms, results from a vitamin C deficiency. Vitamin C is necessary for hydroxylation of proline for proper tropocollagen formation giving rise to fibrils necessary for maintaining teeth in their bony sockets.

CLINICAL CONSIDERATIONS 4-3

Marfan's Syndrome

Patients with Marfan's syndrome, a genetic defect in chromosome 15 that codes for fibrillin, possess undeveloped elastic fibers in their body and are predisposed to rupture of the aorta. Histologically, the aortas of a large portion of individuals with Marfan's syndrome display cystic medial degeneration, a condition in which the fenestrated membranes as well as the smooth muscles of the tunica media are reduced in quantity or are partially absent (Fig. A). In individuals with less severe cystic medial degeneration, the fenestrated membranes are less well organized, the smooth muscle cells are fewer in number, and the connective tissue is richer in ground substance than in normal aortas (Fig. B).

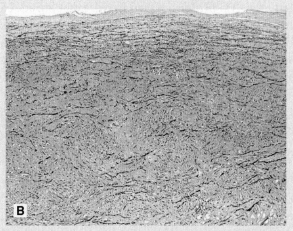

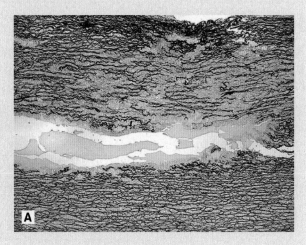

A. Cystic medial degeneration, evident in the media of this aorta from a patient exhibiting Marfan's syndrome, demonstrates that the fenestrated membrane and smooth muscle cells have been replaced by amorphous ground substance. **B.** A less severe case of cystic medial degeneration is displayed in this patient. The tunica media shows disorganized fenestrated membranes and smooth muscle fibers as well as an increase in the amorphous ground substance. (Reprinted with permission from Mills SE, et al., eds. *Sternberg's Diagnostic Surgical Pathology*, 6th ed. Philadelphia: Wolters Kluwer, 2015. p. 1353, Figure 30-1A,B.)

precursor molecules, known as tropoelastin, fill the hollow core of the fibrillin-1 cylinders. As the protoelastins contact the fibrillin-1, they are converted into elastin. In some unknown fashion, fibulin-5 facilitates the formation of elastic fibers. The elasticity of elastin is owing to its lysine content, in that four lysine molecules, each belonging to a different elastin chain, form covalent **desmosine cross-links** with one another. These links are highly deformable and can stretch when tensile forces are applied to them, but the ability to stretch is limited by the inelastic type VIII collagen fibers, which act to protect the elastic fibers from becoming overstretched and breaking. Once the tensile force ceases, the elastic fibers return to their resting length. Elastic fibers do not display periodicity and are found in regions of the body that require considerable flexibility and elasticity, such as large arteries.

Ground Substance

The **amorphous ground substance** constitutes the gel-like matrix in which the fibers and cells are embedded and through which ECF diffuses. Ground substance is composed of **glycosaminoglycans** (GAGs), **proteoglycans**, and **glycoproteins**.

Glycosaminoglycans

GAGs are linear polymers of repeating disaccharides, one of which is always a **hexosamine**, whereas the other is a **hexuronic acid** (Table 4-2). The major GAG constituents are **hyaluronic acid**, **chondroitin-4-sulfate**, **chondroitin-6-sulfate**, **dermatan sulfate**, **keratan sulfate I** and **II**, **heparin**, and **heparan sulfate**. All GAGs, except **hyaluronic acid**, are sulfated and thus possess a predominantly **negative charge**.

Proteoglycans

Proteoglycans are composed of a protein core to which GAGs are covalently bound. Most GAGs are linked to protein cores via **bridge tetrasaccharides** that are added to the serine side chains of the protein cores as they were modified within the Golgi apparatus. Proteoglycans can be relatively small, such as **decorin** (50 kD), or quite large, such as aggrecan (30,000 kDa). Many of these proteoglycan molecules can also be linked to hyaluronic acid via **link proteins**, forming massive molecules, such as **aggrecans aggregate**, forming enormous electrochemical **domains** that attract osmotically active cations (e.g., Na^+). These huge cation-covered proteoglycans attract H_2O molecules, forming hydrated molecules that provide a gel-like consistency to connective tissue proper, thereby resisting compression and slowing down the flow of ECF. This reduced flow rate permits more time for the exchange of materials by the cells and impedes the spread of invading microorganisms. The sulfated GAGs include chondroitin sulfate, dermatan sulfate, heparan sulfate, heparin, and keratan sulfate.

Glycoproteins

Glycoproteins are large polypeptide molecules with attendant carbohydrate side chains. The best characterized are **laminin**, **fibronectin**, chondronectin, osteonectin, entactin, and tenascin. Laminin and entactin are derived from epithelial cells, and tenascin is made by glial cells of the embryo, whereas the remainder are manufactured by cells of connective tissue. Many cells possess **integrins**, transmembrane proteins, with receptor sites for one or more of these glycoproteins. Moreover, glycoproteins also bind to collagen, thus facilitating cell adherence to or migration along the ECM.

The basement membrane, interposed between epithelial and connective tissues, is described in Chapter 3, Epithelium and Glands.

Extracellular Fluid

ECF (tissue or interstitial fluid) is the fluid component of blood, similar to plasma, which percolates throughout the ground substance, carrying nutrients, oxygen, and other blood-borne materials to cells and carbon dioxide and waste products from cells. ECF leaves the capillaries at the arterial end and returns back to the capillaries at the venous end; the excess fluid left in the connective tissue ECM is drained by the lymphatic capillaries.

Cells

A variety of cells are present in connective tissue proper, and their morphology and number can provide valuable information about the tissue function and even the type

Table 4-2   Types of Glycosaminoglycans (GAGs)

GAGs	Sulfated	Repeating Disaccharides	Linked to Core Protein	Location
Hyaluronic acid	No	D-Glucuronic acid-β-1,3-N-acetyl-D-glucosamine	No	Most connective tissue, synovial fluid, cartilage, dermis, vitreous humor, umbilical cord
Keratan sulfate I and II	Yes	Galactose-β-1,4-N-acetyl-D-glucosamine-6-SO₄	Yes	Cornea (keratan sulfate I), cartilage (keratan sulfate II)
Heparan sulfate	Yes	D-Glucuronic acid-β-1,3-N-acetyl galactosamine L-Iduronic acid-2 or-SO₄-β-1,3-N-acetyl-D-galactosamine	Yes	Blood vessels, lung, basal lamina
Heparin (90%)	Yes	L-Iduronic acid-β-1,4-sulfo-D-glucosamine-6-SO₄	No	Mast cell granule, liver, lung, skin
Heparin (10%)		D-Glucuronic acid-β-1,4-N-acetylglucosamine-6-SO₄		
Chondroitin-4-sulfate	Yes	D-Glucuronic acid-β-1,3-N-acetylgalactosamine-6-SO₄	Yes	Cartilage, bone, cornea, blood vessels
Chondroitin-6-sulfate	Yes	D-Glucuronic acid-β-1,3-N-acetylgalactosamine-6-SO₄	Yes	Cartilage, Wharton's jelly, blood vessels
Dermatan sulfate	Yes	L-Iduronic acid-α-1,3-N-acetylglucosamine-4-SO₄	Yes	Heart valves, skin, blood vessels

CLINICAL CONSIDERATIONS 4-4

Edema

Accumulation of excess fluid in the connective tissue ECM is called edema. Two main forces are at play in keeping the ECM fluid volume and content at a constant state, homeostasis. These forces are hydrostatic and osmotic pressures. Hydrostatic pressure, the force generated from the heart contraction, moves the fluid from the capillary at the arterial end into the connective tissue ECM. As this happens, the hydrostatic pressure in the capillary decreases, but the osmotic pressure increases as the capillary approaches the venous end due to solutes in the blood becoming more concentrated. The concentrated solutes in the capillary use osmotic pressure to draw fluid from the connective tissue ECM back to the capillary. Any excess fluid in the ECM is drained via lymphatic channels. An imbalance in this delicate ECM fluid homeostasis, such as weakened hydrostatic pressure and osmotic pressure (as in congestive heart failure), venous blockage (as in deep vein thrombosis), or lymphatic blockage (from lymphatic dissection during surgery), can result in generalized or localized edema.

of injury, repair, or disease processes occurring (Fig. 4-2). Most of these cells are derived from embryonic mesenchymal cells.

- **Fibroblasts**, the predominant cell type, are responsible for the **synthesis** of collagen, elastic and reticular fibers, and much (if not all) of the ground substance.
  - The morphology of these cells results as a function of their synthetic activities; therefore, resting (or inactive fibroblasts) cells are often referred to as fibrocytes, a term that is rapidly disappearing from the literature.

- **Mast cells** are of two types, those located in connective tissue proper in the vicinity of blood vessels (known as **connective tissue mast cells**) and those that reside in the mucosa of the digestive tract (known as **mucosal mast cells**).
  - Both cell types house numerous metachromatic granules containing pharmacologic agents (**primary mediators**, **preformed mediators**) that induce inflammatory responses.
  - Mast cells manufacture additional pharmacologic agents that, instead of being stored in secretory granules, are released as soon as they are formed (**secondary mediators**, **newly synthesized mediators**). Both types of pharmacologic agents and their functions are listed in Table 4-3.
  - The major difference between mucosal and connective tissue mast cells is that mucosal mast cells have **chondroitin sulfate**, and connective tissue mast cells have **heparin** as one of the pharmacologic agents in their granules.
  - All mast cells possess receptors on their cell membranes for the **immunoglobulin E (IgE)**. When antigens enter the body, plasma cells manufacture antibodies against the antigen, among them IgE, which then bind to the **IgE receptors** on the mast cell surface. The next time the same antigen enters the body, they bind to the IgE on the mast cell surface, and, if these antibodies become cross-linked with each other, they precipitate the release of not only the primary mediators but also the secondary mediators, thereby initiating an **inflammatory response**. Unfortunately, in sensitized individuals, these cells may release their granules throughout the body instead of just locally, resulting in **anaphylactic reactions** or even in life-threatening **anaphylactic shock**.

- **Pericytes** are also associated with minute blood vessels, but much more closely than are mast cells, because they share the basal laminae of the endothelial cells.
  - Pericytes are believed to be **contractile cells**, which assist in the regulation of blood flow through the capillaries.
  - Additionally, they may also be **pluripotential cells**, which assume the responsibilities of mesenchymal cells in adult connective tissue. It is now believed that mesenchymal cells are probably not present in the adult (except certain specialized regions, as in the pulps of teeth).

- **Fat cells (adipocytes)** may form small clusters or aggregates in loose connective tissue. They **store lipids** and form adipose tissue, which protects, insulates, and cushions body organs.

- **Leukocytes** (white blood cells [WBCs]) leave the bloodstream and enter the connective tissue spaces. Some differentiate and perform specialized functions, whereas some remain undifferentiated to perform their intended function within their short life span. More detailed leukocyte histology and functions are discussed in Chapters 6 and 10.
  - **Macrophages** are derived from a type of circulating WBCs called monocytes. Once monocytes leave the blood vessels and migrate into connective tissue, they differentiate into macrophages, cells that function in ingesting (**phagocytosing**) foreign particulate matter or any cellular debris from apoptosis or

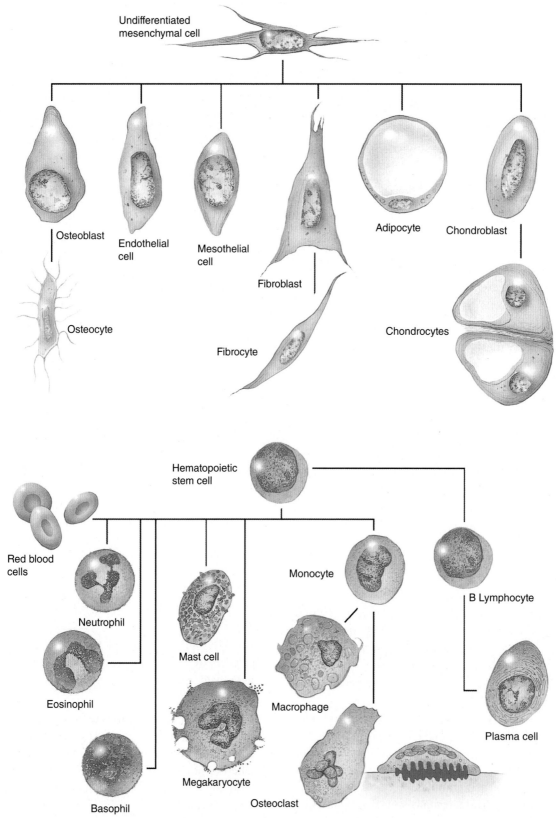

FIGURE 4-2. Connective tissue cells. Note that the cells depicted are not represented in proportion to their actual diameters.

Table 4-3 Mast Cell Factors and Functions

Substance	Intracellular Source	Action
Primary Mediators		
Histamine	Granules	Vasodilator; increases vascular permeability; causes contraction of bronchial smooth muscle; increases mucus production
Heparin	Granules	Anticoagulant; inactivates histamine
Eosinophil chemotactic factor	Granules	Attractant for eosinophils to the site of inflammation
Neutrophil chemotactic factor	Granules	Attractant for neutrophils to the site of inflammation
Aryl sulfate	Granules	Inactivates leukotriene C4, limiting inflammatory response
Chondroitin sulfate	Granules	Binds and inactivates histamine
Neutral proteases	Granules	Protein cleavage to activate complement; increases inflammatory response
Secondary Mediators		
Prostaglandin D2	Membrane lipid	Causes contraction of bronchial smooth muscle; increases mucus secretion; vasoconstriction
Leukotrienes C4, D4, E4	Membrane lipid	Vasodilators; increases vascular permeability; contraction of bronchial smooth muscle
Bradykinins	Membrane lipid	Causes vascular permeability; responsible for pain sensation
Thromboxane A2	Membrane lipid	Causes platelet aggregation; vasoconstriction
Platelet-activating factor	Activated by phospholipase A_2	Attracts neutrophils and eosinophils; causes vascular permeability; contraction of bronchial smooth muscle

CLINICAL CONSIDERATIONS 4-5

Anaphylaxis

The release of histamine and leukotrienes from mast cells during an inflammatory response elicits increased capillary permeability, resulting in an excess accumulation of ECF and, thus, gross swelling (edema). When this reaction is acute, severe, and pervasive throughout much of the body, it can result in anaphylaxis, a medical emergency that results from multiorgan system reaction including edema of the respiratory tract that can close off the airway.

necrosis. These cells also participate in enhancing the immunologic activities of lymphocytes by functioning as antigen-presenting cells (APC). Some of the macrophages in certain organs differentiate into specialized cells:

- **Langerhans cells**: APCs residing in the epidermis of the skin
- **Kupffer cells**: Resident liver macrophages
- **Osteoclasts**: Specialized to break down and release minerals and organic matrix in the bone tissue
- **Dust cells**: Resident lung macrophages in the lungs
- **Microglia**: Resident brain and spinal cord macrophages
- **Plasma cells** are the major cell type present during **chronic inflammation**. These cells are derived from a subpopulation of lymphocytes (B cells), which extravasate into connective tissue and then differentiate into plasma cells. Plasma cells are responsible for the synthesis and release of humoral antibodies.
- **Neutrophils** are the major cell type present during **acute inflammation**. These cells quickly respond to foreign antigens or injury and comprise the major constituent of pus.
- **Eosinophils** are more specialized to respond to parasitic entities and sometimes involved in autoimmune events. They also phagocytose antigen–antibody complexes.
- **Basophils**, the least abundant type of leukocytes, are rarely seen in connective tissues, but appear to have a similar function as mast cells.

Connective Tissue Types

Connective tissue types include **mesenchymal**, **mucous**, **loose (areolar)**, **dense irregular**, **dense regular**, **reticular**, **elastic**, and **adipose**.

Mesenchymal and Mucous Connective Tissues

These connective tissues are limited to the embryo. **Mesenchymal connective tissues** consist of mesenchymal cells and fine reticular fibers interspersed in a semifluid matrix of ground substance (Fig. 4-3A). **Mucous connective tissue** is more viscous in consistency, contains collagen bundles and numerous fibroblasts, and is located deep to the fetal skin and in the umbilical cord (where it is known as Wharton's jelly), surrounding the umbilical vessels (Fig. 4-3B).

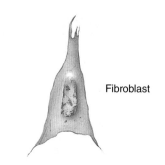

Fibroblast

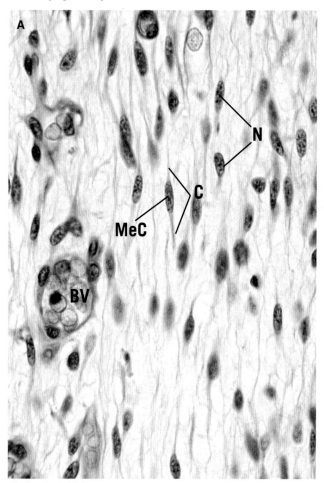

FIGURE 4-3A. Mesenchymal connective tissue. Fetal pig. Paraffin section. ×540.

Mesenchymal connective tissue of the fetus is very immature and cellular. The **mesenchymal cells** (MeC) are stellate shaped to fusiform cells, whose **cytoplasm** (c) can be distinguished from the surrounding matrix. The **nuclei** (N) are pale and centrally located. The ground substance is semifluid in consistency and contains slender reticular fibers. The vascularity of this tissue is evidenced by the presence of **blood vessels** (BV).

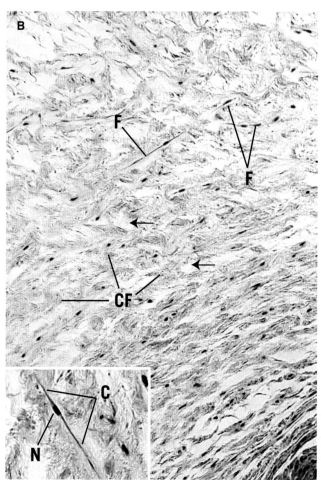

FIGURE 4-3B. Mucous connective tissue. Umbilical cord. Human. Paraffin section. ×132.

This example of mucous connective tissue (Wharton's jelly) was derived from the umbilical cord of a fetus. Observe the obvious differences between the two embryonic tissues. The matrix of mesenchymal connective tissue (see Fig. 4-3A) contains no collagenous fibers, whereas this connective tissue displays a loose network of haphazardly arranged **collagen fibers** (CF). The cells are no longer mesenchymal cells; instead, they are **fibroblasts** (F), although morphologically they resemble each other. The empty-looking spaces (*arrows*) are areas where the ground substance was extracted during specimen preparation.

Inset. Fibroblast. Umbilical cord. Human. Paraffin section. ×270.

Note the centrally placed **nucleus** (N) and the fusiform shape of the **cytoplasm** (c) of this fibroblast.

Loose (Areolar) Connective Tissue

Loose (areolar) connective tissue is distributed widely because it constitutes much of the superficial fascia and invests neurovascular bundles. Further, most epithelia in the body rest on top of the loose connective tissue, separated by the basement membrane. All three fiber types, abundant ground substance, and a variety of cells described above comprise this soft tissue (Fig. 4-4).

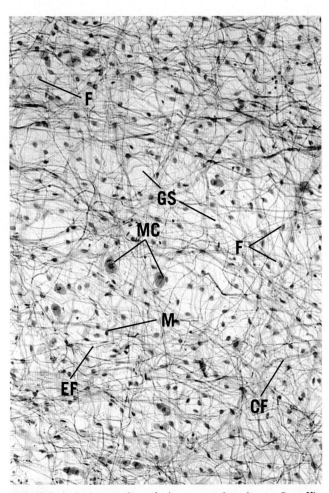

FIGURE 4-4. Loose (areolar) connective tissue. Paraffin section. ×132.

This photomicrograph depicts a whole mount of mesentery, through its entire thickness. The two large **mast cells** (MC) are easily identified because they are the largest cells in the field and possess a granular cytoplasm. Although their cytoplasms are not visible, it is still possible to recognize two other cell types due to their nuclear morphology. **Fibroblasts** (F) possess oval nuclei that are paler and larger than the nuclei of **macrophages** (M). The semifluid **ground substance** (GS) through which tissue fluid percolates is invisible because it was extracted during the preparation of the tissues. However, two types of fibers, the thicker, wavy, ribbon-like, interlacing **collagen fibers** (CF) and the thin, straight, branching **elastic fibers** (EF), are well demonstrated.

Dense Irregular Connective Tissue

Dense irregular connective tissue consists of coarse, almost haphazardly arranged bundles of collagen type I fibers interlaced with few elastic and reticular fibers. The chief cellular constituents are fibroblasts, macrophages, and occasional mast cells. The dermis of the skin and capsules of some organs are composed of dense irregular collagenous connective tissue (Fig. 4-5).

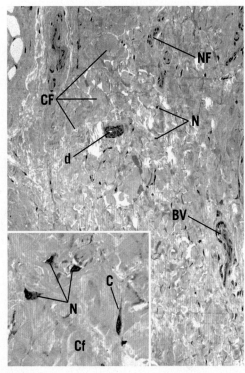

FIGURE 4-5. Dense irregular collagenous connective tissue. Palmar skin. Monkey. Plastic section. ×132.

The dermis of the skin provides a good representation of dense irregular collagenous connective tissue. The thick, coarse, intertwined bundles of **collagen fibers** (CF) are arranged in a haphazard fashion. Although this tissue has numerous **blood vessels** (BV) and **nerve fiber**s (NF) branching through it, it is not a very vascular tissue. Dense irregular connective tissue is only sparsely supplied with cells, mostly fibroblasts and macrophages, whose **nuclei** (N) appear as dark dots scattered throughout the field. At this magnification, it is not possible to identify the cell types with any degree of accuracy. The large epithelial structure in the upper center of the field is the **duct** (d) of a sweat gland.

At higher magnification (Inset, ×540), the coarse bundles of collagen fibers are composed of a conglomeration of **collagen fibrils** (Cf) intertwined around each other. The three cells, whose **nuclei** (N) are clearly evident, cannot be identified with any degree of certainty, even though the cytoplasm (c) of the two on the left-hand side is visible. It is possible that they are macrophages, but without employing special staining techniques, the possibility of their being fibroblasts cannot be ruled out.

Dense Regular Connective Tissue

Dense regular connective tissue may be composed either of thick, parallel arrays of collagen type I fibers, as in tendons and ligaments, or of parallel bundles of elastic fibers, as in the ligamentum nuchae, the ligamentum flavum, and the suspensory ligament of the penis. The cellular constituents of both dense regular collagenous and dense regular elastic connective tissues are almost strictly limited to fibroblasts (Fig. 4-6).

Reticular Connective Tissue

Reticular connective tissue is composed mostly of reticular fibers (type III collagen), which form a network that constitutes the structural framework of bone marrow and many lymphoid structures as well as a framework enveloping certain cells (Fig. 4-7).

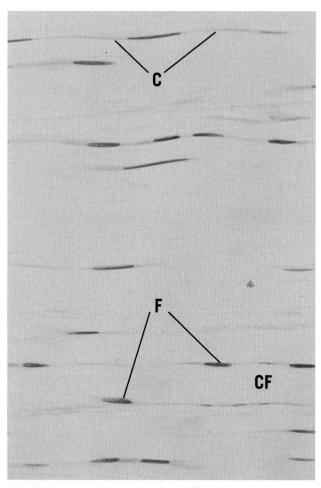

FIGURE 4-6. Dense regular collagenous connective tissue. l.s. Tendon. Monkey. Plastic section. ×270.

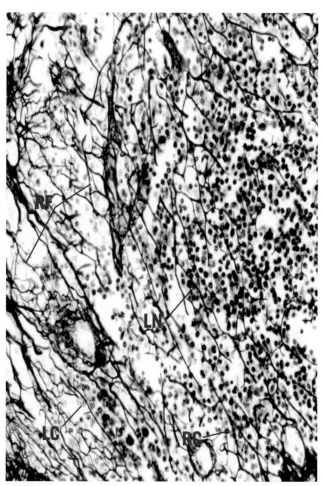

FIGURE 4-7. Reticular connective tissue. Silver stain. Paraffin section. ×270.

Tendons and ligaments present the most vivid examples of dense regular collagenous connective tissue. This connective tissue type is composed of regularly oriented parallel bundles of **collagen fibers** (CF), where individual bundles are demarcated by parallel rows of **fibroblasts** (F). Nuclei of these cells are evident as thin, dark lines, whereas their **cytoplasm** (c) is only somewhat discernible. With hematoxylin and eosin, the collagen bundles stain a more or less light shade of pink with parallel rows of dark blue nuclei of fibroblasts interspersed among them.

Silver stain, used in the preparation of this specimen, was deposited on the carbohydrate coating of the **reticular fibers** (RF). Note that these fibers are thin, long, branching structures that ramify throughout the field. Note that in this photomicrograph of a lymph node, the reticular fibers in the lower right-hand corner are oriented in a circular fashion. These form the structural framework of a cortical **lymphatic nodule** (LN). The small round cells are probably **lymphoid cells** (LC), whereas the larger cells, closely associated with the reticular fibers, may be **reticular cells** (RC), although definite identification is not possible with this stain. It should be noted that reticular connective tissue is characteristically associated with lymphatic tissue.

Elastic Connective Tissue

Elastic connective tissue is composed of abundant elastic fibers admixed with some collagen fibers. This tissue is found in organs such as the aorta and other large arteries that require stretching and recoil to accommodate large volume and pressure change (Fig. 4-8).

Adipose Tissue

Adipose tissue is composed of fat cells, reticular fibers, and a rich vascular supply. There are two types of adipose tissue, white (unilocular) and brown (multilocular).

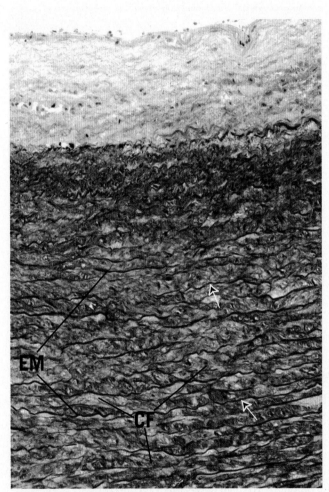

FIGURE 4-8. Elastic connective tissue. Aorta. Paraffin section. ×132.

The wall of the aorta is composed of thick, concentrically arranged **elastic membranes** (EM) composed of elastic fibers. Because these sheet-like membranes wrap around within the wall of the aorta in transverse sections, they present discontinuous, concentric circles, which are represented here by more or less parallel, wavy, dark lines (*arrows*). The connective tissue material between membranes is composed of ground substance, **collagen fibers** (CF), and reticular fibers. Also present are fibroblasts and smooth muscle cells, whose nuclei may be discerned.

Unilocular Adipose Tissue

Unilocular adipose tissue acts as a depot for fat, a thermal insulator, and a shock absorber (Fig. 4-9). Cells of **unilocular adipose tissue** store triglycerides in a single, large fat droplet that occupies most of the cell. Fat cells of adipose tissue make the enzyme **lipoprotein lipase**, which is transported to the luminal surface of the capillary endothelial cell membrane, where it hydrolyzes chylomicrons and very-low-density lipoproteins into fatty acids and monoglycerides, which are transported to the adipocytes, diffuse into their cytoplasm, and are reesterified into triglycerides. **Hormone-sensitive lipase**, activated by **cyclic adenosine monophosphate (cAMP)**, hydrolyzes the stored lipids into fatty acids and glycerol, which are released from the cell as the need arises, to enter the capillaries for distribution to the remainder of the

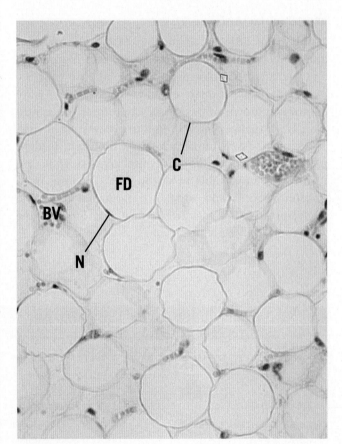

FIGURE 4-9. Adipose tissue. Human. Paraffin section. ×270.

This photograph of adipose tissue is from the fat deposit that surrounds the human suprarenal gland. The **adipocytes** (A), or fat cells, appear empty owing to tissue processing that dissolves fatty material. The **cytoplasm** (C) of these cells is pushed to the periphery, and the **nucleus** (N) is also pressed to the periphery by the single, large **fat droplet** (FD) that occupies most of the space within the cytoplasm. Adipose tissue is subdivided into lobes and lobules by connective tissue septa that carry **blood vessels** (BV) to the adipocytes.

body. Recently, it has been demonstrated that unilocular adipose tissue has certain endocrine functions because its fat cells produce **adipokines** that act as hormones, namely, **leptin**, **adiponectin**, and **retinol-binding protein 4** as well as **apelin**, which has antihypertensive properties, and **vaspin**, whose function in humans is not known (Table 4-4). Additionally, macrophages of unilocular adipose tissue manufacture **tumor necrosis factor-α**, **resistin**, and **interleukin-6**.

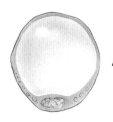

Adipocyte

Multilocular Adipose Tissue

Multilocular adipose tissue (brown fat) releases heat and is especially well represented in hibernating animals and neonates. Multilocular (brown) adipose cells are rare in the adult human, although recent studies have shown that brown adipose tissue can form in older individuals who suffer from various forms of wasting disease. These cells possess numerous droplets of lipid in their cytoplasm and a rich supply of mitochondria. These mitochondria are capable of uncoupling oxidation from phosphorylation, and, instead of producing adenosine triphosphate (ATP), they release heat, thus arousing the animal from hibernation.

CLINICAL CONSIDERATIONS 4-6

Obesity

There are two types of obesity: hypertrophic obesity, which occurs when adipose cells increase in size from storing fat (adult onset), and hyperplastic obesity, which is characterized by an increase in the number of adipose cells resulting from overfeeding a newborn for a few weeks after birth. This type of obesity is usually lifelong.

CLINICAL CONSIDERATIONS 4-7

Systemic Lupus Erythematosus

Systemic lupus erythematosus (SLE) is an autoimmune connective tissue disease that results in inflammation in the connective tissue elements of certain organs as well as of tendons and joints. The symptoms depend on the type and number of antibodies present and can be anywhere from mild to severe, and, owing to a variety of symptoms, SLE may resemble other conditions such as growing pains, arthritis, epilepsy, and even psychologic diseases. The characteristic symptoms include facial and skin rash, sores in the oral cavity, joint pains and inflammation, kidney malfunction, neurologic conditions, anemia, thrombocytopenia, and fluid in the lungs.

Table 4-4	Adipokines Produced by Unilocular Adipose Tissue
Adipokine	**Function**
Manufactured by Adipocytes	
Leptin	Suppresses appetite
Adiponectin trimer	Suppresses appetite
Adiponectin octadecamer	Increases insulin sensitivity of muscle cells; increases liver gluconeogenesis; suppresses glucose release by the liver
Retinol-binding protein 4	Decreases insulin sensitivity of muscle cells; encourages glucose release by liver cells
Apelin	Antihypertensive hormone
Vaspin	Its function in humans is not known
Manufactured by Macrophages in Adipose Tissue	
Tumor necrosis factor-α	Principal cause of insulin resistance; suppresses fatty acid oxidation by hepatocytes
Resistin	In obese individuals, it encourages insulin resistance; increases glucose release by hepatocytes
Interleukin-6	Induces insulin resistance and uptake of glucose in muscle cells

PLATE 4-1 Fibroblasts and Collagen, Transmission Electron Microscopy

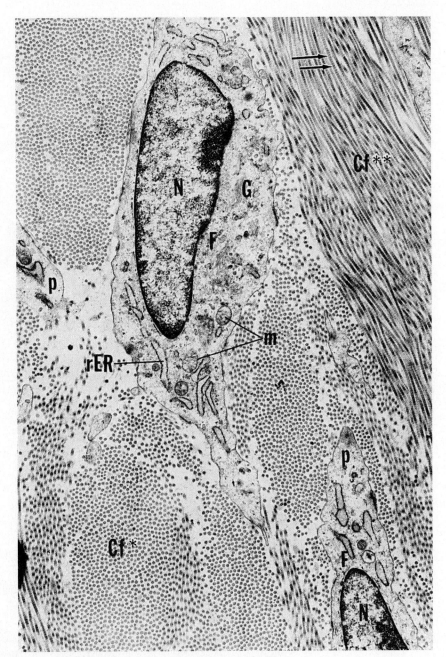

FIGURE 4-1-1. Fibroblast. Baboon. Electron microscopy. ×11,070.

This electron micrograph of **fibroblasts** (F) demonstrates that they are long, fusiform cells whose **processes** (p) extend into the surrounding area between bundles of collagen fibrils. These cells manufacture collagen, reticular and elastic fibers, and the ground substance of connective tissue. Therefore, they are rich in organelles, such as **Golgi apparatus** (G), **rough endoplasmic reticulum** (rER), and **mitochondria** (m); however, in the quiescent stage, as in tendons, where they no longer actively synthesize the intercellular elements of connective tissue, the organelle population of fibroblasts is reduced in number, and the plump, euchromatic **nucleus** (N) becomes flattened and heterochromatic. Note that the bundles of **collagen fibrils** (Cf) are sectioned both transversely (*asterisk*) and longitudinally (*double asterisks*). Individual fibrils display alternating transverse dark and light banding (*arrows*) along their length. The specific banding results from the ordered arrangement of the tropocollagen molecules constituting the collagen fibrils. (From Simpson DM, et al. Histopathologic and ultrastructural features of inflamed gingiva in the baboon. *J Periodontol* 1974;45(7):500–510. Copyright © 1974 American Academy of Periodontology. Reprinted by permission of John Wiley & Sons, Inc.)

KEY					
F	fibroblasts	**rER**	rough endoplasmic	**N**	nucleus
p	processes		reticulum	**Cf**	Collagen fibrils
G	Golgi apparatus	**m**	mitochondria		

PLATE 4-2   Mast Cell, Transmission Electron Microscopy

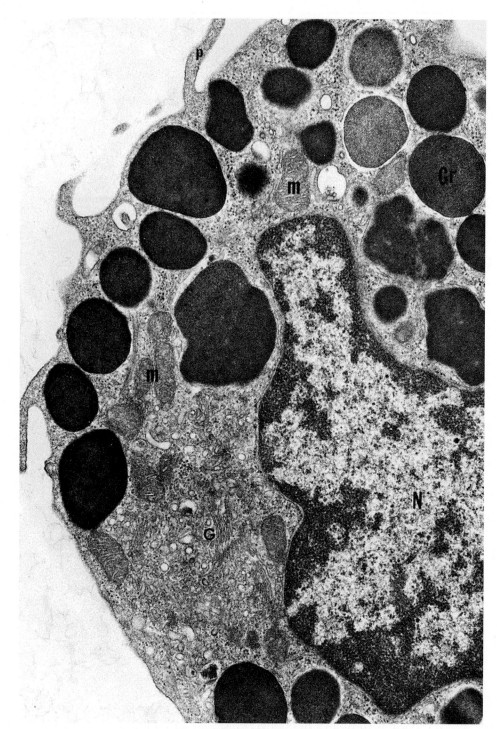

FIGURE 4-2-1. Mast cell. Rat. Electron microscopy. ×14,400.

This electron micrograph of a rat peritoneal mast cell displays characteristics of this cell. Note that the **nucleus** (N) is not lobulated, and the cell contains organelles such as **mitochondria** (m) and **Golgi apparatus** (G). Numerous **processes** (p) extend from the cell. Observe that the most characteristic component of this cell is that it is filled with numerous membrane-bound **granules** (Gr) of more or less uniform density. These granules contain heparin, histamine, and serotonin (although human mast cells do not contain serotonin). Additionally, mast cells release a number of unstored substances that act in allergic reactions. (Reprinted from Lagunoff D. Contributions of electron microscopy to the study of mast cells. *J Invest Dermatol* 1972;58(5):296–311. Copyright © 1972 Elsevier. With permission.)

KEY					
N	nucleus	G	Golgi apparatus	Gr	granules
m	mitochondria	p	processes		

PLATE 4-3   Mast Cell Degranulation, Electron Microscopy

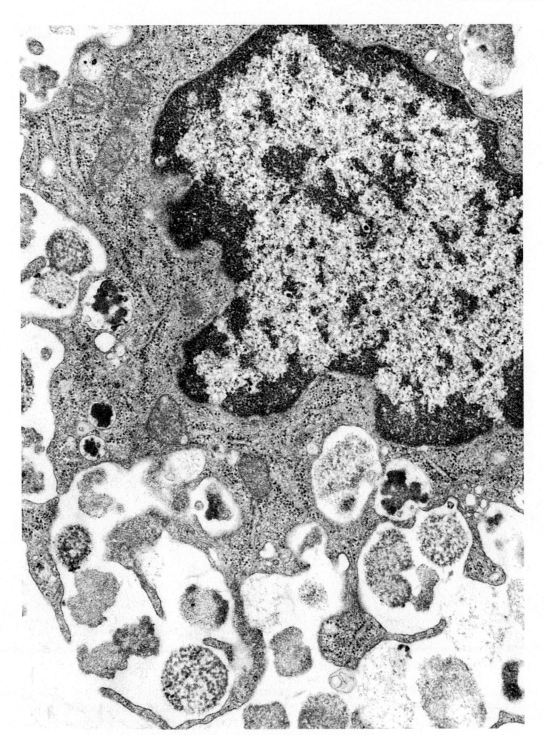

FIGURE 4-3-1. Mast cell degranulation. Rat. Electron microscopy. ×20,250.

Mast cells possess receptor molecules on their plasma membrane, which are specific for the constant region of IgE antibody molecules. These molecules attach to the mast cell surface and, as the cell comes in contact with those specific antigens to which it was sensitized, the antigen binds with the active regions of the IgE antibody. Such antibody–antigen binding on the mast cell surface causes degranulation, that is, the release of granules as well as the unstored substances that act in allergic reactions. Degranulation occurs very quickly but requires both ATP and calcium. Granules at the periphery of the cell are released by fusion with the cell membrane, whereas granules deeper in the cytoplasm fuse with each other, forming convoluted intracellular canaliculi that connect to the extracellular space. Such a canaliculus may be noted in the bottom left-hand corner of this electron micrograph. (Reprinted from Lagunoff D. Contributions of electron microscopy to the study of mast cells. *J Invest Dermatol* 1972;58(5):296–311. Copyright © 1972 Elsevier. With permission.)

PLATE 4-4   Developing Fat Cell, Transmission Electron Microscopy

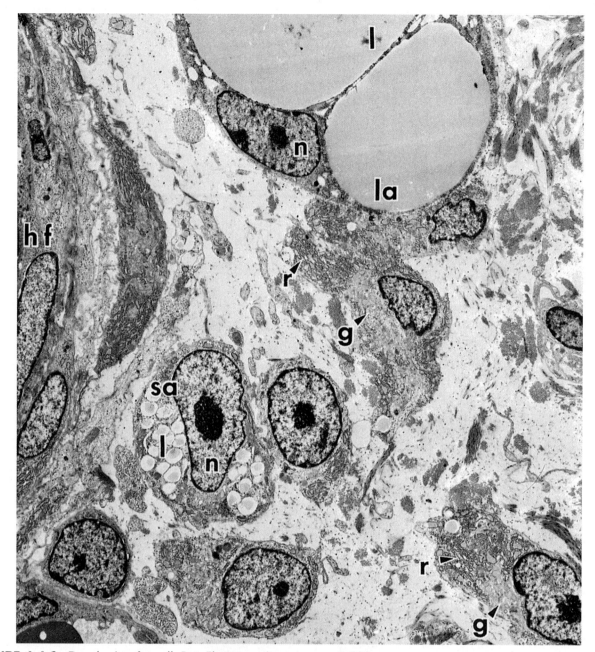

FIGURE 4-4-1. Developing fat cell. Rat. Electron microscopy. ×3,060.

This electron micrograph from the developing rat hypodermis displays a region of the developing **hair follicle** (hf). The peripheral aspect of the hair follicle presents a **small adipocyte** (sa) whose **nucleus** (n) and nucleolus are clearly visible. Although white adipose cells are unilocular, in that the cytoplasm of the cell contains a single, large droplet of lipid, during development lipid begins to accumulate as small **droplets** (l) in the cytoplasm of the small adipocyte. As the fat cell matures to become a **large adipocyte** (la), its **nucleus** (n) is displaced peripherally, and the lipid **droplets** (l) fuse to form several large droplets, which will eventually coalesce to form a single, central fat deposit. The nucleus displays some alterations during the transformation from small to large adipocytes, in that the nucleolus becomes smaller and less prominent. Immature adipocytes are distinguishable because they possess a well-developed **Golgi apparatus** (g) that is actively functioning in the biosynthesis of lipids. Moreover, the **rough endoplasmic reticulum** (r) presents dilated cisternae, indicative of protein synthetic activity. Note the capillary, whose lumen displays a red blood cell in the lower left-hand corner of this photomicrograph. (From Hausman GJ, et al. Adipocyte development in the rat hypodermis. *Am J Anat* 1981;161(1):85–100. Copyright © 1981 Wiley-Liss, Inc. Reprinted by permission of John Wiley & Sons, Inc.)

KEY					
hf	hair follicle	l	lipid droplets	r	rough endoplasmic reticulum
sa	small adipocytes	la	large adipocyte		
n	nucleus	g	Golgi apparatus		

PLATE 4-5 Connective Tissues

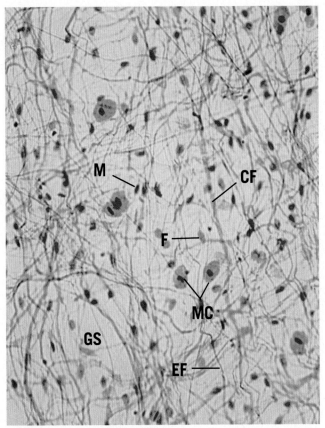

FIGURE 4-5-1. Loose (areolar) connective tissue. Paraffin section. ×540.

Note that in loose (areolar) connective tissue, generally three types of cells are evident. It is easy to differentiate between the oval, paler, and larger nuclei of **fibroblasts** (F) from the smaller and denser nuclei of **macrophages** (M). The large **mast cells** (MC) are clearly evident, and their granular cytoplasm is relatively easy to note. The **collagen fibers** (CF) of loose connective tissue are thicker than the **elastic fibers** (EF). The empty-appearing background is filled with **ground substance** (GS) in the living tissue.

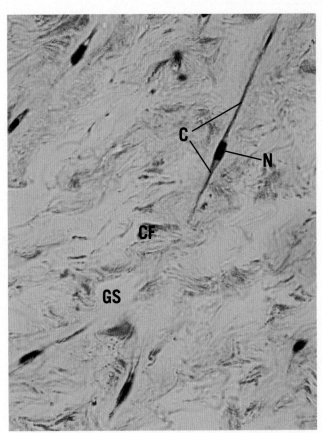

FIGURE 4-5-2. Mucous connective tissue. Umbilical cord. Human. Paraffin section. ×540.

This photomicrograph is a high magnification of mucous connective tissue derived from the umbilical cord. Note that, in section, the **fibroblast** (F) appears as an elongated, spindle-shaped cell with a more or less rectangular-shaped **nucleus** (N) and very little **cytoplasm** (C) filling the narrow cell. Observe the clumps of **collagen fiber** (CF) bundles and the empty-appearing spaces that are filled with **ground substance** (GS) in the living tissue.

 Mast cell

KEY					
C	cytoplasm	F	fibroblast	MC	mast cell
CF	collagen fiber bundles	GS	ground substance	N	nucleus
EF	elastic fibers	M	macrophages		

PLATE 4-6 Connective Tissues

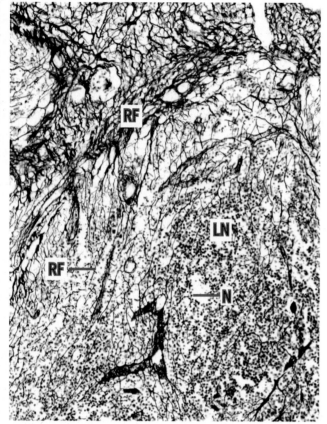

FIGURE 4-6-1. Reticular connective tissue. Silver stain. Human. Paraffin section. ×132.

This specimen was stained with silver to demonstrate the thin **reticular fibers** (RF) composed of type III collagen fibers that form the basic architecture of the spleen and lymph nodes. The circular outline of the **lymphoid nodule** (LN) is evident as are the **nuclei** (N) of lymphocytes that occupy much of this organ.

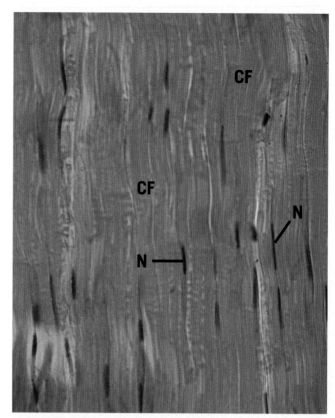

FIGURE 4-6-2. Dense regular collagenous connective tissue. Tendon. Human. Paraffin section. ×540.

Tendons and ligaments present the most vivid examples of dense regular collagenous connective tissue. This connective tissue type is composed of regularly oriented parallel bundles of **collagen fibers** (CF), where individual bundles are demarcated by parallel rows of **fibroblasts** (F). **Nuclei** (N) of these cells are evident as thin, dark lines, whereas their cytoplasm is only somewhat discernible. With hematoxylin and eosin, the collagen bundles stain a more or less light shade of pink with parallel rows of dark blue nuclei of fibroblasts interspersed among them.

KEY			
CF	collagen fiber bundles	**N**	nucleus
F	fibroblast		

PLATE 4-7 Connective Tissues and Cells

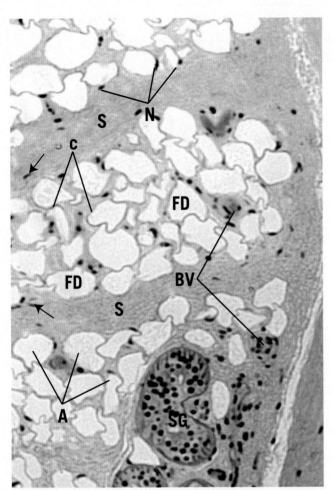

FIGURE 4-7-1. Adipose tissue. Hypodermis. Monkey. Plastic section. ×132.

This photomicrograph of adipose tissue is from monkey hypodermis. The **adipocytes** (A), or fat cells, appear empty because of tissue processing that dissolves fatty material. The **cytoplasm** (c) of these cells appears as a peripheral rim, and the **nucleus** (N) is also pressed to the side by the single, large **fat droplet** (FD) within the cytoplasm. Fat is subdivided into lobules by **septa** (S) of connective tissue conducting **vascular elements** (BV) to the adipocytes. Fibroblast nuclei (*arrows*) are evident in the connective tissue septa. Note the presence of the secretory portions of a **sweat gland** (SG) in the upper aspect of this photomicrograph.

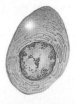

Plasma cell

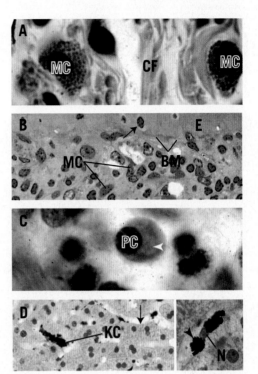

FIGURE 4-7-2. Mast cells, plasma cells, macrophages.

Mast cells (MC) are conspicuous components of connective tissue proper, **A** (Tendon. Monkey. Plastic section. ×540), although they are only infrequently encountered. Note the round to oval nucleus and numerous small granules in the cytoplasm. Observe also, among the bundles of **collagen fibers** (CF), the nuclei of several fibroblasts. Mast cells are very common components of the subepithelial connective tissue (lamina propria) of the digestive tract, **B** (Jejunum. Monkey. Plastic section. ×540). Note the **basement membrane** (BM) separating the connective tissue from the **simple columnar epithelium** (E), whose nuclei are oval in shape. The denser, more amorphous nuclei (*arrows*) belong to lymphoid cells, migrating from the connective tissue into the intestinal lumen. The lamina propria also houses numerous **plasma cells** (PC), as evidenced in **C** (Jejunum. Monkey. Plastic section. ×540). Plasma cells are characterized by clockface ("cartwheel") nuclei, as well as by a clear paranuclear Golgi zone (*arrowhead*). **D** (Macrophage. Liver, injected. Paraffin section. ×270) is a photomicrograph of the liver that was injected with India ink. This material is preferentially phagocytosed by macrophages of the liver, known as **Kupffer cells** (KC). These cells appear as dense, black structures in the liver sinusoids; vascular channels are represented by clear areas (*arrow*). An individual Kupffer cell (Inset. Paraffin section. ×540) displays the **nucleus** (N) as well as the granules of India ink (*arrowhead*) in its cytoplasm.

KEY					
A	adipocytes	**CF**	collagen fiber	**MC**	mast cell
BM	basement membrane	**E**	simple columnar	**N**	nucleus
BV	blood vessel (vascular		epithelium	**PC**	plasma cells
	elements)	**FD**	fat droplet	**S**	septa
C	cytoplasm	**KC**	Kupffer cells	**SG**	sweat gland

Selected Review of Histologic Images

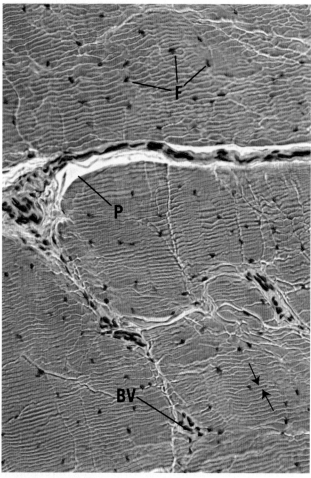

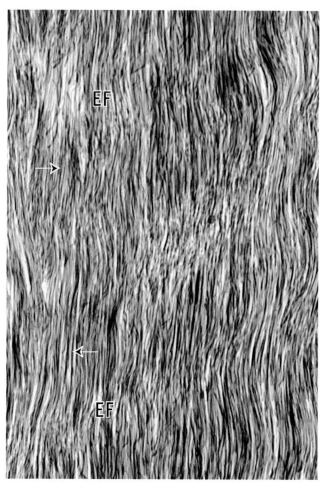

REVIEW FIGURE 4-1-1. Dense regular collagenous connective tissue. x.s. Tendon. Paraffin section. ×270.

Transverse sections of the tendon present a typical appearance. Tendon is organized into fascicles that are separated from each other by the **peritendineum** (P) surrounding each fascicle. **Blood vessels** (BV) may be observed in the peritendineum. Collagen bundles within the fascicles are regularly arranged; however, shrinkage owing to preparation causes an artifactual layering (*arrows*), although in some preparations swelling of the tissue results in a homogenous appearance. The nuclei of **fibroblasts** (F) appear to be strewn about in a haphazard manner.

REVIEW FIGURE 4-1-2. Elastic connective tissue. l.s. Paraffin section. ×132.

This longitudinal section of elastic connective tissue demonstrates that the **elastic fibers** (EF) are arranged in parallel arrays. However, the fibers are short and are curled at their ends (*arrows*). The white spaces among the fibers represent the loose connective tissue elements that remain unstained. The cellular elements are composed of parallel rows of flattened fibroblasts. These cells are also unstained and cannot be distinguished in this preparation.

KEY					
BV	blood vessels	**F**	fibroblasts	**P**	peritendineum
EF	elastic fibers				

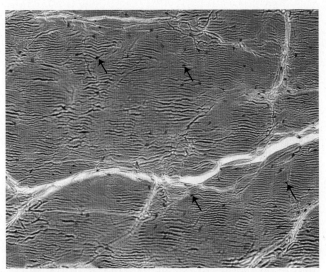

REVIEW FIGURE 4-1-3. Dense regular connective tissue, transverse section.

A cross section of the dense regular connective tissue reveals abundant, eosinophilic collagen type I fibers cut in transverse to oblique plane. The dark dots (*arrows*) are the nuclei of the fibroblasts present in between the fibers.

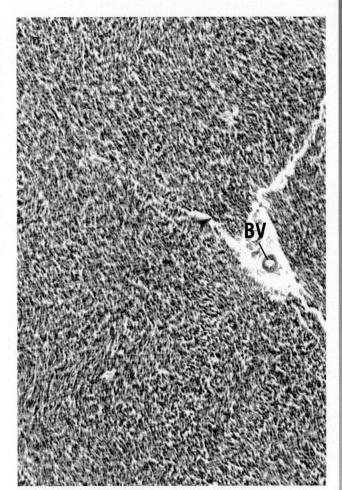

REVIEW FIGURE 4-1-4. Elastic connective tissue. x.s. Paraffin section. ×132.

A transverse section of elastic connective tissue displays a characteristic appearance. In some areas, the fibers present precise cross-sectional profiles as dark dots of various diameters (*arrows*). Other areas present oblique sections of these fibers, represented by short linear profiles (*arrowhead*). As in the previous figure, the white spaces represent the unstained loose connective tissue elements. The large clear area (**middle left**) is also composed of loose connective tissue surrounding **blood vessels** (BV).

KEY

BV	blood vessels

Summary of Histologic Organization

I. EMBRYONIC CONNECTIVE TISSUE

A. Mesenchymal Connective Tissue (Mesenchyme)

1. Cells

Stellate to spindle-shaped **mesenchymal cells** have processes that touch one another. Pale scanty cytoplasm with large clear nuclei. Indistinct cell membrane.

2. Extracellular Matrix

Mostly empty-looking matrix owing to abundant ground substance, with fine **reticular fibers** forming a delicate network. Small blood vessels are evident.

B. Mucous Connective Tissue

1. Cells

Fibroblasts, with their numerous flattened processes and oval nuclei, constitute the major cellular component. In section, these cells frequently appear spindle-shaped and resemble or are identical with mesenchymal cells when viewed with a light microscope.

2. Extracellular Matrix

When compared with mesenchymal connective tissue, the intercellular space is filled with coarse **collagen bundles**, irregularly arranged, in a matrix of precipitated jelly-like ground substance.

II. CONNECTIVE TISSUE TYPES

A. Loose (Areolar) Connective Tissue

1. Cells

The most common cell types are **fibroblasts**, whose spindle-shaped morphology closely resembles the next most numerous cells, the **macrophages**. The oval nuclei of macrophages are smaller, darker, and denser than those of fibroblasts. **Mast cells**, located in the vicinity of blood vessels, may be recognized by their size, the numerous small granules in their cytoplasm, and their large, round, centrally located nuclei. Occasional **fat cells** resembling round, empty spaces bordered by a thin rim of cytoplasm may also be present. When sectioned through, its peripherally squeezed, flattened nucleus may give a fat cell a signet ring-like appearance.

Additionally, in certain regions such as the subepithelial connective tissue (lamina propria) of the intestines, plasma cells and leukocytes are commonly found. **Plasma cells** are small, oval cells with round, eccentric nuclei, whose chromatin network presents a clockface (cartwheel) appearance. These cells also display a clear, paranuclear Golgi zone. **Lymphocytes**, **neutrophils**, and occasional **eosinophils** also contribute to the cellularity of loose connective tissue.

2. Extracellular Matrix

Slender bundles of long, ribbon-like bands of **collagen fibers** are intertwined by numerous thin, straight, long, branching **elastic fibers** embedded in a watery matrix of **ground substance**, most of which is extracted by dehydration procedures during preparation. **Reticular fibers**, also present, are usually not visible in sections stained with hematoxylin and eosin.

B. Reticular Connective Tissue

1. Cells

Reticular cells are specialized fibroblasts in reticular connective tissue. They are stellate in shape and envelop the reticular fibers, which they also manufacture. They possess large, oval, pale nuclei, and their cytoplasm is not easily visible with the light microscope. The other cells in the interstitial spaces are **lymphocytes**, **macrophages**, and other **lymphoid cells**.

2. Extracellular Matrix

Reticular fibers constitute the major fiber component of the ECM suspended in ground substance. With the use of a silver stain, they are evident as dark, thin, branching fibers.

C. Adipose Tissue

1. Cells

Unlike other connective tissues, adipose tissue is mostly composed of adipose cells (adipocytes) so closely packed together that the normal spherical morphology of these cells becomes distorted. Groups of fat cells are subdivided into lobules by thin sheaths of loose connective tissue septa housing **mast cells**, blood vessels lined by **endothelial cells**, and other components of **neurovascular elements**.

III. Extracellular Matrix

Each fat cell is invested by **reticular fibers**, which, in turn, are anchored to the **collagen fibers** of the connective tissue septa.

A. Dense Irregular Connective Tissue

1. Cells

Fibroblasts, **macrophages**, and cells associated with **neurovascular bundles** constitute the chief cellular elements.

2. Extracellular Materials

Haphazardly oriented thick, wavy bundles of **collagen fibers** as well as occasional **elastic** and **reticular fibers** are found in dense irregular connective tissue.

B. Dense Regular Connective Tissue

1. Cells

Parallel rows of flattened **fibroblasts** are essentially the only cells found here. Even these are few in number.

2. Extracellular Materials

Parallel fibers of densely packed **collagen fibers** comprise most of the ECM with much less ground substance.

C. Elastic Connective Tissue

1. Cells

Parallel rows of flattened fibroblasts, specialized to produce elastic fibers, are usually difficult to distinguish in preparations that use stains specific for elastic fibers. Smooth muscle cells may be interspersed between bundles of elastic fibers.

2. Extracellular Materials

Parallel bundles of **elastic fibers**, surrounded by slender elements of loose connective tissue, constitute the intercellular components of elastic connective tissue.

Chapter Review Questions

4-1. Which cells in the connective tissue are responsible for anaphylaxis?

   A. Fibroblasts

   B. Macrophages

   C. Mast cells

   D. Plasma cells

4-2. A mutation resulting in defective fibrillin may render the affected person susceptible to which medical condition?

   A. Aortic dissection

   B. Generalized edema

   C. Keloids

   D. Obesity

   E. Systemic lupus erythematosus

4-3. Which collagen types are the predominant ECM component of the lymph node?

   A. I

   B. II

   C. III

   D. IV

4-4. Which tissue is best suited for withstanding frequent and substantial force applied from multiple directions?

   A. Loose connective tissue

   B. Dense irregular connective tissue

   C. Dense regular connective tissue

   D. Mesenchymal tissue

   E. Reticular connective tissue

4-5. Which ECM component is largely responsible for attracting water molecules, thereby keeping the ECM hydrated?

   A. Fibrillins

   B. Glycoproteins

   C. Glycosaminoglycans

   D. Tropocollagens

CARTILAGE AND BONE

Cartilage and bone form the supporting tissues of the body. In these specialized connective tissues, as in other connective tissues, the extracellular elements dominate their microscopic appearance, whereas the cellular elements are proportionately smaller in number and variety.

Cartilage

Cartilage forms the supporting framework of certain organs, the articulating surfaces of bones, and the greater part of the fetal skeleton, although most of that will be replaced by bone. Unlike a typical connective tissue, cartilage is avascular; therefore, it is unable to thicken beyond the reach of nearby nutritional supply, most commonly the vasculature within the surrounding dense connective tissue called **perichondrium**. The extracellular matrix (ECM) of cartilage contains an abundance of **proteoglycans** whose **glycosaminoglycan (GAG)** components attract water, which provides rigidity to this tissue. The cartilage matrix also serves as a conduit for nutrients and waste products that travel between blood vessels of the perichondrium and the cells of cartilage, known as **chondrocytes**. The prominent fiber component of the ECM is type II collagen, which forms fine fibrils rather than thick fiber bundles and imparts a homogeneous "glassy" appearance to cartilage (Fig. 5-1).

Cartilage Extracellular Matrix

The ground substance of the ECM is composed of the GAG, **hyaluronic acid**, to which proteoglycans are bound, forming very large molecules called **aggrecan aggregates**. The GAG components of the proteoglycans are mainly **heparan sulfate**, **chondroitin-4-sulfate**, and **chondroitin-6-sulfate**. The acidic nature, combined with the enormous size, of aggrecan aggregates results in these molecules possessing large **domains** and a tremendous capacity for binding cations, principally Na^+ ions, which, in turn, attract water. The well-hydrated ground substance is primarily responsible for the rigidity of the cartilage. Additionally, the matrix contains **glycoproteins**, specifically **chondronectin**, that help the cells maintain contact with the matrix. Chondrocytes are scattered throughout the matrix, occupying small spaces known as **lacunae**. Each lacuna is surrounded by a 50-μm-wide collagen-poor matrix, known as the **territorial matrix**; the remaining matrix outside the territorial matrix is known as the **interterritorial matrix**. A narrow region (3- to 5-μm wide) of the territorial matrix, just adjacent to the lacuna, is known as the **pericellular capsule**, which is believed to be rich in type IX, X, and XI collagen.

The primary fiber component of the cartilage matrix is **type II collagen**; small amounts of type IX, X, and XI collagen are also present. In elastic cartilage and fibrocartilage, in addition to type II collagen, elastic fibers and type I collagen bundles, respectively, provide added functional characteristics to each.

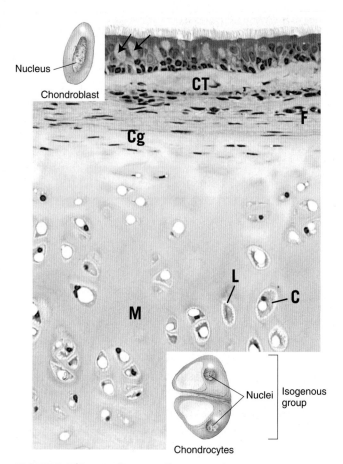

FIGURE 5-1. Hyaline cartilage. Trachea. Monkey. Plastic section. ×270.

The structural framework of trachea is the hyaline cartilage, deep to the pseudostratified ciliated columnar epithelium, which displays numerous goblet cells (*arrows*). The cilia, appearing at the free border of the epithelium, are evident. Note how the subepithelial **connective tissue** (CT) merges with the **fibrous perichondrium** (F). The **chondrogenic layer** of the perichondrium (Cg) houses chondrogenic cells and chondroblasts. As chondroblasts surround themselves with matrix, they become trapped in **lacunae** (L) and are referred to as **chondrocytes** (C). At the periphery of the cartilage, the chondrocytes are flattened, whereas toward the interior, they are round to oval. Owing to various histologic procedures, some of the chondrocytes fall out of their lacunae, which then appear as empty spaces. The **matrix** (M) contains many type II collagen fibrils masked by the glycosaminoglycans; hence, the matrix appears homogeneous and smooth. The proteoglycan-rich lining of the **lacunae** (L) is responsible for the more intense staining of the territorial matrix.

Cartilage Cellular Component

Unlike connective tissue proper, which contains diverse cell types, cartilage is limited to a few specialized cell types (see Fig. 5-1). **Chondroblasts** and **chondrogenic** cells are relatively fewer in number, and both are located in the surrounding **perichondrium** as a reserve for new chondrocytes. Chondrogenic cells have a dual capability. During low oxygen tension (as in poorly vascularized tissues), chondrogenic cells can give rise to chondroblasts; however, if the tissue's oxygen tension is high (as in well-vascularized tissue), they can differentiate into osteoprogenitor cells that give rise to osteoblasts.

Chondrocytes are the predominant type of cells and are housed in small spaces known as **lacunae**, interspersed within the matrix. The **chondrocytes** of hyaline and elastic cartilage resemble each other, in that they may be arranged individually in their **lacunae** or in **cell nests** (in young cartilage). Peripherally located chondrocytes are lenticular in shape, whereas those located centrally are round. The cells completely fill their lacunae. They possess an abundance of glycogen, frequent large lipid droplets, and a well-developed protein synthetic machinery (rough endoplasmic reticulum, Golgi apparatus, *trans*-Golgi network), as well as mitochondria, because these cells continuously turn over the cartilage matrix. In order for these cells to manufacture type II collagen and the other components of the cartilage matrix, these cells need **Sox9**, a transcription factor.

Perichondrium

The perichondrium is the dense, irregular connective tissue membrane that surrounds most hyaline and elastic cartilage. It has an outer fibrous layer and an inner chondrogenic layer (see Fig. 5-1). The **fibrous layer**, although poor in cells, is composed mostly of fibroblasts and collagen fibers. The inner cellular or **chondrogenic layer** is composed of chondroblasts and chondrogenic cells. The latter give rise to chondroblasts, cells that are responsible for secreting the **cartilage matrix**.

Cartilage Growth

Cartilage may grow or thicken in two ways: appositionally or interstitially (Fig. 5-2). **Appositional growth** (outside in) occurs when chondrogenic cells differentiate into chondroblasts and start to elaborate cartilaginous matrix around themselves, thus adding new cartilage onto already existing cartilage tissue. As the chondroblasts secrete matrix and fibers around themselves, they become incarcerated by their own secretions and are then termed **chondrocytes**.

Interstitial growth occurs in young cartilage, in which chondrocytes within the cartilage matrix possess the capacity to undergo mitosis. When this occurs, a single lacuna may house several daughter chondrocytes, and each cell will start to secrete cartilaginous matrix

around itself and eventually the daughter cells become separated from each other. A single lacuna containing several chondrocytes or a small cluster of lacunae with chondrocytes in close proximity is referred to as a cell nest (**isogenous group**), which is indicative of interstitial growth.

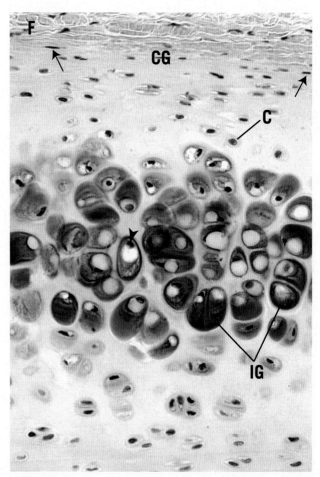

FIGURE 5-2. Hyaline cartilage. Rabbit. Paraffin section. ×270.

The two modes of cartilage growth are well demonstrated. The perichondrium is composed of **fibrous** (F) and **chondrogenic** (CG) layers. The former is composed of mostly collagenous fibers with a few fibroblasts, whereas the latter is more cellular, consisting of **chondroblasts** and **chondrogenic cells** (*arrows*). In appositional growth, chondroblasts in the **chondrogenic layer** (CG) secrete matrix and are surrounded by the intercellular substance and become **chondrocytes** (C). In interstitial growth, chondrocytes in the center of the cartilage undergo mitosis, and the daughter cells, initially in tight clusters called **isogenous groups** (IG), will eventually separate from each other as each cell secretes its own matrix surrounding it in its own lacuna. Note that chondrocytes at the periphery of the cartilage are small and elongated, whereas those at the center are large and ovoid to round (*arrowhead*).

Cartilage Types

Hyaline Cartilage

Hyaline cartilage is present at the articulating surfaces of most bones; the C rings of the trachea; and the laryngeal, costal, and nasal cartilages, among others. It is the most common type of cartilage and is surrounded by a well-defined **perichondrium**, except for those regions that form the articular surfaces supported by the synovial fluid. The predominant fiber in the matrix of hyaline cartilage is type II collagen. These fibers do not form thick bundles; they are mostly very fine and are, therefore, fairly well-masked by the surrounding **glycosaminoglycans**, giving the matrix a smooth, glassy appearance (see Figs. 5-1 and 5-2).

Elastic Cartilage

Elastic cartilage, as its name implies, possesses a great deal of elasticity, which is due to the elastic fibers embedded in its matrix. This cartilage forms the structural cores of the epiglottis, the Eustachian tube, external ear and ear canal, and some of the smaller laryngeal cartilages.

Elastic cartilage also possesses a perichondrium. The matrix, in addition to the type II collagen fibers, contains a wealth of coarse elastic fibers that impart to it a characteristic appearance (Fig. 5-3A,B). Elastic fibers are also responsible for the unique functional characteristics of elastic cartilage in its ability to not only bend or stretch but also recoil back to its original shape to provide structural support to organs such as the epiglottis, auditory tubes, and external ear.

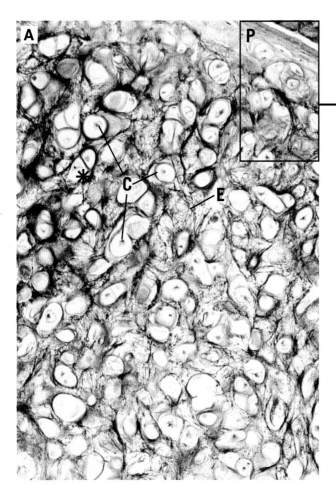

FIGURE 5-3A. Elastic cartilage. Epiglottis. Human. Paraffin section. ×132.

Elastic cartilage, like hyaline cartilage, is enveloped by a **perichondrium** (P). **Chondrocytes** (C), which are housed in lacunae, have shrunk away from the walls, giving the appearance of empty spaces. Occasional lacunae display two chondrocytes (*asterisk*), indicative of interstitial growth. The matrix has a rich **elastic fiber** (E) component that gives elastic cartilage its characteristic appearance as well as contributing to its elasticity.

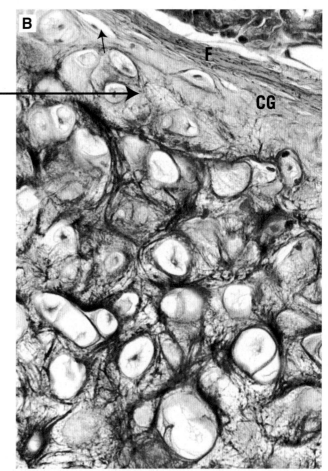

FIGURE 5-3B. Elastic cartilage. Epiglottis. Human. Paraffin section. ×270.

This higher magnification of the perichondrial region of Figure 3A displays the outer **fibrous** (F) and inner **chondrogenic** (CG) regions of the perichondrium. Note that the chondrocytes (*arrow*) immediately deep to the chondrogenic layer are more or less flattened and smaller than those deeper in the cartilage. Additionally, the amount and coarseness of the elastic fibers increase adjacent to the large cells.

Fibrocartilage

Fibrocartilage is present in only a few places, namely, in some symphyses, intervertebral (and some articular) discs, and certain areas where tendons insert into bone. **Fibrocartilage** differs from elastic and hyaline cartilage in that it has no perichondrium. Additionally, the chondrocytes are smaller and are usually oriented in parallel longitudinal rows (Fig. 5-4). The matrix of this cartilage contains, in addition to type II collagen fibrils, a large number of thick type I collagen fiber bundles between the rows of chondrocytes.

The characteristics and locations of the three types of cartilage are presented in Table 5-1.

Bone

Bone has many functions, including support, protection, mineral storage, and hemopoiesis. At the specialized cartilage-covered ends, it permits articulation or movement. Bone, a vascular connective tissue consisting of cells and calcified extracellular materials, may be structurally dense (compact) or sponge-like (cancellous; Fig. 5-5).

Cancellous (**spongy, medullary**) **bone**, like that present inside the epiphyses (heads) of long bones, is always surrounded by compact bone. Cancellous bone has large, open spaces surrounded by thin, anastomosing plates of bone. The large spaces are **marrow spaces**, and the plates of bones are known as **spicules** (if smaller) or **trabeculae** (if larger).

Compact (**cortical**) **bone** is much denser than cancellous bone.

Histologically, both compact and cancellous bones can comprise woven (primary, immature) or lamellar (secondary, mature) bone tissues.

• **Woven** (**primary, immature**) **bone** is characterized by irregularly organized collagen fibers within a calcified matrix, where the arrangement of the fibers resembles that of dense irregular connective tissue. Woven bones form compact and cancellous bones of infants and young children. In adults, woven bones are limited

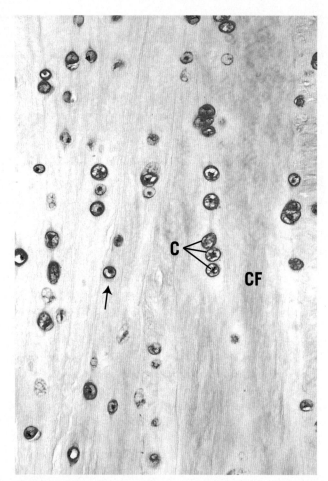

FIGURE 5-4. Fibrocartilage. Intervertebral disc. Human. Paraffin section. ×132.

The **chondrocytes** (C) of fibrocartilage are aligned in parallel rows, lying singly in individual lacunae. The nuclei of these chondrocytes are easily observed, whereas their cytoplasm is not as evident (*arrow*). The matrix contains thick bundles of **collagen fibers** (CF), which are arranged in a more or less regular fashion between the rows of cartilage cells. Unlike elastic and hyaline cartilages, fibrocartilage is not enveloped by a perichondrium.

to regions where frequent remodeling occurs, such as alveolar bones surrounding teeth, tendon attachment sites, or healing of bone fractures.

Table 5-1	Cartilage Types, Characteristics, and Locations		
Type	**Characteristics**	**Perichondrium**	**Locations (Major Samples)**
Hyaline	Chondrocytes in lacunae are in clusters (in young cartilage) or evenly spaced (in mature cartilage) within a basophilic matrix containing type II collagen	Usually present except at articular surfaces	Articular ends of long bones, ventral rib cartilage, templates for endochondral bone formation
Elastic	Chondrocytes in lacunae compacted in matrix containing type II collagen and elastic fibers	Present	Pinna of the ear, auditory canal, epiglottis
Fibrocartilage	Chondrocytes in lacunae arranged in rows in an acidophilic matrix containing, in addition to type II collagen, bundles of type I collagen arranged in rows	Absent	Intervertebral discs, pubic symphysis

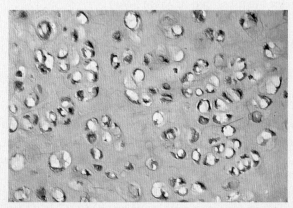
- **Lamellar (secondary, mature) bone** is characterized by well-organized layers of collagen fibers within a calcified matrix where the fiber orientation is a function of the direction of the forces applied to the bone. Most of the bones in the adult body are lamellar bones.

Bone Extracellular Matrix

Calcified bone matrix is composed of 50% minerals (mostly **calcium hydroxyapatite**) and 50% organic matter and bound water. The organic matrix of bone is composed mainly of **type I collagen** (as much as 90% of the organic components), sulfated **GAGs**, **proteoglycans**, and some **glycoproteins**. The matrix of collagen is calcified with **calcium hydroxyapatite** crystals, making bone one of the hardest substances in the body. The presence of these crystals makes bone the body's storehouse of calcium, phosphate, and other inorganic ions. Thus, bone is in a dynamic state of flux, continuously gaining and losing inorganic ions to maintain the body's calcium and phosphate homeostasis.

Bone matrix is produced by **osteoblasts** and as they elaborate bone matrix, they become trapped, and as the matrix calcifies, the trapped osteoblasts in small lenticular cavities, called **lacunae**, become known as **osteocytes**. Because nutrients or waste materials cannot be transferred through the calcified bone matrix, tiny channels known as **canaliculi** are present in which slender processes of osteocytes contact each other and are bathed in interstitial fluid to convey nutrients, hormones, and other necessary substances.

In an adult body, the bony lamellae of compact bone are organized into four lamellar systems (see Fig. 5-5):

- **external (outer)** and **internal (inner) circumferential lamellae,**
- **interstitial lamellae,** and
- **concentric lamellae** forming the **osteons.**

Osteons are cylindrical structures constituting the bulk of compact bone. They are formed by several layers of concentric lamellae whose **central canal** (osteonic or haversian canal) transports neurovascular elements that serve bone (Fig. 5-6). Perforating (Volkmann's) canals

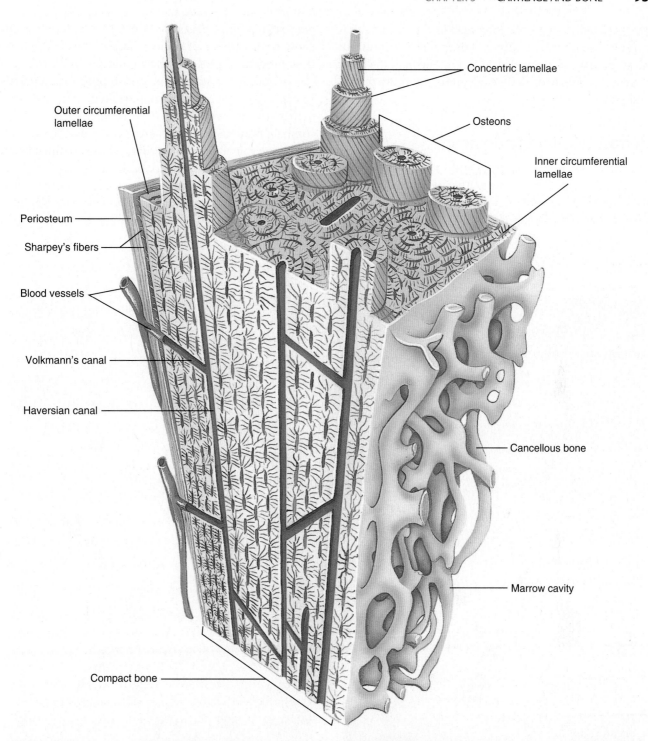

FIGURE 5-5. Compact bone is surrounded by dense, irregular collagenous connective tissue, the **periosteum**, which is attached to the **outer circumferential lamellae** by **Sharpey's fibers**. Blood vessels of the periosteum enter the bone via larger nutrient canals or small **Volkmann's canals**, which not only convey blood vessels to the **haversian canals** of **osteons** but also interconnect adjacent haversian canals. Each osteon is composed of concentric lamellae of bone whose collagen fibers are arranged so that they are perpendicular to those of contiguous lamellae. The **inner circumferential lamellae** are lined by endosteum, and are connected to the endosteum-lined cancellous bone that protrudes into the marrow cavity.

run perpendicular to the long axis of the osteons that connect neighboring central canals, permitting communication between them (Fig. 5-7). Canaliculi in the bony matrix are directly or indirectly connected to the central and perforating canals.

Periosteum and Endosteum

Bone is covered on its external and internal surfaces by uncalcified connective tissues. The **periosteum** covers the external bone surface and is composed of an **outer fibrous layer** consisting mainly of collagen fibers and populated by fibroblasts (see Fig. 5-6). The **inner osteogenic layer** consists of some collagen fibers and mostly osteoprogenitor cells and their progeny, the osteoblasts. The periosteum is strongly affixed to bone via **Sharpey's fibers**, collagenous bundles trapped in the calcified bone matrix during ossification. The internal surface of the compact bone facing the marrow cavity and the cancellous bone spicules and trabeculae within are lined by an **endosteum** composed of a delicate, uncalcified connective tissue layer populated with **osteoprogenitor cells**, **osteoblasts**, and occasional **osteoclasts** (Fig. 5-8; also see Fig. 5-6).

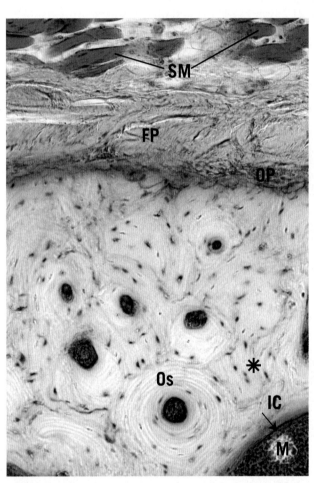

FIGURE 5-6. Decalcified compact bone. Human. Paraffin section. ×132.

Cross section of decalcified bone, displaying **skeletal muscle** (SM) fibers that will insert a short distance from this site. The outer **fibrous periosteum** (FP) and the inner **osteogenic periosteum** (OP) are distinguishable because of the fibrous component of the former and the cellularity of the latter. Note the presence of the **inner circumferential** (IC) **lamellae, osteons** (Os), and interstitial lamellae (*asterisk*). Also observe the **marrow** (M) occupying the marrow cavity, as well as the endosteal lining (*arrow*).

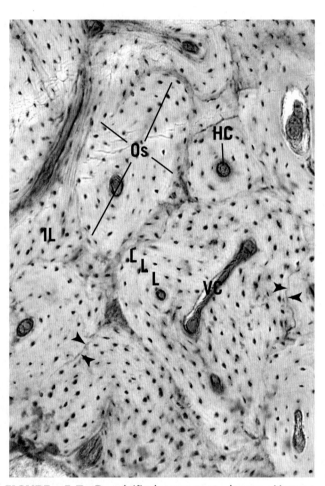

FIGURE 5-7. Decalcified compact bone. Human. Paraffin section. ×132.

This is a cross section of decalcified compact bone, displaying **osteons** or **haversian canal systems** (Os), as well as **interstitial lamellae** (IL). Each osteon possesses a central **haversian canal** (HC), surrounded by several **lamellae** (L) of bone. The boundary of each osteon is visible and is referred to as a cementing line (*arrowheads*). Neighboring haversian canals are connected to each other by **Volkmann's canals** (VC), through which blood vessels of osteons are interconnected.

Bone Cells

Osteoprogenitor Cells

Osteoprogenitor cells are undifferentiated, flattened cells located in the inner osteogenic layer of the periosteum, in the endosteum, and lining the haversian canals. They give rise to osteoblasts under the influence of **transforming growth factor-β** and **bone morphogenic protein-6 (BMP-6)**. However, under hypoxic conditions, osteoprogenitor cells become **chondrogenic cells**; therefore, these two cells are really the same cells that express different factors under differing oxygen tension.

Osteoblasts

Osteoblasts, when active, are cuboidal to low columnar cells with euchromatic nuclei and basophilic cytoplasm, responsible for the synthesis of bone matrix (see Fig. 5-8). As they elaborate bone matrix, they become surrounded by the matrix and then become osteocytes trapped in their lacunae. The bone matrix is calcified because of the seeding of the matrix via **matrix vesicles** derived from osteoblasts. When osteoblasts are quiescent, they lose much of their protein synthetic machinery and resemble fusiform osteoprogenitor cells. Osteoblasts function in the control of bone matrix mineralization and are also responsible for the formation, recruitment, and maintenance of osteoclasts as well as for the initiation of bone resorption. Osteoblasts possess **parathyroid hormone receptors** on their cell membrane, and in the presence of **parathyroid hormone**, they release **macrophage colony–stimulating factor** that induces the formation of osteoclast precursors.

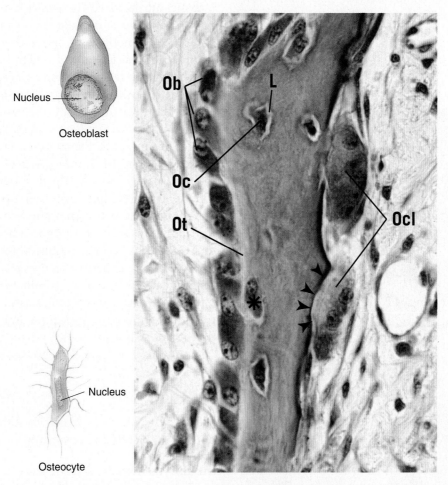

Nucleus

Osteoblast

Nucleus

Osteocyte

FIGURE 5-8. Cells of bone tissues. Pig skull. Paraffin section. ×540.

This photomicrograph is taken from an area of active bone formation and remodeling. The **osteoblasts** (Ob) cover the entire surface on one side of the trabecula, actively secreting organic bone matrix, **osteoid** (Ot), on top of the calcified matrix. Additionally, note that the osteoblast marked with the *asterisk* is apparently trapping itself in the matrix it is elaborating. Once this entrapment is complete, osteoblasts become the **osteocytes** (Oc) within the **lacunae** (L). Finally, note the large, multinuclear cells, **osteoclasts** (Ocl), which are in the process of resorbing bone. The activity of these large cells results in the formation of Howship's lacunae (*arrowheads*), which are shallow depressions on the bone surface. The interactions between osteoclasts and osteoblasts are very finely regulated in the normal formation and remodeling of bone.

Osteoclast-stimulating factor, also released by osteoblasts, activates osteoclasts to begin resorbing bone.

Osteocytes

Osteocytes are derived from osteoblasts that have surrounded themselves with the bone matrix that they produced. Osteocytes are flattened, discoid cells with numerous thin cellular processes, responsible for the maintenance of bone (see Fig. 5-8). The bulk of the cell containing most organelles are located in **lacunae**, whereas thin cell processes occupy the **canaliculi** (Fig. 5-9). It is here that an osteocyte cell process contacts the process of a neighboring osteocyte and they form **gap junctions** with each other; thus, these cells sustain a communication network, so that a large population of osteocytes are able to respond to blood calcium levels as well as to **calcitonin** and **parathyroid hormones**, released by the thyroid and parathyroid glands, respectively. Thus, these cells are responsible for the short-term calcium and phosphate homeostasis of the body.

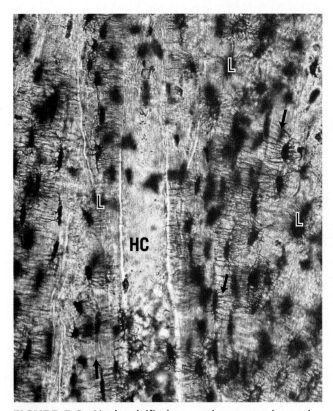

FIGURE 5-9. Undecalcified ground compact bone. l.s. Human. ×270.

This longitudinal section of undecalcified ground compact bone displays a **haversian canal** (HC) with parallel arrays of **lamellae** (L) whose lacunae demonstrate canaliculi (*arrows*), tunnel-like spaces through which nutrients and oxygen can be exchanged for the by-products and waste materials of osteocytes.

Osteoclasts

Osteoclasts are large, multinucleated cells derived from monocyte precursors that are responsible for the resorption of bone (see Fig. 5-8). As they remove bone, they appear to occupy a shallow cavity called **Howship's lacuna**. Osteoclasts have four regions: the basal zone, ruffled border, vesicular zone, and clear zone. The **basal zone** houses nuclei and organelles of the cell; the **ruffled border** is composed of finger-like processes that are suspended in the subosteoclastic compartment where the resorption of bone is actively proceeding. The ruffled border possesses many **proton pumps** that deliver hydrogen ions from the osteoclast into the subosteoclastic compartment. Additionally, **aquapores** and **chloride channels** permit the delivery of water and chloride ions, respectively, forming a concentrated solution of HCl in the subosteoclastic compartment, thus decalcifying bone. Enzymes are delivered via vesicles into the subosteoclastic compartment to degrade the organic components of bone. The by-products of degradation are endocytosed by endocytic vesicles and are used by the osteoclast or are exocytosed into the extracellular space (away from Howship's lacuna) where they enter vascular system for distribution to the rest of the body. The **vesicular zone** houses numerous vesicles that ferry material both in and out of the cell from and to the subosteoclastic compartment. The **clear zone**, the fourth region of the cell, is where the osteoclast forms a seal with the bone, isolating the subosteoclastic compartment from the external milieu.

The osteoclast **cell membrane** also possesses **calcitonin receptors**. When calcitonin is bound to the receptors, osteoclasts become inhibited, stop bone resorption, leave the bone surface, and dissociate into individual cells or disintegrate and are eliminated by macrophages.

Cooperation between osteoclasts and osteoblasts is responsible not only for the formation, remodeling, and repair of bone but also for the long-term maintenance of calcium and phosphate homeostasis of the body.

Osteogenesis

Histogenesis of bone occurs via either **intramembranous** or **endochondral ossification**.

Intramembranous Ossification

Intramembranous bone arises in a richly vascularized mesenchymal membrane where **mesenchymal cells** differentiate into osteoblasts (possibly via osteoprogenitor cells), which begin to elaborate bone matrix, thus forming spicules and trabeculae of bone (Fig. 5-10).

As more and more trabeculae form in the same vicinity, they will become interconnected. As they fuse with each other, they form **cancellous bone**, the peripheral regions of which will be remodeled to form **compact**

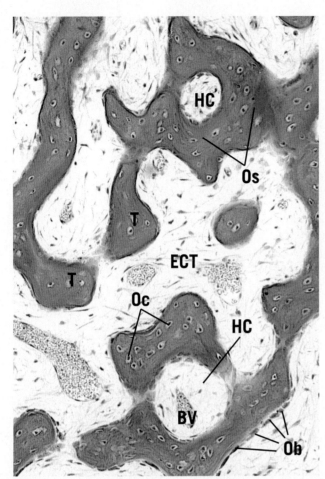

FIGURE 5-10. Intramembranous ossification. Pig skull. Paraffin section. ×132.

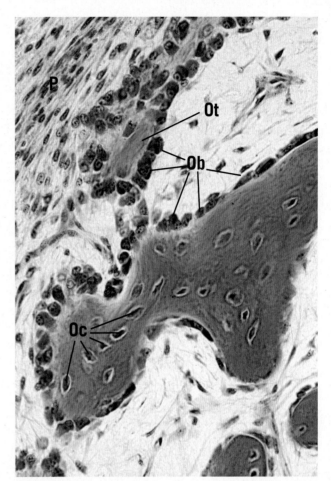

FIGURE 5-11. Intramembranous ossification. Pig skull. Paraffin section. ×270.

The anastomosing **trabeculae** (T) of forming bone appear darkly stained in a background of **embryonic connective tissue** (ECT), the mesenchyme. Observe that this connective tissue is highly vascular and that the bony trabeculae are forming primitive **osteons** (Os) surrounding large, primitive haversian canals (HC), whose center is occupied by **blood vessels** (BV). Observe that the **osteocytes** (Oc) are arranged somewhat haphazardly. Every trabecula is covered by **osteoblasts** (Ob).

bone. The surfaces of these trabeculae are populated with osteoblasts; frequently, **osteoclasts** may also be present. These large, multinucleated cells, derived from **monocyte precursors**, are found in shallow depressions on the trabecular surface (**Howship's lacunae**) and function to resorb bone. Bone is remodeled through the integrated interactions of osteoclasts and osteoblasts.

The region of the mesenchymal membrane that does not participate in the ossification process will remain the soft tissue component of bone (i.e., periosteum, endosteum; Fig. 5-11).

Endochondral Ossification

Long, short, and some parts of irregular bones arise from endochondral ossification, which relies on the presence of a hyaline cartilage model that is used as a template on

This photomicrograph of intramembranous ossification is taken from the periphery of the bone-forming region. Note the developing **periosteum** (P) in the upper left-hand corner. Just deep to this primitive periosteum, **osteoblasts** (Ob) are differentiating and are elaborating **osteoid** (Ot), as yet uncalcified bone matrix. As the osteoblasts surround themselves with bone matrix, they become trapped in their lacunae and are known as **osteocytes** (Oc). These osteocytes are more numerous, larger, and more ovoid than those of mature bone, and the organization of the collagen fibers of the bony matrix is less precise than that of mature bone. Hence, this bone is referred to as immature (primary) bone, and it will be replaced by mature bone later in life.

and within which bone is made (Fig. 5-12). However, cartilage does not become bone. Instead, a **bony subperiosteal collar** is formed (via intramembranous ossification) around the midriff of the cartilaginous template. This collar increases in width and length.

The **chondrocytes** in the center of the template hypertrophy and resorb some of their matrix, thus enlarging their lacunae so much that some lacunae become confluent. The **hypertrophied chondrocytes**, after assisting in calcification of the cartilage, degenerate and die. The newly

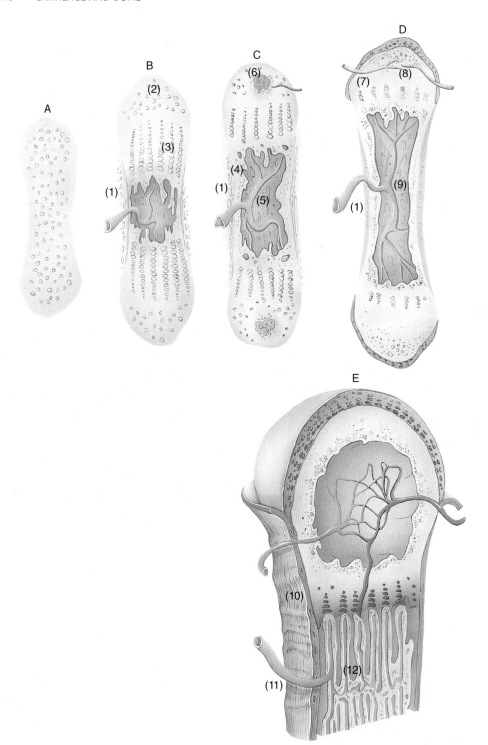

FIGURE 5-12. Endochondral bone formation. **A**. Endochondral bone formation requires the presence of a hyaline cartilage model. **B**. Vascularization of the diaphysis perichondrium (1) results in the transformation of chondrogenic cells to osteogenic cells, resulting in the formation of a **subperiosteal bone collar** (1) (via intramembranous bone formation), which quickly becomes perforated by osteoclastic activity. Although hyaline cartilage in the epiphysis (2) remains unchanged, chondrocytes in the center of the cartilage hypertrophy (3), and their lacuna becomes confluent. **C**. The subperiosteal bone collar increased in length and width, the confluent lacunae are invaded by the **periosteal bud** (4), and osteoclastic activity forms a primitive marrow cavity (5) whose walls are composed of calcified cartilage–calcified bone complex. The epiphyses display the beginning of **secondary ossification centers** (6). **D** and **E**. The subperiosteal bone color has become sufficiently large to support the developing long bone, so that much of the cartilage has been resorbed, with the exception of the **epiphyseal plate** (7) and the covering of the epiphyses. Ossification bone of the epiphyses occurs from the center (8); thus, the vascular periosteum does not cover the cartilaginous surface. Blood vessels enter the **epiphyses**, without vascularizing the cartilage. In the diaphysis, deep to the periosteum-lined cortical bone (10), blood vessels (11) ramify to form the vascular network (12) around which spongy bone will be formed.

CLINICAL CONSIDERATIONS 5-3

Vitamin Deficiency

Deficiency in vitamin A inhibits proper bone formation and growth, whereas an excess accelerates ossification of the epiphyseal plates producing small stature. **Deficiency in vitamin D**, which is essential for absorption of calcium from the intestine, results in poorly calcified (soft) bone—rickets in children and osteomalacia in adults. When in excess, bone is resorbed. **Deficiency in vitamin C**, which is necessary for collagen formation, produces scurvy—resulting in poor bone growth and repair.

CLINICAL CONSIDERATIONS 5-4

Paget Disease of the Bone

Paget disease of the bone is a generalized skeletal disease that usually affects older people. Often, the disease has a familial component and it results in thickened but softer bones of the skull and extremities. It is usually asymptomatic and is frequently discovered after radiographic examination prescribed for other reasons or as a result of blood chemistry showing elevated alkaline phosphatase levels.

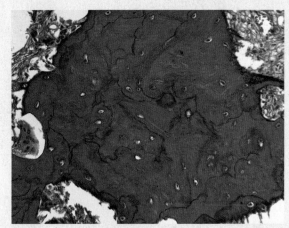

Note that the cement lines that surround haversian canal systems are well-defined but irregular in morphology. The osteocytes in their lacunae as well as the peripheral osteoblasts, along with the large osteoclasts in their Howship's lacunae, are clearly evident. (Reprinted with permission from Strayer DS, et al., eds. *Rubin's Pathology: Mechanisms of Human Disease*, 8th ed. Philadelphia: Wolters Kluwer, 2020. Figure 30-33A.)

formed spaces are invaded by the **periosteal bud** (composed of blood vessels, mesenchymal cells, and osteoprogenitor cells). Osteoprogenitor cells differentiate into osteoblasts, and these cells elaborate a bony matrix on the surface of the calcified cartilage. As the subperiosteal bone collar increases in thickness and length, osteoclasts resorb the calcified cartilage–calcified bone complex, leaving an enlarged space, the future marrow cavity (which will be populated by marrow cells). The entire process of ossification will spread away from this primary ossification center, and eventually, most of the cartilage template will be replaced by bone, forming the **diaphysis** of a long bone. The formation of the **bony epiphyses** (secondary ossification center) occurs in a modified fashion so that a cartilaginous covering may be maintained at the articular surface.

The growth in length of a long bone is due to the presence of **epiphyseal (growth) plates** of cartilage located between the epiphysis and the diaphysis. The epiphyseal plate exhibits five histologically distinct zones (Fig. 5-13A,B):

- **Zone of rest**, closest to the epiphysis, appears as typical hyaline cartilage.
- **Zone of proliferation** is where chondrocytes undergo mitosis in interstitial growth; however, the isogenous groups of chondrocytes form linear stacks rather than circular clusters.
- **Zone of hypertrophy** is characterized by enlarging chondrocytes and their lacunae.
- **Zone of calcification** has calcifying cartilage matrix and remnants of empty lacunae.
- **Zone of ossification**, closest to the diaphysis, has active osteoblasts elaborating bone matrix while osteoclasts are resorbing partially calcified cartilage matrix.

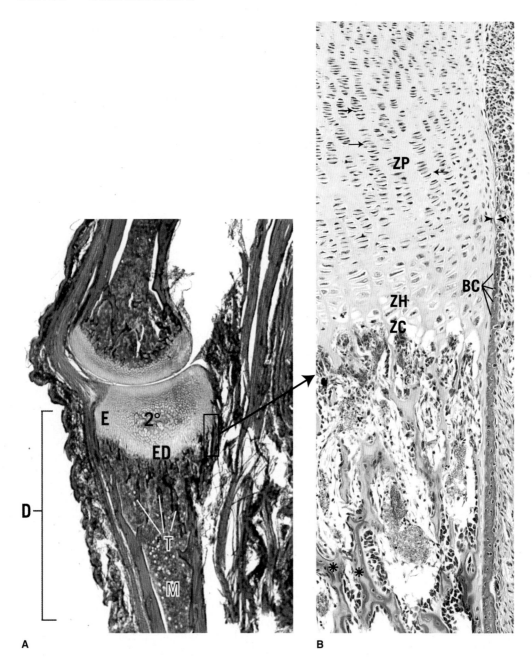

A

B

FIGURE 5-13A. Epiphyseal ossification center. Monkey. Paraffin section. ×14.

Most long bones are formed by the endochondral method of ossification, which involves the replacement of a cartilage model by bone. In this low-power photomicrograph, the **diaphysis** (D) of the lower phalanx has been replaced by bone, and the medullary cavity is filled with **marrow** (M). The **epiphysis** (E) of the same phalanx is undergoing ossification and is the **secondary center of ossification** (2°), thereby establishing the **epiphyseal plate** (ED). The **trabeculae** (T) are clearly evident on the diaphyseal side of the epiphyseal plate.

FIGURE 5-13B. Endochondral ossification. Monkey. Paraffin section. ×132. This montage is a higher magnification of the *boxed area* of Figure 5-13A. The region where the periosteum and perichondrium meet is evident (*arrowheads*). Deep to the periosteum is the **subperiosteal bone collar** (BC), which was formed via intramembranous ossification. Endochondral ossification is evident within the cartilage template. Starting at the top of the montage, note how the chondrocytes are lined up in long columns (*arrows*), indicative of their intense mitotic activity at the future epiphyseal plate region. In the epiphyseal plate, this will be the **zone of cell proliferation** (ZP). The chondrocytes increase in size in the **zone of cell maturation and hypertrophy** (ZH) and resorb some of their lacunar walls, enlarging them to such an extent that some of the lacunae become confluent. The chondrocytes die in the **zone of calcifying cartilage** (ZC). The presumptive medullary cavity is being populated by bone marrow, osteoclastic and osteogenic cells, and blood vessels. The osteogenic cells are actively differentiating into osteoblasts, which are elaborating bone on the calcified walls of the confluent lacunae. At the bottom of the photomicrograph, observe the bone-covered trabeculae of calcified cartilage (*asterisks*).

CLINICAL CONSIDERATIONS 5-5

Osteoporosis, Osteopetrosis, and Osteomalacia

Osteoporosis is a decrease in bone mass arising from lack of bone formation or from increased bone resorption. It occurs commonly in old age because of decreased growth hormone and in postmenopausal women because of decreased estrogen secretion. In the latter, estrogen binding to receptors on osteoblasts stimulates the secretion of bone matrix. Without sufficient estrogen, osteoclastic activity reduces bone mass without the concomitant formation of bone, therefore making the bones more liable to fracture.

Osteopetrosis is a constellation of heritable disorders that result in denser bones with possible skeletal malformations. The disease may be the early-onset type or the delayed-onset type. The early-onset type may begin in infancy and can result in early death because of anemia, uncontrollable bleeding, and rampant infection. The delayed-onset type of osteopetrosis may be quite mild, exhibiting no clinical symptoms, but thickening of the bones and slight facial deformities may be evident. As the bones become thicker, the diameters of the foramina become smaller and nerves passing through those constricted openings may become compressed and cause considerable pain.

Osteomalacia is a condition in the adult that resembles rickets, which occur in children who have depressed vitamin D levels and, consequently, cannot absorb enough calcium in their gastrointestinal tract. This condition is difficult to diagnose because initially the patient presents with nonspecific symptoms that range from aches and pains to muscle weakness. Once advanced stages of osteomalacia are reached, the symptoms include deep bone pain, difficulty in walking, and bone fractures. Histologic pictures of cancellous bone present overly thin trabeculae of bone with prominent Howship's lacunae occupied by osteoclasts and the presence of exceptionally thick osteoid over the thin calcified bony trabeculae and spicules.

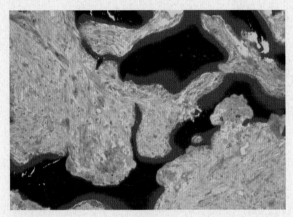

Observe the large marrow spaces and the thin calcified bone (black) in the histologic image of osteomalacia. Note the very thick osteoid (magenta-colored homogeneous material) covering the calcified bony trabeculae. Osteoclastic activity is apparent in the scalloped indentation on the middle right of the image. (Reprinted with permission from Strayer DS, et al., eds. *Rubin's Pathology: Mechanisms of Human Disease*, 8th ed. Philadelphia: Wolters Kluwer, 2020. Figure 30-30B.)

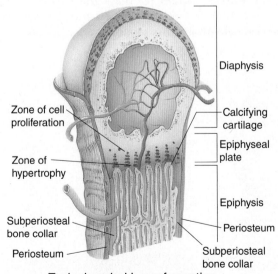

Endochondral bone formation

Labels: Diaphysis, Calcifying cartilage, Epiphyseal plate, Epiphysis, Periosteum, Subperiosteal bone collar, Zone of cell proliferation, Zone of hypertrophy, Subperiosteal bone collar, Periosteum

Hormonal Influences on Bone

Calcitonin inhibits bone matrix resorption by altering osteoclast function, thus preventing calcium release. **Parathyroid hormone** activates osteoblasts to secrete **osteoclast-stimulating factor**, thus activating osteoclasts to increase bone resorption resulting in increased blood calcium levels. If in excess, bones become brittle and are susceptible to fracture.

PLATE 5-1A Cartilage

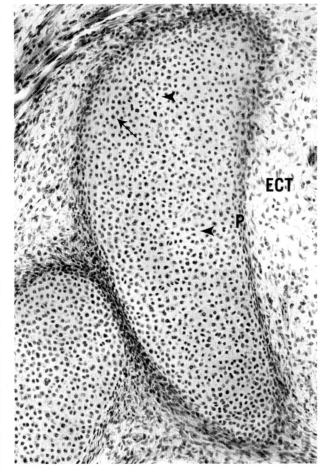

FIGURE 5-1-1. Embryonic hyaline cartilage. Pig. Paraffin section. ×132.

The developing hyaline cartilage is surrounded by **embryonic connective tissue** (ECT), the mesenchyme. Mesenchymal cells have participated in the formation of this cartilage. Note that the developing **perichondrium** (P), investing the cartilage, merges both with the embryonic connective tissue and with the cartilage. The chondrocytes in their lacunae are round, small cells packed closely together (*arrow*), with little intervening homogeneously staining matrix (*arrowheads*).

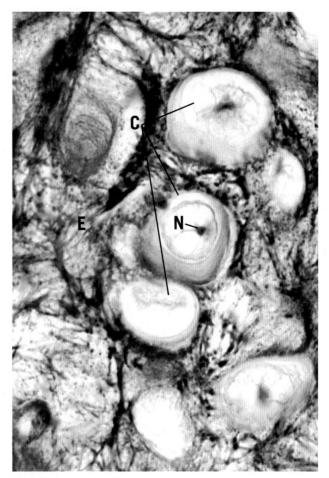

FIGURE 5-1-2. Elastic cartilage. Epiglottis. Human. Paraffin section. ×540.

A high-magnification view of elastic cartilage. The **chondrocytes** (C) are large, oval to round cells with acentric **nuclei** (N). The cells accumulate lipids in their cytoplasm, often in the form of lipid droplets, thus imparting to the cell a "vacuolated" appearance. Note that the **elastic fibers** (E) mask the matrix in some areas and that the fibers are of various thicknesses, especially evident in cross sections.

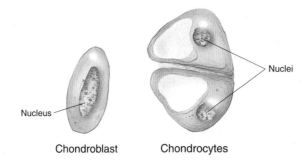

Chondroblast   Chondrocytes

KEY					
N	nuclei	**ECT**	embryonic connective	**P**	perichondrium
E	elastic fibers		tissue		
C	chondrocyte				

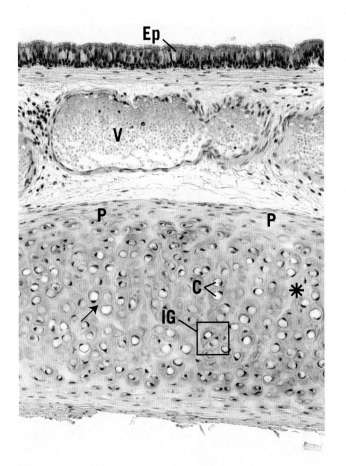

FIGURE 5-1-3. Hyaline cartilage. Trachea. Monkey. Paraffin section. ×132.

The trachea is lined by a **pseudostratified ciliated columnar epithelium** (Ep). Deep to the epithelium, observe the large, blood-filled **vein** (V). The lower half of the photomicrograph presents hyaline cartilage whose **chondrocytes** (C) are disposed in **isogenous groups** (IG) indicative of interstitial growth. Chondrocytes are housed in spaces known as lacunae. Note that the territorial matrix (*arrow*) in the vicinity of the lacunae stains darker than the interterritorial matrix (*asterisk*). The entire cartilage is surrounded by a **perichondrium** (P).

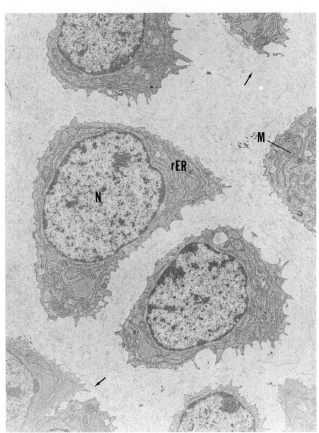

FIGURE 5-1-4. Hyaline cartilage. Mouse. Electron microscopy. ×6,120.

The hyaline cartilage of a neonatal mouse trachea presents chondrocytes, whose centrally positioned **nuclei** (N) are surrounded with a rich **rough endoplasmic reticulum** (rER) and numerous **mitochondria** (M). The matrix displays fine collagen fibrils (*arrows*). (Reprinted from Seegmiller R, et al. Studies on cartilage: VI. A genetically determined defect in tracheal cartilage. *J Ultrastruct Res* 1972;38(3):288–301. Copyright © 1972 Elsevier. With permission.)

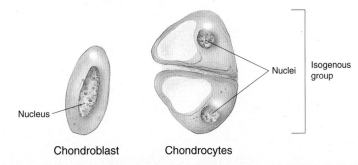

KEY					
C	chondrocyte	**IG**	isogenous groups	**rER**	rough endoplasmic
E	elastic fiber	**M**	mitochondria		reticulum
Ep	pseudostratified ciliated	**N**	nuclei	**V**	vein
	columnar epithelium	**P**	perichondrium		

PLATE 5-2A   Bone

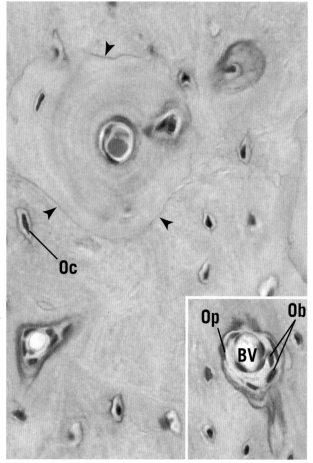

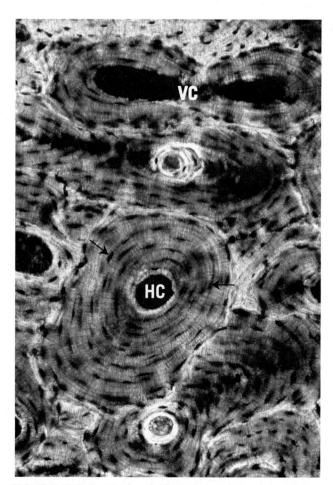

FIGURE 5-2-1. Decalcified compact bone. Human. Paraffin section. ×540.

FIGURE 5-2-2. Undecalcified ground compact bone. x.s. Human. Paraffin section. ×132.

A small osteon is delineated by its surrounding cementing line (*arrowheads*). The lenticular-shaped **osteocytes** (Oc) occupy flattened spaces, known as lacunae. The lacunae are lined by uncalcified osteoid matrix. *Inset.* **Decalcified compact bone. Human. Paraffin section**. **×540**. A haversian canal of an osteon is shown to contain a small **blood vessel** (BV) supported by slender connective tissue elements. The canal is lined by flattened **osteoblasts** (Ob) and, perhaps, **osteogenic cells** (Op).

This specimen was treated with India ink to accentuate some of the salient features of compact bone. The **haversian canals** (HC) as well as the lacunae (*arrows*) appear black in the figure. Note the connection between the HC of two osteons at top center, known as **Volkmann's canal** (VC). The canaliculi appear as fine, narrow lines leading to the HC as they anastomose with each other and with lacunae of other osteocytes of the same osteon.

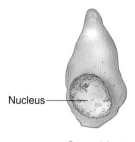

Nucleus

Osteoblast

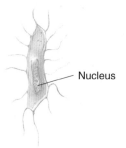

Nucleus

Osteocyte

KEY					
BV	blood vessel	**Ob**	osteoblast	**Op**	osteogenic cell
HC	haversian canal	**Oc**	osteocyte	**VC**	Volkmann's canal

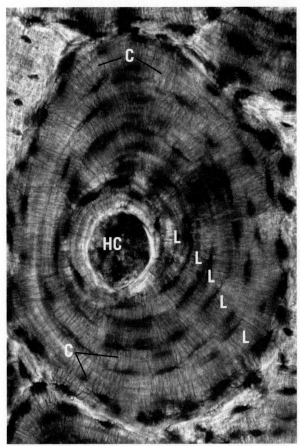

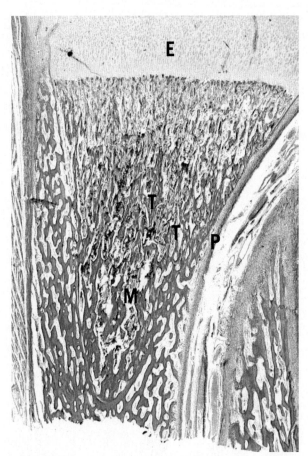

FIGURE 5-2-3. Undecalcified ground bone. x.s. Human. Paraffin section. ×270.

This transverse section of an osteon clearly displays the **lamellae** (L) of bone surrounding the **haversian canal** (HC). The cementing line acts to delineate the periphery of the osteon. Note that the **canaliculi** (C) arising from the peripheral-most lacunae usually do not extend toward other osteons. Instead, they lead toward the HC. Canaliculi, which appear to anastomose with each other and with lacunae, house long osteocytic processes in the living bone.

FIGURE 5-2-4. Endochondral ossification. l.s. Monkey. Paraffin section. ×14.

Much of the cartilage has been replaced in the diaphysis of this forming bone. Note the numerous **trabeculae** (T) and the developing **bone marrow** (M) of the medullary cavity. Ossification is advancing toward the **epiphysis** (E), in which the secondary center of ossification has not yet appeared. Observe the **periosteum** (P), which appears as a definite line between the subperiosteal bone collar and the surrounding connective tissue.

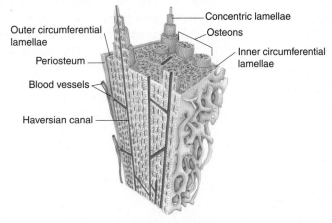

Concentric lamellae
Osteons
Outer circumferential lamellae
Inner circumferential lamellae
Periosteum
Blood vessels
Haversian canal

Compact bone

KEY					
C	canaliculi	**L**	lamellae	**P**	periosteum
E	epiphysis	**M**	bone marrow	**T**	trabeculae
HC	haversian canal				

PLATE 5-2C Bone

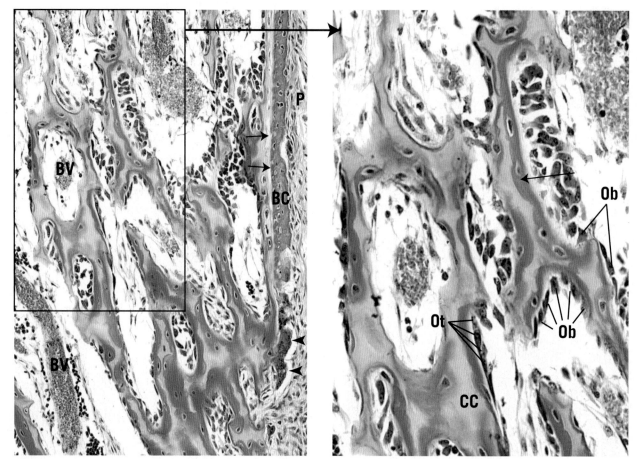

FIGURE 5-2-5. Endochondral ossification. Monkey. Paraffin section. ×132.

Observe the multinucleated osteoclast (*arrowheads*) resorbing the bone-covered trabeculae of calcified cartilage. The **subperiosteal bone collar** (BC) and the **periosteum** (P) are clearly evident, as is the junction between the bone collar and the cartilage (*arrows*). The medullary cavity is being established and is populated by **blood vessels** (BV), osteogenic cells, osteoblasts, and hematopoietic cells.

FIGURE 5-2-6. Endochondral ossification. Monkey. Paraffin section. ×270.

This photomicrograph is a higher magnification of the *boxed area* in Figure 5-2-5. Note that the trabeculae of calcified cartilage are covered by a thin layer of bone. The darker staining bone (*arrow*) contains osteocytes, whereas the lighter staining **calcified cartilage** (CC) is acellular, because the chondrocytes of this region have died, leaving behind empty lacunae that are confluent with each other. Observe that **osteoblasts** (Ob) line the trabecular complexes and that they are separated from the calcified bone by thin intervening **osteoid** (Ot). As the subperiosteal bone collar increases in thickness, the trabeculae of bone-covered calcified cartilage will be resorbed so that the cartilage template will be replaced by bone. The only cartilage that will remain will be the epiphyseal plate and the articular covering of the epiphysis.

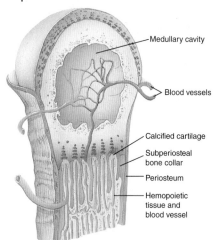

Medullary cavity

Blood vessels

Calcified cartilage

Subperiosteal bone collar

Periosteum

Hemopoietic tissue and blood vessel

Endochondral bone formation

KEY					
BC	bone collar	**CC**	calcified cartilage	**Ot**	osteoid
BV	blood vessels	**Ob**	osteoblasts	**P**	periosteum

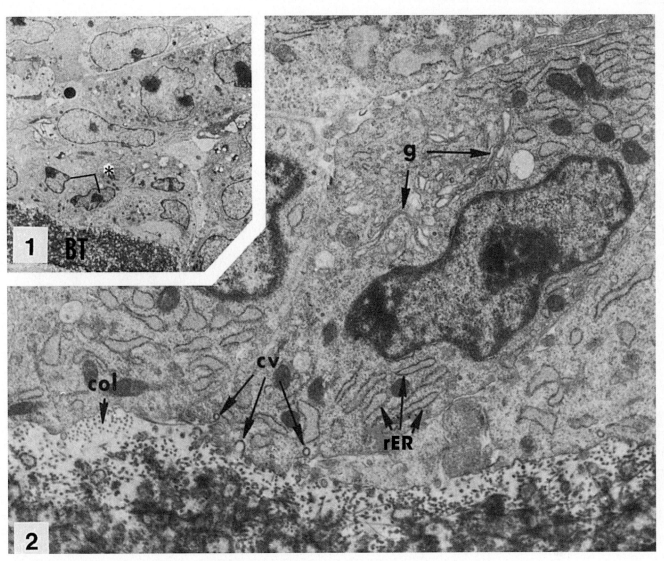

FIGURE 5-3-1. Osteoblasts from long bone. Rat. Electron microscopy. ×1,350.

This low-magnification electron micrograph displays numerous fibroblasts and osteoblasts in the vicinity of a **bony trabecula** (BT). The osteoblasts (*asterisk*) are presented at a higher magnification in Figure 2. (From Ryder MI, et al. The adherence to bone by cytoplasmic elements of osteoclast. *J Dent Res* 1981;60(7):1349–1355. Copyright © 1981 SAGE Publications. Reprinted by permission of SAGE Publications, Inc.)

FIGURE 5-3-2. Osteoblasts. Rat. Electron microscopy. ×9,450.

Osteoblasts, at higher magnification, present well-developed **Golgi apparatus** (g), extensive **rough endoplasmic reticulum** (rER), and several **coated vacuoles** (cv) at the basal cell membrane. Observe the cross sections of **collagen fibers** (col) in the bone matrix. (From Ryder MI, et al. The adherence to bone by cytoplasmic elements of osteoclast. *J Dent Res* 1981;60(7):1349–1355. Copyright © 1981 SAGE Publications. Reprinted by permission of SAGE Publications, Inc.)

KEY					
BT	bony trabecula	**cv**	coated vacuoles	**rER**	rough endoplasmic
col	collagen fibers	**G**	Golgi apparatus		reticulum

PLATE 5-3B Cells of the Bone

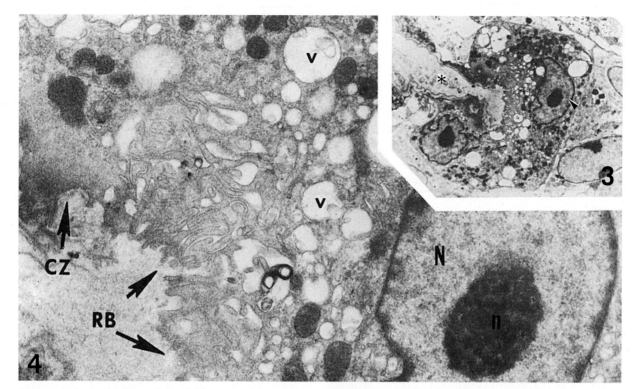

FIGURE 5-3-3. Osteoclast from long bone. Rat. Electron microscopy. ×1,800.

Two nuclei of an osteoclast are evident in this section. Observe that the cell is surrounding a bony surface (*asterisk*). The region of the nucleus marked by an *arrowhead* is presented at a higher magnification in Figure 5-3-4.

FIGURE 5-3-4. Osteoclast. Rat. Electron microscopy. ×10,800.

This is a higher magnification of a region of Figure 5-3-3. Note the presence of the **nucleus** (N) and its **nucleolus** (n), as well as the **ruffled border** (RB and *arrows*) and **clear zone** (CZ and *arrow*) of the osteoclast. Numerous **vacuoles** (v) of various sizes may be observed throughout the cytoplasm. (From Ryder MI, et al. The adherence to bone by cytoplasmic elements of osteoclast. *J Dent Res* 1981;60(7):1349–1355. Copyright © 1981 SAGE Publications. Reprinted by permission of SAGE Publications, Inc.)

KEY					
N	nucleus	**RB**	ruffled border	**v**	vacuoles
n	nucleolus	**CZ:**	clear zone		

PLATE 5-3B   Cells of the Bone

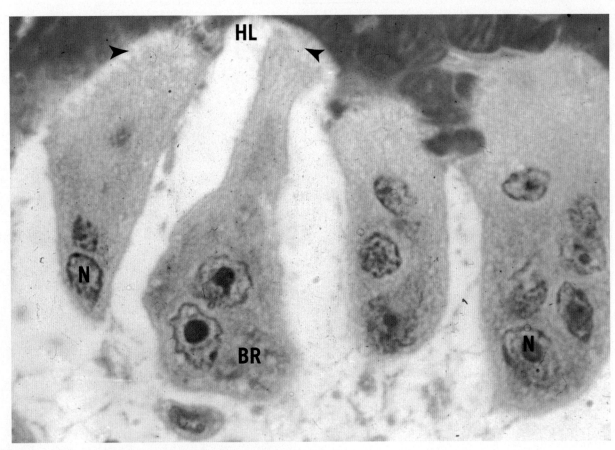

FIGURE 5-3-5. Osteoclasts. Human. Paraffin section. ×600.

The **nuclei** (N) of these multinuclear cells are located in their **basal region** (BR), away from **Howship's lacunae** (HL). Note that the **ruffled border** (RB) (*arrowheads*) is in intimate contact with HL. (Courtesy of Dr. J. Hollinger.)

KEY					
BR	basal region	**N**	nucleus	**RB**	ruffled border
HL	Howship's lacunae				

Selected Review of Histologic Images

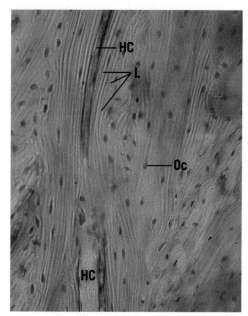

REVIEW FIGURE 5-1-1. Decalcified compact bone. Human. l.s. Paraffin section. ×270.

Longitudinal section of decalcified bone displays parallel arrays of **lamellae** (L) and the long **haversian canal** (HC) in the center of the osteon. Nuclei of **osteocytes** (Oc) are clearly evident.

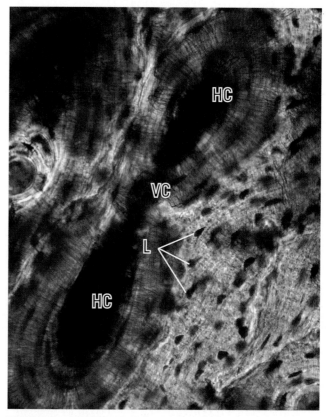

REVIEW FIGURE 5-1-2. Undecalcified ground compact bone. x.s. Human. ×270.

This transverse section of undecalcified ground compact bone displays a cross section of two **haversian canals** (HC) connected to each other by a **Volkmann's canal** (VC). Blood vessels that nourish compact bone travel via haversian canals, and it is through VC that they are able to penetrate bone and provide branches to adjacent HC. Observe the **lamellae** (L) whose lacunae are occupied by osteocytes in the living bone.

KEY					
HC	haversian canal	**Oc**	osteocytes	**VC**	Volkmann's canal
L	lamellae				

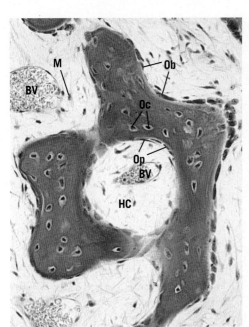

REVIEW FIGURE 5-1-3. Intramembranous ossification. Pig skull. Paraffin section. ×270.

This is a figure displaying a developing osteon whose **haversian canal** (HC) houses a centrally located **blood vessel** (BV) surrounded by mesenchymal connective tissue. Note that the HC is lined by flat **osteoprogenitor cells** (Op) and the developing osteon contains round, immature **osteocytes** (Oc) in large lacunae. **Osteoblasts** (Ob) cover the developing osteon, which is being formed in mesenchymal connective tissue rich in BV and **mesenchymal cells** (M) of osteocytes are clearly evident.

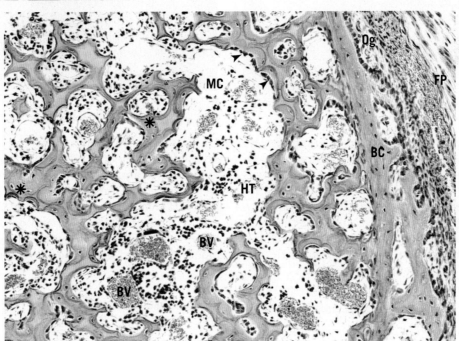

REVIEW FIGURE 5-1-4. Endochondral ossification. x.s. Monkey. Paraffin section. ×196.

A cross section of the region of endochondral ossification presents many round spaces in calcified cartilage that are lined with bone (*asterisks*). These spaces represent confluent lacunae in the cartilage template, where the chondrocytes have hypertrophied and died. Subsequently, the cartilage calcified, and the invading osteogenic cells have differentiated into osteoblasts (*arrowheads*) and lined the calcified cartilage with bone. Because neighboring spaces were separated from each other by calcified cartilage walls, bone was elaborated on the sides of the walls. Therefore, these trabeculae, which in longitudinal section appear to be stalactite-like structures of bone with a calcified cartilaginous core, are, in fact, spaces in the cartilage template that are lined with bone. The walls between the spaces are the remnants of cartilage between lacunae that became calcified and form the substructure upon which bone was elaborated. Observe the forming **medullary cavity** (MC), housing **blood vessels** (BV), **hematopoietic tissue** (HT), osteogenic cells, and osteoblasts (*arrowheads*). The **subperiosteal bone collar** (BC) is evident and is covered by a periosteum, whose two layers, **fibrous** (FP) and **osteogenic** (Og), are clearly discernible.

KEY					
BC	bone collar	**HT**	hematopoietic tissue	**Oc**	osteocytes
BV	blood vessel	**M**	mesenchymal cells	**Og**	osteogenic periosteum
FP	fibrous periosteum	**MC**	medullary cavity	**Op**	osteoprogenitor cells
HC	haversian canal	**Ob**	osteoblasts		

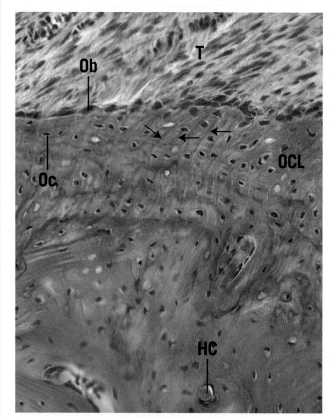

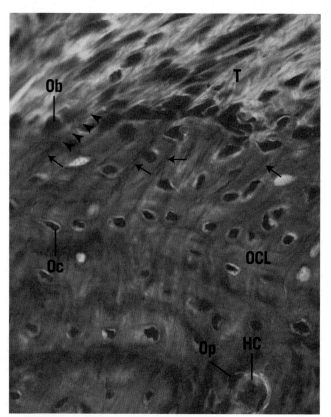

REVIEW FIGURE 5-2-1. Decalcified compact bone. Rib. Sharpey's fibers. x.s. Human. ×270.

This medium-magnification photomicrograph displays the **tendon** (T) attaching to the rib via **Sharpey's fibers** (*arrows*), continuation of the type I collagen fibers from the tendon into the **outer circumferential lamellae** (OCL) of the compact bone. Note the presence of **osteoblasts** (Ob) covering the surface of the outer circumferential lamellae and the **osteocytes** (Oc) in their lacunae. A **haversian canal** (HC) of the HC system housing a blood vessel is clearly evident.

REVIEW FIGURE 5-2-2. Decalcified compact bone. Rib. Sharpey's fibers. x.s. Human. ×540.

This is a higher magnification of the upper right-hand side of Review Figure 5-2-1. Note that type I collagen fibers of the **tendon** (T) can be followed (arrowheads) as it inserts into the **outer circumferential lamellae** (OCL), where they are known as **Sharpey's fibers** (*arrows*). **Osteoblasts** (Ob) and **osteocytes** (Oc) are labeled, as well as a **haversian canal** (HC) with its blood vessels and **osteoprogenitor cells** (Op).

KEY					
HC	haversian canal	**Oc**	osteocytes	**T**	tendon
Ob	osteoblast	**OCL**	outer circumferential lamellae	**Op**	osteoprogenitor cells

Summary of Histologic Organization

I. CARTILAGE

A. Embryonic Cartilage

1. Perichondrium

The **perichondrium** is very thin and cellular.

2. Matrix

The **matrix** is scanty and smooth in appearance.

3. Cells

Numerous, small, round **chondrocytes** are housed in small spaces in the matrix.

These spaces are known as **lacunae**.

B. Hyaline Cartilage

1. Perichondrium

The perichondrium has two layers: an outer **fibrous layer**, which contains collagen and fibroblasts, and an inner **chondrogenic layer**, which contains **chondrogenic cells** and **chondroblasts**.

2. Matrix

The **matrix** is smooth and basophilic in appearance. It has two regions: the **territorial (capsular) matrix**, which is darker and surrounds **lacunae**, and the **interterritorial (intercapsular) matrix**, which is lighter in color. The collagen fibrils are masked by the ground substance.

3. Cells

Either **chondrocytes** are found individually in **lacunae** or there may be two or more chondrocytes (**isogenous group**) in a lacuna. The latter case signifies **interstitial growth**. **Appositional growth** occurs just deep to the perichondrium and is attributed to **chondroblasts**.

C. Elastic Cartilage

1. Perichondrium

The perichondrium is the same in elastic cartilage as in hyaline cartilage.

2. Matrix

The **matrix** contains numerous dark **elastic fibers** in addition to the **collagen fibrils**.

3. Cells

The cells are **chondrocytes**, **chondroblasts**, and **chondrogenic cells**, as in hyaline cartilage.

D. Fibrocartilage

1. Perichondrium

The perichondrium is usually absent.

2. Matrix

The **ground substance** of matrix is very scanty. In addition to type II collagen, many thick type I collagen bundles are located between parallel rows of chondrocytes.

3. Cells

The **chondrocytes** in fibrocartilage are smaller than those in hyaline or elastic cartilage, and they are arranged in parallel longitudinal rows between bundles of thick collagen fibers.

II. BONE

A. Compact Bone

1. Periosteum

The **periosteum** has two layers: an outer **fibrous layer**, containing **collagen fibers** and **fibroblasts**, and an inner **osteogenic layer**, containing **osteoprogenitor cells** and **osteoblasts**. It is anchored to bone by **Sharpey's fibers**.

2. Lamellar Systems

In newly forming bones, the bone matrix comprises unorganized **woven (immature, primary) bone** tissues. Through remodeling, the woven bone is replaced with **lamellar (mature, secondary) bone**.

Lamellar organization consists of **outer** and **inner circumferential lamellae**, **concentric lamellae** comprising **osteons (haversian canal systems)**, and **interstitial lamellae**. Lacunae, containing osteocytes, are found in between the layers of lamellae. **Canaliculi** radiate from **lacunae**, which allow osteocytic processes to communicate with each other via gap junctions, eventually opening to the central **haversian canal**. **Cementing lines** demarcate the peripheral extent of each osteon. **Volkmann's canals** interconnect neighboring haversian canals.

3. Endosteum

The **endosteum** is a thin, cellular membrane comprising inactive osteoblasts, osteoprogenitor cells, and occasional osteoclasts. Endosteum lines the **inner circumferential lamellae**, and the external surfaces of spongy bone **spicules** and **trabeculae**, thus lining the **medullary cavity**, which contains **yellow** or **white bone marrow**.

4. Cells

Osteocytes are housed in small spaces called **lacunae**. **Osteoblasts** and **osteoprogenitor cells** are found in the osteogenic layer of the periosteum, in the endosteum, and in the lining of the haversian canals. **Osteoclasts** are located in **Howship's lacunae** along resorptive surfaces of bone. **Osteoid**, noncalcified bone matrix, is interposed between the cells of bone and the calcified tissue.

5. Vascular Supply

Blood vessels are found in the periosteum, in the marrow cavity, and in the haversian canals of osteons. Haversian canals are connected to each other by Volkmann's canals.

B. Cancellous (Spongy, Medullary) Bone

1. Endosteum

All external surface of the cancellous bone spicules and trabeculae are covered by the delicate endosteum.

2. Lamellar Systems

Similar to compact bone, the forming cancellous bone **spicules** and **trabeculae** bone matrix are comprised of unorganized **woven (immature, primary) bone** tissues. Through remodeling, the woven bone is replaced with the well-organized **lamellar (mature, secondary) bone**. However, there are no osteons in the small spicules and trabeculae.

3. Cells

Osteocytes are housed in lacunae with osteocytic processes in canaliculi. **Osteoblasts**, as a part of endosteum, line all trabeculae and spicules. Occasionally, multinuclear, large **osteoclasts** occupy **Howship's lacunae**. **Osteoid**, noncalcified bone matrix, is interposed between the cells of bone and the calcified tissue.

    Bone marrow, comprising hematopoietic tissue or adipose tissue, occupies the **marrow cavity**, the spaces among and between **trabeculae**.

C. Osteogenesis

1. Intramembranous Ossification

Ossification centers form within the vascularized areas of **mesenchymal connective tissue** where **mesenchymal cells** probably differentiate into **osteoprogenitor cells**, which differentiate into **osteoblasts**. Networks of **spicules** and **trabeculae** coalesce to form primitive osteons surrounding blood vessels in the **cortical (compact) bone** regions.

2. Endochondral Ossification

a. Primary Ossification Center

The **perichondrium** of the **diaphysis** of the cartilage template becomes vascularized, followed by **hypertrophy** of the centrally located chondrocytes, confluence of contiguous lacunae, calcification of the cartilage remnants, and subsequent **chondrocytic death**. Concomitant with these events, the **chondrogenic cells** of the perichondrium become **osteoprogenitor cells**, which, in turn, differentiate into **osteoblasts**. The osteoblasts form the **subperiosteal bone collar**, thus converting the overlying **perichondrium** into a **periosteum**. A **periosteal bud** invades the diaphysis, entering the confluent **lacunae** left empty by the death of chondrocytes. Osteogenic cells give rise to osteoblasts, which elaborate bone on the **trabeculae of calcified cartilage**. Hemopoiesis begins in the primitive medullary cavity; **osteoclasts** (and, according to some, chondroclasts) develop, which resorb the bone-covered trabeculae of calcified cartilage as the subperiosteal bone collar becomes thicker and elongated.

b. Secondary Ossification Center

The **epiphyseal (secondary) center of ossification** is initiated somewhat after birth. It begins in the center of the epiphysis and proceeds radially from that point, leaving cartilage only at the **articular surface** and at the interface between the epiphysis and the diaphysis, the future **epiphyseal plate**.

c. Epiphyseal Plate

The **epiphyseal plate** is responsible for the future lengthening of a long bone. It is divided into five zones: (1) **zone of rest**, a region of reserve hyaline cartilage; (2) **zone of proliferation**, where isogenous groups of chondrocytes are arranged in rows whose longitudinal axis parallels that of the growing bone; (3) **zone of hypertrophy**, where cells enlarge and the matrix between adjoining cells becomes very thin; (4) **zone of calcification**, where lacunae become confluent and the matrix between adjacent rows of chondrocytes becomes calcified, causing subsequent chondrocytic death; and (5) **zone of ossification**, where osteoblasts deposit bone on the calcified cartilage remnants between the adjacent rows. Osteoclasts (and, according to some, chondroclasts) resorb the calcified complex.

Chapter Review Questions

5-1. Which component of the cartilage matrix is directly responsible for its rigidity?

A. Chondrocytes

B. Hyaluronic acid

C. Type II collagen

D. Water

5-2. The zone of proliferation in the epiphyseal plate demonstrates which mode of tissue growth?

A. Appositional

B. Hypertrophy

C. Interstitial

D. Intramembranous

5-3. Which organ would be most adversely affected by vitamin C deficiency in adults?

A. Alveolar bones

B. Articulating joint surfaces

C. Epiglottis

D. Trachea

5-4. Which cells have parathyroid hormone receptors?

A. Chondroblasts

B. Chondrocytes

C. Osteoblasts

D. Osteoclasts

5-5. Which structures allow direct cell–cell communication in the bone tissue?

A. Canaliculi

B. Haversian canals

C. Territorial matrix

D. Volkmann's canals

CHAPTER OUTLINE

The total volume of blood in an average person is ~5 L; it is a **specialized type of connective tissue**, composed of cells and cell fragments, collectively referred to as **formed elements**, suspended in an extracellular fluid called **plasma**. Blood circulates throughout the body and is well adapted for its manifold functions in transporting nutrients, oxygen, waste products, carbon dioxide, electrolytes, hormones, cells, and other substances. Moreover, blood also functions in the maintenance of body temperature and regulates acid–base balance and osmotic balance. The formed elements of blood must be replaced constantly as they reach the end of their life span; this process of replacement is referred to as **hemopoiesis**.

Blood

The formed elements of blood are **erythrocytes (red blood cells [RBCs])**, **leukocytes (white blood cells [WBCs])**, and **platelets (thrombocytes)**; see Table 6-1.

Formed Elements of Blood

The nomenclature developed for these formed elements is based on their colorations with Wright or Giemsa's modification of the Romanowsky-type stains as applied to blood and marrow smears used in hematology.

Erythrocytes

Erythrocytes, the most numerous cells of the blood, are biconcave, anucleated disks with no organelles that function entirely within the circulatory system. The biconcave shape is caused by the interactions between the integral and peripheral proteins of the erythrocyte plasmalemma and the cytoskeletal proteins, such as **actin**, **spectrin**, **ankyrin**, and other proteins.

Erythrocytes are packed with **hemoglobin**, the protein that transports oxygen and carbon dioxide to and from the tissues of the body (exchange of gases is described in Chapter 13, Respiratory System). Additionally, several soluble enzymes, such as **carbonic anhydrase** and those necessary for glycolysis and adenosine triphosphate (ATP) synthesis, are also well represented.

RBCs vary in number by biologic sex, with males living at sea level having ~5 million, and females living at sea level having ~4.5 million erythrocytes/mm^3 of blood. They are 7 to 8 µm in diameter in blood smears and 6 to 7 µm in histologic sections. They stain salmon pink in color (Figs. 6-1 and 6-2) and have a life span of ~120 days. Old erythrocytes are destroyed by **macrophages** of the spleen, liver, and bone marrow.

The plasmalemma of erythrocytes presents **hereditary antigenic** carbohydrate groups on its external surface that represent the **ABO blood groups (blood types)**. Although they are very similar, they must be considered

Table 6-1	Formed Elements of Blood						
Element	**Diameter (µm)** Smear	Section	**No./mm³**	**% of Leukocytes**	**Granules**	**Function**	**Nucleus**
Erythrocyte	7–8	6–7	5 × 10⁶ (males) 4.5 × 10⁶ (females)		None	Transport of O₂ and CO₂	None
Lymphocyte	8–10	7–8	1,500–2,500	20–25	Azurophilic only	Immunologic response	Large, round, acentric
Monocyte	12–15	10–12	200–800	3–8	Azurophilic only	Phagocytosis	Large, kidney-shaped
Neutrophil	9–12	8–9	3,500–7,000	60–70	Azurophilic and small specific (neutrophilic)	Phagocytosis	Polymorphous
Eosinophil	10–14	9–11	150–400	2–4	Azurophilic and large specific (eosinophilic)	Phagocytosis of antigen–antibody complexes and control of parasitic diseases	Bilobed (sausage-shaped)
Basophil	8–10	7–8	50–100	0.5–1	Azurophilic and large specific (basophilic) granules (heparin and histamine)	Perhaps assists in initiating the inflammatory response	Large, S-shaped
Platelets	2–4	1–3	250,000–400,000		Granulomere	Agglutination and clotting	None

CLINICAL CONSIDERATIONS 6-1

Sickle Cell Anemia

Sickle cell anemia, a hereditary disease, is the result of a point mutation in the gene that codes for hemoglobin. A single amino acid substitution of alanine replacing glutamine occurs in some individuals who are descendants of the indigenous population of tropical and subtropical regions of Africa, especially from the Sub-Saharan area. Approximately 2/1,000 African Americans are afflicted with this disease, and 10% of that population carry one copy of the gene and are therefore carriers of the trait but not afflicted by the disease. The RBCs of patients with two copies of the mutated gene are susceptible to hypoxic stress and become easily misshapen into a sickle shape. Because of their shape, the erythrocytes are fragile, can only carry a reduced amount of oxygen, and do not pass easily through small capillaries. This causes blockage and, frequently, downstream tissue damage. The abnormal RBCs have deleterious effects on the kidneys, brain, bones, and spleen, among other organs. Depending on the severity of the condition, the patient's symptoms may vary from slight to severe, and, in the latter case, it may result in death at an early age. Because sickle cell anemia is incurable, it is treated with avoidance of strenuous physical exertions, avoiding high altitudes, and instructing patients to seek treatment for even minor infections.

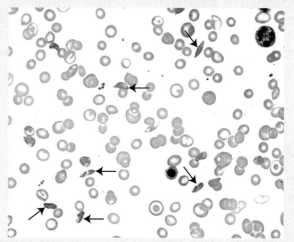

This blood smear, from a patient suffering from sickle cell anemia, displays numerous RBCs distorted so that they appear spindle-shaped (*arrows*).

CLINICAL CONSIDERATIONS 6-2

Polycythemia Vera

Polycythemia vera (**primary polycythemia**) is a rare disorder of the blood that manifests itself by an excess production of RBCs and, frequently, platelets, resulting in greater blood volume and an increase in the viscosity of blood. It mainly involves individuals in their early 60s, although occasionally it occurs in patients in their early 20s. Symptoms may be absent for several years after the onset of the condition, but patients suffering from this disorder may exhibit headaches, vertigo, fatigue, shortness of breath, enlarged liver and spleen, burning sensation in the extremities, and visual disorders as well as gingival bleeding and generalized itching. If left untreated, the patient may die within 2 years; with proper treatment, the life span can be extended by 10 to 20 years.

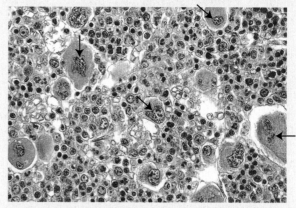

This is a bone marrow biopsy from a middle-aged woman suffering from polycythemia vera. Observe that the marrow is hypercellular, exhibiting abnormally high numbers of erythrocyte precursors and megakaryocytes (*arrows*). (Reprinted with permission from Mills SE, et al., eds. *Sternberg's Diagnostic Surgical Pathology*, 6th ed. Philadelphia: Wolters Kluwer, 2015. p. 698, Figure 16-21.)

prior to blood transfusion to prevent the death of the individual receiving the blood (Table 6-2). There are four major blood types, based on the three alleles of the *ABO* gene (I^A, I^B, and i), namely A, B, AB, and O. All three antigens that determine these blood types are identical except that

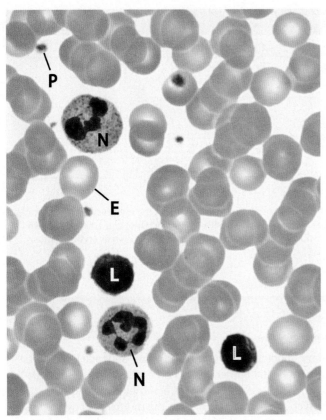

FIGURE 6-1. Erythrocytes (E), lymphocytes (L), neutrophils (N), and platelets (P). ×1,325.

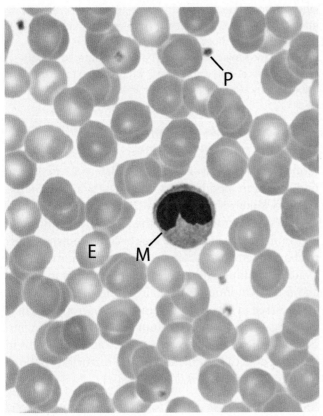

FIGURE 6-2. Monocyte (M), erythrocytes (E), and platelets (P). ×1,325.

- types A and B have one additional sugar molecule in their carbohydrate chain (located at their free terminus) than type O and

- the extra terminal sugar molecule of type A antigen differs from that of the type B antigen.

It should be noted that all type O antigens are identical; all type A antigens are identical because they possess the same terminal sugar molecule; and all type B antigens are identical because they possess the same terminal sugar molecule. Both I^A and I^B are dominant over i but not over each other.

Leukocytes

Leukocytes (WBCs) perform their functions outside the circulatory system and use the bloodstream as a mode of transportation to reach their destinations. The two major categories of WBCs are agranulocytes and granulocytes. Lymphocytes and monocytes compose the first group, whereas neutrophils, eosinophils, and basophils compose the latter and are recognizable by their distinctive **specific granules** (see Table 6-1).

Lymphocytes

Lymphocytes, somewhat larger than erythrocytes, are approximately 8 to 10 μm in diameter in blood smears. They are round cells with a relatively large, heterochromatic nucleus that occupies most of the cell's volume (see Fig. 6-1 and Table 6-1). There are three types of lymphocytes: T lymphocytes (T cells), B lymphocytes (B cells), and null cells, and they are morphologically indistinguishable from each other. It is customary to speak of **T cells** as being responsible for **cell-mediated immune response** and **B cells** as functioning in **humorally mediated immune response**. T cells are also responsible for the formation of cytokines that facilitate the initiation of most humorally mediated immune responses. **Null cells** are few in number, possess no determinants on their cell membrane, and are of two types: **pluripotential hemopoietic stem cells** (PHSC; responsible for the formation of all of the formed elements of blood) and **natural killer cells** (NK cells).

- T-cell precursors are formed in the bone marrow and migrate to the **thymic cortex** to become immunocompetent cells. They recognize **epitopes** (antigenic determinants) that are displayed by cells possessing **major histocompatibility complex (MHC) molecules**, also known as **human leukocyte antigen (HLA)**. There are various subtypes of T cells, each possessing a **T-cell receptor (TCR)** surface determinant and a **cluster of differentiation determinants (CD molecules)**. The former recognizes the epitope, whereas the latter recognizes the type of MHC molecule on the displaying cell surface. The various subtypes of T cells

Blood Group	Genotype*	Surface Antigens	Can Accept Blood From
A	*I^A* and *I^A* or *I^A* and *i*	A antigen	Both A and O
B	*I^B* and *I^B* or *I^B* and *i*	B antigen	Both B and O
AB	*I^A* and *I^B*	Both A and B antigens	A, B, AB, and O (Universal acceptor)
O	*i* and *i*	O antigen	Only O (Universal donor)

Table 6-2 ABO Blood Groups

*Note that this is a simplified explanation of the possible genotypes.

In addition to the ABO antigens, the **D antigen (Rh factor)** is important to mention because it is present on the erythrocyte plasmalemma of almost 85% of the world population. Therefore, it is said that 85% of the world population is **Rh+ (Rh positive)** and 15% is **Rh− (Rh negative)**. This is not a problem in transfusions, but it is the cause of a possibly fatal condition of the newborn, known as erythroblastosis fetalis.

CLINICAL CONSIDERATIONS 6-3

Erythroblastosis Fetalis

Erythroblastosis fetalis is a very serious condition caused by **Rh factor (antigen D) incompatibility** between an Rh− pregnant woman and the Rh+ fetus that she is carrying. After the second trimester, there is a strong possibility of some fetal blood crossing the placental barrier, causing the mother to manufacture antibodies (see Chapter 10, Lymphoid (Immune) System for a discussion of the types of antibodies) against the fetal RBCs. Fortunately, in the first such pregnancy, immunoglobulin M (IgM) molecules are produced initially, which are unable to cross the placental barrier and, therefore, the fetus's RBCs are not attacked. However, after the formation of the IgM, the mother's immune system switches isotype, producing immunoglobulin G (IgG), and these antibodies can cross the placental barrier. By this time, the baby is usually delivered. However, in case of a subsequent pregnancy, in which the fetus is again Rh+, the mother already has IgG molecules against antigen D, and these antibodies cross the placental barrier. The IgG molecules attack the Rh factor on the fetal RBC surface, causing widespread hemolysis (erythroblastosis fetalis), possibly killing the fetus. In 1968, **anti-D globulin (RhoGAM)** was developed which, when given to the pregnant woman, binds with, thereby masking, antigen D so that the mother's immune system disregards it and does not mount an immune response. RhoGAM (or similar substances) are administered at various intervals during subsequent pregnancies to prevent the occurrence of erythroblastosis fetalis.

are described in Chapter 10, Lymphoid (Immune) System.

- **B cells** bear MHC type II (also known as HLA II) surface markers and **surface immunoglobulins (sIgs)** on their plasmalemma. They are formed in and become immunocompetent in the bone marrow. They are responsible for the humoral response and, under the direction of T$_H$2 cells and in response to an antigenic challenge, will differentiate into antibody-manufacturing **plasma cells** and **B memory cells** as described in Chapter 10.

- **NK cells** belong to the null cell population. They possess F$_C$ receptors but no cell surface determinants and are responsible for **nonspecific cytotoxicity** against virus-infected and tumor cells. They also function in **antibody-dependent cell-mediated cytotoxicity (ADCC)**, as described in Chapter 10.

Monocytes

Monocytes are large cells, approximately 12 to 15 μm in diameter in blood smears, that possess a single, large, acentric, kidney-shaped nucleus (see Fig. 6-2 and Table 6-2). When **monocytes** leave the bloodstream and enter the connective tissue spaces, they become known as **macrophages**, cells that phagocytose particulate matter, activate the immune response, present epitopes to T cells, and assist lymphocytes in their immunologic activities, as discussed in Chapter 10. Recall that macrophages may have organ-specific names; Kupffer cells in the liver, microglia in the central nervous system, Langerhans cells in the skin, dust cells in the lungs, and osteoclasts in bone (refer to Chapter 4, Connective Tissue).

Neutrophils

Neutrophils, the most abundant type of leukocytes, are 9 to 12 μm in diameter in smears, have multilobed

CLINICAL CONSIDERATIONS 6-4

Multiple Myeloma

Multiple myeloma is a relatively uncommon malignant neoplasm with greater incidence in males than females. Its origin is the bone marrow, and it is characterized by the presence of large numbers of malignant plasma cells that may also be abnormal in morphology. These cells accumulate in the bone marrow of various regions of the skeletal system. Frequently, cell proliferation is so great in the marrow that the huge number of cells places pressure on the walls of the marrow cavity causing bone pain and even fracture of bones such as the ribs. These cells also produce abnormal proteins such as Bence-Jones proteins that enter the urine, where they can be detected to provide a diagnosis for multiple myeloma.

CLINICAL CONSIDERATIONS 6-5

Infectious Mononucleosis

Infection with the Epstein-Barr virus causes **infectious mononucleosis**, also referred to as the "kissing disease," because it is common among adolescents and is frequently spread by saliva. Patients suffering from infectious mononucleosis present with symptoms such as sore throat, swollen and painful lymph nodes, low energy, and an elevated lymphocyte count (lymphocytosis). The disease can be life-threatening in immunosuppressed individuals.

nuclei, generate ATP via an anaerobic pathway, and possess three types of granules—specific, azurophilic, and tertiary. These granules possess very limited affinity to stains. Neutrophils are usually the first responders to bacterial infection or tissue damage and function in **phagocytosis** of bacteria. They are frequently referred to as microphages.

- **Specific granules** (0.1 μm in diameter) contain pharmacologic agents and enzymes that permit the neutrophils to perform their antimicrobial roles.
- **Azurophilic granules** (0.5 μm in diameter) are lysosomes, containing the various lysosomal hydrolases, as well as myeloperoxidase, bacterial permeability–increasing protein, lysozyme, and collagenase.
- **Tertiary granules** house glycoproteins dedicated for insertion into the cell membrane as well as gelatinase and cathepsins.

Neutrophils use the contents of the three types of granules to perform their antimicrobial function. When neutrophils arrive at their site of action, they exocytose the contents of their granules.

- **Gelatinase** increases the neutrophil's ability to migrate through the endothelial basal lamina, and the glycoproteins of the tertiary granules aid in the recognition and phagocytosis of bacteria into phagosomes of the neutrophil.
- Azurophilic granules and specific granules fuse with and release their hydrolytic enzymes into the phagosomes, thus initiating the enzymatic degradation of the microorganisms.

In addition to enzymatic degradation, microorganisms are destroyed by the capability of neutrophils to undergo a sudden increase in O_2 utilization, known as a **respiratory burst**, whereby O_2 is converted by the enzyme NADPH oxidase into **superoxides** (O_2^-).

- The superoxide is converted into hydrogen peroxide by superoxide dismutase, and the enzyme myeloperoxidase combines chloride ions and hydrogen peroxide into hypochlorous acid.
- All three of these highly reactive compounds also destroy bacteria within the phagosomes.
- Frequently, the avid response of neutrophils results in the release of some of these highly potent compounds into the surrounding connective tissue, precipitating tissue damage.
- Neutrophils also produce leukotrienes from plasmalemma arachidonic acids to aid in the initiation of an inflammatory response.
- After performing these functions, the neutrophils die and become a major component of pus.

Eosinophils

Eosinophils, big cells ~10 to 14 μm in diameter in smears, possess a large, bilobed nucleus (Fig. 6-3). Their specific granules, which occupy a large percentage of their cytoplasm, stain a reddish-orange color. Eosinophils participate in antiparasitic activities and phagocytose antigen–antibody complexes.

Basophils

Basophils, comprising 1% or less of the leukocytes, are approximately the same size as lymphocytes, 8 to 10 μm

CLINICAL CONSIDERATIONS 6-6

NADPH Oxidase Deficiency

Certain individuals suffer from persistent bacterial infection caused by a hereditary **NADPH oxidase deficiency**. The neutrophils of these individuals are unable to effect a respiratory burst and, therefore, are incapable of forming highly reactive compounds, such as hypochlorous acid, hydrogen peroxide, and superoxide that assist in the killing of bacteria within their phagosomes.

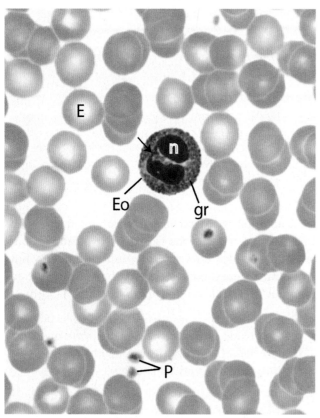

FIGURE 6-3. Eosinophil (Eo) with its bilobed nucleus (N) displaying the connection (*arrow*) between the lobes, and its numerous, large granules (gr), erythrocytes (E), and platelets (P). ×1,325.

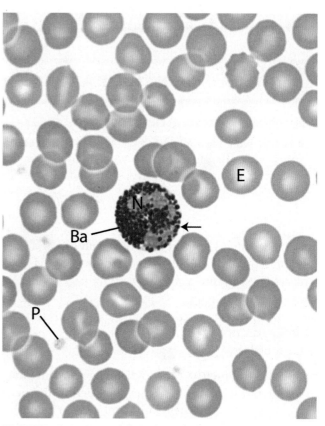

FIGURE 6-4. Basophil (Ba) with its large nucleus (N), and numerous large, dark granules (*arrow*). Also observe the platelets (P) and the numerous erythrocytes (E). ×540.

in diameter in smears. They possess abundant specific granules and stain dark blue (Fig. 6-4). Although the precise function of basophils is unknown, the contents of their granules are like those of mast cells, and they also release the same pharmacologic agents via degranulation. Additionally, basophils, just as mast cells, produce and release other pharmacologic agents derived from the arachidonic acid in their membranes.

Platelets

Circulating blood also contains cell fragments known as **platelets (thrombocytes)**. These small, oval-to-round structures, 2 to 4 μm in diameter, are derived from **megakaryocytes** of the bone marrow and function in hemostasis, the clotting mechanism of blood. Each platelet membrane is coated by a **glycocalyx**, containing glycoproteins, glycosaminoglycans, and several

CLINICAL CONSIDERATIONS 6-7

Eosinophilia

Eosinophilia is a disorder in which the number of eosinophils in a blood smear is >7% of the leukocytes. As long as it is <30% of circulating WBCs, the condition is not treated as a malignancy, a very rare condition. Usually, eosinophilia is caused either by parasitic (or fungal) infections or by an allergic reaction.

coagulation factors, that, when exposed to ATP and Ca^{+2} ions, enhances the adherence of platelets to one another. Platelets have two regions, as determined by light microscopy, an outer clear region, the **hyalomere**, containing cytoskeletal components, and a darker central region, the **granulomere**, containing lysosomes and vesicles with coagulation factors and enzymes involved in coagulation.

Coagulation

Coagulation is the result of the exquisitely controlled interaction of several plasma proteins and coagulation factors. The regulatory mechanisms are in place so that coagulation typically occurs only if the endothelial lining of the vessel becomes injured.

- In the intact blood vessel, the endothelium manufactures inhibitors of platelet aggregation (nitrous oxide and prostacyclins) as well as display agents, thrombomodulin, and heparin-like molecule on their luminal plasmalemmae that block coagulation.

- However, if the wall of the blood vessel and the endothelium or the endothelium only is damaged, the endothelial cells switch from producing and displaying anti-aggregation and anticoagulation agents and release **tissue factor** (tissue thromboplastin is released also by the connective tissue cells that are exposed to blood), **von Willebrand factor**, and **endothelins**, which initiate a cascade of clotting pathways that ultimately lead to the conversion of fibrinogen to fibrin, the insoluble fibrous mesh.

Plasma and Serum

Plasma, the fluid component of blood, comprises ~55% of the total blood volume. Plasma contains electrolytes and ions, such as calcium, sodium, potassium, and bicarbonate; larger molecules, namely, albumins, globulins, complement proteins, and clotting factors; as well as organic compounds as varied as amino acids, lipids, vitamins, hormones, and cofactors.

- **Albumins** are small proteins, ~60,000 molecular weight, whose major function is to maintain the proper **colloid osmotic pressure** within the circulatory system, thereby conserving normal blood volume by preventing the movement of plasma into the extracellular space.

- **Globulins** are of three major types: γ-globulins, α-globulins, and β-globulins. γ-Globulins are antibodies, whereas α- and β-globulins function in ferrying metal ions and lipids in the bloodstream.

- **Complement proteins** belong to the innate immune system (see Chapter 10).

- **Clotting factors**, such as fibrinogen and prothrombin, are activated during the process of coagulation.

After clotting, a straw-colored **serum** is expressed from blood. This fluid is identical to plasma but contains neither fibrinogen nor other components necessary for the clotting reaction.

Hemopoiesis

Circulating blood cells have relatively short life spans and must be replaced continuously by newly formed cells. This process of blood cell replacement is known as **hemopoiesis** (hematopoiesis). The location of hemopoiesis begins in the yolk sac of the embryo and then progresses to the liver and spleen; by the 6th month of gestation, it occurs mostly in the bone marrow. By the time of birth, bone marrow is the exclusive location because hemopoiesis ceases in the liver and spleen. Postnatally, the bone marrow remains the sole location for hemopoiesis, although, in case of an emergency, both the liver and the spleen can resume blood cell formation. There are two types of bone marrow, **red bone marrow** (Fig. 6-5), which actively manufactures blood cells and **white** (or **yellow**) **bone marrow**, housing an abundance of lipid, that no longer is active in hemopoiesis (although, if the need arises, it can convert to red marrow). Most adult hemopoietic stem cells are located in the **red bone marrow** of short and flat bones. The marrow of long bones is red in young individuals, but when it becomes infiltrated by fat in the adult, it takes on a yellow to white appearance and is known as yellow or white marrow.

Although it was once believed that adipose cells accumulated the fat, it is now known that the cells responsible for storing fat in the marrow are the **adventitial reticular cells**. These cells also form long processes that contact processes of other adventitial reticular cells, thus partitioning the bone marrow volume into smaller spaces, thereby isolating the bone marrow cell population into small **islands of hemopoietic cells**.

- All blood cells develop from a single pluripotential precursor cell known as the **pluripotential hemopoietic stem cell (PHSC)**. These cells are able to replicate themselves and give rise to all **blood cell lineages**.

- PHSCs undergo mitotic activity, whereby they give rise to two types of **multipotential hemopoietic stem cells: colony-forming unit-granulocyte, erythrocyte, monocyte, megakaryocyte (CFU-GEMM)**, previously known as CFU-S, and colony-forming unit-lymphocyte (**CFU-Ly**). These cells cannot be differentiated by Wright or Giemsa's stains as giving rise to a particular type of blood cell.

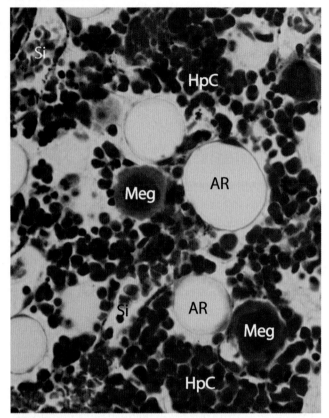

FIGURE 6-5. Red marrow displaying megakaryocytes (Meg), adventitial reticular cells (AR), and various hemopoietic cells (HpC) as well as blood vessels and sinusoids (Si). ×540.

- CFU-GEMM and CFU-Ly give rise to **progenitor cells** dedicated to give rise to a single cell lineage. These cells cannot be recognized by Wright or Giemsa's stains as giving rise to a particular type of blood cell.

- Progenitor cells give rise to **precursor cells** that can be recognized by light microscopy to give rise to a particular type of blood cell (e.g., erythrocytes, eosinophils, or lymphocytes). Precursor cells are committed, in that they are unable to differentiate into a different line of precursor cells.

- Stem cells, in response to various hemopoietic growth factors, undergo cell division and maintain the population of circulating erythrocytes, leukocytes, and platelets.

Erythrocytic Series

Erythrocyte development proceeds from CFU-GEMM, which, in response to elevated levels of erythropoietin, gives rise to cells known as burst-forming unit-erythroid (BFU-E), which, in response to lower erythropoietin levels, then give rise to colony-forming unit-erythroid (CFU-E). Later generations derived from CFU-E are recognizable histologically as proerythroblasts.

These cells give rise to **basophilic erythroblasts** (whose basophilic staining is attributed to the abundant rER), which, in turn, undergo cell division to form:

- **Polychromatophilic erythroblasts**, whose mixture of basophilic and eosinophilic staining is attributed to abundant rough endoplasmic reticulum (rER) and accumulating hemoglobins. These cells will divide mitotically to form:

- **Orthochromatophilic erythroblasts (normoblasts)** that are characterized by a smaller size, eosinophilic cytoplasm, and a condensed nucleus. Cells of this stage no longer divide.

- Orthochromatophilic erythroblasts will extrude their nuclei and most organelles and differentiate into **reticulocytes** (immature RBCs not to be confused with reticular cells of connective tissue), which, in turn, become mature RBCs.

- Reticulocytes are stained with methylene blue for manual or thiazole orange for automated counting. On average, reticulocytes comprise ~1% to 2% of circulating RBCs, which equals the amount of old or deformed RBCs that are in the process of being destroyed. An increased percentage of reticulocytes (reticulocytosis) may indicate a variety of conditions, such as anemia, increased oxygen demand in high altitude, or other situations that require the body to produce more RBCs.

Granulocytic Series

The development of the granulocytic series is initiated from the multipotential **CFU-GEMM**.

The first histologically distinguishable member of this series is the **myeloblast**, which gives rise mitotically to:

- **Promyelocytes**, which also undergo cell division to yield myelocytes.

- **Myelocytes** are the first cells of this series to possess specific granules; therefore, neutrophilic, eosinophilic, and basophilic myelocytes may be recognized.

- **Metamyelocytes** are next in the series and no longer divide, but differentiate into band cells.

- **Band (stab) cells**, the juvenile form, will become mature granulocytes that enter the bloodstream.

Lymphoid Series

The development of the lymphoid series is initiated from the multipotential **CFU-Ly**, the lymphoid stem cell, a progenitor cell. CFU-Ly gives rise to three precursor cells: CFU-LyB (B cells), CFU-LyT (T cells), and CFU-NK (NK cells).

Hemopoietic Growth Factors

Several **hemopoietic growth factors** activate and promote hemopoiesis. These act by binding to plasma membrane receptors of their target cell, controlling their mitotic rate, as well as the number of mitotic events. Additionally, they stimulate cell differentiation and enhance the survival of the progenitor cell population (Table 6-3). If the stem cell factor and even some other factors fail to contact PHSCs, the stem cells undergo apoptosis. The best-known factors are as follows:

- **Stem cell factor**: stimulates proliferation of pluripotential and multipotential stem cells;

- **Erythropoietin**: acts on BFU-E and CFU-E;

- **Interleukin-1**: (along with IL-3 and IL-6) acts on PHSC, CFU-GEMM, and CFU-Ly and suppresses erythroid precursors;

- **Interleukin-7**: acts on CFU-LyB, CFU-LyT, promotes NK cell differentiation;

- **Granulocyte colony-stimulating factor**: acts on granulocyte progenitor cells;

- **Macrophage colony-stimulating factor**: acts on monocyte progenitor cells; and

- **Granulocyte-macrophage colony-stimulating factor**: activates CFU-GM proliferation.

CLINICAL CONSIDERATIONS 6-8

B-Cell Prolymphocytic Leukemia

B-cell prolymphocytic leukemia is a relatively rare form of leukemia that arises relatively late in life, around 60 years of age, and affects males more frequently than females. The histopathologic picture presents bone marrow smears and blood smears with medium to large prolymphocytes. Usually, the disease is accompanied by an enlargement of the spleen. The prognosis is not good because this type of leukemia is quite aggressive and treatment modalities are not very effective; in fact, they are mostly palliative and usually the patient succumbs in 2 to 3 years.

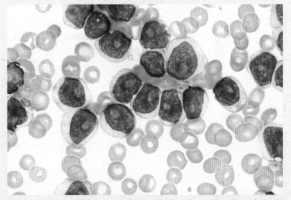

This blood smear, from a patient suffering from B-cell prolymphocytic leukemia, displays numerous large prolymphocytes whose nucleus presents a coarse chromatin network and large vesicles. (Reprinted with permission from Mills SE, et al., eds. *Sternberg's Diagnostic Surgical Pathology*, 5th ed. Philadelphia: Wolters Kluwer Health//Lippincott Williams & Wilkins, 2010. p. 644.)

Table 6-3	Hemopoietic Growth Factors	
Factors	**Principal Action**	**Site of Origin**
Stem cell factor (steel factor, c-kit ligand)	Stimulates proliferation of pluripotential and multipotential stem cells and the formation of mast cells	Stromal cells of bone marrow
GM-CSF	Promotes CFU-GM mitosis and differentiation; facilitates granulocyte activity	T cells; endothelial cells
G-CSF	Promotes CFU-G mitosis and differentiation; facilitates neutrophil activity	Macrophages; endothelial cells
M-CSF	Promotes CFU-M mitosis and differentiation	Macrophages; endothelial cells
IL-1	In conjunction with IL-3 and IL-6, it promotes proliferation of PHSC, CFU-GEMM, and CFU-Ly; suppresses erythroid precursors	Monocytes; macrophages and endothelial cells
IL-2	Stimulates activated T- and B-cell mitosis; induces differentiation of NK cells	Activated T cells

(continued)

Table 6-3	Hemopoietic Growth Factors (continued)	
Factors	**Principal Action**	**Site of Origin**
IL-3	In conjunction with IL-1 and IL-6, it promotes proliferation of PHSC, CFU-GEMM, and CFU-Ly as well as all unipotential precursors (except for LyB and LyT); also promotes the formation of BFU-E	Activated T and B cells
IL-4	Stimulates T- and B-cell activation and development of mast cells and basophils; also promotes the formation of BFU-E	Activated T cells
IL-5	Promotes CFU-Eo mitosis and activates eosinophils	T cells
IL-6	In conjunction with IL-1 and IL-3, it promotes proliferation of PHSC, CFU-GEMM, and CFU-Ly; also facilitates CTL and B-cell differentiation	Monocytes and fibroblasts
IL-7	Promotes differentiation of CFU-LyB and CFU-LyT, and enhances differentiation of NK cells	Stromal cells
IL-8	Induces neutrophil migration and degranulation	Leukocytes, endothelial cells, and smooth muscle cells
IL-9	Induces mast cell activation and proliferation; modulates IgE production; promotes T helper cell proliferation	T helper cells
IL-10	Inhibits cytokine production by macrophages, T cells, and NK cells; facilitates CTL differentiation and proliferation of B cells and mast cells	Macrophages and T cells
IL-12	Stimulates NK cells; enhances CTL and NK cell function	Macrophages
IL-15	Stimulates NK cell maturation	Macrophages
γ-Interferons	Activate B cells and monocytes; enhance CTL differentiation; augment the expression of class II HLA	T cells and NK cells
Erythropoietin	CFU-E differentiation; BFU-E mitosis	Endothelial cells of the peritubular capillary network of the kidney; hepatocytes
Thrombopoietin	Proliferation and differentiation of CFU-meg and megakaryoblasts	Hepatocytes and liver sinusoidal lining cells; kidney proximal tubule cells and stromal cells of bone marrow
GATA3 transcription factor	Differentiation of B and T lymphocytes	Expressed in the relevant cells
Ikaros family of transmission factors	Differentiation of B and T lymphocytes	Expressed in the relevant cells
Pax5 transcription factor	B lymphocyte maturation	Expressed in the relevant cells
PU.1 transcription factor	Development of granulocytes, macrophages, and B lymphocytes	Expressed in the relevant cells

BFU-E, burst-forming unit-erythrocyte; CFU-E, colony-forming unit-erythrocyte; CFU, colony-forming unit (Eo, eosinophil; G, granulocyte; GEMM, granulocyte, erythrocyte, monocyte, megakaryocyte; GM, granulocyte-monocyte; Ly, lymphocyte); CSF, colony-stimulating factor (G, granulocyte; GM, granulocyte-monocyte; M, monocyte); CTL, cytotoxic T cell; HLA, human leukocyte antigen; IL, interleukin; NK, natural killer; PHSC, pluripotential hemopoietic stem cell.

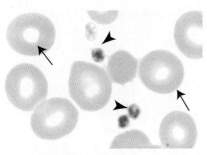

FIGURE 6-1-1. Red blood cells. Human. ×1,325.

Red blood cells (*arrows*) display a central clear region that represents the thinnest area of the biconcave disk. Note that the platelets (*arrowheads*) possess a central dense region, the granulomere, and a peripheral light region, the hyalomere.

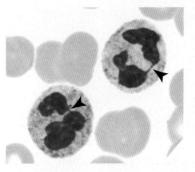

FIGURE 6-1-2. Neutrophils. Human. ×1,325.

Neutrophils display a somewhat granular cytoplasm and lobulated (*arrowheads*) nuclei.

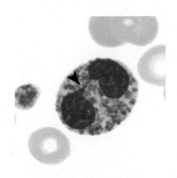

FIGURE 6-1-3. Eosinophils. Human. ×1,325.

Eosinophils are recognized by their large, pink granules and their sausage-link-shaped nucleus. Observe the slender connecting link (*arrowhead*) between the two lobes of the nucleus.

PLATE 6-1A   Circulating Blood

PLATE 6-1B Circulating Blood

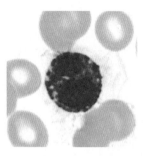

FIGURE 6-1-4. Basophils. Human. ×1,325.

Basophils are characterized by their dense, dark, large granules.

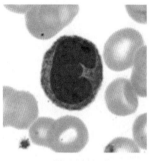

FIGURE 6-1-5. Monocytes. Human. ×1,325.

Monocytes are characterized by their large size, acentric, kidney-shaped nucleus, and lack of specific granules.

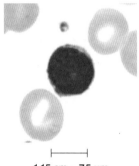

1.15 cm = 7.5 µm

FIGURE 6-1-6. Lymphocytes. Human. ×1,325.

Lymphocytes are small cells that possess a single, large, acentrically located nucleus and a narrow rim of light blue cytoplasm.

PLATE 6-2 Circulating Blood (Drawing)

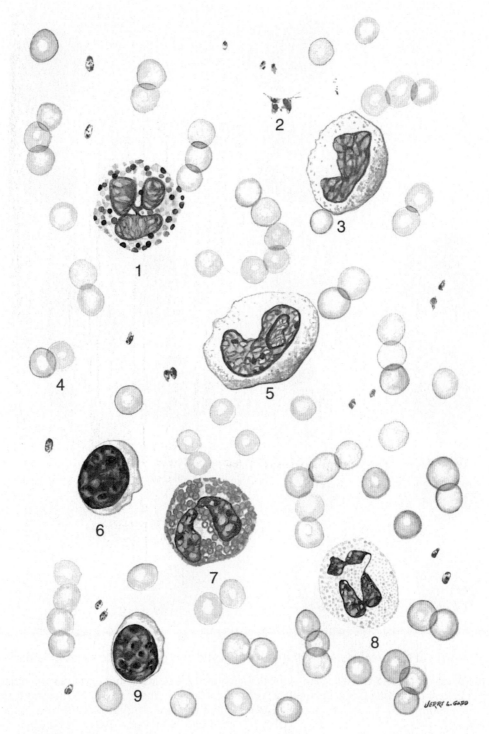

FIGURE 6-2-1. A drawing of the formed elements of circulating blood (not drawn to scale).

KEY					
1.	Basophil	4.	Erythrocytes	7.	Eosinophil
2.	Platelets	5.	Monocyte	8.	Neutrophil
3.	Monocyte	6.	Lymphocyte	9.	Lymphocyte

PLATE 6-3   Blood and Hemopoiesis

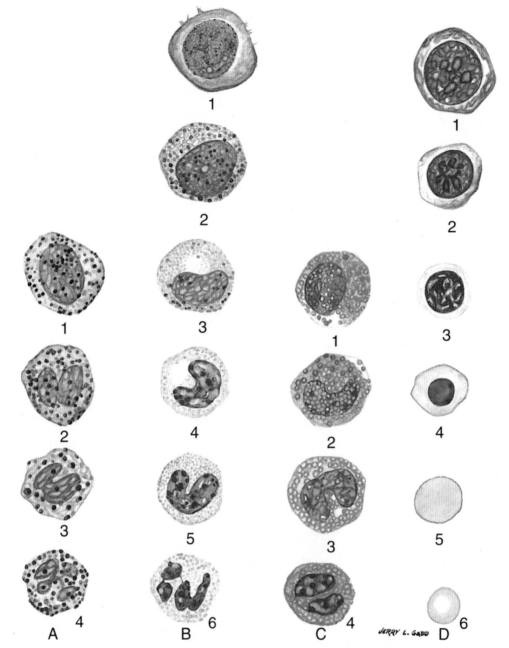

FIGURE 6-3-1. Drawing of the precursor cells of the granulocytic and erythrocytic series of hemopoiesis.

Note: that using the Wright or Giemsa's modification of the Romanovsky-type stains cannot distinguish whether the myeloblast or the promyelocyte belong to the basophilic, neutrophilic, or eosinophilic line. Therefore, in this drawing these two cell types are added only to the neutrophilic cell line with the understanding that they are identical with the ones in the basophilic and eosinophilic cell lines.

KEY					
A		**4.**	Neutrophilic metamyelocyte	**D**	
1.	Basophilic myelocyte	**5.**	Neutrophilic stab cell	**1.**	Proerythroblast
2.	Basophilic metamyelocyte	**6.**	Neutrophil	**2.**	Basophilic erythroblast
3.	Basophil stab cell	**C**		**3.**	Polychromatophilic erythroblast
4.	Basophil	**1.**	Eosinophilic myelocyte	**4.**	Orthochromatophilic erythroblast
B		**2.**	Eosinophilic metamyelocyte	**5.**	Reticulocyte
1.	Myeloblast			**6.**	Erythrocyte
2.	Promyelocyte	**3.**	Eosinophil stab cell		
3.	Neutrophilic myelocyte	**4.**	Eosinophil		

PLATE 6-4A Bone Marrow

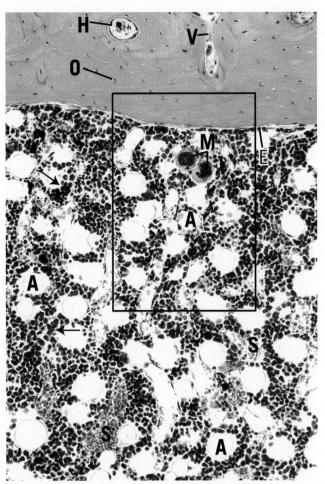

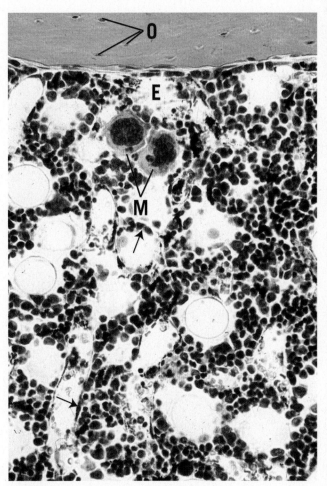

FIGURE 6-4-1. Bone marrow. Human. Paraffin section. ×132.

This transverse section of a decalcified human rib displays the presence of **haversian canals** (H), **Volkmann's canals** (V), **osteocytes** (O) in their lacunae, and the **endosteum** (E). The marrow presents numerous **adventitial reticular cells** (A), blood vessels, and **sinusoids** (S). Moreover, the forming blood elements are also evident as small nuclei (*arrows*). Note the large **megakaryocytes** (M), cells that are the precursors of platelets. The *boxed area* is represented in Figure 6-4-2.

FIGURE 6-4-2. Bone marrow. Human. Paraffin section. ×270.

This photomicrograph is a higher magnification of the *boxed area* of Figure 6-4-1. Observe the presence of **osteocytes** (O) in their lacunae as well as the flattened cells of the **endosteum** (E). The endothelial lining of the sinusoids (*arrows*) is evident, as are the numerous cells that are in the process of hemopoiesis. Two large **megakaryocytes** (M) are also discernible.

KEY					
A	adventitial reticular cell	**E**	endosteum	**H**	haversian canal
M	megakaryocyte	**O**	osteocyte	**V**	Volkmann's canal
S	sinusoid				

PLATE 6-4B Blood Smear and Bone Marrow Smear

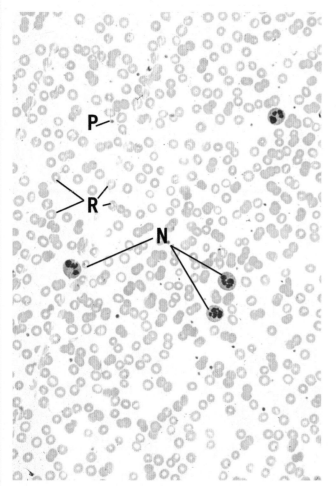

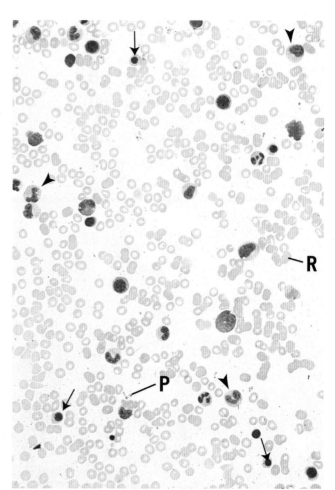

FIGURE 6-4-3. Blood smear. Human. Wright stain. ×270.

This normal blood smear presents **erythrocytes** (R), **neutrophils** (N), and **platelets** (P). The apparent holes in the centers of the erythrocytes represent the thinnest areas of the biconcave disks. Note that the erythrocytes far outnumber the platelets, and they in turn are much more numerous than the white blood cells. Because neutrophils constitute the highest percentage of white blood cells, they are the ones most frequently encountered in the white blood cell population.

FIGURE 6-4-4. Bone marrow smear. Human. Wright stain. ×270.

This normal bone marrow smear presents forming blood cells as well as **erythrocytes** (R) and **platelets** (P). In comparison with a normal peripheral blood smear (Figure 6-4-3), marrow possesses many more nucleated cells. Some of these are of the erythrocytic series (*arrows*), whereas others are of the granulocytic series (*arrowheads*).

KEY					
N	neutrophil	**P**	platelet	**R**	erythrocyte

PLATE 6-5   Erythropoiesis

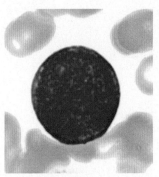

FIGURE 6-5-1. Human marrow smear. ×1,325.

Proerythroblast.

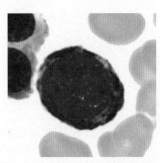

FIGURE 6-5-2. Human marrow smear. ×1,325.

Basophilic erythroblast.

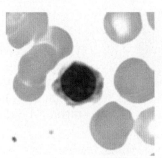

FIGURE 6-5-3. Human marrow smear. ×1,325.

Polychromatophilic erythroblast.

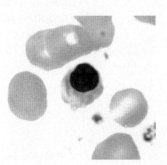

FIGURE 6-5-4. Human marrow smear. ×1,325.

Orthochromatophilic erythroblast.

FIGURE 6-5-5. Human marrow smear. Methylene blue stain. ×1,325.

Reticulocyte.

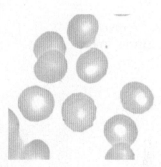

FIGURE 6-5-6. Human marrow smear. ×1,325.

Erythrocyte.

1.15 cm = 7.5 µm

PLATE 6-6   Granulocytopoiesis

FIGURE 6-6-1. Myeloblast. Human bone marrow smear. ×1,325.

FIGURE 6-6-2. Promyelocyte. Human bone marrow smear. ×1,325.

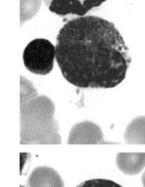

FIGURE 6-6-3A. Eosinophilic myelocyte. Human bone marrow smear. ×1,325.

FIGURE 6-6-3B. Neutrophilic myelocyte. Human bone marrow smear. ×1,325.

FIGURE 6-6-4A. Eosinophilic metamyelocyte. Human bone marrow smear. ×1,325.

FIGURE 6-6-4B. Neutrophilic metamyelocyte. Human bone marrow smear. ×1,325.

FIGURE 6-6-5A. Eosinophilic stab cell. Human bone marrow smear. ×1,325.

FIGURE 6-6-5B. Neutrophilic stab cell. Human bone marrow smear. ×1,325.

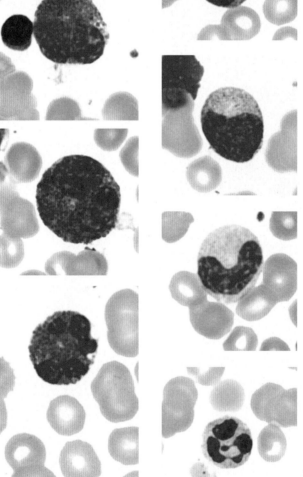

FIGURE 6-6-6. Neutrophil. Human bone marrow smear. ×1,325.

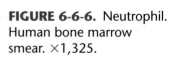

1.15 cm = 7.5 μm

Selected Review of Histologic Images

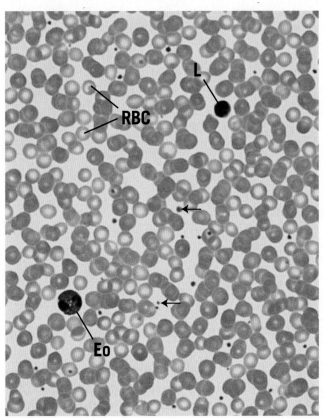

REVIEW FIGURE 6-1-1. Blood smear. Human. Wright's stain. ×540.

This blood smear from a healthy individual demonstrates the presence of numerous **red blood cells** (RBC) and **platelets** (*arrows*) as well as the less abundant **lymphocytes** (L) and even fewer **eosinophils** (Eo) present in circulating blood.

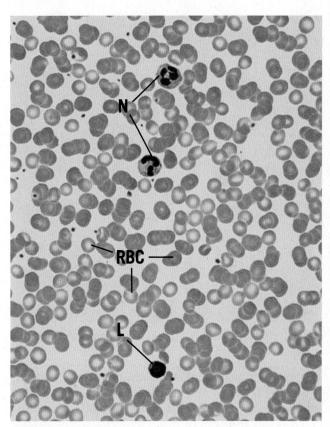

REVIEW FIGURE 6-1-2. Blood smear. Human. Wright's stain. ×540.

This blood smear from a healthy individual demonstrates the copious **erythrocytes** (RBC), plentiful platelets (not labeled), **neutrophils** (N), and **lymphocytes** (L).

KEY					
Eo	eosinophil	**N**	neutrophil	**RBC**	red blood cell
L	lymphocyte				(erythrocyte)

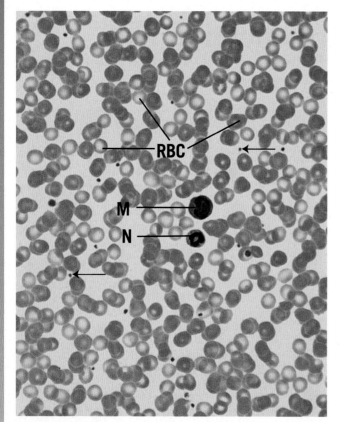

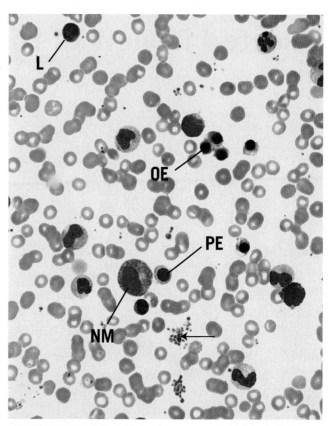

REVIEW FIGURE 6-1-3. Blood smear. Human. Wright's stain. ×540.

This blood smear from a healthy individual demonstrates the presence of **red blood cells** (RBC), **platelets** (*arrows*), as well as a **neutrophil** (N) and the much larger **monocyte** (M). Observe that the monocyte resembles a lymphocyte but is much larger and has an indented nucleus.

REVIEW FIGURE 6-1-4. Bone marrow smear. Human. Wright's stain. ×540.

This bone smear from a healthy individual demonstrates the presence of an abundance of erythrocytes (not labeled) as well as clusters of **platelets** (*arrow*). Note that the obvious difference between the bone marrow smear and the circulating blood smear is that bone marrow displays many more nucleated leukocytes in various stages of development. A **lymphocyte** (L), **neutrophilic myelocyte** (NM), **polychromatophilic erythroblast** (PE), and **orthochromatophilic erythroblast** (OE) are shown.

KEY					
L	lymphocyte	**OE**	orthochromatophilic erythroblast	**RBC**	red blood cell (erythrocyte)
M	monocyte				
N	neutrophil	**PE**	polychromatophilic erythroblast		
NM	neutrophilic myelocyte				

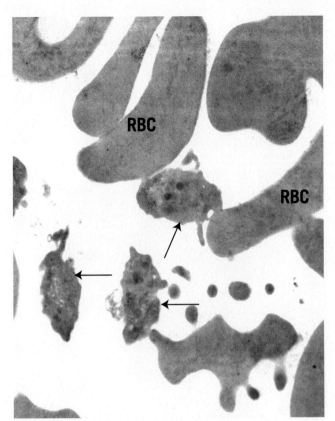

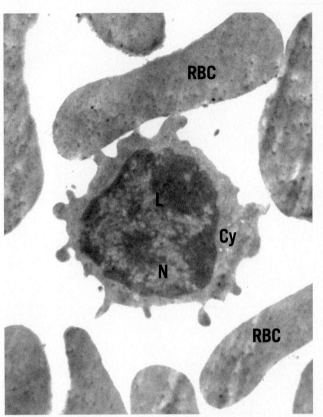

REVIEW FIGURE 6-2-1. Erythrocytes and platelets. Electron microscopy. ×5,600.

This electron micrograph of circulating blood displays both **erythrocytes** (RBC) and **platelets** (*arrows*). Note that the RBCs are mostly homogeneous in appearance, whereas the platelets possess various vesicles. (Courtesy of Dr. Zulmarie Franco.)

REVIEW FIGURE 6-2-2. Lymphocyte and erythrocytes. Electron microscopy. ×5,600.

This electron micrograph of circulating blood displays both **erythrocytes** (RBC) and a **lymphocyte** (L). Observe that the lymphocyte is approximately the same size in diameter as the RBCs and that the **nucleus** (N) occupies most of the cell, leaving a rim of **cytoplasm** (Cy). (Courtesy of Dr. Zulmarie Franco.)

KEY					
Cy	cytoplasm	**N**	nucleus	**RBC**	red blood cell
L	lymphocyte				(erythrocyte)

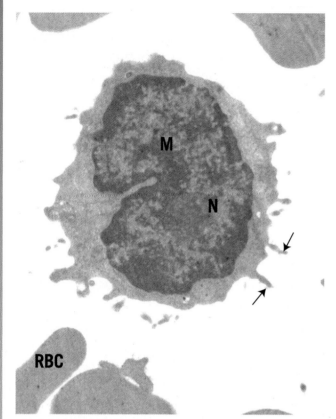

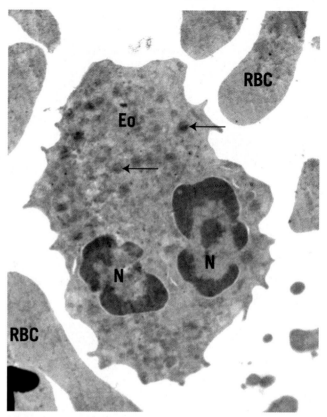

REVIEW FIGURE 6-2-3. Monocyte and erythrocytes. Electron microscopy. ×4,600.

This electron micrograph of circulating blood displays both **erythrocytes** (RBC) and a **monocyte** (M). Observe that the diameter of the monocyte is much greater than that of erythrocytes. Note that the **nucleus** (N) has an indentation and that the cytoplasm has **filopodia** (*arrows*) along its rim. (Courtesy of Dr. Zulmarie Franco.)

REVIEW FIGURE 6-2-4. Eosinophil and erythrocytes. Electron microscopy. ×5,600.

This electron micrograph of circulating blood displays both **erythrocytes** (RBC) and an **eosinophil** (Eo). Observe that the diameter of the eosinophil is much greater than that of erythrocytes. Note that the bilobed **nucleus** (N) appears as if it were two separate nuclei and that the cytoplasm has large **specific granules** (*arrows*) whose center is darker than the periphery. (Courtesy of Dr. Zulmarie Franco.)

KEY					
Eo	eosinophil	**N**	nucleus	**RBC**	red blood cell
M	monocyte				(erythrocyte)

Summary of Histologic Organization

I. CIRCULATING BLOOD*

A. Erythrocytes (RBC)

RBCs are pink, biconcave disks that are 7 to 8 μm in diameter. They are filled with hemoglobin and possess no nuclei.

B. Agranulocytes

1. Lymphocytes

Histologically, **lymphocytes** may be **small**, **medium**, or **large** (this bears no relationship to T cells, B cells, or null cells). Most lymphocytes are small (8 to 10 μm in diameter) and possess a dense, blue, acentrically positioned nucleus that occupies most of the cell, leaving a thin rim of light blue, peripheral cytoplasm. Azurophilic granules (lysosomes) may be evident in the cytoplasm.

2. Monocytes

Monocytes are the largest of all circulating blood cells (12 to 15 μm in diameter). There is a considerable amount of **grayish-blue cytoplasm** containing numerous azurophilic granules. The **nucleus** is acentric and kidney-shaped and possesses a coarse chromatin network with clear spaces. Lobes of the nucleus are superimposed on themselves, and their outlines appear to be distinctly demarcated.

C. Granulocytes

1. Neutrophils

Neutrophils are the most populous of the leukocytes, are 9 to 12 μm in diameter, and display a light pink cytoplasm housing many azurophilic and smaller specific granules. The specific granules do not stain well, hence the name of these cells. The nucleus is dark blue, coarse, and multilobed, with most being two- to three-lobed with thin connecting strands.

2. Eosinophils

Eosinophils are 10 to 14 μm in diameter and possess numerous refractive, spherical, large, reddish-orange specific granules. Azurophilic granules are also present. The nucleus, which is brownish-black, is bilobed, resembling sausage links united by a thin connecting strand.

3. Basophils

Basophils, the least numerous of all leukocytes, are 8 to 10 μm in diameter. Frequently, their cytoplasm is so filled with dark, large, basophilic specific granules that they appear to press against the cell membrane, giving it an angular appearance. The specific granules usually mask the azurophilic granules, as well as the S-shaped, light blue nucleus.

D. Platelets

Platelets, occasionally called **thrombocytes**, are small, round (2 to 4 μm in diameter) cell fragments. As such, they possess no nuclei, are frequently clumped together, and present with a dark blue, central granular region, the **granulomere**, and a light blue, peripheral, clear region, the **hyalomere**.

1. Hemopoiesis*

During the maturation process, hemopoietic cells undergo evident morphologic alterations. As the cells become more mature, they decrease in size. Their nuclei also become smaller, the chromatin network appears coarser, and their nucleoli (which resemble pale grayish spaces) disappear. The granulocytes first acquire azurophilic and then specific granules, and their nuclei become segmented. Cells of the erythrocytic series never display granules and eventually lose their nuclei.

E. Erythrocytic Series

1. Proerythroblast

a. Cytoplasm

Light blue to deep blue clumps in a pale grayish-blue background.

b. Nucleus

Round with a fine chromatin network; it is a rich burgundy red with 3 to 5 pale gray nucleoli.

2. Basophilic Erythroblast

a. Cytoplasm

Bluish clumps in a pale blue cytoplasm with a hint of grayish pink in the background.

b. Nucleus

Round, somewhat coarser than the previous stage; burgundy red. A nucleolus may be present.

---

* All colors designated in this summary are based on the Wright or Giemsa's modification of the Romanowsky-type stains as applied to blood smears.

3. Polychromatophilic Erythroblast

a. Cytoplasm

Yellowish pink with a bluish tinge.

b. Nucleus

Small and round with a condensed, coarse chromatin network; dark, reddish black. No nucleoli are present.

4. Orthochromatophilic Erythroblast

a. Cytoplasm

Pinkish with a slight tinge of blue.

b. Nucleus

Dark, condensed, round structure that may be in the process of being extruded from the cell.

5. Reticulocyte

a. Cytoplasm

Appears just like a normal, circulating RBC; if stained with supravital dyes (e.g., methylene blue), however, a bluish reticulum—composed mostly of rough endoplasmic reticulum—is evident.

b. Nucleus

Not present.

F. Granulocytic Series

The first two stages of the granulocytic series, the myeloblast and promyelocyte, possess no specific granules. These make their appearance in the myelocyte stage, when the three types of myelocytes (neutrophilic, eosinophilic, and basophilic) may be distinguished. Because they only differ from each other in their specific granules, only the neutrophilic series is described in this summary, with the understanding that myelocytes, metamyelocytes, and stab (band) cells occur in these three varieties.

1. Myeloblast

a. Cytoplasm

Small blue clumps in a light blue background. No granules. Cytoplasmic blebs extend along the periphery of the cell.

b. Nucleus

Reddish-blue, round nucleus with fine chromatin network. Two or three pale gray nucleoli are evident.

2. Promyelocyte

a. Cytoplasm

The cytoplasm is bluish and displays numerous, small, dark, azurophilic granules.

b. Nucleus

Reddish-blue, round nucleus whose chromatin strands appear coarser than in the previous stage. A nucleolus is usually present.

3. Neutrophilic Myelocyte

a. Cytoplasm

Pale blue cytoplasm containing dark azurophilic and smaller neutrophilic (specific) granules. A clear, paranuclear Golgi region is evident.

b. Nucleus

Round, usually somewhat flattened, acentric nucleus, with a somewhat coarse chromatin network. Nucleoli are not distinct.

4. Neutrophilic Metamyelocyte

a. Cytoplasm

Similar to the previous stage except that the cytoplasm is paler in color and the Golgi area is nestled in the indentation of the nucleus.

b. Nucleus

Kidney-shaped, acentric nucleus with a dense, dark chromatin network. Nucleoli are not present.

5. Neutrophilic Stab (Band) Cell

a. Cytoplasm

A little bluer than the cytoplasm of a mature neutrophil. Both azurophilic and neutrophilic (specific) granules are present.

b. Nucleus

The nucleus is horseshoe-shaped and dark blue, with a very coarse chromatin network. Nucleoli are not present.

Chapter Review Questions

6-1. Sickle cell anemia, characterized by altered shape of erythrocytes, is caused by mutations in which of the following molecules?

A. Spectrin

B. Hemoglobin

C. Actin

D. D antigen

E. Ankyrin

6-2. The multipotential hemopoietic stem cells arise from which of the following cells?

A. BFU-E

B. CFU-Ly

C. PHSC

D. CFU-GEMM

E. CFU-E

6-3. Interleukin-7, a hemopoietic growth factor, stimulates the formation of which of the following cells?

A. Neutrophils

B. Eosinophils

C. Basophil

D. Monocytes

E. Lymphocytes

6-4. Colloid osmotic pressure within the circulatory system is maintained by which of the following molecules?

A. α-Globulins

B. β-Globulins

C. γ-Globulins

D. Albumins

E. von Willebrand factor

6-5. A patient with parasitic invasion is likely to have an elevated count of which of the following leukocytes?

A. Lymphocytes

B. Neutrophils

C. Neutrophils

D. Eosinophils

E. Basophils

CHAPTER

7

MUSCLE

CHAPTER OUTLINE

REVIEW PLATE 7-2A

Review Figure 7-2-1   Smooth muscle. l.s. Human. Paraffin section. ×270

Review Figure 7-2-2   Smooth muscle. l.s. Human. Paraffin section. ×540

REVIEW PLATE 7-3A

Review Figure 7-3-1   Cardiac muscle. l.s. Human. Paraffin section. ×270

Review Figure 7-3-2   Cardiac muscle. l.s. Human. Paraffin section. ×540

REVIEW PLATE 7-2B

Review Figure 7-2-3   Smooth muscle. x.s. Human. Paraffin section. ×70

Review Figure 7-2-4   Smooth muscle. x.s. Human. Paraffin section. ×540

REVIEW PLATE 7-3B

Review Figure 7-3-3   Cardiac muscle. x.s. Human. Paraffin section. ×270

Review Figure 7-3-4   Cardiac muscle. x.s. Human. Paraffin section. ×540

Animals' ability to move is due to the presence of specific cells that have become highly differentiated, so that they function almost exclusively in contraction. The contractile process has been harnessed by the organism to permit various modes of movement and other activities for its survival. Some of these activities depend on quick contractions of short duration. Others depend on long-lasting contractions without the necessity for rapid actions. Still others depend on powerful, rhythmic contractions that must be repeated in rapid sequences.

These varied needs are accommodated by three types of muscles—namely, skeletal, smooth, and cardiac.

There are basic similarities among the three muscle types (Table 7-1). Almost all muscles are **mesodermally derived** and are elongated parallel to their axis of contraction; they possess numerous mitochondria to accommodate their high energy requirements, and all contain **contractile elements** known as **myofilaments**, in the form of **actin** and **myosin**, as well as additional contractile-associated proteins. Myofilaments of skeletal and cardiac muscles are arranged in a specific ordered array that gives rise to a repeated sequence of uniform banding along their length—hence their collective name, **striated muscle**.

Table 7-1 Comparison of Skeletal, Smooth, and Cardiac Muscle			
Characteristics	**Skeletal Muscle**	**Smooth Muscle**	**Cardiac Muscle**
Location	Generally attached to skeleton	Generally in hollow viscera, iris, blood vessels	Myocardium, major blood vessels as they enter or leave the heart
Shape	Long, cylindrical parallel fibers	Short, spindle shaped	Branched and blunt ended
Striations	Yes	No	Yes
Number and location of nucleus	Numerous, peripherally	Single, central	One or two, central
T tubules	Present at A–I junctions	No, but caveolae	Present at Z disks
Sarcoplasmic reticulum	Complex surrounds myofilaments forming meshwork; forms triads with T tubules	Some smooth sarcoplasmic reticulum but poorly developed	Less developed than in skeletal muscle; forms dyads with T tubules
Gap junctions	No	Yes	Yes, within intercalated disks
Control of contraction	Voluntary	Involuntary	Involuntary
Sarcomere	Yes	No	Yes
Regeneration	Restrictive	Extensive	Perhaps some but limited
Histologic distinction	Multiple striations and numerous peripherally located nuclei	No striations, central nucleus	Intercalated disks

Because muscle cells are much longer than they are wide, they are commonly referred to as **muscle fibers**. However, it must be appreciated that these fibers are living entities, unlike the nonliving fibers of connective tissue. Neither are they analogous to nerve fibers, which are living extensions of nerve cells. Often, the prefix "sarco-," referring to flesh, is used to specify structures of muscle cells; thus, the muscle cell membrane is **sarcolemma** (although earlier use of this term included the attendant basal lamina and reticular fibers), cytoplasm is **sarcoplasm**, mitochondria are **sarcosomes**, and endoplasmic reticulum is **sarcoplasmic reticulum**.

Skeletal Muscle

An entire skeletal muscle (Fig. 7-1), such as the biceps, is invested by dense irregular collagenous connective tissue known as the **epimysium**, which penetrates the substance of the gross muscle, separating it into groups of muscle cells, known as **fascicles**. Each fascicle is surrounded by **perimysium**, a looser, but still dense irregular collagenous connective tissue. Finally, each individual muscle fiber within a fascicle is enveloped by fine reticular fibers, the **endomysium**. The vascular and nerve supplies of the muscle travel in these interrelated connective tissue compartments.

There are three types of skeletal muscle fibers: **red (type I/slow-twitch)**, **white (type IIb/fast-twitch)**, and **intermediate (type IIa)** depending on their contraction velocities, mitochondrial and myoglobin content, and types of enzymes the cell contains (See Table 7-2).

Each gross muscle, such as the biceps, usually possesses all three types of muscle cells, but the proportion of the three types can vary from person to person. In general terms, however, muscles of the arms and legs tend to have a greater proportion of white muscle fibers, whereas postural muscles that maintain prolonged contraction tend to have a greater proportion of red muscle fibers. The innervation of a particular muscle cell determines whether it is red, white, or intermediate. Regardless of the type, each skeletal muscle fiber is roughly cylindrical in shape, possessing numerous elongated nuclei located at the periphery of the cell, just deep to the sarcolemma (Figs. 7-2 and 7-3).

Longitudinally sectioned muscle fibers display intracellular contractile elements, which are the parallel arrays of longitudinally disposed **myofibrils**. Each myofibril is essentially a chain of contractile units called the **sarcomeres**. Each sarcomere, in turn, is composed of two types of myofilaments: the thick, myosin fibers in the middle and the thin, actin fibers in the periphery. This arrangement of myofibrils produces an overall effect of **cross-banding** of alternating light and dark bands traversing each skeletal muscle cell (Fig. 7-2). The dark bands are **A bands**, and the light bands are **I bands**. Each I band is bisected by a thin dark **Z disk** (Z band), and the region of the myofibril extending from Z disk to Z disk, the **sarcomere**, is the contractile unit of the skeletal muscle cell. The A band is bisected by a paler **H zone**, the center of which is marked by the dark **M disk**.

Myofilaments

Banding is the result of interdigitation of thick and thin myofilaments. The I band consists solely of thin filaments, whereas the A band, with the exception of its H and M components, consists of both thick and thin

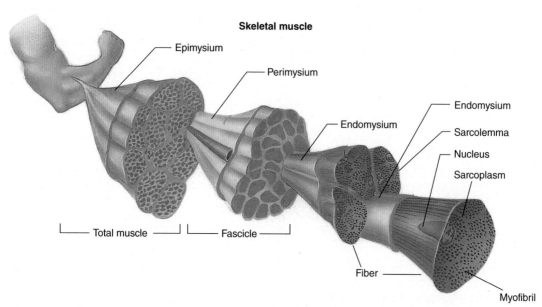

FIGURE 7-1. Diagram displaying the connective tissue components of skeletal muscle.

Table 7-2   Characteristics of Skeletal Muscle Fibers

Muscle Type	Myoglobin Content	Mitochondrial Population	Enzyme Content	ATP Generation	Contraction Characteristics	Relative Diameter of Muscle Fibers
Red (type I/ slow-twitch)	High	Abundant	High in oxidative enzymes, low ATPase	Oxidative phosphorylation	Slow and repetitive; not easily fatigued	Smallest
Intermediate (type IIa)	Intermediate	Intermediate	Intermediate-oxidative enzymes and ATPase	Oxidative phosphorylation and anaerobic glycolysis	Fast but not easily fatigued	Intermediate
White (type IIb/ fast-twitch)	Low	Sparse	Low oxidative enzymes; high ATPase and phosphorylases	Anaerobic glycolysis	Fast and easily fatigued	Largest

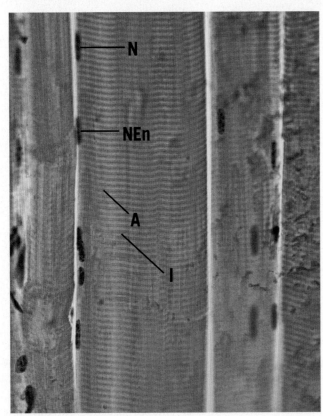

FIGURE 7-2. Note that the **nucleus** (N) of the skeletal muscle cell is clearly deep to the sarcolemma, whereas the **nucleus of the cells of the endomysium** (NEn) is clearly outside the sarcolemma. The **A bands** (A) and **I bands** (I) are clearly distinguishable from each other.

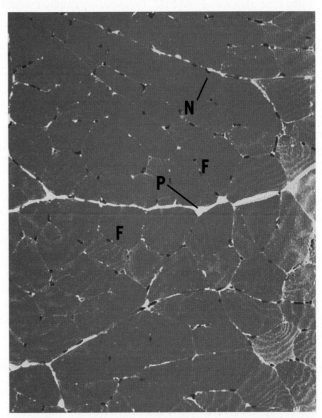

FIGURE 7-3. This transverse section of **skeletal muscle fibers** (F) demonstrates that the cells are cylindrical in shape, and their **nuclei** (N) are located peripherally just underneath the sarcolemma. In addition to the endomysium that envelops each muscle fiber, bundles of skeletal muscle fibers are surrounded by a thicker connective tissue element, known as the **perimysium** (P).

filaments. During contraction, the thick and thin filaments slide past each other (see below), and the Z disks are brought near the ends of the thick filaments (Figs. 7-4 and 7-5).

Thin Filaments

Thin filaments (7 nm in diameter and 1 μm in length) are composed of **F actin**, double-helical polymers of **G actin** molecules, resembling a pearl necklace twisted upon itself. Each groove of the helix houses linear **tropomyosin**

molecules (each 40 nm in length) positioned end to end. Associated with each tropomyosin molecule is a **troponin** molecule composed of three polypeptides: **troponin T (TnT)**, **troponin I (TnI)**, and **troponin C (TnC)**. TnI binds to actin, masking its active site (where it is able to interact with myosin II); TnT binds to tropomyosin; and TnC (a molecule similar to **calmodulin**) has a high affinity for calcium ions (Table 7-3).

CLINICAL CONSIDERATIONS 7-1

Duchenne Muscular Dystrophy

Duchenne muscular dystrophy is a muscle degenerative disease that is caused by an x-linked genetic defect that strikes 1 in 30,000 males. The defect results in the absence of dystrophin molecules in the muscle cell membrane. Dystrophin is a protein that functions in the interconnection of the cytoskeleton to transmembrane proteins that interact with the extracellular matrix as well as in providing structural support for the muscle plasmalemma. Individuals afflicted with Duchenne muscular dystrophy experience muscle weakness by the time they are seven years of age and are usually wheelchair-bound by the time they are 12 years old. These patients rarely survive into their early 20s.

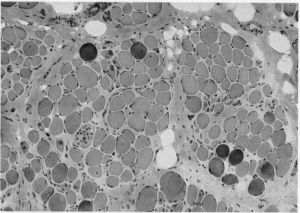

This photomicrograph of a biopsy from the vastus lateralis muscle of a patient suffering from Duchenne muscular dystrophy was stained by a modified Gomori trichrome stain. Note the numerous necrotic muscle cells and the presence of fibrosis evidenced by the thickened endomysium and perimysium. (Reprinted with permission from Strayer DS, et al., eds. *Rubin's Pathology: Mechanisms of Human Disease*, 8th ed. Philadelphia: Wolters Kluwer, 2020. Figure 31-9.)

Thick Filaments

Thick filaments (15 nm in diameter and 1.5 μm in length) are composed of 200 to 300 **myosin II molecules** arranged in an antiparallel fashion (Table 7-4). Each myosin molecule is composed of two pairs of light chains and two identical heavy chains. Each **myosin heavy chain** resembles a golf club, with a linear tail and a globular head, where the tails are wrapped around each other in a helical fashion. The enzyme **trypsin** cleaves each heavy chain into a linear (most of the tail) segment (**light meromyosin**) and a globular segment with the remainder of the tail (**heavy meromyosin**). Another enzyme, papain, cleaves heavy meromyosin into a short tail region (**S2 fragment**) and a pair of globular regions (S1 fragments). A pair of myosin light chains is associated with each S1 fragment. S1 fragments have **ATPase activity** but require the association with actin for this activity to be manifest.

Sliding Filament Model of Skeletal Muscle Contraction

Nerve impulses, transmitted at the myoneural junction across the synaptic cleft by acetylcholine (ACh), cause a wave of depolarization of the sarcolemma, with the eventual result of muscle contraction. This wave of depolarization is distributed throughout the depth of muscle fiber by transverse tubules (T tubules), tubular invaginations of the sarcolemma. The T tubules become closely associated with the terminal cisterns of the SR, so that each T tubule is flanked by two of these elements of the SR, forming a **triad. Voltage-sensitive** integral proteins, **dihydropyridine-sensitive receptors (DHSRs)**, located in the T tubule membrane are in contact with **calcium channels (ryanodine receptors)** in the terminal cisternae of the **sarcoplasmic reticulum (SR)**. This complex is visible with the electron microscope and is referred to as **junctional feet.**

During depolarization of the skeletal muscle sarcolemma, the DHSRs of the T tubule undergo voltage-induced conformational change, causing the calcium channels of the terminal cisternae to open, permitting the influx of Ca^{2+} ions into the sarcoplasm. **Troponin C** of the thin filament binds the calcium ions and by changing its conformation, presses the **tropomyosin** deeper into the grooves of the F actin filament, thus exposing the **active site** (myosin-binding site) on the actin molecule. **Adenosine triphosphate (ATP)**, bound to the globular head (**S1 fragment**) of the myosin II molecule, is hydrolyzed, but both **adenosine diphosphate (ADP)** and **inorganic phosphate (Pi)** remain attached on the S1. The myosin II molecule swivels so that the myosin head approximates the active site on the actin molecule. The Pi moiety is released, and in the presence of calcium, a link is formed between the actin and myosin. The bound ADP is freed, and the myosin head alters its

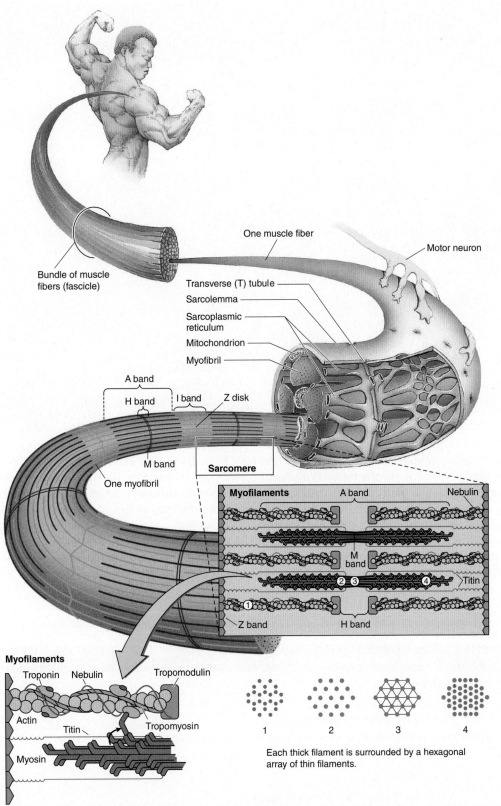

One muscle fiber

Motor neuron

Bundle of muscle
fibers (fascicle)

Transverse (T) tubule

Sarcolemma

Sarcoplasmic
reticulum

Mitochondrion

Myofibril

A band

H band   I band   Z disk

M band

One myofibril

Sarcomere

Myofilaments   A band   Nebulin

M
band

Titin

Z band   H band

Myofilaments

Troponin   Nebulin   Tropomodulin

Actin

Titin   Tropomyosin

Myosin

1   2   3   4

Each thick filament is surrounded by a hexagonal
array of thin filaments.

FIGURE 7-4. Structural components of skeletal muscle, including the morphology of the sarcomere. Striations of skeletal muscle are resolved into **A bands** and **I bands**. I bands are divided into two equal halves by a **Z disk**, and each A band has a light zone, the **H band**. The center of each H band is a dark **M band**. Adjacent myofibrils are secured to each other by the intermediate filaments desmin and vimentin. The basic contractile unit of the skeletal muscle cell is the sarcomere, a precisely ordered collection of **myofilaments (thick and thin filaments)**. Tubular invaginations, **T tubules (transverse tubules)**, of the muscle cell membrane penetrate deep into the sarcoplasm and surround myofibrils in such a manner that at the junction of each A and I band, these tubules become associated with the dilated **terminal cisternae** of the SR (smooth ER), forming triads.

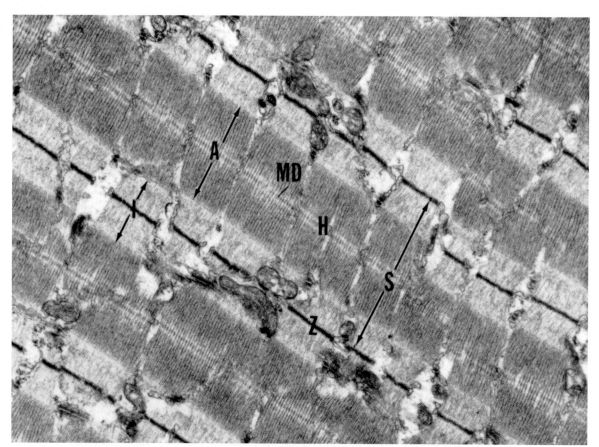

FIGURE 7-5. This moderately low-power electron micrograph of skeletal muscle was sectioned longitudinally. Perpendicular to its longitudinal axis, note the dark and light cross-bandings. The **A band** (A) in this view extends from the upper left-hand corner to the lower right-hand corner and is bordered by an **I band** (I) on either side. Each I band is traversed by a **Z disk** (Z). Observe that the Z disk has the appearance of a dashed line because individual myofibrils are separated from each other by sarcoplasm. Note that the extent of a **sarcomere** (S) is from Z disk to Z disk and that an almost precise alignment of individual myofibrils ensures the specific orientation of the various bands within the sarcomere. The **H zone** (H) and the **M disk** (MD) are clearly defined in this electron micrograph. Mitochondria are preferentially located in mammalian skeletal muscle, occupying the region at the level of the I band as they wrap around the periphery of the myofibril. Several sarcomeres are presented at a higher magnification in Review Figure 7-2-1. (Courtesy of Dr. J. Strum.)

Table 7-3	Proteins Associated with the Thin Myofilament
Protein	**Function**
G actin	Monomers assemble to form the F actin component of the thin myofilament; interacts with myosin II during skeletal muscle contraction
Tropomyosin	Linear molecules that assemble head to tail and occupy the grooves in the F actin
Troponin	A complex of three molecules (TnC, TnT, and TnI) that is associated with each tropomyosin molecule
TnC	Binds calcium ions
TnT	Binds the troponin complex to tropomyosin
TnI	Binds to actin, masking its active site, thus inhibiting myosin II–actin interaction
Cap Z	That portion of the Z disk that forms a cap on the plus end of the F actin preventing it from adding or deleting G actins from the thin myofilament
α-Actinin	Fastens the thin myofilament's plus end to the Z disk
Nebulin	An inelastic protein that, along with its counterpart, anchors each thin myofilament to the Z disk, stabilizing its length and position in the sarcomere
Tropomodulin	Forms a cap on the minus end of the F actin preventing it from adding or deleting G actins from the thin myofilament

Table 7-4	Proteins Associated with the Thick Myofilament
Protein	**Function**
Myosin II	The principal protein of the thick myofilament; it is composed of two heavy chains and four light chains; interacts with the actin of the thin myofilament to achieve shortening of the sarcomere
Titin	Elastic protein that fastens the thick filament to the Z disk thereby fixing its place in the sarcomere
Myomesin	Protein that cross-links adjacent myosin II molecules to each other at the M line
C protein	Assists myomesin in cross-linking adjacent myosin II molecules to each other at the M line

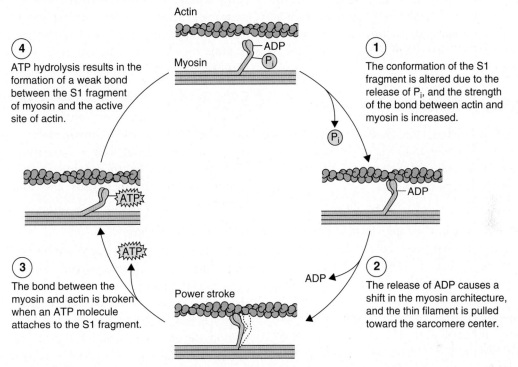

FIGURE 7-6. Contraction cycle in skeletal muscle cells. This sequence of steps is repeated many times, leading to an extensive overlay of thick and thin filaments, which shortens the sarcomere and consequently the entire skeletal muscle fiber. (Adapted from Alberts B, et al., eds. *Molecular Biology of the Cell*, 3rd ed. New York: Garland Publishing, 1994. p. 852. Copyright © 1983, 1989, 1994 by Bruce Alberts, Dennis Bray, Julian Lewis, Martin Raff, Keith Roberts, and James D. Watson. Used by permission of W. W. Norton & Company, Inc.)

CLINICAL CONSIDERATIONS 7-2

Pompe's Disease

Pompe's disease is one of the inherited metabolic glycogen storage diseases in which the cells of the patient are unable to degrade glycogen owing to an **acid maltase deficiency**. The inability to degrade glycogen results in the accumulation of glycogen in the lysosomes. There are two types of this disease, the early onset that occurs in the infant and the late onset that occurs either in childhood or in the adult. The early onset is fatal, and children do not usually live past age 2 years; the symptoms are enlargement of the heart and liver, generalized weakness, and lack of muscle tone. Death results from cardiac and respiratory failure. The late-onset form differs from the juvenile condition in that the cardiac complications are not as assiduous, but muscle weakness, especially of the legs, is more pronounced. Recent advancement in the treatment of Pompe's disease appears to decrease the mortality rate as well as the severity of the condition.

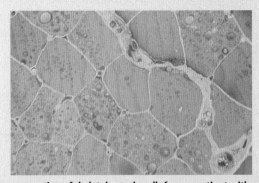

This cross section of skeletal muscle cells from a patient with adult-onset Pompe's disease, stained with toluidine blue, displays enlarged lysosomes filled with pinkish-colored glycogen. (Reprinted with permission from Rubin R, et al., eds. *Rubin's Pathology: Clinicopathologic Foundations of Medicine*, 5th ed. Philadelphia: Wolters Kluwer Health/Lippincott Williams & Wilkins, 2008. Figure 27-27.)

conformation, moving the thin filament toward the center of the sarcomere. A new ATP attaches to the globular head, and the myosin dissociates from the active site of the actin. This cycle is repeated 200 to 300 times for complete contraction of the sarcomere (Fig. 7-6).

Relaxation ensues when the calcium pump of the SR transports calcium from the sarcoplasm into the SR cisterna, where it is bound by **calsequestrin**. The decreased cytosolic Ca^{2+} induces TnC to lose its bound calcium ions, the TnC molecule returns to its previous conformational state, the tropomyosin molecule returns to its original location, and the active site of the actin molecule is once again masked.

Skeletal Muscle Motor Innervation

The innervation of skeletal muscle is composed of a motor element, myoneural junction (neuromuscular junction), and two sensory elements, Golgi tendon organs and muscle spindles.

Myoneural Junction

A **myoneural junction** is a synapse formed between a motor nerve **axon terminal (end-foot)** and a specialized region of a skeletal muscle cell (Fig. 7-7). The axon terminal, covered on its nonsynaptic surface by a Schwann cell but no myelin, houses ACh-containing vesicles, known as **synaptic vesicles**, smooth endoplasmic reticulum (SER), and mitochondria. The cytoplasmic aspect of its synaptic surface houses receptors for the synaptic vesicles as well as voltage-gated calcium channels; this region of the axon terminal membrane is referred to as the **presynaptic membrane**. The sarcolemma of the skeletal muscle cell that participates in the formation of the synapse, referred to as the **motor end plate (postsynaptic membrane)**, forms numerous infoldings, known as **junctional folds**, to increase the surface area to accommodate a high concentration of **acetylcholine receptors**. The space between the presynaptic and postsynaptic membranes is known as the **synaptic cleft**. The mechanism of how a nerve impulse is conducted across the synaptic cleft to induce muscle contraction is discussed in Chapter 8, Nervous Tissue.

A single motor neuron can innervate a varying number of skeletal muscle fibers, which all contract together as a unit in response to the neural impulse from a single neuron. The number of skeletal muscle fibers innervated by a single motor neuron, therefore, determines the strength of contraction. A large motor unit (hundreds of skeletal muscle fibers innervated by a single neuron) generates a strong contraction, whereas a small motor unit (only a handful of muscle fibers innervated by a single neuron) generates a weak but fast and fine-tuned contraction. Typically, muscles of the limbs are composed of large motor units, whereas those in the fingers and extrinsic eye muscles are in small motor units.

Golgi Tendon Organ and Muscle Spindle

As a protective mechanism against muscle fiber tears from overstretching and to provide information concerning the position of the body in three-dimensional space, tendons and muscles are equipped with specialized receptors, **Golgi tendon organs** and **muscle spindles**, respectively.

Golgi Tendon Organ

Golgi tendon organs, situated within tendons, are collagen fibers that are encapsulated and are surrounded by a special type of sensory nerve fiber, known as **type Ib** sensory nerves. If the skeletal muscle of the tendon contracts too forcefully, causing possible damage to the tendon, the type Ib neuron inhibits the motor neuron of the muscle, thus preventing continued contraction.

Muscle Spindle

Muscle spindles are modified skeletal muscle cells (**intrafusal fibers**) encapsulated in a connective tissue capsule within skeletal muscles. The skeletal muscle cells that immediately surround the intrafusal fibers are known as **extrafusal fibers**. The muscle spindle is attached to the endomysium and the perimysium of the extrafusal fibers. This attachment provides information to the intrafusal fibers concerning the rate and the duration of the muscle stretching. If the muscle is being stretched for too long or with too much frequency, the muscle spindle induces muscle contraction protecting it from being overstretched.

CLINICAL CONSIDERATIONS 7-3

Myasthenia Gravis

Myasthenia gravis is an autoimmune disease characterized by incremental weakening of skeletal muscles. Antibodies formed against ACh receptors of skeletal muscle fibers bond to and, thus, block these receptors. The number of sites available for the initiation of depolarization of the muscle sarcolemma is decreased. The gradual weakening affects the most active muscles first (muscles of the face, eyes, and tongue), but eventually the muscles of respiration become compromised and the individual dies of respiratory insufficiency.

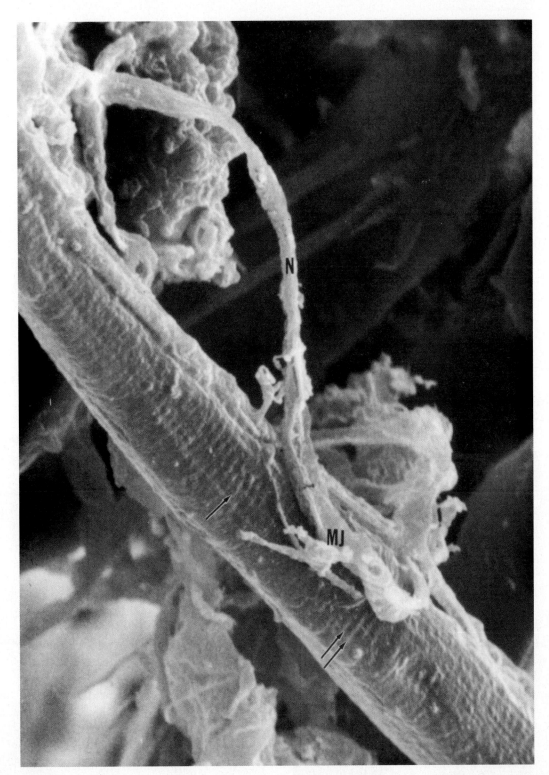

FIGURE 7-7. Scanning electron micrograph of a cat tongue myoneural junction, ×2,610. The striations (*arrows*) of an isolated skeletal muscle fiber are evident in this scanning electron micrograph. Note the **nerve** "twig" (N), which loops up and makes contact with the muscle at the **myoneural junction** (MJ). (Courtesy of Dr. L. Litke.)

Cardiac Muscle

Cardiac muscle cells (Figs. 7-8 through 7-10) are also striated, but each cell usually contains only one centrally placed nucleus. These cells form specialized junctions known as **intercalated disks** as they interdigitate with each other. These intercalated disks act as Z disks as well as regions of intercellular adhering and communication junctions because they have **transverse portions** that specialize in cell–cell attachments by forming numerous desmosomes and fasciae adherentes and **lateral portions** that are rich in gap junctions, thus permitting cell to cell communications for cardiac muscle cells forming a functional syncytium.

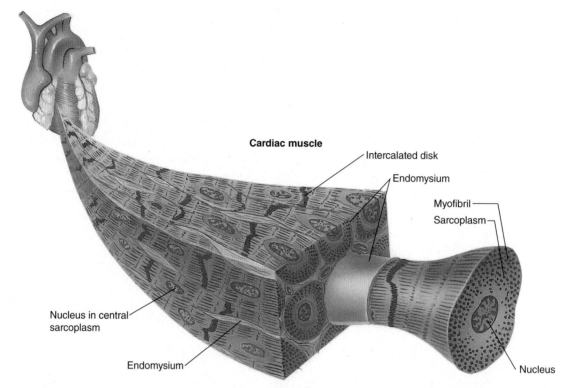

FIGURE 7-8. Schematic diagram of cardiac muscle.

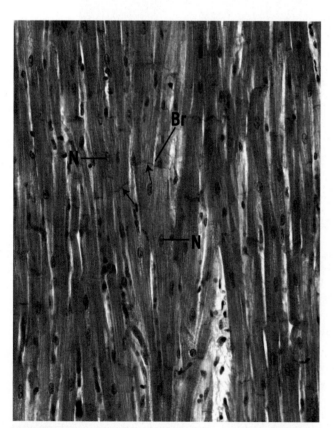

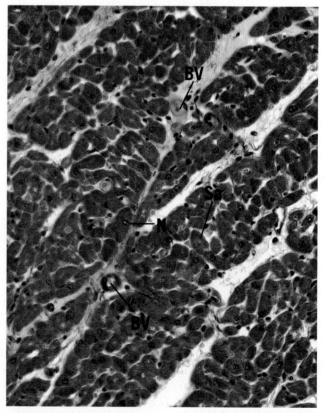

FIGURE 7-9. This longitudinal section of cardiac muscle from the human heart exhibits that the **muscle cells branch** (Br) and the individual cells are separated from one another by specialized intercellular junctions known as intercalated disks (*arrows*). Each cardiac muscle cell has a centrally positioned **nucleus** (N). ×270.

FIGURE 7-10. This transverse section of cardiac muscle from the human heart exhibits that these cells possess a rich **blood supply** (BV). Observe that the **nuclei** (N) of cardiac muscle cells are located at the center of the cell, and, at either end of the nucleus, a clear area of the **sarcoplasm** (Sa) represents a glycogen deposit that was removed during processing. ×270.

CLINICAL CONSIDERATIONS 7-4

Viral Myocarditis

Viral myocarditis is supposed to be a virally caused inflammation of the myocardium, even though the viral nature of the pathology is not always evident. Early in the onset of the disease, there is very little cardiac muscle cell necrosis with a minimal amount of lymphocytic and macrophage infiltration. As the disease progresses, the infiltration becomes more prominent and the patient experiences heart failure and the histopathology displays foci of necrotic cardiomyocytes. If the necrosis is limited in scope, neutrophils are rarely present; however, in widespread necrosis, neutrophilic infiltration becomes evident. The condition is rarely lethal, and most patients recover with minor medical intervention.

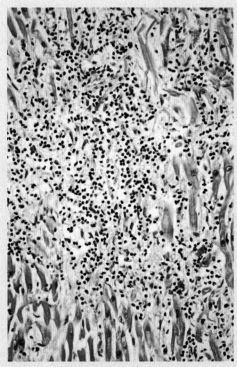

Accumulation of neutrophils and lymphocytes disrupts the normal arrangement of the cardiac muscle cells in viral myocarditis. (Reprinted with permission from Strayer DS, et al., eds. *Rubin's Pathology: Mechanisms of Human Disease*, 8th ed. Philadelphia: Wolters Kluwer, 2020. Figure 17-40.)

Heart muscle contraction is involuntary, and the cells have an inherent rhythm. The heart possesses a group of specialized cardiac muscle cells that form the **sinoatrial (SA) node**, which initiates contraction of the atrial muscles, thereby establishing the rate of heart contraction. The SA node receives input from the sympathetic and parasympathetic components of the autonomic nervous system; the former increases and the latter decreases the rate of heart contraction. The impulse is transmitted from the SA node to another group of specialized cardiac muscle cells, the **atrioventricular (AV) node** that holds up the impulse for a few milliseconds and then the impulse travels along the **bundle of His** to the **Purkinje fibers** (both of which are modified cardiac muscle cells) to cause contraction of the ventricles.

Morphologic Components of Cardiac Muscle Cells

The morphologic components of cardiac muscle cells resemble those of skeletal muscle cells in that they both possess very similar arrangements of **thin** and **thick filaments** and **Z disks** that form sarcomeres, and the thin and thick filaments slide past each other during muscle contraction. The actin–myosin interaction is regulated by calcium ions and, just as in skeletal muscle, when the calcium binds the TnC moiety of troponin the change in its conformation forces tropomyosin deeper into the groove of the actin filaments, unmasking the **myosin-binding sites** on actin.

Both skeletal and cardiac muscle cells have an abundant mitochondrial population, although cardiac muscle cells have a richer supply of mitochondria than skeletal muscle cells. The system of **T tubules** differs because those of cardiac muscle cells have a larger diameter, and, unlike those of skeletal muscle cells, they are lined by an **external lamina**.

The **sarcoplasmic reticulum** of cardiac muscle cells is scant and instead of forming triads with the T tubules, they form **dyads**, in that a single T tubule is associated with a single SR profile. The cardiac muscle T tubule also possesses voltage-gated calcium channels through which calcium enters the cardiac muscle cell from the extracellular milieu, supplementing the calcium released from the SR. Phosphorylation and de-phosphorylation of **phospholamban**, an integral protein of the SR membrane, regulate the activity of the sarcoplasmic calcium pump, thereby controlling the movement of calcium ions into or out of the SR. When phosphorylated, this protein causes the sarcoplasmic calcium channels to open permitting calcium ions to enter the SR, causing relaxation of cardiac muscle cells. Dephosphorylated phospholamban is an inhibitor of the sarcoplasmic calcium channels, causing the contraction of cardiac muscle cells.

Smooth Muscle

Smooth muscle (Figs. 7-11 through 7-13) is also involuntary. Each fusiform smooth muscle cell houses a single, centrally placed nucleus, which becomes corkscrew-shaped during contraction of the cell. Smooth muscle cells contain an apparently haphazard arrangement of thick and thin filaments which are anchored to intermediate filaments. These intermediate filaments, desmin and vimentin, form dense bodies where they cross each other and at points of attachment to the cytoplasmic aspect of the sarcolemma. Although the **thick** and **thin myofilaments** of smooth muscle are not arranged into sarcomeres and myofibrils, they are organized so that they are aligned obliquely to the longitudinal axis of the cell. **Myosin II molecules** of smooth muscle are unusual because the **light meromyosin moiety** is folded in such a fashion that its free terminus binds to a "sticky region" of the globular S1 portion. The thin filaments, composed of actin, possess tropomyosin as well as two additional proteins: **caldesmon**, which masks the active site of the actin monomers, and **calponin**, whose function resembles that of troponin of skeletal muscle, in that it obstructs the ATPase activity of myosin II.

It is interesting to note that although the thin filaments of smooth muscle possess F actin and tropomyosin, troponin is absent, and its function is assumed by calmodulin which becomes complexed with calcium. The cytosol is rich in calmodulin and the enzyme myosin light-chain kinase, whereas troponin is absent.

Smooth muscle may be of the multiunit type, in which each cell possesses its own nerve supply, or of the unitary (visceral) smooth muscle type, in which nerve impulses are transmitted via nexus (gap junctions) from one muscle cell to its neighbor.

Smooth Muscle Contraction

For smooth muscle contraction to occur, calcium ions, released from **caveolae**, permit the phosphorylation of calponin, and the phosphorylated calponin cannot inhibit contraction from occurring. Calcium ions also bind to calmodulin, and the Ca^{2+}–**calmodulin complex** binds to caldesmon, causing it to unmask the active site of actin and activates **myosin light-chain kinase**, which phosphorylates one of the **myosin II light chains**, altering its conformation. The phosphorylation causes the free terminus of the light meromyosin to be released from the S1 moiety. ATP binds to the S1, and the resultant interaction between actin and myosin is like that of skeletal (and cardiac) muscle. If calcium and ATP are present, the smooth muscle cell will remain contracted. Smooth muscle contraction lasts longer but develops slower than cardiac or skeletal muscle contraction. It should be noted that, unlike in skeletal muscle where the myosin II molecules are assembled in an antiparallel fashion, where the center of the thick filament has only light meromyosin in its middle, in smooth muscle the heavy meromyosin heads are present even along the middle of the thick filament. Because of this arrangement of the myosin II molecules in the thick filament, contraction in smooth muscle lasts longer than in skeletal muscle.

CLINICAL CONSIDERATIONS 7-5

Leiomyomas and Leiomyosarcomas

Leiomyomas are benign tumors of smooth muscle cells, usually involving the uterus, arrector pili muscles, scrotum, labia, and nipples. They are usually solitary (but can be multiple in the arrector pili), 1 to 2 cm in diameter, where they usually present as painful, well-defined, yellow nodules that are firm to the touch. Their histopathology presents with normal-appearing spindle-shaped muscle cells that criss-cross each other. Fortunately, solitary leiomyomas are easily treated by surgical removal.

Leiomyosarcomas are more common in females than in males. They are painless malignant tumors of smooth muscle located mostly in the dermis of the skin and retroperitoneal connective tissues in the abdominal region. Histopathology of these tumors presents with smooth muscle-like cells. They are usually detected early in their development when in the dermis and are treated by simple surgical excision; however, because they are painless, they are rarely detected in the retroperitoneal areas until they have become not only enlarged but also metastasized, leading to poor prognosis.

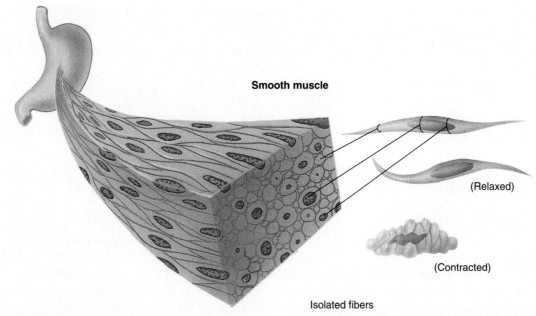

Smooth muscle

(Relaxed)

(Contracted)

Isolated fibers

FIGURE 7-11. Schematic diagram of smooth muscle.

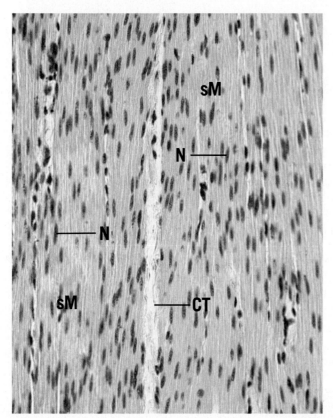

FIGURE 7-12. This longitudinal section of smooth muscle from the human duodenum exhibits that the spindle-shaped **smooth muscle cells** (sM) are arranged so that they mostly obliterate the spaces between the cells. The **nuclei** (N) of smooth muscle cells are also spindle shaped and are located in the center of the longitudinal extent of the muscle fiber but pressed to the periphery of the cell. **Connective tissue elements** (CT) subdivide the entire muscle into bundles of muscle cells. ×270.

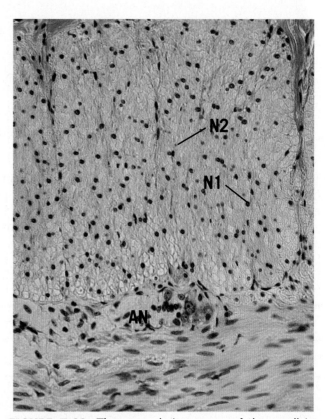

FIGURE 7-13. The muscularis externa of the small intestine is composed of an inner circular and an outer longitudinal layer of smooth muscle with **autonomic plexuses** (AN) positioned between them. A transverse section of the small intestine exhibits the outer longitudinal layer of smooth muscle in cross section. Recalling that smooth muscle cells are spindle shaped and their nuclei, also spindle shaped, are much shorter than the muscle cell, it becomes intuitive that, in a random section, some cells will appear without nuclei, others appear whose **nuclei** (N1) are sectioned at their narrowed tips, whereas other **nuclei** (N2) are sectioned near their center, widest region and appear as large circular profiles. ×270.

PLATE 7-1A   Skeletal Muscle

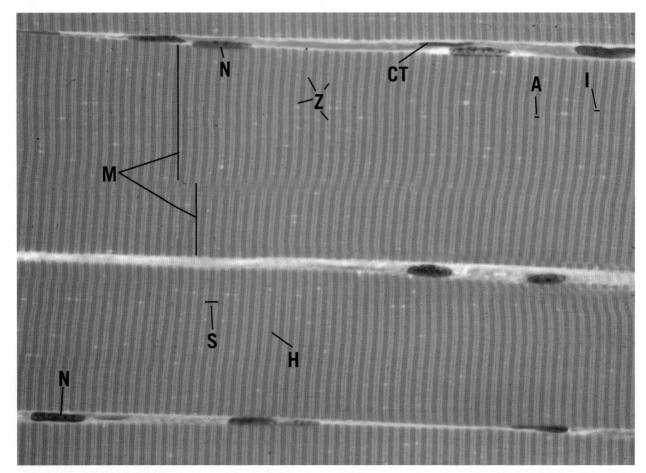

FIGURE 7-1-1. Skeletal muscle. l.s. Monkey. Plastic section. ×800.

This photomicrograph displays several of the characteristics of skeletal muscle in the longitudinal section. The muscle fibers are long, and their numerous **nuclei** (N) are peripherally located. The intercellular space is occupied by endomysium, with its occasional flattened **connective tissue cells** (CT) and reticular fibers. Two types of striations are evident: longitudinal and transverse. The longitudinal striations represent **myofibrils** (M) that are arranged in almost precise register with each other. This ordered arrangement is responsible for the dark and light transverse banding that gives this type of muscle its name. Note that the **light band** (I) is bisected by a narrow, dark line, the **Z disk** (Z). The **dark band** (A) is also bisected by the clear **H zone** (H). The center of the H zone is occupied by the M disk, appearing as a faintly discernible dark line in a few regions. The basic contractile unit of skeletal muscle is the **sarcomere** (S), extending from one Z disk to its neighboring Z disk. During muscle contraction, the myofilaments of each sarcomere slide past one another, pulling Z disks closer to each other, thus shortening the length of each sarcomere. During this movement, the width of the A band remains constant, whereas the I band and H zone disappear.

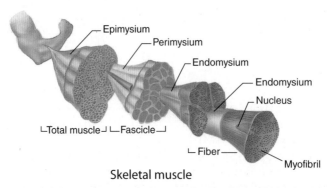

Skeletal muscle

KEY							
A	A band		**I**	light band		**S**	sarcomere
CT	connective tissue cells		**M**	myofibrils		**Z**	Z disk
H	H zone		**N**	nucleus			

PLATE 7-1B Skeletal Muscle

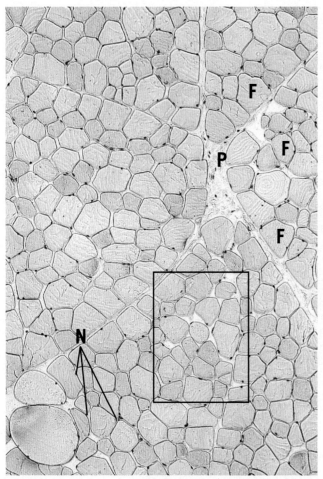

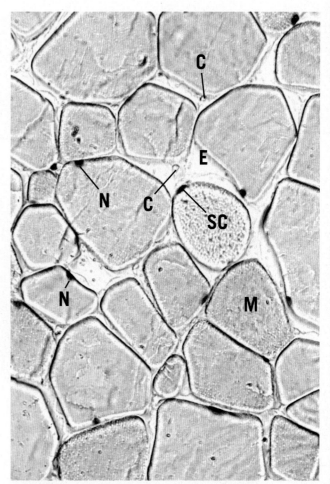

FIGURE 7-1-2. Skeletal muscle. x.s. Monkey. Paraffin section. ×132.

FIGURE 7-1-3. Skeletal muscle. x.s. Monkey. Paraffin section. ×540.

Portions of a few fascicles are presented in this photomicrograph. Each fascicle is composed of numerous **muscle fibers** (F) that are surrounded by connective tissue elements known as the **perimysium** (P), which houses nerves and blood vessels supplying the fascicles. The nuclei of endothelial, Schwann, and connective tissue cells are evident as black dots in the perimysium. The peripherally placed **nuclei** (N) of the skeletal muscle fibers appear as black dots; however, they are all within the muscle cell. Nuclei of satellite cells are also present, just external to the muscle fibers, but their identification at low magnification is questionable. The *boxed area* is presented at a higher magnification in Figure 7-1-3.

This is a higher magnification of the *boxed area* of Figure 7-1-2. Transverse sections of several muscle fibers demonstrate that these cells appear to be polyhedral, that they possess peripherally placed **nuclei** (N), and that their **endomysia** (E) house numerous **capillaries** (C). Many of the capillaries are difficult to see because they are collapsed in a resting muscle. The pale sarcoplasm occasionally appears granular owing to the transversely sectioned myofibrils (M). Occasionally, nuclei that appear to belong to **satellite cells** (SC) may be observed, but definite identification cannot be expected. Moreover, the well-defined outline of each fiber was believed to be owing to the sarcolemma, but now it is known to be due more to the adherent basal lamina and endomysium.

KEY					
C	capillaries	F	muscle fibers	P	perimysium
E	endomysia	N	nuclei	SC	satellite cells

PLATE 7-2   Skeletal Muscle, Electron Microscopy

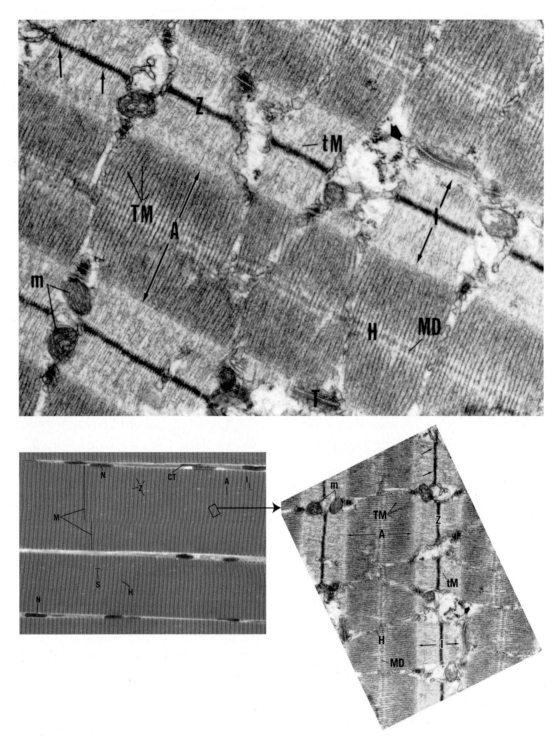

FIGURE 7-2-1. Skeletal muscle. l.s. Rat. Electron microscopy. ×28,800.

This is a higher-power electron micrograph presenting several sarcomeres. The box in the *inset* H&E micrograph demonstrates the approximate location and orientation of the electron micrograph. Note that the **Z disks** (Z) possess projections (*arrows*) to which the **thin myofilaments** (tM) are attached. The **I band** (I) is composed only of thin filaments. **Thick myofilaments** (TM), comprising the **A band** (A), interdigitate with the thin filaments from either end of the sarcomere. However, the thin filaments in a relaxed muscle do not extend all the way to the center of the A band; therefore, the **H zone** (H) is composed only of thick filaments. The center of each thick filament appears to be attached to its neighboring thick filament, resulting in localized thickenings, collectively comprising the **M disk** (MD). During muscle contraction, the thick and thin filaments slide past each other, thus pulling the Z disks toward the center of the sarcomere. Because of the resultant overlapping of thick and thin filaments, the I bands and H zones disappear, but the A bands maintain their width. The sarcoplasm houses **mitochondria** (m) peripherally located, glycogen granules (*arrowhead*) as well as a specialized system of sarcoplasmic reticulum and T tubules, forming **triad**s (T). In mammalian skeletal muscle, triads are positioned at the junction of the I and A bands. (Courtesy of Dr. J. Strum.)

PLATE 7-3A   Myoneural Junction, Light Microscopy

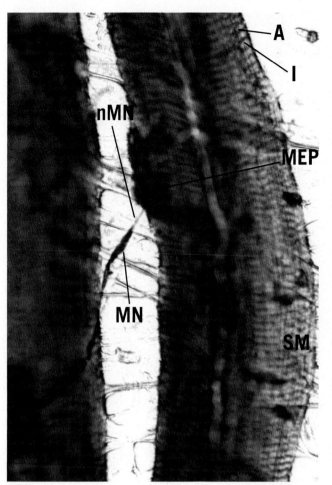

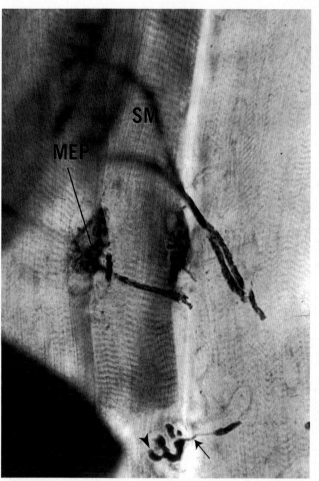

FIGURE 7-3-1. Myoneural junction. Lateral view. Paraffin section. ×540.

This view of the myoneural junction clearly displays the **myelinated nerve fiber** (MN) approaching the **skeletal muscle fiber** (SM). The **A bands** (A) and **I bands** (I) are well delineated, but the Z disks are not observable in this preparation. As the axon nears the muscle cell, it loses its myelin sheath and continues as a **nonmyelinated axon** (nMN) but retains its Schwann cell envelope. As the axon reaches the muscle cell, it terminates as the end-foot overlying the **motor end plate** (MEP) of the muscle fiber. Although the sarcolemma is not visible in light micrographs, such as this one, its location is clearly approximated because of its associated basal lamina and reticular fibers.

FIGURE 7-3-2. Myoneural junction. Surface view. Paraffin section. ×540.

This view of the myoneural junction demonstrates, as in Figure 7-3-1, that as the axon reaches the vicinity of the **skeletal muscle fiber** (SM), it loses its myelin sheath. The axon terminates as the end-foot overlying the **motor end plate** (MEP) of the skeletal muscle fiber. Although it is not apparent in this light micrograph, the motor end plate is a slight depression of the skeletal muscle fiber. The plasma membranes of the end-foot and the muscle fiber do not contact each other. Figure 7-3-3 clearly demonstrates the morphology of such a synapse.

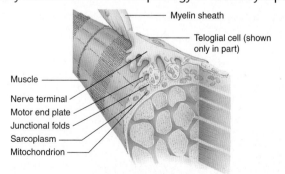

Myoneural junction

KEY					
A	A band	MEP	motor end plate	nMN	nonmyelinated nerve fiber
I	I band	MN	myelinated nerve fiber	SM	skeletal muscle fiber

PLATE 7-3B Myoneural Junction, Electron Microscopy

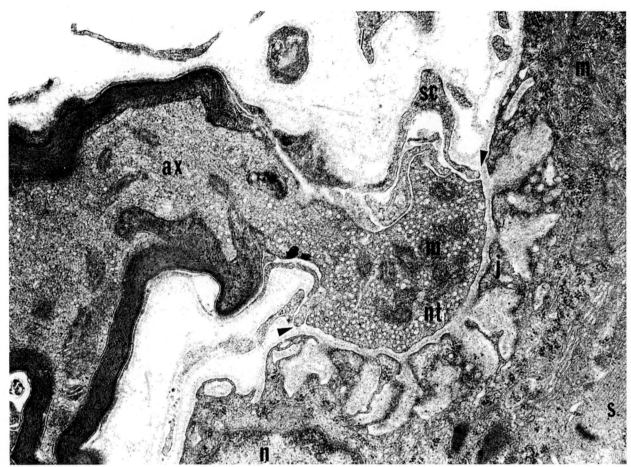

FIGURE 7-3-3. Myoneural junction. Rat. Electron microscopy. ×15,353.

This electron micrograph is of a myoneural junction taken from the diaphragm muscle of a rat. Observe that the **axon** (ax) loses its myelin sheath, but the Schwann cell (sc) continues, providing a protective cover for the nonsynaptic surface of the end-foot or **nerve terminal** (nt). The myelinated sheath ends in typical paranodal loops at the terminal heminode. The nerve terminal possesses **mitochondria** (m) and numerous clear synaptic vesicles. The margins of the 50-nm primary synaptic cleft are indicated by *arrowheads*. Postsynaptically, the **junctional folds** (j), many **mitochondria** (m), and portions of a **nucleus** (n) and **sarcomere** (s) are apparent in the skeletal muscle fiber. (Courtesy of Dr. C. S. Hudson.)

KEY					
ax	axon	**n**	nucleus	**s**	sarcomere
j	junctional folds	**nt**	nerve terminal	**sc**	Schwann cell
m	mitochondria				

PLATE 7-4   Muscle Spindle, Light and Electron Microscopy

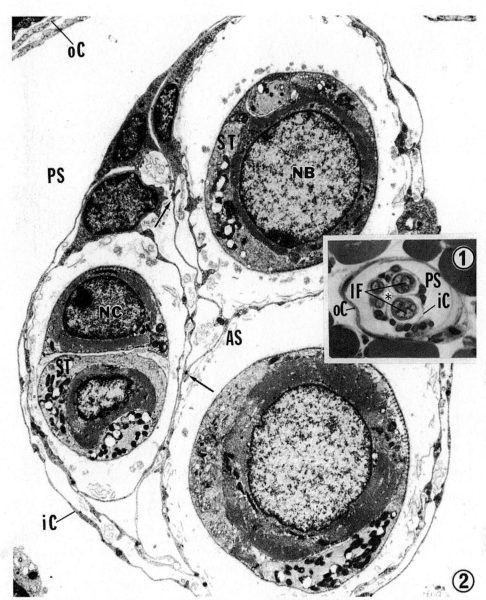

FIGURE 7-4-1. Muscle spindle. Mouse. Plastic section. ×436.

Observe that the **outer** (oC) and **inner** (iC) **capsules** of the muscle spindle define the outer **peraxial space** (PS) and the inner **axial space** (*asterisk*). The inner capsule forms an envelope around the **intrafusal fibers** (IF). (From Ovalle WK, et al. Comparative ultrastructure of the inner capsule of the muscle spindle and the tendon organ. *Am J Anat* 1983;166(3):343–357. Copyright © 1983 Wiley-Liss, Inc. Reprinted by permission of John Wiley & Sons, Inc.)

FIGURE 7-4-2. Muscle spindle. Mouse. Electron microscopy. ×6,300.

Parts of the **outer capsule** (oC) may be observed at the corners of this electron micrograph. The **periaxial space** (PS) surrounds the slender **inner capsule** (iC), whose component cells form attenuated branches, subdividing the **axial space** (AS) into several compartments for the **nuclear chain** (NC) and **nuclear bag** (NB) intrafusal fibers and their corresponding **sensory terminals** (ST). Note that the attenuated processes of the inner capsule cells establish contact with each other (*arrows*). (From Ovalle WK, et al. Comparative ultrastructure of the inner capsule of the muscle spindle and the tendon organ. *Am J Anat* 1983;166(3):343–357. Copyright © 1983 Wiley-Liss, Inc. Reprinted by permission of John Wiley & Sons, Inc.)

PLATE 7-5A Smooth Muscle

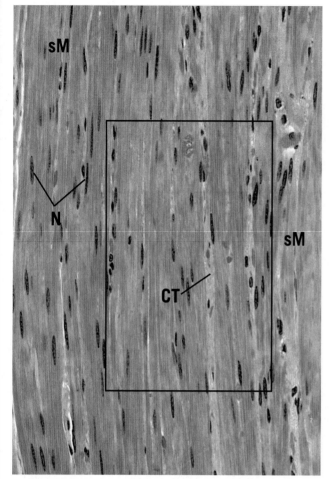

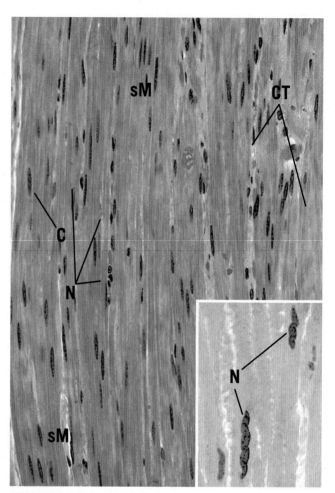

FIGURE 7-5-1. Smooth muscle. l.s. Monkey. Plastic section. ×270.

FIGURE 7-5-2. Smooth muscle. l.s. Monkey. Plastic section. ×540.

The longitudinal section of smooth muscle in this photomicrograph displays long fusiform **smooth muscle cells** (sM) with centrally located, elongated **nuclei** (N). Because the muscle fibers are arranged in staggered arrays, they can be packed very closely, with only a limited amount of intervening **connective tissue** (CT). Using hematoxylin and eosin, the nuclei appear bluish, whereas the cytoplasm stains a light pink. Each smooth muscle cell is surrounded by a basal lamina and reticular fibers, neither of which is evident in this figure. Capillaries are housed in the connective tissue separating bundles of smooth muscle fibers. The *boxed area* is presented at higher magnification in Figure 7-5-2.

This photomicrograph is a higher magnification of the *boxed area* of Figure 7-5-1. Observe that the **nuclei** (N) of the smooth muscle fibers are long, tapered structures located in the center of the cell. The widest girth of the nucleus is almost as wide as the muscle fiber. However, the length of the fiber is much greater than that of the nucleus. Note also that any line drawn perpendicular to the direction of the fibers will intersect only a few of the nuclei. Observe the difference between the **connective tissue** (CT) and **smooth muscle** (sM). The sM cytoplasm stains darker and appears smooth relative to the paleness and rough-appearing texture of the connective tissue. Observe **capillaries** (C) located in the connective tissue elements between bundles of muscle fibers. *Inset.* **Smooth muscle. Contracted. l.s. Monkey. Plastic section.** ×540. This longitudinal section of smooth muscle during contraction displays the characteristic corkscrew-shaped **nuclei** (N) of these cells.

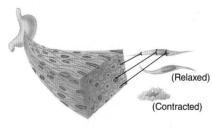

(Relaxed)

(Contracted)

Smooth muscle

KEY					
C	capillaries	N	nuclei	sM	smooth muscle cells
CT	connective tissue				

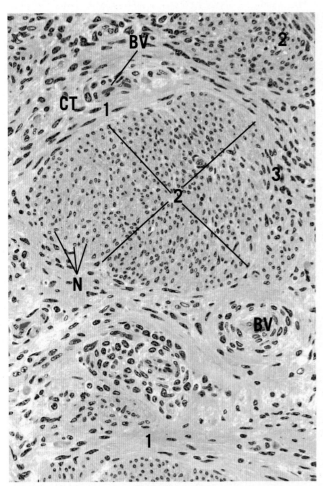

FIGURE 7-5-3. Smooth muscle. Uterine myometrium. x.s. Monkey. Plastic section. ×270.

The myometrium of the uterus consists of interlacing bundles of smooth muscle fibers, surrounded by **connective tissue** (CT) elements. Note that some of these bundles are cut in longitudinal section (1), others are sectioned transversely (2), and still others are cut obliquely (3). At low magnifications, such as in this photomicrograph, the transverse sections present a haphazard arrangement of dark **nuclei** (N) in a lightly staining region. With practice, it will become apparent that these nuclei are intracellular and that the pale circular regions represent smooth muscle fibers sectioned transversely. Note the numerous **blood vessels** (BV) traveling in the connective tissue between the smooth muscle bundles.

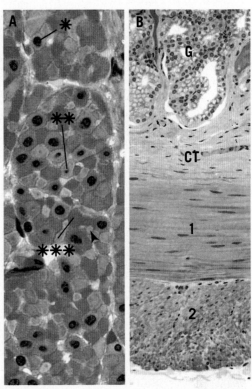

FIGURE 7-5-4A. Smooth muscle. x.s. Monkey. Plastic section. ×540.

To understand the three-dimensional morphology of smooth muscle as it appears in two dimensions, refer to Figure 7-5-2. Once again note that the muscle fibers are much longer than their nuclei and that both structures are spindle shaped, being tapered at both ends. Recall also that at its greatest girth, the nucleus is almost as wide as the cell. In transverse section, this would appear as a round nucleus surrounded by a rim of **cytoplasm** (*asterisk*). If the nucleus is sectioned at its tapered end, merely a small dot of it would be present in the center of a large **muscle fiber** (*double asterisks*). Sectioned anywhere between these two points, the nucleus would have varying diameters in the center of a large muscle cell. Additionally, the cell may be sectioned in a region away from its nucleus, where only the **sarcoplasm** of the large muscle cell would be evident (*triple asterisks*). Moreover, if the cell is sectioned at its tapered end, only a small circular profile of sarcoplasm is distinguishable (*arrowhead*). Therefore, in transverse sections of smooth muscle, one would expect to find only a few cells containing nuclei of various diameters. Most of the field will be closely packed profiles of sarcoplasm containing no nuclei.

FIGURE 7-5-4B. Smooth muscle. Duodenum. Monkey. Plastic section. ×132.

This photomicrograph of the duodenum demonstrates the **glandular portion** (G) with its underlying **connective tissue** (CT). Deep to the connective tissue, note the two smooth muscle layers, one of which is sectioned longitudinally (1) and the other transversely (2).

KEY			
CT	connective tissue	BV	blood vessels
N	nuclei	G	glandular portion

PLATE 7-6   Smooth Muscle, Electron Microscopy

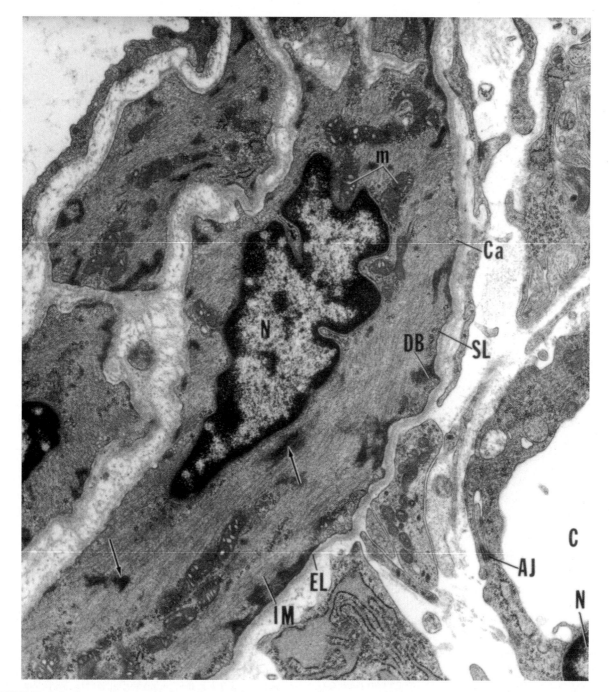

FIGURE 7-6-1. Smooth muscle. l.s. Mouse. Electron microscopy. ×15,120.

Smooth muscle does not display cross-bandings, transverse tubular systems, or the regularly arranged array of myo-filaments characteristic of striated muscle. However, smooth muscle does possess myofilaments that, along with a system of intermediate filaments, are responsible for its contractile capabilities. Moreover, the plasma membrane appears to possess the functional, if not the structural, aspects of the T tubule. Observe that each smooth muscle is surrounded by an **external lamina** (EL), which is similar in appearance to the basal lamina of epithelial cells. The **sarcolemma** (SL) displays the presence of numerous pinocytotic-like invaginations, the **caveolae** (Ca), which are believed to act as T tubules of striated muscles in conducting impulses into the interior of the fiber. Some suggest that they may also act in concert with the sarcoplasmic reticulum in modulating the availability of calcium ions. The cytoplasmic aspect of the sarcolemma also displays the presence of **dense bodies** (DB), which are indicative of the attachment of **intermediate microfilaments** (IM) at that point. Dense bodies, composed of α-actinin (Z disk protein present in striated muscle), are also located in the sarcoplasm (*arrows*). The **nucleus** (N) is centrally located, and, at its pole, mitochondria (m) are evident. Actin and myosin are also present in smooth muscle but cannot be identified with certainty in longitudinal sections. Parts of a second smooth muscle fiber may be observed to the left of the cell described. A small **capillary** (C) is evident in the lower right-hand corner. Note the **adherens junctions** (AJ) between the two epithelial cells, one of which presents a part of its **nucleus** (N).

PLATE 7-7A Cardiac Muscle

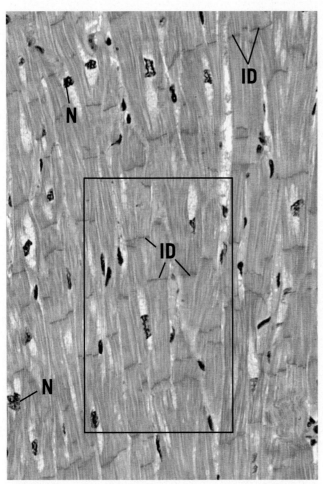

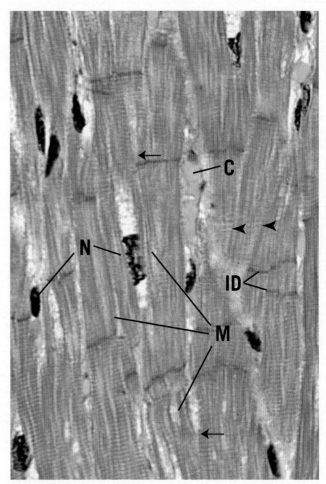

FIGURE 7-7-1. Cardiac muscle. l.s. Human. Plastic section. ×270.

FIGURE 7-7-2. Cardiac muscle. l.s. Human. Plastic section. ×540.

This medium magnification of longitudinally sectioned cardiac muscle displays many of the characteristics of this muscle type. The branching of the fibers is readily apparent, as are the dark and light bands running transversely along the length of the fibers. Each muscle cell possesses a large, centrally located, oval **nucleus** (N), although occasional muscle cells may possess two nuclei. The **intercalated disks** (ID), indicating intercellular junctions between two cardiac muscle cells, clearly delineated in this photomicrograph, are not easily demonstrable in sections stained with hematoxylin and eosin. The intercellular spaces of cardiac muscle are richly endowed by blood vessels, especially capillaries. Recall that, in contrast to cardiac muscle, the long skeletal muscle fibers do not branch, their myofilaments parallel one another, their many nuclei are peripherally located, and they possess no intercalated disks. The *boxed area* appears at a higher magnification in Figure 7-7-2.

This is a higher magnification of the *boxed area* of Figure 7-7-1. The branching of the fibers (*arrows*) is evident, and the cross-striations, I and A bands (*arrowheads*), are clearly distinguishable. The presence of **myofibrils** (M) within each cell is well displayed in this photomicrograph, as is the "steplike" appearance of the **intercalated disks** (ID). The oval, centrally located **nucleus** (N) is surrounded by a clear area usually occupied by organelles and other substances. The intercellular areas are richly supplied by **capillaries** (C) supported by slender connective tissue elements.

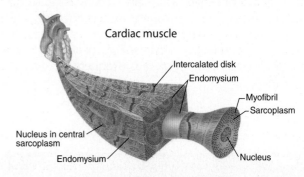

Cardiac muscle

Intercalated disk
Endomysium
Myofibril
Sarcoplasm
Nucleus in central sarcoplasm
Endomysium
Nucleus

KEY					
C	capillary	**M**	myofibril	**N**	nucleus
ID	intercalated disk				

PLATE 7-7B Cardiac Muscle

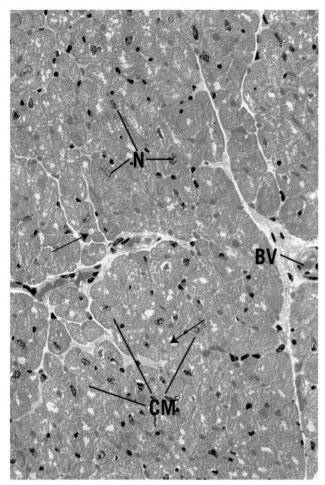

FIGURE 7-7-3. Cardiac muscle. x.s. Human. Plastic section. ×270.

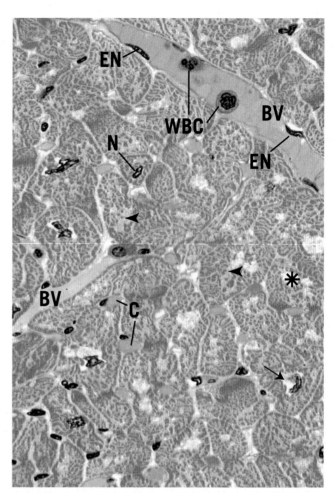

FIGURE 7-7-4. Cardiac muscle. x.s. Human. Plastic section. ×540.

Cross sections of cardiac muscle demonstrate polygon-shaped areas of **cardiac muscle fibers** (CM) with relatively large intercellular spaces whose rich **vascular supply** (BV) is readily evident. Note that the **nucleus** (N) of each muscle cell is located in the center, but not all cells display a nucleus. The clear areas in the center of some cells (*arrows*) represent the perinuclear regions at the poles of the nucleus. These regions are rich in sarcoplasmic reticulum, glycogen, lipid droplets, and an occasional Golgi apparatus. The numerous smaller nuclei in the intercellular areas belong to endothelial and connective tissue cells. In contrast to cardiac muscle, cross sections of skeletal muscle fibers display a homogeneous appearance with peripherally positioned nuclei. The connective tissue spaces between skeletal muscle fibers display numerous (frequently collapsed) capillaries.

At high magnifications of cardiac muscle in cross section, several aspects of this tissue become apparent. Numerous **capillaries** (C) and larger **blood vessels** (BV) abound in the connective tissue spaces. Note the **endothelial cell nuclei** (EN) of these vessels as well as the **white blood cells** (WBC) within the venule in the upper right-hand corner. **Nuclei** (N) of the muscle cells are centrally located, and the perinuclear clear areas (*arrow*) are evident. The central clear zones at the nuclear poles are denoted by *asterisks*. Cross sections of myofibrils (*arrowheads*) are recognizable as numerous small dots of varying diameters within the sarcoplasm.

KEY					
BV	blood vessel	**EN**	endothelial nucleus	**N**	nucleus
C	capillary	**ID**	intercalated disk	**WBC**	white blood cell
CM	cardiac muscle fiber	**M**	myofibril		

PLATE 7-8   Cardiac Muscle, Electron Microscopy

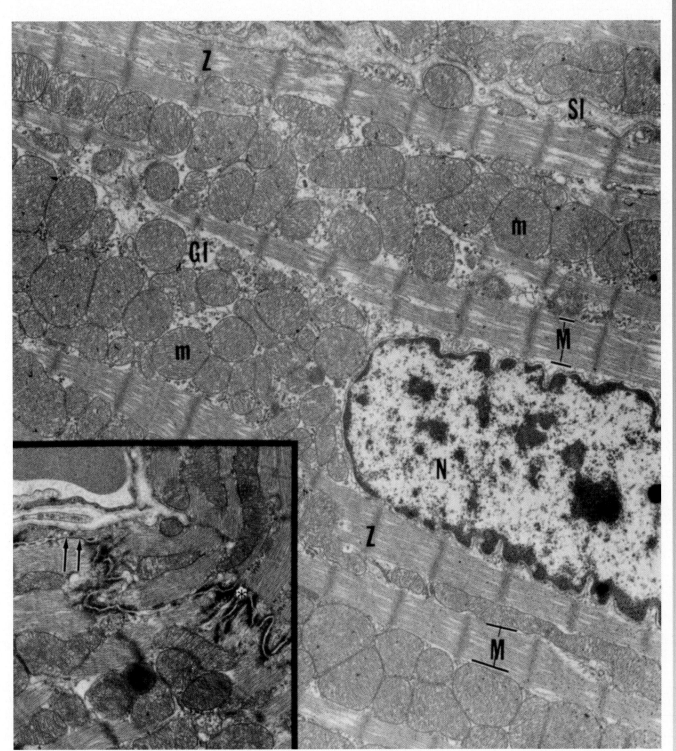

FIGURE 7-8-1. Cardiac muscle, l.s. Mouse. Electron microscopy. ×11,700.

The **nucleus** (N) of cardiac muscle cells is located in the center of the cell, as is evident from the location of the **sarcolemma** (Sl) in the upper part of the photomicrograph. The sarcoplasm is well endowed with **mitochondria** (m) and **glycogen** (Gl) deposits. Because this muscle cell is contracted, the I bands are not visible. However, the **Z disks** (Z) are clearly evident, as are the individual **myofibrils** (M). *Inset.* **Cardiac muscle. l.s. Mouse. Electron microscopy.** ×20,700. An intercalated disk is presented in this electron micrograph. Note that this intercellular junction has two zones, the transverse portion (*asterisk*), composed mostly of desmosome-like junctions, and a longitudinal portion that displays extensive gap junctions (*arrows*).

Selected Review of Histologic Images

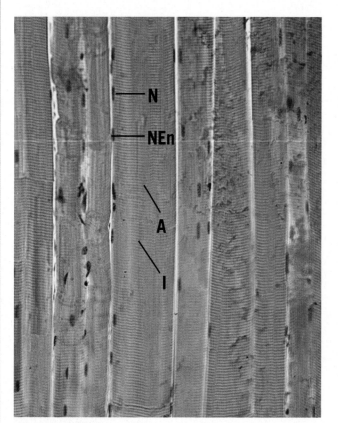

REVIEW FIGURE 7-1-1. Skeletal muscle. l.s. Human. Paraffin section. ×270.

This longitudinal section of skeletal muscle fibers demonstrates that the fibers are cylindrical in shape and their **nuclei** (N) are located peripherally just underneath the cell membrane. Each skeletal muscle cell is enveloped by an endomysium, and the **nuclei** (NEn) **belonging to cells of the endomysium** are outside the skeletal muscle fibers. The **dark bands** (A) and **light bands** (I) of the sarcomere are just about visible.

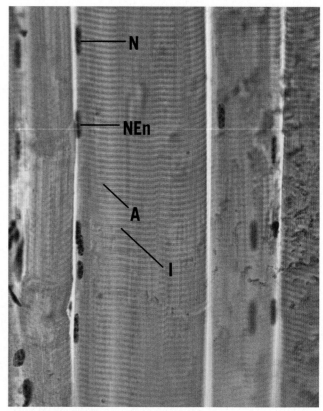

REVIEW FIGURE 7-1-2. Skeletal muscle. l.s. Human. Paraffin section. ×540.

This is a higher magnification of the *labeled area* of Review Figure 7-1-1. Note that the **nucleus** (N) of the skeletal muscle cell is clearly deep to the sarcolemma, whereas the **nucleus** (NEn) **of the cells of the endomysium** is clearly outside the sarcolemma. The **A bands** (A) and **I bands** (I) are clearly distinguishable from each other.

KEY					
A	A bands, dark bands	**N**	nucleus	**NEn**	nucleus of the cells of
I	I bands, light bands				the endomysium

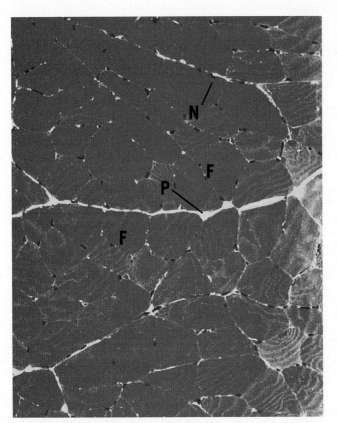

REVIEW FIGURE 7-1-3. Skeletal muscle. x.s. Human. Paraffin section. ×270.

This transverse section of **skeletal muscle fibers** (F) demonstrates that the cells are cylindrical in shape, and their **nuclei** (N) are located peripherally just underneath the sarcolemma. In addition to the endomysium that envelops each muscle fiber, bundles of skeletal muscle fibers are surrounded by a thicker connective tissue element, known as the **perimysium** (P).

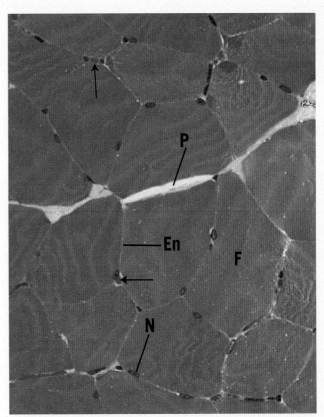

REVIEW FIGURE 7-1-4. Skeletal muscle. x.s. Human. Paraffin section. ×540.

This transverse section of **skeletal muscle fibers** (F) is a higher magnification of Review Figure 7-1-3. Observe that the **endomysium** (En) is very slender, whereas the **perimysium** (P) is more substantial. Observe that the **skeletal muscle nuclei** (N) are clearly evident, and note that capillary profiles (*arrows*) abound in skeletal muscle.

KEY					
En	endomysium	**N**	nucleus	**P**	perimysium
F	skeletal muscle fibers				

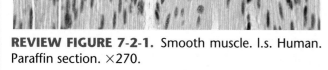

REVIEW FIGURE 7-2-1. Smooth muscle. l.s. Human. Paraffin section. ×270.

This longitudinal section of smooth muscle from the human duodenum exhibits that the spindle-shaped **smooth muscle cells** (sM) are arranged so that they mostly obliterate the spaces between the cells. The **nuclei** (N) of smooth muscle cells are also spindle shaped and are located in the center of the longitudinal extent of the muscle fiber but pressed to the periphery of the cell. **Connective tissue elements** (CT) subdivide the entire muscle into bundles of muscle cells.

REVIEW FIGURE 7-2-2. Smooth muscle. l.s. Human. Paraffin section. ×540.

This is a higher magnification of the right half of Review Figure 7-2-1 providing a better appreciation of the spindle shape of the smooth muscle cells. Observe the elongated **cytoplasm** (Cy) and the centrally placed **nucleus** (N).

KEY					
CT	connective tissue elements	Cy	cytoplasm	sM	smooth muscle cells
		N	nucleus		

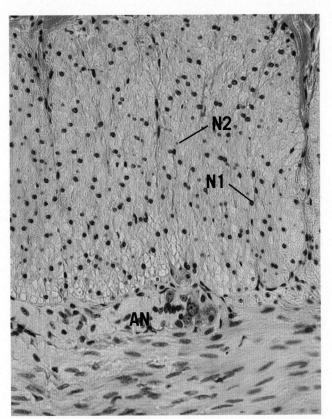

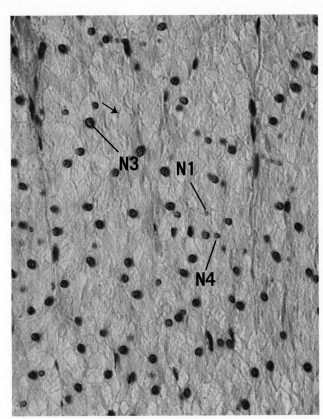

REVIEW FIGURE 7-2-3. Smooth muscle. x.s. Human. Paraffin section. ×70.

REVIEW FIGURE 7-2-4. Smooth muscle. x.s. Human. Paraffin section. ×540.

The muscularis externa of the small intestine is composed of an inner circular and an outer longitudinal layer of smooth muscle with **autonomic plexuses** (AN) positioned between them. A transverse section of the small intestine exhibits the outer longitudinal layer of smooth muscle in cross section. Recalling that smooth muscle cells are spindle shaped and their nuclei, also spindle shaped, are much shorter than the muscle cell, it becomes intuitive that, in a random section, some cells will appear without nuclei, others appear whose **nuclei** (N1) are sectioned near their center, widest region and appear as large circular profiles, whereas other **nuclei** (N2) are sectioned at their narrowed tips.

This image is a higher magnification of Review Figure 7-2-3, demonstrating that some of the **nuclei** are sectioned at their widest region (N3), other **nuclei** are sectioned at their narrowed tips (N1), whereas still other **nuclei** are sectioned in between these two regions (N4). It is evident that most smooth muscle cells are transected in regions to which the nuclei do not extend (*arrow*).

KEY					
AN	autonomic plexuses	**N2**	nucleus sectioned near its center	**N3**	nucleus sectioned between its narrowest and widest regions
N1	nucleus sectioned at its widest region				

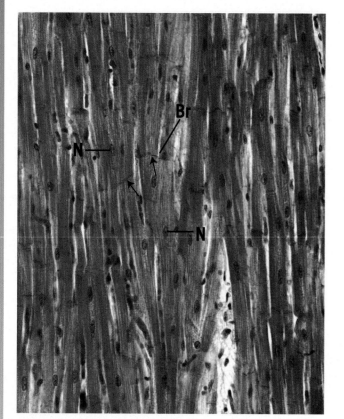

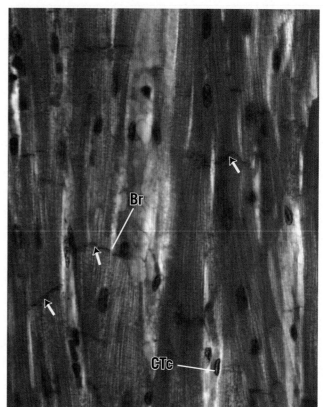

REVIEW FIGURE 7-3-1. Cardiac muscle. l.s. Human. Paraffin section. ×270.

This longitudinal section of cardiac muscle from the human heart exhibits that the **muscle cells branch** (Br) and that individual cells are separated from one another by specialized intercellular junctions known as intercalated disks (*arrows*). Each cardiac muscle cell has a centrally positioned **nucleus** (N).

REVIEW FIGURE 7-3-2. Cardiac muscle. l.s. Human. Paraffin section. ×540.

This image is a higher magnification of the region of Review Figure 7-3-1 where the **branching muscle cell** (Br) is identified. Note the evident intercalated disks (*arrows*) as well as the **connective tissue cells** (CTc) located between adjacent cardiac muscle cells.

KEY					
Br	branching muscle cells	**CTc**	connective tissue cells	**N**	nucleus

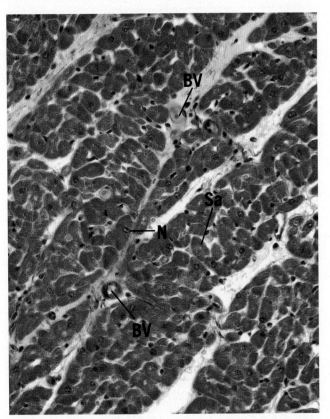

REVIEW FIGURE 7-3-3. Cardiac muscle. x.s. Human. Paraffin section. ×270.

This transverse section of cardiac muscle from the human heart exhibits that these cells possess a rich **blood supply** (BV). Observe that the **nuclei** (N) of cardiac muscle cells are located at the center of the cell, and, at either end of the nucleus, a clear area of the **sarcoplasm** (Sa) represents organelles as well as a glycogen deposit that was removed during processing.

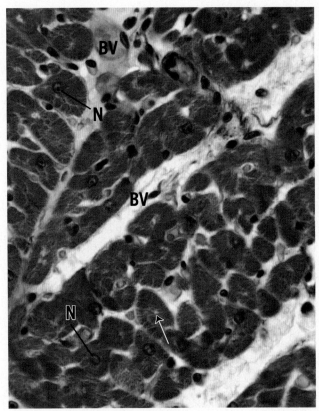

REVIEW FIGURE 7-3-4. Cardiac muscle. x.s. Human. Paraffin section. ×540.

This transverse section of cardiac muscle is a higher magnification of the previous image. Observe the presence of the centrally positioned **nucleus** (N) in each cell as well as the rich **vascular supply** (BV) of cardiac muscle. The *arrow* points to a region of the cell near either end of the nucleus that, in the live cell, was occupied by organelles as well as by a glycogen deposit.

KEY					
BV	blood (vascular) supply	**N**	nucleus	**Sa**	sarcoplasm

Summary of Histologic Organization

I. SKELETAL MUSCLE

A. Longitudinal Section

1. Connective Tissue Elements

Connective tissue elements of perimysium contain nerves, blood vessels, collagen, fibroblasts, and occasionally other cell types. Endomysium is composed of fine reticular fibers and basal lamina, neither of which are normally evident with the light microscope.

2. Skeletal Muscle Cells

Skeletal muscle cells appear as long, parallel, cylindrical fibers of almost uniform diameter. Nuclei are numerous and peripherally located. Satellite cell nuclei may be evident. Cross-striations, A, I, and Z, should be clearly noted at higher magnifications, and with oil immersion (or even high dry), the H zone and M disk may be distinguished in good preparations.

B. Transverse Section

1. Connective Tissue Elements

Connective tissue elements may be noted, especially nuclei of fibroblasts, cross sections of capillaries, other small blood vessels, and nerves.

2. Skeletal Muscle Cells

Muscle cells appear as irregular polygon-shaped sections of fibers of more or less uniform size. Myofibrils present a stippled appearance inside the fiber, frequently clustered into distinct but artifactual groups known as Cohnheim's fields. Peripherally, a nucleus or two may be noted in many fibers. Fasciculi are closely packed, but the delicate endomysium clearly outlines each cell.

II. CARDIAC MUSCLE

A. Longitudinal Section

1. Connective Tissue Elements

Connective tissue elements are clearly identifiable because of the presence of nuclei that are considerably smaller than those of cardiac muscle cells. The connective tissue is rich in vascular components, especially capillaries. The endomysium is present but indistinct.

2. Cardiac Muscle Cells

Cardiac muscle cells form long, branching, and anastomosing muscle fibers. Bluntly oval nuclei are large, are centrally located within the cell, and appear somewhat vesicular. A and I bands are present but are not as clearly defined as in skeletal muscle. Intercalated disks, marking the boundaries of contiguous cardiac muscle cells, may be indistinct unless special staining techniques are used. Purkinje fibers are occasionally evident.

B. Transverse Section

1. Connective Tissue Elements

Connective tissue elements separating muscle fibers from each other are obvious because nuclei of these cells are much smaller than those of cardiac muscle cells.

2. Cardiac Muscle Cells

Cross-sectional profiles of muscle fibers are irregularly shaped and vary in size. Nuclei are infrequent but are large and located in the center of the cell. Myofibrils are clumped as Cohnheim's fields (an artifact of fixation) in a radial arrangement. Occasionally, Purkinje fibers are noted, but they are present only in the subendocardium of the ventricles.

III. SMOOTH MUSCLE

A. Longitudinal Section

1. Connective Tissue Elements

Connective tissue elements between individual muscle fibers are scant and consist of fine reticular fibers. Larger bundles or sheets of muscle fibers are separated by loose connective tissue housing blood vessels and nerves.

2. Smooth Muscle Cells

Smooth muscle cells are tightly packed, staggered, fusiform structures, whose centrally located nuclei are oblong in shape. When the muscle fibers contract, their nuclei assume a characteristic corkscrew shape.

B. Transverse Section

1. Connective Tissue Elements

A very limited amount of connective tissue, mostly reticular fibers, may be noted in the intercellular spaces. Sheets and bundles of smooth muscle are separated from each other by loose connective tissue in which neurovascular elements are evident.

2. Smooth Muscle Cells

Because smooth muscle cells are tightly packed, staggered, fusiform structures, transverse sections produce circular, homogeneous-appearing profiles of various diameters. Only the widest profiles contain nuclei; therefore, in transverse section, only a limited number of nuclei will be present.

Chapter Review Questions

7-1. Which ultrastructure is unique to skeletal muscle cells and distinguishes it from the cardiac muscle cells?

A. Dyads

B. Triads

C. Calmodulin

D. Caveolae

E. Desmin

7-2. A patient presented with several firm, painful, yellowish nodules, each approximately 1 cm in diameter, in the dermis of her arm. The histopathology revealed spindle-shaped cells that appeared to criss-cross each other. Which of the following is the possible diagnosis?

A. Lipoma

B. Rhabdomyosarcoma

C. Leiomyoma

D. Fibrosarcoma

E. Leiomyosarcoma

7-3. A 2-year-old child succumbed to a glycogen storage disease. Which of the following is the possible disease that caused the child's death?

A. Duchenne muscular dystrophy

B. Myasthenia gravis

C. Rhabdomyosarcoma

D. Leiomyoma

E. Pompe's disease

7-4. Which of the following is considered a characteristic of myasthenia gravis?

A. It weakens visceral smooth muscles.

B. Antibodies are formed against acetylcholine.

C. Antibodies are formed against acetylcholine receptors.

D. It interferes with calmodulin.

E. It prevents the formation of intercalated disks.

7-5. During skeletal muscle contraction which of the following remains the same width as in the relaxed muscle?

A. I band

B. A band

C. H band

D. Sarcomere

E. Intercalated disk

CHAPTER

8

NERVOUS TISSUE

CHAPTER OUTLINE

Nervous System

More than a trillion **neurons** and perhaps 10 times as many supporting **neuroglia** constitute the nervous tissue, one of the four basic tissues of the body. In nervous tissue, the abundant neuroglia and numerous neuronal processes, collectively called the **neuropil**, form most of the structural framework instead of connective tissue fibers, as elsewhere. Nervous tissue specializes in receiving information from the external and internal milieu. The incoming information is processed, integrated, and compared with stored experiences and/or predetermined (reflex) responses, to select and effect an appropriate reaction.

Anatomically, the nervous system is divided into the central nervous system (CNS) and the peripheral nervous system (PNS).

- The **CNS**, comprising the brain and spinal cord, integrates and analyzes information that it receives and responds to it appropriately.

- The **PNS**, comprising the nerve roots, rami, nerves, and ganglia, transmits sensory information to the CNS and relays the response to the effector organ.

Because sensory and motor neurons extend into and from the CNS, the PNS is merely a physical extension of the CNS, and the separation of the two should not imply a strict dichotomy.

The nervous system may also be divided functionally into somatic and autonomic nervous systems (ANS).

- The **somatic nervous system** exercises conscious control over voluntary functions.

- The **ANS** controls involuntary functions. It regulates the motor functions of smooth muscles, cardiac muscles, and some glands. Its three components, sympathetic, parasympathetic, and enteric nervous systems, usually act in concert to maintain homeostasis.
    - The **sympathetic nervous system** prepares the body for action as in a "fight or flight or freeze" mode.
    - The **parasympathetic system** functions to calm the body and provides secretomotor innervation to most exocrine glands.
    - The **enteric nervous system** is more or less a stand-alone system responsible for the process of digestion. Interestingly, the ENS is very large; it has about the same number of neurons as does the spinal cord. Its actions are modulated by the sympathetic and parasympathetic components of the ANS.

The CNS is protected by a bony housing, consisting of the skull and vertebral column, as well as by the **meninges**, a triple-layered connective tissue sheath (Fig. 8-1).

- The outermost meninx is the thick fibrous **dura mater**.

- Deep to the dura mater is the **arachnoid**, a thin avascular connective tissue membrane.

- The innermost vascular **pia mater** is the most intimate and delicate investment of the CNS.

- The space between the arachnoid and the pia mater, the subarachnoid space, is filled with **cerebrospinal fluid (CSF)**.

Neurons

The structural and functional unit of the nervous system is the **neuron**. These morphologically complex and highly specialized cells perform two major functions: irritability and conductivity. Each neuron is composed of a **cell body (soma, perikaryon)** and processes of varying lengths, known as **axons** and **dendrites**, usually located on opposite sides of the cell body (Fig. 8-2A).

- A typical neuron has a single **axon** that transmits information away from the cell body, but it usually has numerous **dendrites** that receive excitatory and inhibitory stimuli from other neurons.

- The neuron cell body is large with euchromatic nuclei containing a punctate nucleolus or two, well-defined Golgi bodies and an abundance of rough endoplasmic reticulum (rER) in the cytoplasm, which appear as basophilic aggregates called **Nissl bodies** when stained by hematoxylin and eosin (H&E). The rich presence of these organelles indicates vigorous translation activities involved in the production of neurotransmitters and/or neuromodulators (Fig. 8-2B).

- The incoming stimuli from the dendrites travel through the cell membrane of the soma and are summated at the **axon hillock**, the region of the cell body from which the axon originates.

- When the summated stimuli are excitatory, the action potential travels down the length of the axon membrane to the **axon terminal**, which forms branches and synapses with other neurons or effector organs. The core of the axon houses numerous microtubules, which, along with dynein and kinesin, are essential in intracellular transport of vesicles between the cell body and the axon terminals. Axons can be quite long, and, in the case of some motor neurons, the portion of the axon residing in the CNS is myelinated by oligodendrocytes, whereas the remainder may extend into the PNS where it is myelinated by Schwann cells.

Morphologically, neurons may be categorized into three types, depending on the total number of processes emanating from the cell body:

- **Unipolar (pseudounipolar)** neurons have a single, short process emerging from the cell body that divides into distal and proximal branches. The proximal branches project to the CNS, whereas distal branches travel with nerves to reach sensory organs in the body. Most unipolar neuron cell bodies reside in ganglia throughout the body (Fig. 8-3A).

- **Bipolar** neurons have two cellular processes from the cell body, an axon, and one dendrite. These types of neurons are limited to neural networks transmitting

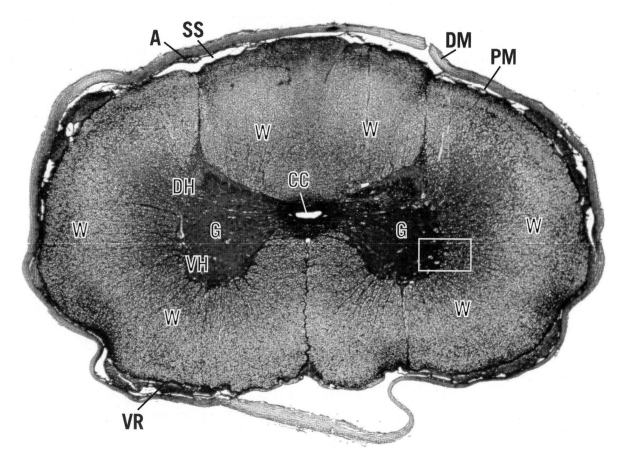

FIGURE 8-1. Spinal cord. x.s. Cat. Silver stain. Paraffin section. ×21.

The spinal cord is invested by a protective coating, the three-layered meninges. Its outermost fibrous layer, the **dura mater** (DM), is surrounded by epidural fat, not present in this photomicrograph. Deep to the dura is the **arachnoid** (A) with its **subarachnoid space** (SS), which is closely applied to the most intimate layer of the meninges, the vascular **pia mater** (PM). The spinal cord itself is organized into **white matter** (W) and **gray matter** (G). The former, which is peripherally located and does not contain nerve cell bodies, is composed of axons, most of which are myelinated, that travel up and down the cord. The centrally positioned gray matter contains the cell bodies of the neurons, dendrites as well as the initial and terminal ends of their axons, many of which are not usually myelinated. The dendrites and axons, along with processes of the numerous glial cells form an intertwined network of structural framework that is referred to as the neuropil. The gray matter is subdivided into regions, namely, the **dorsal horn** (DH), the **ventral horn** (VH), and the gray commissure. The **central canal** (CC) of the spinal cord passes through the gray commissure, dividing it into dorsal and ventral components. Processes of neurons leave and enter the spinal cord as **ventral roots** (VR) and dorsal roots, respectively.

special sensory information such as vision, taste, smell, and hearing (Fig. 8-3B).

- **Multipolar** neurons are the most common type of neurons that possess one axon and numerous dendrites (see Fig. 8-2A).

Neurons also may be classified according to their function:

- **Sensory neurons** receive stimuli from either the internal or external environment and then transmit these impulses toward the CNS for processing. Unipolar and bipolar neurons generally provide sensory functions.

- **Interneurons** act as connectors between neurons in a chain or typically between sensory and motor neurons within the CNS. Interneurons tend to be multipolar

neurons and usually possess axons shorter than those of motor neurons.

- **Motor neurons** conduct impulses from the CNS to the target cells (muscles, glands, and other neurons). Motor neurons are almost always multipolar in morphology and possess long axons and numerous axon terminals.

Synapses

Information is transferred from one neuron to another across an intercellular space or gap, the **synapse** (Fig. 8-4). Depending on the regions of the neurons participating in the formation of the synapse, it could be axodendritic, axosomatic, axoaxonic, or dendrodendritic.

Most synapses are axodendritic and involve one of many **neurotransmitter substances** (such as

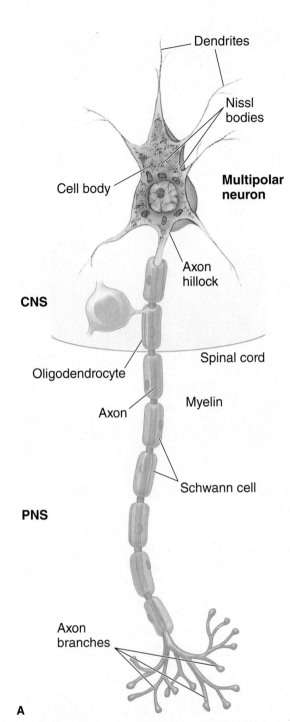

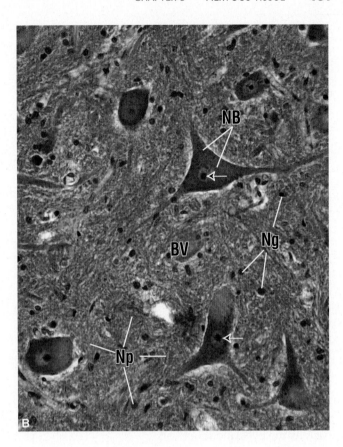

FIGURE 8-2. **A**. Multipolar neuron with numerous dendrites and a long axon demonstrates the large soma with its Nissl bodies and euchromatic nucleus with distinct nucleolus. Although the cell body, dendrites, and a portion of the axon may reside in the CNS, the remainder of the axon may exit the CNS and become a part of a nerve fiber nerve in the PNS. The axon is myelinated by oligodendrocytes in the CNS and by Schwann cells in the PNS. **B**. Spinal cord. x.s. Gray matter. Human. Paraffin section. ×270. Large cell bodies of multipolar neurons, each with its large **nucleolus** (*arrow*) and the clearly visible **Nissl bodies** (NB), are evident as are the cellular processes emanating from them. **Blood vessels** (BV) and nuclei of **neuroglia cells** (Ng) are observed. The fibrous network comprising the **neuropil** (Np) is well demonstrated.

acetylcholine [ACh]) that are released by the axon of the first (presynaptic) neuron into the synaptic cleft. When the neurotransmitter binds the receptors on the second (postsynaptic) neuron's dendrites, it momentarily destabilizes the plasma membrane, and a wave of depolarization passes along the plasma membrane of the second neuron, which can trigger the release of a neurotransmitter substance at the terminus of its axon. At this point, the second neuron is now the presynaptic neuron, and the cell it synapses with is now the

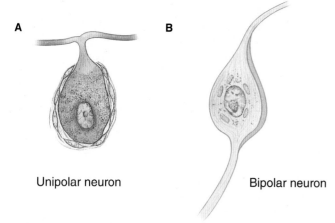

A

B

Unipolar neuron

Bipolar neuron

FIGURE 8-3. A. The unipolar neuron has one short process extending from the cell body, which then branches into proximal and distal branches. These types of neurons generally relay somatosensory information to the CNS, and the cell bodies reside in the dorsal root ganglia as well as in the sensory ganglia of cranial nerves. **B.** Bipolar neurons have two cellular projections extending from the cell body, one serving as a dendrite and the other as an axon. Bipolar neurons relay specialized sensory information to the CNS, and the cell bodies are found in the ganglia near the special sensory organs such as the eyes and inner ears.

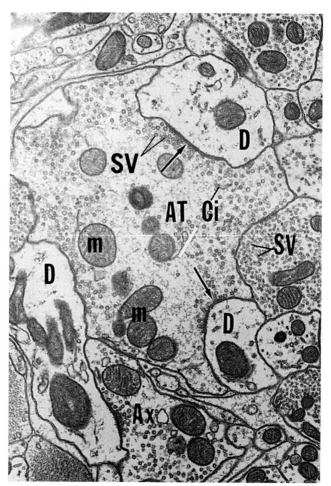

FIGURE 8-4. Synapse. Afferent terminals. Electron microscopy. ×16,200.

The **axon terminal** (AT) is forming multiple synapses with **dendrites** (D) and **axons** (Ax). Observe the presence of **synaptic vesicles** (SV) in the pre- and postsynaptic axon terminals as well as the thickening of the membrane of the presynaptic axon terminal (*arrows*). This terminal also houses **mitochondria** (m) and **cisternae** (Ci) for the synaptic vesicles. (From Meszler RM. Fine structure and organization of the infrared receptor relays: lateral descending nucleus of V in Boidae and nucleus reticularis caloris in the rattlesnake. *J Comp Neurol* 1983;220(3):299–309. Copyright © 1983 Wiley-Liss, Inc. Reprinted by permission of John Wiley & Sons, Inc.)

postsynaptic neuron. This type of chemical synapse is an **excitatory synapse**, which results in the transmission of an impulse.

Another type of synapse may stop the transmission of an impulse by stabilizing the plasma membrane of the second neuron and is called an **inhibitory synapse**.

Neuroglia

Neuroglial cells function in the metabolism and the support of neurons. To prevent spontaneous or accidental depolarization of the neuron's cell membrane, specialized neuroglial cells provide a physical covering over its entire surface. There are four types of neuroglial cells in the CNS:

- **Astrocytes** are the most numerous and contribute to the neuropil with many cellular extensions. They provide physical and microenvironmental support to the neurons and support the blood–brain barrier. In H&E stain, astrocytes can be recognized by the nuclear staining pattern, which exhibits a mixture of heterochromatin and euchromatin that some describe as the "salt-and-pepper" pattern. The cytoplasmic boundaries cannot be observed because of the elaborate cell projections (Fig. 8-5A).

- **Oligodendrocytes** have many cytoplasmic extensions, each of which wraps around a segment of a

different axon. These segments of the axon are known as internodes. A single oligodendrocyte can provide myelination for internodes of as many as 50 axons. Oligodendrocytes can be identified in H&E stain by their smaller and mostly heterochromatic nuclei (see Fig. 8-5A).

- **Microglia**, macrophages derived from monocytes, may be recognized by their spindle-shaped nuclei (Fig. 8-5B).

- **Ependymal cells** are the cuboidal cells lining the ventricles of the brain and the central canal of the spinal

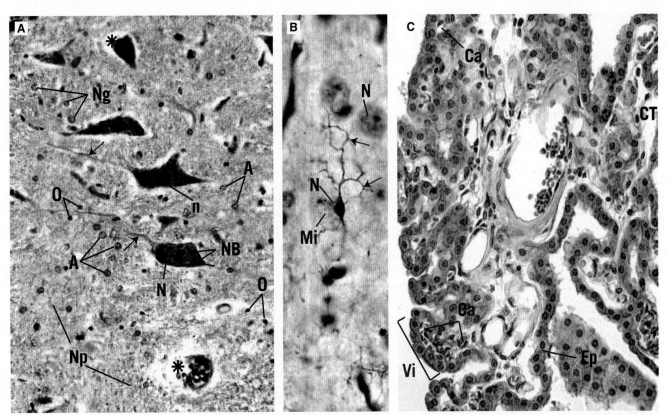

FIGURE 8-5. Glial cells in the CNS. **A**. Spinal cord. x.s. Ventral horn. Human. Paraffin section. ×270. In addition to the large multipolar neuron cell bodies and their various processes (*arrows*), two types of glial cells can be identified by their nuclear features. Small round nuclei with a mixture of euchromatin and heterochromatin belong to **astrocytes** (A) and smaller, heterochromatic nuclei belong to **oligodendrocytes** (O). In the cell bodies of neurons, note the large **nucleus** (N) and dense **nucleolus** (n), and the cytoplasmic clumps of basophilic material called **Nissl bodies** (NB). The dendrites, axons, and processes of the neuroglia compose the **neuropil** (Np), the structural framework of neural tissues. The white spaces (*asterisks*) surrounding the soma and blood vessels are caused by shrinkage artifacts. **B**. Microglia. Silver stain. Paraffin section. ×540. This photomicrograph is of a section of the cerebral cortex, demonstrating **nuclei** (N) of nerve cells as well as the **microglia** (Mi). Microglia are CNS-residing macrophages, derived from monocytes. They are small and possess a dense, sometimes fusiform **nucleus** (N) as well as numerous cell processes (*arrows*). **C**. Choroid plexus. Paraffin section. ×270. The choroid plexus, located within the ventricles of the brain, is composed of **capillary** (Ca)-rich **connective tissue** (CT) **villi** (Vi), lined by the cuboidal **ependymal cells** (Ep). The clear spaces surrounding the choroid plexus belong to the ventricle of the brain.

CLINICAL CONSIDERATIONS 8-1

Neuroglial Tumors

Almost 50% of the intracranial tumors are caused by proliferation of neuroglial cells. Some of the **neuroglial tumors**, such as oligodendroglioma, are of mild severity, whereas others, such as glioblastoma that are neoplastic cells derived from astrocytes, are highly invasive and usually fatal.

CLINICAL CONSIDERATIONS 8-2

Huntington Chorea

Huntington's chorea is a hereditary condition that becomes evident in the third and fourth decades of life. Initially, this condition affects only the joints but later is responsible for motor dysfunction and dementia. It is thought to be caused by the loss of neurons of the CNS that produce the neurotransmitter **GABA** (γ-aminobutyric acid). The advent of dementia is thought to be related to the loss of ACh-secreting cells.

CLINICAL CONSIDERATIONS 8-3

Parkinson's Disease

Parkinson's disease is related to the loss of the neurotransmitter **dopamine** in the brain. This crippling

disease causes muscular rigidity, tremor, slow movement, and progressively difficult voluntary movement.

CLINICAL CONSIDERATIONS 8-4

Axon Injury

When an axon is injured and severed, several changes occur. The region of the axon distal to the injury degenerates and their associated Schwann cells disassemble to permit macrophages to clear the axonal debris. After the removal of the axonal debris, Schwann cells reassemble and form a solid cellular column, extending from the site of the injury to the effector organ. As this is occurring, the cell body of the injured neuron becomes edematous, Nissl bodies disassemble (a process known as **chromatolysis**) and the

nucleus is displaced to the periphery. The cut end of the axon proximal to the site of injury forms branches, and, if one of these branches penetrates the Schwann cell column, it grows down the length of the column to the effector organ. If none of the axon branches establish contact with the Schwann cell column, or if the Schwann cell column does not form, the neural connection to the effector organ is permanently lost. In such a case, effector organs such as skeletal muscles atrophy in the absence of neural impulse, but they remain alive while they have an intact vascular supply.

cord. In the ventricles, ependymal cells form a part of the **choroid plexus** that produces **CSF** (Fig. 8-5C).

There are two types of neuroglial cells in the PNS:

- **Satellite** cells are limited to the areas in the PNS, called **ganglia**, where neuron cell bodies are present as a collection. Satellite cells surround the neuron cell body and perform similar roles as the astrocytes in the CNS (Fig. 8-6A).

- **Schwann cells** myelinate axons in the PNS. Although oligodendrocytes in the CNS can myelinate internodes of multiple axons by sending out several cell extensions, a Schwann cell can myelinate an internode of just one axon, as the entire cell wraps around an axon segment (Fig. 8-6B).

The region where the myelin sheath of one Schwann cell or oligodendrocyte ends and the next one begins is referred to as the **node of Ranvier**.

Histologic Basis for Neuroanatomy

Macroscopically, the CNS is organized into **gray matter** and **white matter** based on the relative color of the brain and the spinal cord when cut in cross sections (Fig. 8-7; also see Fig. 8-1). Histologically, gray matter is where neuron cell bodies are concentrated, whereas white matter is where myelinated axons are abundant.

Myelin sheaths being repeated wrapping of oligodendrocyte plasmalemma, rich in phospholipid, appear white and glistening en masse. In the brain, gray matter is present in the outer layer, and it surrounds the white matter (inner layer) (see Fig. 8-7A); however, in the spinal cord, gray matter is the inner layer and is surrounded by white matter (outer layer), as shown in Figure 8-7B (also see Fig. 8-1).

In addition to the gray matter, several groups of neuron cell bodies are dispersed throughout the white matter of the brain, and each of these groups is called a **nucleus** with an additional specific name (e.g., nucleus ambiguus, superior olivary nucleus). A collection of axons traversing the white matter in the same direction in the CNS is called a **tract** (or **fasciculus** or **column**).

In the PNS, a collection of neuron cell bodies is called a **ganglion**, and a bundle of axons traveling together is called a **nerve (peripheral nerve)**. Ganglia are surrounded by dense irregular connective tissue capsules of various thicknesses, depending on locations in the body (Fig. 8-8).

The nerves are composed of a mixture of myelinated and nonmyelinated axons (Table 8-1) organized into fascicles (bundles), and several fascicles form a nerve (Fig. 8-9).

A nerve is supported by connective tissues organized into similar patterns as skeletal muscles:

- The **epineurium** is the dense irregular connective tissue surrounding a collection of fascicles that provides

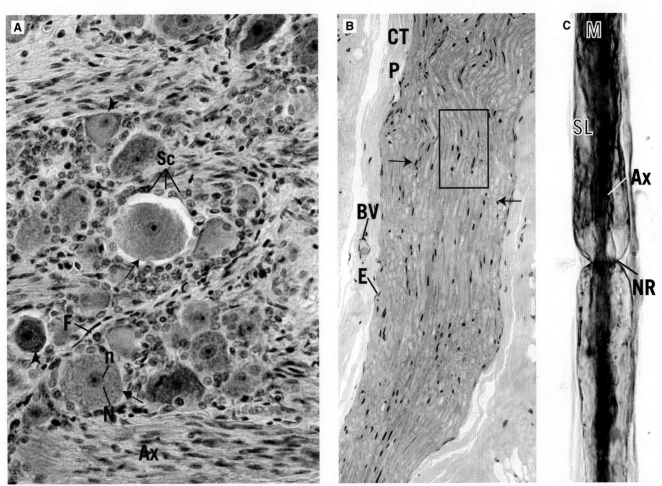

FIGURE 8-6. **A**. Sensory ganglion. l.s. Human. Paraffin section. ×270. The large spherical cell bodies with centrally located **nuclei** (N) and **nucleoli** (n) belong to the unipolar neurons. Observe that both small (*arrowheads*) and large (*arrows*) somata are present in the field and that the nuclei are not always in the plane of section. Surrounding the unipolar neuron somata are the small **satellite cells** (Sc) with clearly evident nuclei and cytoplasm. Moreover, the small, elongated, densely staining nuclei of **fibroblasts** (F) are also noted to surround somata, just peripheral to the satellite cells. Myelinated **axons** (Ax) in the vicinity belong to the unipolar neurons. **B**. Peripheral nerve. l.s. Monkey. Plastic section. ×132. The longitudinal section of the peripheral nerve fascicle is enveloped by a **connective tissue layer** (CT), the **perineurium** (P), which conducts small **blood vessels** (BV). The peripheral nerve is composed of numerous nonmyelinated and myelinated axons. The myelinated axons are surrounded by pale staining regions representing the myelinating Schwann cells. The dense nuclei (*arrows*) within the nerve fascicle belong to Schwann cells surrounded by endoneurium (E). **C**. Teased, myelinated nerve fiber. Paraffin section. l.s. ×540. This longitudinal segment of a single myelinated nerve fiber displays its **axon** (Ax) and the remnants of the dissolved **myelin** (M). Note the **node of Ranvier** (NR), a nonmyelinated region between two Schwann cells. Here, the axon membrane has a high concentration of Na$^+$/K$^+$ pumps, facilitating saltatory conduction of the action potential. Observe that **Schmidt-Lanterman incisures** (SL) are clearly evident. These are regions where the cytoplasm of Schwann cells is trapped in the myelin sheath.

CLINICAL CONSIDERATIONS 8-5

Guillain-Barré Syndrome

Guillain-Barré syndrome is a form of immune-mediated condition resulting in rapidly progressing weakness with possible paralysis of the extremities and, occasionally, even of the respiratory and facial muscles. This demyelinating disease is often associated with a recent respiratory or gastrointestinal infection; the muscle weakness reaches its greatest point within 3 weeks of the initial symptoms, and 5% of the afflicted individuals die of the disease. Early recognition of the disease is imperative for complete (or nearly complete) recovery.

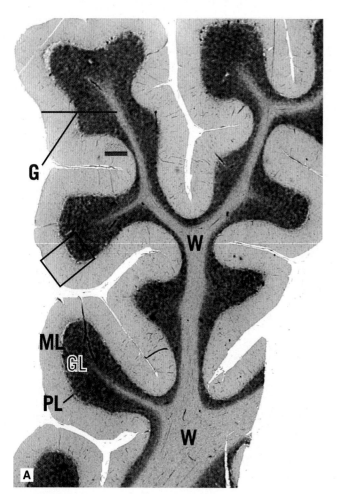

FIGURE 8-7A. Cerebellum. Human. Paraffin section. ×14.

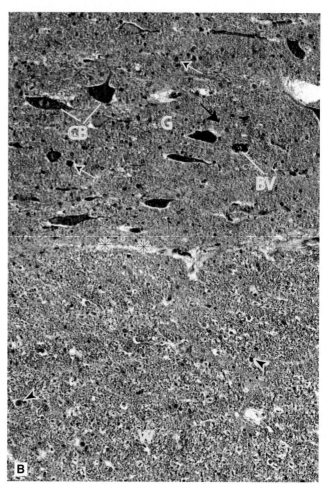

FIGURE 8-7B. Spinal cord. x.s. White and gray matter. Human. Paraffin section. ×132.

The cerebellum consists of a core of **white matter** (W) and superficially located **gray matter** (G). Although it is difficult to tell from this low-magnification photomicrograph, the gray matter is subdivided into three layers, the outer **molecular layer** (ML), a middle **Purkinje cell layer** (PL), and the inner **granular layer** (GL), each layer consisting of high concentration of cell bodies belonging to neurons of specialized morphologies and functions. The less-dense appearance of the molecular layer is because of the sparse arrangement of nerve cell bodies, whereas the darker appearance of the granular layer is a function of the great number of darkly staining nuclei packed closely together.

structural strength to the delicate neural tissue as well as conveying blood vessels to enter the neural tissue (see Fig. 8-9).

- Each fascicle within the epineurium is surrounded by a **perineurium** consisting of an outer connective tissue layer and an inner layer of flattened epithelioid cells.

- Each nerve fiber and associated Schwann cell has its own slender connective tissue sheath, the **endoneurium**, whose components include fibroblasts, an occasional macrophage, and type I and type III collagen fibers (reticular fibers).

Here, the interface between the outer **white matter** (W) and a core of **gray matter** (G) is readily evident (*asterisks*). The numerous nuclei (*arrowheads*) present in white matter belong to the various neuroglia, which supports the axons traveling up and down the spinal cord. The large neuron **cell bodies** (CB) in the gray matter possess euchromatic nuclei with dense, dark nucleoli. **Blood vessels** (BV), which penetrate deep into the gray matter, are surrounded by processes of neuroglial cells, forming the blood–brain barrier, not visible in this photomicrograph. Small nuclei (*arrows*) in gray matter belong to the neuroglial cells, whose cytoplasm and cellular processes are not evident.

Membrane Resting Potential

The normal concentration of K^+ is about 20 times greater inside the cell than outside, whereas the concentration of Na^+ is 10 times greater outside the cell than inside. Along with minor contributions from other charged ions, there is an electrical charge difference (**potential difference**) across the neuron cell membrane. This difference is maintained by the presence of **potassium leak channels** in the plasmalemma.

- These potassium leak channels are always open, and it is through these channels that K^+ ions diffuse from

CLINICAL CONSIDERATIONS 8-6

Ischemic Injury

Ischemia, the reduction of blood supply to an organ, such as the brain, results in hypoxia and subsequent cell death. The cause of ischemia could be blockage of a blood vessel that serves the area or of another vessel farther away whose responsibility is to supply blood flow to the vessels in question. Other causes of diminished blood supply could be lowered blood pressure, cardiac insufficiency, accidental injury to a vessel, and myriad other factors. Ischemia in the brain is evidenced by the presence of necrotic neurons (different from apoptotic neurons) whose cytoplasm displays a high degree of eosinophilia. These necrotic neurons are known as red neurons.

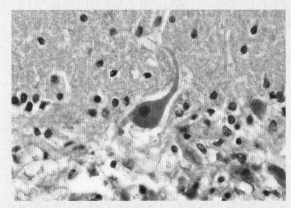

This Purkinje cell from the cerebellum of a patient displays a high degree of eosinophilia and is considered a red neuron. The presence of such cells indicates that the patient had an ischemic injury of a region of the cerebellum. Note that the cell is reduced in size, its nucleus is pyknotic, and the nucleolus is not evident. If this cell had died because of an apoptotic event, its cytoplasm would be basophilic. (Reprinted with permission from Mills SE, ed. *Histology for Pathologists*, 5th ed. Philadelphia: Wolters Kluwer, 2020. Figure 9-34.)

CLINICAL CONSIDERATIONS 8-7

Alzheimer's Disease

Alzheimer's disease (AD) is one of the most common forms of dementia that affects ~5 million people in the United States and more than 30 million people globally. This devastating condition begins, on average, around the age of 65 but may affect individuals at a much younger age. The early onset of AD is often masked as symptoms of stress or "senior moments"; however, it progresses to include the incapacity to remember newly acquired information. Additional symptoms develop as the disease continues its progress, namely, personality changes to a more hostile and petulant behavior accompanied by uncertainty and language difficulty. Moreover, the patient experiences an inability to remember previously known personal and general information, and the patient eventually becomes unable to take care of bodily functions, resulting in muscle loss and immobility. Individuals diagnosed with AD usually die within 7 to 10 years. Although the cause of the disease is not known, it has been suggested that the intraneuronal presence of neurofibrillary tangles, formed by coalescence of modified τ proteins, and the extracellular deposits of β-amyloid-like protein interfere with neuronal function.

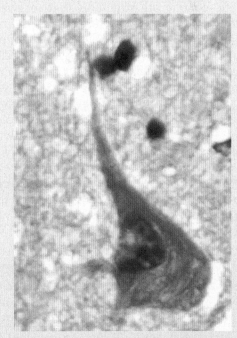

The neuron depicted in this photomicrograph is from a patient who died from AD. Note the presence of neurofibrillary tangles in its cytoplasm. (Reprinted with permission from Mills SE, et al., eds. *Sternberg's Diagnostic Surgical Pathology*, 6th ed. Philadelphia: Wolters Kluwer, 2015. p. 479, Figure 10-138A.)

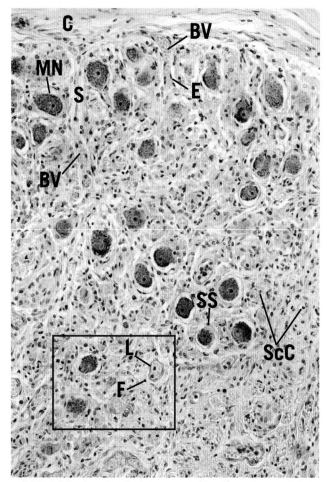

FIGURE 8-8. Sympathetic ganglion. l.s. Paraffin section. ×132.

Sympathetic ganglia are structures that receive axons of presynaptic cells, whose somata are within the CNS. Located within the ganglion are somata of postsynaptic neurons upon which the presynaptic cell axons synapse. These ganglia are enveloped by a dense irregular connective tissue **capsule** (C), which sends **septa** (S) containing **blood vessels** (BV) within the substance of the ganglion. The arrangement of the cell bodies of the **multipolar neurons** (MN) within the ganglion appears to be haphazard. This very vascular structure contains numerous nuclei that belong to **endothelial cells** (E), intravascular **leukocytes** (L), **fibroblasts** (F), **Schwann cells** (ScC), and those of the **supporting cells** (SS) surrounding the nerve cell bodies.

inside the cell to the outside (down the concentration gradient), thus establishing a **positive charge on the outer** aspect and a **negative (less positive) charge on the internal** aspect of the cell membrane, with a steady potential difference, known as the **resting potential**, of approximately -70 mV.

- Sodium leak channels also allow Na^+ ions to move into the cell, but at a 100-fold slower rate than the outward movement of K^+ ions caused by the much fewer number of these channels.

- Although most of the establishment of the resting membrane potential is because of the potassium leak channels, the action of the Na^+–K^+ **pumps** of the cell membrane, which pump these ions against the concentration gradient, also makes a minor contribution.

Action Potential

The **action potential** is electrical activity in which charges move along the membrane surface. It is an **all-or-none response**, whose duration and amplitude are constant. Some axons can sustain up to 1,000 impulses/sec.

- **Generation of an action potential** begins when a region of the plasma membrane is **depolarized**.

- As the resting potential diminishes, a **threshold level** is reached, voltage-gated Na^+ channels open, and Na^+ rushes into the cell. At that point, the **resting potential is reversed**, so that the inside of the membrane becomes positive with respect to the outside.

- In response to this reversal of the resting potential, the voltage-gated Na^+ channel closes and, for the next 1 to 2 msec, cannot be opened (the **refractory period**).

- The reason why these voltage-gated Na^+ channels cannot be opened immediately is that they have two gates, one on the extracellular opening, known as the **activation gate**, and the other on the intracellular opening, known as the **inactivation gate**. Both must be open for Na^+ ions to traverse it. The activation gate opens when the resting potential is disturbed and does not close while the cell membrane is depolarized. The inactivation gate also opens upon membrane depolarization; however, it closes within a few 10,000ths of a

Table 8-1	Nerve Fiber Classification and Conduction Velocities		
Fiber Group	**Diameter (μm)**	**Conduction Velocity (μ/s)**	**Function**
A fibers Thick myelin sheath	1–20	15–120	Motor: skeletal muscles Sensory: pain, touch, temperature, proprioception
B fibers Thin myelin sheath	1–3	3–15	Mostly visceral afferents; preganglionic autonomic fibers; pain fibers; pressure sensation
C fibers Nonmyelinated	0.5–1.5	0.5–2	Chronic pain fibers and postganglionic autonomic fibers

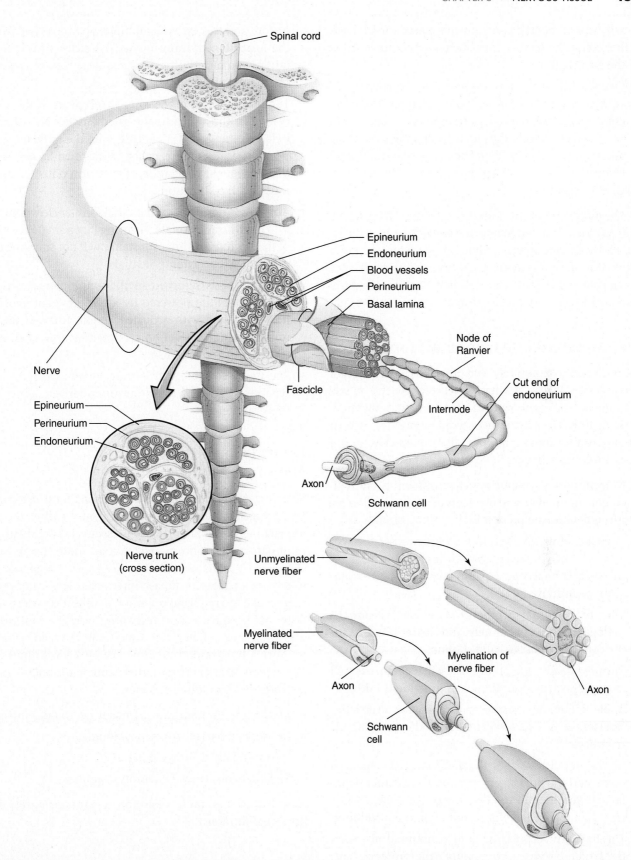

FIGURE 8-9. A nerve is a collection of myelinated and unmyelinated axons organized into fascicles outside the CNS. The nerve is supported structurally and metabolically by the connective tissue network, endoneurium around each axon and Schwann cell unit, perineurium surrounding each fascicle, and epineurium surrounding the entire nerve. The inset demonstrates the difference between the myelinated and unmyelinated axons. Although unmyelinated axons do not have oligodendrocyte (within the CNS) or Schwann cell wrappings (outside the CNS), they are surrounded and supported by these neuroglial cells' membrane infoldings.

second after opening and remains closed for ~2 msec, impeding the further movement of Na^+ ions across the Na^+ channel.

- Depolarization also causes the **opening** of voltage-gated K^+ channels (note that these are different from the potassium leak channels) through which K^+ ions exit the cell, thus repolarizing the membrane and ending not only the refractory period of the Na^+ channel but also causing the closure of the voltage-gated K^+ channel.

The movement of Na^+ ions that enter the cell causes depolarization of the cell membrane toward the axon terminal (**orthodromic spread**). Although Na^+ ions also move away from the axon terminal (**antidromic spread**), they are unable to affect Na^+ channels in the antidromic direction because those channels are in their refractory period.

Neuromuscular (Myoneural) Junction

Neurons also communicate with other effector cells at synapses. A special type of synapse, between skeletal muscle cells and neurons, is known as a **neuromuscular (myoneural) junction**. The axon forms a terminal swelling, known as the **axon terminal (end-foot)** that comes close to but does not contact the muscle cell's sarcolemma (Fig. 8-10).

- Mitochondria, synaptic vesicles containing the neurotransmitter ACh, and elements of smooth endoplasmic reticulum are present in the axon terminal.

- The axolemma involved in the formation of the synapse is known as the **presynaptic membrane**, whereas the sarcolemmal counterpart is known as the **postsynaptic membrane**.

- The presynaptic membrane has Na^+ **channels**, **voltage-gated Ca^+ channels**, and **carrier proteins** for the cotransport of Na^+ and choline.

- The postsynaptic membrane has **ACh receptors** as well as slight invaginations known as **junctional folds**.

- A basal lamina containing the enzyme **acetylcholinesterase** is also associated with the postsynaptic membrane.

- As the impulse reaches the end-foot, Na^+ channels open, and the presynaptic membrane becomes depolarized, resulting in the opening of the voltage-gated Ca^+ channels and the influx of Ca^+ into the end-foot.

- The high intracellular calcium concentration causes the synaptic vesicles, containing **ACh**, proteoglycans, and adenosine triphosphate (ATP), to fuse with the presynaptic membrane and release their contents into the synaptic cleft.

- After the contents of the synaptic vesicle are released, the presynaptic membrane is larger than prior to fusion, and this excess membrane will be recycled via the formation of clathrin-coated vesicles, thus maintaining the morphology and requisite surface area of the presynaptic membrane.

- The released ACh binds to **ACh receptors** of the sarcolemma, thus opening the sarcolemma's Na^+ **channels**, resulting in Ca^+ influx into the muscle cell, depolarization of the postsynaptic membrane, and the subsequent generation of an action potential and muscle cell contraction.

- **Acetylcholinesterase** of the basal lamina cleaves ACh into **choline** and acetate, ensuring that a single release of the neurotransmitter substance will not continue to generate excess action potentials.

- The choline is returned to the end-foot via carrier proteins that are powered by a Na^+ gradient, where it is combined with activated acetate (derived from mitochondria), a reaction catalyzed by **acetylcholine transferase**, to form ACh.

- The newly formed ACh is transported into forming synaptic vesicles by a proton pump–driven, antiport carrier protein.

Neurotransmitters and Neuromodulators

Signaling molecules released by neurons form two major categories: **neurotransmitters** that act directly on ion channels (and are **primary messengers**) and **neuromodulators** (neurohormones) that act indirectly on ion channels by utilizing **second messenger systems** (via G protein or receptor kinase intermediaries). Although both evoke the requisite response, neurotransmitters act faster but produce a short response (usually in millisecond durations), whereas neuromodulators act slower but produce a long response (some lasting a few minutes). The at least 100 neurotransmitters and neuromodulators are classified into four categories:

- Small molecule transmitters (mostly neurotransmitters)
- Neuropeptides (mostly neuromodulators)
- Gases (mostly neuromodulators)
- Miscellaneous (mostly neurotransmitters)

A list of the most common neurotransmitters is presented in Table 8-2.

Blood–Brain Barrier

The selective barrier that exists between the neuronal tissue of the CNS and many blood-borne substances is termed the **blood–brain barrier**. This barrier is formed by the **fasciae occludentes** of contiguous endothelial

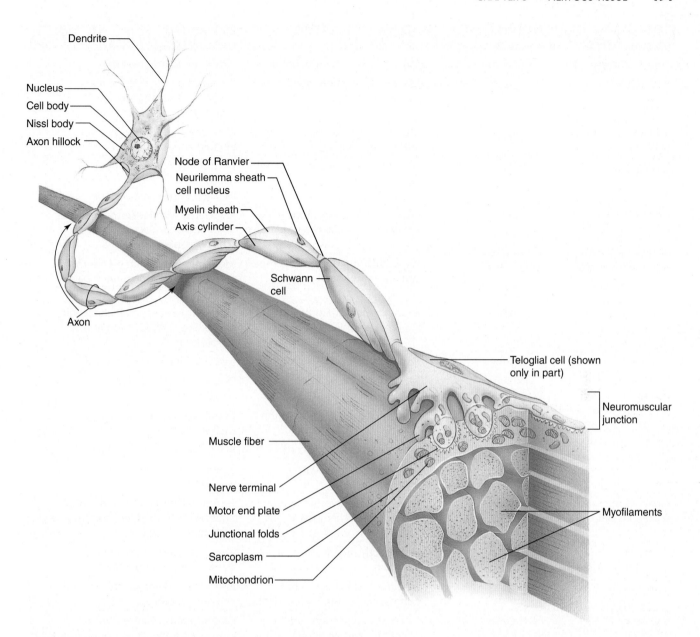

Dendrite

Nucleus

Cell body

Nissl body

Axon hillock

Node of Ranvier

Neurilemma sheath cell nucleus

Myelin sheath

Axis cylinder

Schwann cell

Axon

Teloglial cell (shown only in part)

Neuromuscular junction

Muscle fiber

Nerve terminal

Motor end plate

Junctional folds

Sarcoplasm

Mitochondrion

Myofilaments

FIGURE 8-10. A motor neuron has its cell body in the ventral horn of the gray matter in the spinal cord. A portion of the axon, myelinated by oligodendrocytes, travels through the cortex (outer layer) of the spinal cord, contributing to the white matter. Once the axon emerges from the spinal cord, it is myelinated by Schwann cells and becomes a part of the spinal nerve. The axon terminals form synapses with skeletal muscle fibers at the neuromuscular junction. When an action potential reaches the axon terminal, acetylcholine (ACh) neurotransmitters located in the synaptic vesicles are released into the synaptic cleft and bind to ACh receptors on the sarcolemma, initiating depolarization of the muscle cell membrane, and the impulse travels along the T tubules to trigger a contraction of the muscle cell.

cells lining the continuous capillaries that course through the neural tissues. Certain substances (i.e., O_2, H_2O, CO_2, and selected small lipid-soluble substances and some drugs) can penetrate the barrier, usually because of the presence of **aquaporins** of the endothelial cell plasma membranes. However, others, including glucose, certain vitamins, amino acids, and drugs, access passage only by **receptor-mediated transport** and/or via active transport-driven **carrier proteins**. Certain ions are also transported via **active transport**. It is also believed

that the basal lamina investing the capillary endothelium, pericytes, and the end-feet of perivascular neuroglia (**perivascular glia limitans**) may play roles in the maintenance of the barrier that regulates the transport of materials between the brain and its vascular supply. The combination of the blood–brain barrier, perivascular glia limitans, and pericytes has been referred to in the recent literature as the **neurovascular unit**, and it is this complex that regulates the movement of molecules between the CNS and the blood vessels that supply it.

Table 8-2	Alphabetical List of the Most Common Neurotransmitters and Their Function			
Neurotransmitter	**Major Function**	**Location in Nervous System**	**Additional Information**
Acetylcholine	Excitatory/inhibitory	Myoneural junction; autonomic nervous system; striatum	Removed by the enzyme acetyl-cholinesterase; cholinergic neurons degenerate in Alzheimer's disease
Adenosine triphosphate (ATP)	Excitatory	Motor neurons of the spinal cord; autonomic ganglia	Also coreleased with numerous neurotransmitters
β-Endorphin	Inhibitory	Hypothalamus; nucleus solitarius	Least numerous of the opioid neurotransmitter-containing cells; function in pain suppression
Dopamine	Excitatory	Neurons of the substantia nigra, arcuate nucleus, and tegmentum	Associated with Parkinson's disease; inhibition of prolactin release; schizophrenia
Dynorphin	Inhibitory	Hypothalamus; amygdala; limbic system	More numerous than β-endorphin–containing cells; function in pain suppression
Enkephalins	Inhibitory	Raphe nuclei; striatum; limbic system; cerebral cortex	More numerous than β-endorphin–containing cells; function in pain suppression
Epinephrine	Excitatory	Rostral medulla	Not commonly present in the CNS
γ-Aminobutyric acid (GABA)	Inhibitory	Mostly local circuit interneurons	Decreased GABA synthesis in vitamin B_6 deficiency
Glutamate	Excitatory	Most excitatory neurons of the CNS	Glutamate–glutamine cycle; excitotoxicity
Glycine	Inhibitory	Neurons of the spinal cord	Activity blocked by strychnine
Nitric oxide (NO)	Inhibitory	Cerebellum; hippocampus; olfactory bulb	Smooth muscle relaxant, thus strong vasodilator
Norepinephrine (noradrenaline)	Excitatory	Postganglionic sympathetic neurons; locus ceruleus	Associated with mood and mood disorders (mania, depression, anxiety, and panic)
Serotonin (5-hydroxytryptamine)	Excitatory	Pineal body; raphe nuclei of midbrain, pons, and medulla	Associated with sleep modulation; arousal, cognitive behaviors
Somatostatin	Inhibitory	Amygdala, small dorsal root ganglion cells, and hypothalamus	Also known as somatotropin release–inhibiting factor
Substance P	Excitatory	Dorsal root and trigeminal ganglia (C and Aδ fibers)	Composed of 11 amino acids; associated with transmission of pain

CNS, central nervous system.

CLINICAL CONSIDERATIONS 8-8

Therapeutic Circumvention of the Blood–Brain Barrier

The selective nature of the blood–brain barrier prevents certain therapeutic drugs and neurotransmitters conveyed by the bloodstream from entering the CNS. For example, the perfusion of mannitol into the bloodstream changes the capillary permeability by altering the tight junctions, thus permitting the administration of therapeutic drugs. Other therapeutic drugs can be attached to antibodies developed against transferrin receptors located on the luminal aspect of the plasma membranes of these endothelial cells that will permit transport into the CNS.

PLATE 8-1 Central Nervous System

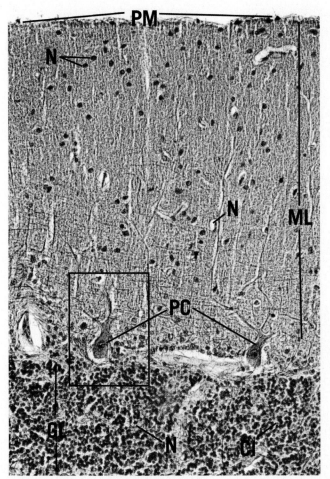

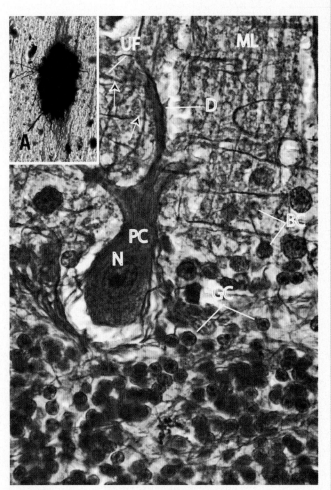

FIGURE 8-1-1. Cerebellum. Human. Paraffin section. ×132.

This is the cortex (gray matter) of the cerebellum with three distinctive layers. The **granular layer** (GL) is composed of closely packed **neurons** (Nr), which, at first glance, resemble lymphocytes owing to their dark, round nuclei. Interspersed among these cells are clear spaces where synapses occur between axons entering the cerebellum from outside and dendrites of granular layer cells. The **Purkinje cells** (PC) send their axons into the granular layer; their dendrites arborize in the **molecular layer** (ML). The ML contains unmyelinated fibers from the granular layer as well as two types of **neurons**. The surface of the cerebellum is invested by **pia mater** (PM), just barely evident in this photomicrograph. The *boxed area* is presented at a higher magnification in Figure 8-1-2.

FIGURE 8-1-2. Purkinje cell. Human cerebellum. Paraffin section. ×540.

This is a higher magnification of the *boxed area* of Figure 8-1-1. The **granular layer** (GL) of the cerebellum is composed of small neurons. The flask-shaped **Purkinje cell** (PC) displays its large **nucleus** (N) and **dendritic tree** (D). Nuclei of numerous basket cells (BC) of the **molecular layer** (ML) as well as the **unmyelinated fibers** (UF) of the granular layer cells are well defined in this photomicrograph. These fibers make synaptic contact (*arrows*) with the dendritic processes of the Purkinje cells. *Inset.* **Astrocyte. Human cerebellum. Golgi stain. Paraffin section.** ×132. Note the numerous processes of this **fibrous astrocyte** (A) in the white matter of the cerebellum.

KEY					
A	fibrous astrocyte	**ML**	molecular layer	**PM**	pia mater
D	dendrite	**N**	nucleus	**UF**	unmyelinated fiber
GL	granular layer	**PC**	Purkinje cell		

PLATE 8-2 | Cerebrum and Neuroglial Cells

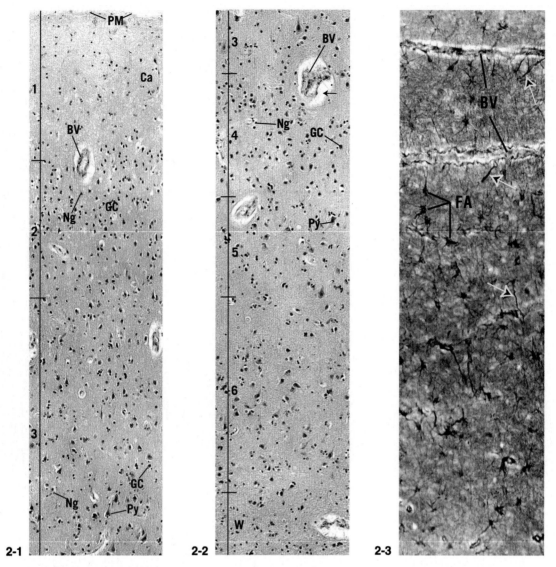

2-1 2-2 2-3

FIGURES 8-2-1 AND 8-2-2. Cerebrum. Human. Paraffin section. ×132.

FIGURE 8-2-3. Astrocytes. Silver stain. Paraffin section. ×132.

These figures represent a montage of the entire human cerebral cortex, the gray matter (1 to 6), and some of the underlying **white matter** (W) at low magnification. Observe that the numerous **blood vessels** (BV) that penetrate the entire cortex are surrounded by a clear area (*arrow*), which is because of shrinkage artifact. The cerebral cortex is comprised of six ill-defined layers approximated by brackets. These six layers are marked by different types of neuron cell bodies including those of pyramidal cells (Py) present. The neuropil is comprised of cellular processes from neurons as well as the **neuroglial cells** (Ng). The **pia mater** (PM), covering the surface of the cortex, is a vascular tissue that provides larger blood vessels as well as **capillaries** (Ca) that penetrate the brain tissue. The **white matter** (W) appears very cellular because of the nuclei of the numerous neuroglial cells supporting the cell processes derived from and traveling to the cortex. This photomicrograph of the white matter of the cerebrum presents a matted appearance owing to the interweaving of various neuronal and glial cell processes. Note also the presence of two **blood vessels** (BV) passing horizontally across the field. The long processes of the **fibrous astrocytes** (FA) approach the blood vessels (*arrows*).

KEY					
BV	blood vessel	**FA**	fibrous astrocyte	**W**	white matter
Ca	capillary	**PM**	pia mater		

PLATE 8-3 Sympathetic Ganglia and Sensory Ganglia

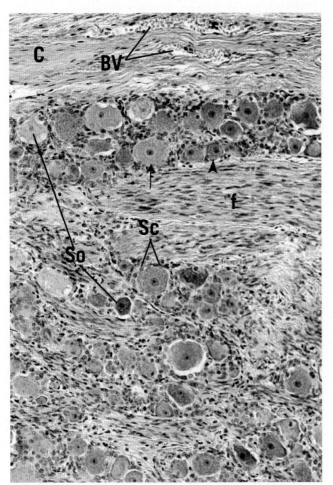

FIGURE 8-3-1. Dorsal root ganglion. l.s. Human. Paraffin section. ×132.

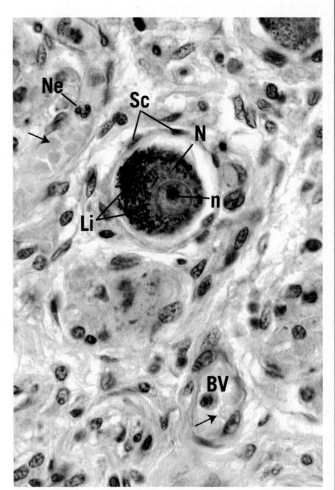

FIGURE 8-3-2. Sympathetic ganglion. l.s. Paraffin section. ×540.

A **vascular** (BV) connective tissue **capsule** (C) envelops the dorsal root ganglion. The neurons of the dorsal root ganglion are unipolar in morphology; therefore, their **somata** (So) appear spherical in shape. The **fibers** (f), many of which are myelinated, alternate with rows of cell bodies. Note that some somata are large (*arrow*), whereas others are small (*arrowhead*). Each soma is surrounded by neuroectodermally derived **satellite cells** (Sc).

Neurons of the sympathetic ganglion are multipolar, but their processes are not evident in this specimen stained with hematoxylin and eosin. The **nucleus** (N), with its prominent **nucleolus** (n), is clearly visible. The cytoplasm contains **lipofuscin** (Li), a yellowish pigment that is prevalent in neurons of older individuals. The clear space between the soma and the **satellite cells** (Sc) is a shrinkage artifact. Note the numerous **blood vessels** (BV) containing red blood cells (*arrows*) and a **neutrophil** (Ne).

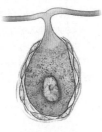

Unipolar cell (pseudounipolar cell from dorsal root ganglion)

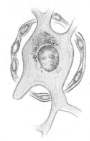

Multipolar cell (autonomic ganglia)

KEY					
BV	blood vessel	Li	lipofuscin	Ne	neutrophil
C	capsule	n	nucleolus	Sc	satellite cell
f	nerve fiber	N	nucleus	So	somata

PLATE 8-4   Peripheral Nerve

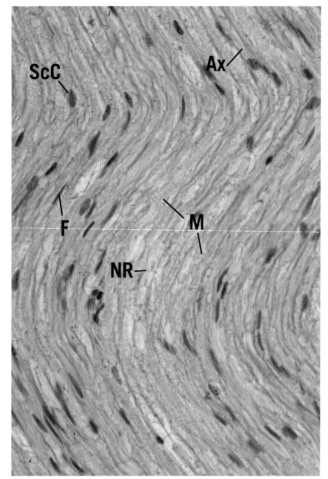

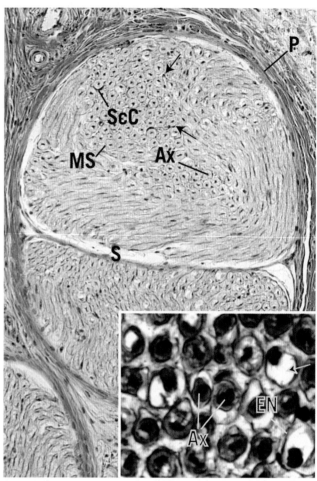

FIGURE 8-4-1. Peripheral nerve. l.s. Paraffin section. ×270.

FIGURE 8-4-2. Peripheral nerve. x.s. Paraffin section. ×132.

A distinguishing characteristic of longitudinal sections of peripheral nerves is that they appear to follow a zigzag course, particularly evident in this photomicrograph. The sinuous course of these fibers is accentuated by the presence of nuclei of **Schwann cells** (ScC), **fibroblasts** (F), and endothelial cells of capillaries belonging to the endoneurium. Many of these nerve fibers are **myelinated** (M) as corroborated by the presence of the **nodes of Ranvier** (NR) and myelin proteins around the **axons** (Ax).

This transverse section presents portions of two fascicles, each surrounded by **perineurium** (P). The intervening loose connective tissue of the epineurium with its blood vessels is clearly evident. The perineurium forms a **septum** (S), which subdivides this fascicle into two compartments. Note that the **axons** (Ax) are in the center of the **myelin sheath** (MS) and occasionally a crescent-shaped nucleus of a **Schwann cell** (ScC) is evident. The denser, smaller nuclei (*arrows*) belong to endoneurial cells. *Inset.* **Peripheral nerve. x.s. Silver stain. Paraffin section.** ×540. Silver-stained sections of myelinated nerve fibers have large, clear spaces (*arrow*) that indicate the dissolved myelin. The **axons** (Ax) stain well as dark, dense structures, and the delicate **endoneurium** (En) is also evident.

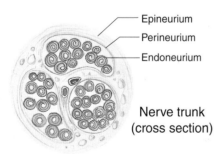

Epineurium

Perineurium

Endoneurium

Nerve trunk
(cross section)

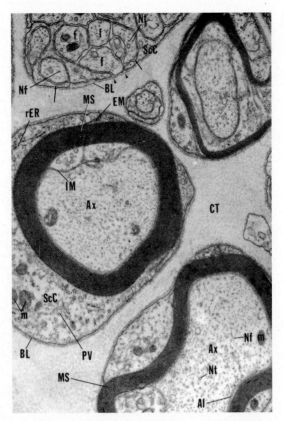

FIGURE 8-5-1. Peripheral nerve. x.s. Mouse. Electron microscopy. ×33,300.

This electron micrograph presents a cross section of three myelinated and several unmyelinated nerve fibers. Note that the **axons** (Ax) (although they may be the afferent fibers of pseudounipolar neurons) are surrounded by a thick **myelin sheath** (MS), peripheral to which is the bulk of the **Schwann cell cytoplasm** (ScC) housing **mitochondria** (m), **rough endoplasmic reticulum** (rER), and **pinocytotic vesicles** (PV). The Schwann cell is surrounded by a **basal lamina** (BL) isolating this cell from the **endoneurial connective tissue** (CT). The myelin sheath is derived from the plasma membrane of the Schwann cell, which presumably wraps spirally around the axon. The **axolemma** (Al) is separated from the Schwann cell membrane by a narrow cleft, the periaxonal space. The axoplasm houses **mitochondria** (m) as well as **neurofilaments** (Nf) and **neurotubules** (Nt). Occasionally, the myelin wrapping is surrounded by Schwann cell cytoplasm on its outer and inner aspects, as in the nerve fiber in the upper right-hand corner. The unmyelinated nerve **fibers** (f) at the top of this electron micrograph display their relationship to the **Schwann cell** (ScC). The fibers are positioned in such a fashion that each lies in a complicated membrane-lined groove within the Schwann cell. Some fibers are situated superficially, whereas others are positioned more deeply within the grooves. However, a periaxonal (or peridendritic) space (*arrows*) is always present. **Mitochondria** (m), **neurofilaments** (Nf), and **neurotubules** (Nt) are also present. Note that the entire structure is surrounded by a **basal lamina** (BL), which covers but does not extend into the grooves (*arrowheads*) housing the nerve fibers. (Courtesy of Dr. J. Strum.)

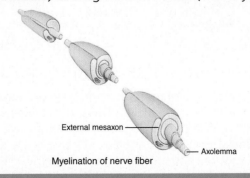

External mesaxon

Axolemma

Myelination of nerve fiber

KEY						
Al	axolemma	**f**	nerve fiber	**Nt**	neurotubule
Ax	axon	**m**	mitochondrion	**PV**	pinocytotic vesicle
BL	basal lamina	**MS**	myelin sheath	**rER**	rough ER
CT	endoneurial connective tissue	**Nf**	neurofilament	**ScC**	Schwann cell cytoplasm

PLATE 8-6   Neuron Cell Body, Electron Microscopy

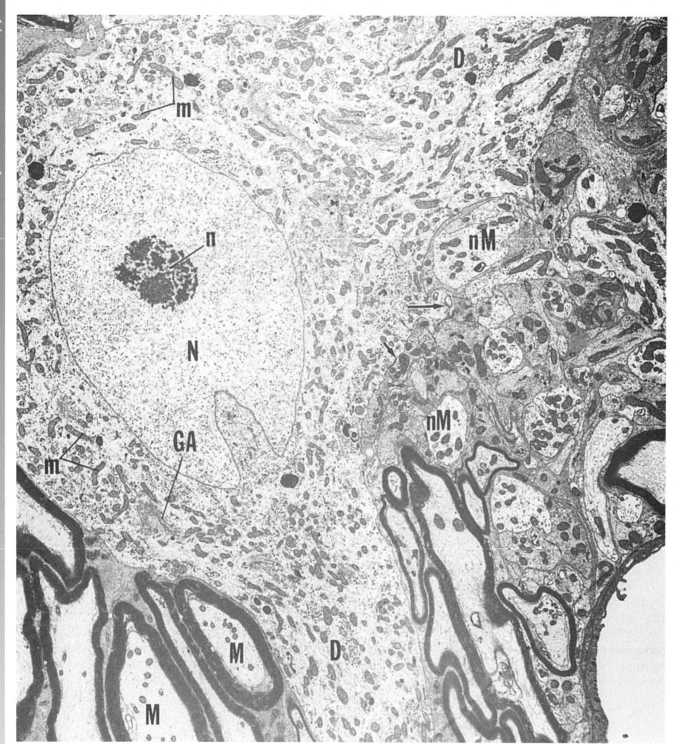

FIGURE 8-6-1. Neuron. Lateral descending nucleus. Electron microscopy. ×3,589.

The soma of this neuron presents a typical appearance. Note the large **nucleus** (N) and **nucleolus** (n) surrounded by a considerable amount of cytoplasm rich in organelles. Observe the extensive **Golgi apparatus** (GA), numerous **mitochondria** (m), and elements of rough endoplasmic reticulum, which extend into the **dendrites** (D). **Myelinated** (M) and **nonmyelinated** (nM) fibers are also present, as are synapses (*arrows*) along the cell surface. (From Meszler RM, et al. Fine structure and organization of the infrared receptor relay, the lateral descending nucleus of the trigeminal nerve in pit vipers. *J Comp Neurol* 1981;196(4):571–584. Copyright © 1981 Alan R. Liss, Inc. Reprinted by permission of John Wiley & Sons, Inc.)

KEY

D	dendrites	**M**	myelinated fibers	**N**	nucleus
Ga	Golgi apparatus	**n**	nucleolus	**nM**	nonmyelinated fibers
m	mitochondria				

Selected Review of Histologic Images

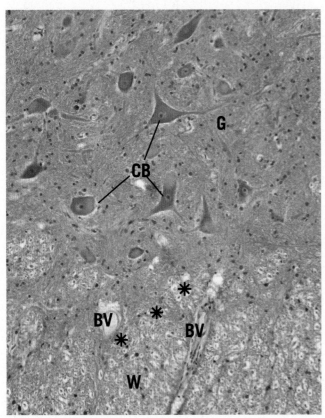

REVIEW FIGURE 8-1-1. Spinal cord. x.s. Gray and white matter. Human. Paraffin section. ×132.

Note the numerous multipolar neuron **cell bodies** (CB) that occupy the **gray matter** (G) of the spinal cord. The boundary between the gray matter and the **white matter** (W) is demarcated by the three *asterisks*. The rich **vascular supply** (BV) is clearly evident.

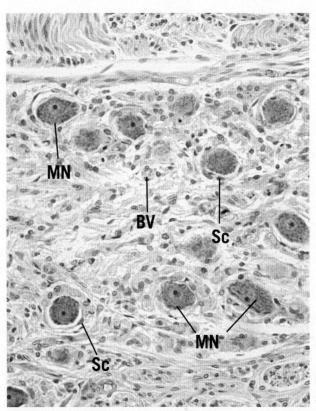

REVIEW FIGURE 8-1-2. Sympathetic ganglion. l.s. Human. Paraffin section. ×270.

Presynaptic axons from the lateral horns of the spinal cord enter the sympathetic ganglia to *synapse* there with the postganglionic sympathetic soma. The ganglia are encapsulated by a connective tissue that sends septa, carrying **blood vessels** (BV), into the ganglia. The cell bodies of these **multipolar neurons** (MN) are surrounded and protected by neuroectodermally derived **satellite cells** (Sc).

KEY					
BV	blood vessel (vascular supply)	**G**	gray matter	**Sc**	satellite cell
CB	cell body	**MN**	multipolar neuron	**W**	white matter

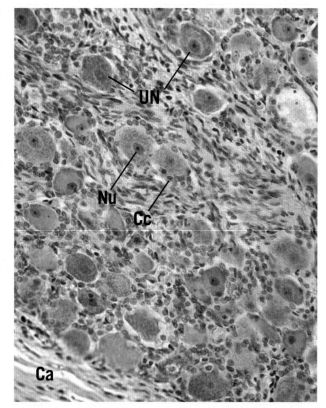

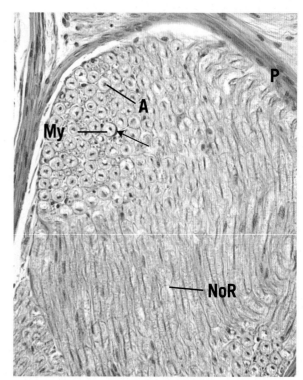

REVIEW FIGURE 8-2-1. Sensory ganglion (dorsal root ganglion). l.s. Human. Paraffin section. ×270.

Sensory ganglia are **encapsulated** (Ca) structures that house the cell bodies of **unipolar (pseudounipolar) neurons** (UN). Each soma, whose **nucleus** (Nu) and nucleolus are clearly evident, is surrounded by neuroectodermally derived **satellite cells** (Cc).

REVIEW FIGURE 8-2-2. Peripheral nerve xs and ls. Human. Paraffin section. ×270.

This transverse section of a nerve fiber is composed of several fascicles, each surrounded by its **perineurium** (P). Because of the way this particular fascicle was sectioned, some of its nerve fibers are cut in cross section (top left, bottom right, and bottom left), whereas the top right and central regions are sectioned longitudinally. Each fiber is surrounded by **Schwann cells** (*arrow* points to the nucleus of the cell). The center of the fiber houses the **axon** (A), which is surrounded by its **myelin sheath** (My). The longitudinally sectioned region of the fascicle displays the presence of **nodes of Ranvier** (NoR).

KEY					
A	axon	**NoR**	node of Ranvier	**Cc**	satellite cells
Ca	encapsulated structures	**Nu**	nucleus	**UN**	unipolar (pseudounipolar) neurons
My	myelin sheath	**P**	perineurium		

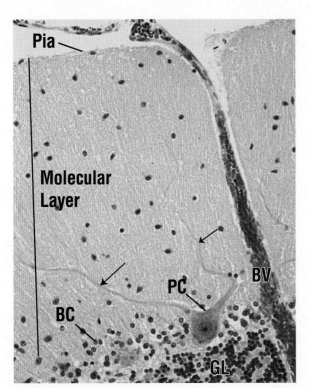

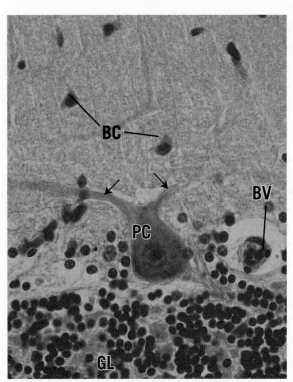

REVIEW FIGURE 8-2-3. Cerebellum. Human. Paraffin section. ×270.

Unlike the spinal cord, where the gray matter is surrounded by white matter, in the cerebellum, the gray matter surrounds the white matter. In this photomicrograph, only the gray matter with its three regions, outermost molecular layer, middle **Purkinje cell layer** (PC), and inner **granular layer** (GL) are presented. Note that the outermost aspect of the molecular layer is covered by the vascular **pia mater** (Pia), and its **blood vessels** (BV) penetrate the substance of the cerebellum. The middle layer of the cerebellar gray matter is composed solely of **Purkinje cells** (PC), whose **dendritic tree** (*arrows*) penetrates far into the molecular layer. The axon of the Purkinje cell enters the **granular layer** (GL) of the cerebellum.

REVIEW FIGURE 8-2-4. Cerebellum. Human. Paraffin section. ×540.

This higher magnification of the **Purkinje cell** labeled in Review Figure 8-2-3 displays its flask-shaped cell body (PC) with its large "owl eye–resembling" nucleus. **Basket cells** (BC) are shown to be multipolar neurons, and the **dendrites** of the Purkinje cells are indicated by the *arrows*. As in the previous photomicrograph, the rich **vascular supply** (BV) is quite evident. Granule cells of the **granular layer** (GL) resemble clusters of lymphocytes because of their dark, round nuclei. The clear areas among these clusters of granule cells are known as cerebellar islands, where dendrites of granule cells synapse with axons entering the region.

KEY					
BV	blood vessel (vascular supply)	BC	basket cells	PC	Purkinje cell (layer)
		GL	granular layer	Pia	pia mater

Summary of Histologic Organization

I. Neurons

A. Cell Body/Soma/Perikaryon

The largest part of the cell with a euchromatic nucleus and punctate nucleolus, large cytoplasm with **Nissl bodies** (aggregates of rER), and a tapered region called **axon hillock** from which axon originates. The soma is the site of **neurotransmitter** production. Collections of cell bodies are called **gray matter** and **nucleus** in the CNS, and **ganglion** in the PNS.

B. Dendrite

Thin and numerous extensions from the cell body, specialized to receive information from other neurons or receptor cells and conduct the signals to the cell body.

C. Axon

Single projection from the cell body specialized to conduct summated impulses from the cell body to the next neuron or effector organ. It possesses numerous **microtubules** for intracellular transport of neurotransmitter vesicles from the cell body to the axon terminal via **kinesin** (anterograde transport) and vesicles with recycled or endocytosed products from the axon terminal to the cell body via **dynein** (retrograde transport). The axon may be myelinated or unmyelinated. The **axon terminal** serves as the dilated storage site for neurotransmitter vesicles for rapid release and the formation of the presynaptic component of the synapse. Collections of axons are called **white matter** and **tract** in the CNS, and **nerve** (**peripheral nerve**) in the PNS. In the PNS, the nerve is supported by a network of connective tissues, **endoneurium**, **perineurium**, **and epineurium**.

II. Neuroglia

A. CNS

1. **Astrocytes** are the most numerous glial cells in the CNS and provide structural and metabolic support to the neurons.
2. **Oligodendrocytes** myelinate axons in the CNS. Unlike their counterparts in the PNS, a single oligodendrocyte can myelinate internodes of more than one axon.
3. **Microglia** are the specialized macrophages in the CNS, derived from monocytes.

4. **Ependymal cells** line all the ventricles of the brain and central canal of the spinal cord. In the ventricles, they form a part of the choroid plexus and produce CSF.

B. PNS

1. **Schwann cells** myelinate axons in the PNS. Unlike their counterparts in the CNS, a single Schwann cell can myelinate only a single internode of only one axon.
2. **Satellite cells** surround neuron cell bodies in the PNS and perform similar functions as astrocytes perform in the CNS.

III. Spinal Cord

A. White Matter (Outer Layer)

White matter, comprised of **ascending** and **descending tracts**, forms the outer layer of the spinal cord. The axons in the tracts are mostly **myelinated** (by **oligodendrocytes**), accounting for the whitish coloration in live tissue.

B. Gray Matter (Core)

Gray matter, in the shape of an H, forms the center of the spinal cord, which is subdivided into two **dorsal horns** and two **ventral horns**. Ventral horns house numerous **multipolar neuron cell bodies** performing a motor function, whereas dorsal horns house numerous multipolar neuron cell bodies that function as **interneurons** for the sensory axons synapsing here. The right and left halves of the gray matter are connected by the **gray commissure**, which houses the **central canal** lined by **ependymal cells**.

IV. Brain

A. Gray Matter (Outer Layer)

Gray matter forms the outer layer of the brain which undulates with the contours of the numerous folds called the **gyri**. The position of the gray matter on the surface with folds increases surface area and volume to house neuron cell bodies. The **cerebral cortex** is subdivided into six ill-defined layers, with each housing neurons with characteristic morphology. The **cerebellar cortex** has three well-defined layers with the outermost **molecular layer**, **Purkinje cell layer**, and the innermost **granular layer**.

B. White Matter (Core)

White matter comprising of **tracts** predominates the core of the brain; however, there are several **nuclei** throughout the white matter of the cerebrum and brainstem.

C. Ventricles

Ventricles are the fluid-filled cavities within the brain, lined by **ependymal cells**. Each ventricle also houses **choroid plexus**, delicate infoldings of capillary-rich pia and arachnoid matter, lined by ependymal cells. Choroid plexus continuously produces **cerebrospinal fluid (CSF)** which circulates throughout the ventricles, subarachnoid space, and central canal of the spinal cord and suspends the brain and the spinal cord within the meningeal casing.

D. Meninges

The **meninges** are the connective tissue coverings of the brain and the spinal cord. The innermost layer investing the brain and spinal cord is the **pia mater**, surrounded by the **arachnoid**, which, in turn, is invested by the thick and tough **dura mater**, comprised of dense irregular collagenous connective tissue.

V. Dorsal Root Ganglia

Dorsal root ganglia (DRGs) are positioned just outside of the spinal cord and house the **cell bodies** of **unipolar neurons** conducting sensory information from the periphery to the spinal cord. The cell bodies contain large nuclei with punctate nucleoli and **Nissl bodies**. **Lipofuscin** may accumulate in the cell body over time and is evident in the DRGs from older individuals. Surrounding each soma are **satellite cells**, recognized by their small, round nuclei. Distal and proximal neuron cell processes (fibers) are mostly myelinated and travel in bundles through the DRG. Synapses do not occur in the DRG. The DRG is surrounded by **dense irregular collagenous connective tissue**, whose septa penetrate the substance of the ganglion.

VI. Peripheral Nerve

A **nerve**, a collection of myelinated and nonmyelinated axons outside the CNS, is supported by a network of connective tissues organized into **endoneurium**, surrounding exterior of axons or Schwann cells, **perineurium**, surrounding nerve fascicles, and **epineurium**, surrounding the entire nerve.

A. Longitudinal Section

The parallel axons stain pale pink with hematoxylin and eosin, although **Schwann cells** and occasional **fibroblast nuclei** are evident. The most characteristic feature is the apparent wavy, zigzag course of the nerve fibers. At low magnification, the **perineurium** is distinguishable, whereas at high magnification, the **nodes of Ranvier** may be recognizable.

B. Transverse Section

The most characteristic feature of transverse sections of nerve fibers is the numerous, small, irregular circles with a centrally located dot. Thin spokes appear to traverse the empty-looking space between the dot and the circumference of the circle. These represent the **neurolemma**, the extracted **myelin (myelin proteins)**, and the central **axon**. Occasionally, crescent-shaped nuclei hug the myelin; these belong to **Schwann cells**. The **endoneurium** may show evidence of **nuclei of fibroblasts** also. At lower magnification, the **perineuria** of several fascicles of nerve fibers are clearly distinguishable. When stained with OsO_4, the **myelin sheath** stands out as dark, round structures with lightly staining centers.

Chapter Review Questions

8-1. What is the site of neurotransmitter synthesis?

A. Axon

B. Axon hillock

C. Axon terminal

D. Dendrite

E. Soma

8-2. Chromatolysis of the neuron cell bodies observed in the ventral horn of the spinal cord may indicate which functional deficit?

A. Impulse relay

B. Motor

C. Sensory

D. Special sensory

8-3. Which cellular structure is responsible for the long-lasting adverse effect of certain neurotoxins that are introduced at the axon terminal?

A. Dynein

B. Kinesin

C. Microtubule

D. Neuropil

8-4. Which cell population plays a role in cerebrospinal fluid production?

A. Astrocytes

B. Ependymal cells

C. Microglia

D. Oligodendrocytes

E. Satellite cells

8-5. Which neuroglial cell type myelinates axon fibers traversing through the dorsal root ganglia?

A. Astrocytes

B. Microglia

C. Oligodendrocytes

D. Satellite cells

E. Schwann cells

CIRCULATORY SYSTEM

CHAPTER OUTLINE

The circulatory system is composed of two separate but connected components: the **cardiovascular system** that transports blood and the **lymphatic vascular system** that collects and returns excess extracellular fluid (lymph) to the cardiovascular system after filtering through lymphoid tissues. Lymphoid tissue is presented in Chapter 10.

Cardiovascular System

The **cardiovascular system**, consisting of the heart and blood vessels, functions in propelling and transporting blood and its various constituents throughout the body. The **heart**, acting as a pump, forces blood at high pressure into large, elastic arteries that carry the blood away from the heart. **Arteries** give way to increasingly smaller muscular arteries. Eventually, the smallest arteries called **arterioles** deliver blood to the thin-walled capillaries, and small venules (postcapillary venules), where exchange of materials with the tissues occurs. It is mostly here that certain cells, oxygen, nutrients, hormones, certain proteins, and additional materials leave the bloodstream, whereas carbon dioxide, waste products, certain cells, and various secretory products enter the bloodstream.

Almost all capillary beds are drained by the **venous components** of the circulatory system, which return blood to the heart, increasing in size from **venules** to **medium veins** to **large veins** as they approach the heart.

Anatomically, the cardiovascular system is subdivided into the pulmonary and systemic circuits, which originate from the right and left sides of the heart, respectively. The **pulmonary circuit** takes oxygen-poor blood to the lungs to become oxygenated and returns it to the left side of the heart. The oxygen-rich blood is propelled via the **systemic circuit** to the remainder of the body to be returned to the right side of the heart, completing the cycle.

Histologic Layers of Blood Vessels

Blood vessels are composed of three concentric layers: tunica intima, tunica media, and tunica adventitia (Fig. 9-1):

- The **tunica intima** (the innermost layer) is composed of a continuous sheet of simple squamous endothelial cells (**endothelium**) lining the lumen and of various amounts of **subendothelial connective tissue (CT)**. The **internal elastic lamina**, a thin layer of elastic fibers, forms the outermost boundary of the tunica intima.

- The **tunica media**, usually the thickest of the three layers in the arterial leg of the circulatory system, is composed of circularly arranged smooth muscle cells and fibroelastic CT, whose elastic content increases greatly with the size of the vessel. The **external elastic lamina**, an elastic fiber-rich layer, forms the outermost boundary of the tunica media.

- The **tunica adventitia** is the outermost layer of the vessel wall, consisting of dense irregular CT. In larger vessels, the tunica adventitia houses **vasa vasorum**, small blood vessels that supply the tunica adventitia and media of that vessel. In the venous leg of the circulatory system, the tunica adventitia is the thickest of the three layers.

Heart

The heart is a four-chambered organ composed of two atria and two ventricles. The atria, after receiving blood from the pulmonary veins, venae cavae, and coronary sinus, discharge it into the ventricles. Contractions of the ventricles then propel the blood from the right ventricle into the pulmonary trunk for distribution to the lungs (pulmonary circuit) and from the left ventricle into the aorta for distribution to the remainder of the body (systemic circuit). Although the walls of the ventricles are thicker than those of the atria, these chambers possess common characteristics in that they are composed of three layers: epicardium, myocardium, and endocardium.

- **Epicardium**, the outermost layer, is covered by a simple squamous epithelium (mesothelium) deep to which is a fibroelastic CT. The deepest aspect of the epicardium is composed of adipose tissue that houses nerves and the coronary vessels.

- Most of the wall of the heart is composed of **myocardium**, consisting of bundles of cardiac muscle (Fig. 9-2) that are attached to the thick collagenous CT skeleton of the heart.

- The **endocardium** forms the lining of the atria and ventricles and is composed of a simple squamous epithelium (endothelium) as well as a subendothelial fibroelastic CT. The endocardium participates in the formation of the heart valves, which control the direction of blood flow through the heart.
  - **Atrioventricular (AV) valves** between the atria and ventricles prevent regurgitation of blood from the ventricles into the atria.
  - Similarly, **semilunar valves** located in the pulmonary trunk and the aorta prevent regurgitation of blood from these vessels back into their respective ventricles. The closing of these valves is responsible for the sounds associated with the heartbeat.

Some cardiac muscle fibers are modified and specialized to regulate the sequence of atrial and ventricular contractions. These are the sinoatrial (SA) and atrioventricular

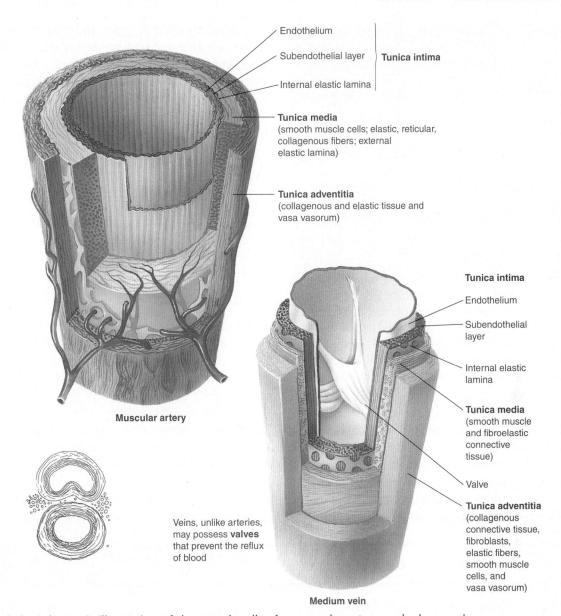

Endothelium
Subendothelial layer
Internal elastic lamina
Tunica intima

Tunica media
(smooth muscle cells; elastic, reticular,
collagenous fibers; external
elastic lamina)

Tunica adventitia
(collagenous and elastic tissue and
vasa vasorum)

Muscular artery

Tunica intima
Endothelium
Subendothelial
layer
Internal elastic
lamina

Tunica media
(smooth muscle
and fibroelastic
connective
tissue)

Valve

Tunica adventitia
(collagenous
connective tissue,
fibroblasts,
elastic fibers,
smooth muscle
cells, and
vasa vasorum)

Veins, unlike arteries,
may possess **valves**
that prevent the reflux
of blood

Medium vein

FIGURE 9-1. Schematic illustration of the vessel walls of a muscular artery and a large vein.

(AV) nodes and the bundle of His and Purkinje fibers, collectively known as the conduction system of the heart.

The **sinoatrial (SA) node**, the pacemaker of the heart, is located at the junction of the superior vena cava and the right atrium. The SA node generates impulses that result in the contraction of the atrial muscles; blood from the atria then enters the ventricles. Impulses generated at the SA node are then conducted to the **atrioventricular (AV) node**, which is located on the medial wall of the right ventricle near the tricuspid valve, as well as to the atrial myocardium. Arising from the AV node is the **bundle of His**, which extends into and bifurcates in the membranous interventricular septum to serve both ventricles. As these fibers reach the subendocardium of the muscular interventricular septum, they ramify and are known as **Purkinje fibers** (Fig. 9-3). Purkinje fibers are larger and stain paler than typical cardiomyocytes because of abundant glycogen stored in the sarcoplasm; however, as they

travel further down, they eventually merge with and become indistinguishable from other cardiac muscle cells.

The inherent rhythm of the SA node can be modulated by the autonomic nervous system, in that parasympathetic fibers derived from the vagus nerve synapse with postganglionic parasympathetic neurons (located in small ganglia) whose postganglionic parasympathetic fibers decrease the rate of the heartbeat. In contrast, postganglionic sympathetic nerve fibers originating in the sympathetic ganglia increase it. Cardiac muscles in the atria and the ventricles are conductively insulated from each other by the dense CT rings, known as the fibroskeleton of the heart, where cardiac muscles and valves attach. After the SA node initiates an impulse, the cardiomyocytes of the atria contract as a syncytium, then the impulse is delayed at the AV node for a period of 0.09 seconds before it is transmitted to the bundle of His, which penetrates through the fibroskeleton and carries

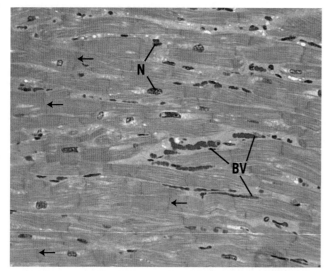

FIGURE 9-2. This high-magnification photomicrograph of a longitudinal section of the myocardium displays the centrally placed **nucleus** (N) of cardiac muscle cells as well as the intercalated disks (*arrows*) that connect individual muscle fibers to each other. Note the presence of a rich **vascular supply** (BV).×540.

the impulse down to the Purkinje fibers in the ventricles. This time lag permits the complete contraction of the atria and the delivery of the entire atrial blood volume into the ventricles before they begin their contraction. In this fashion, blood from the atria can enter the ventricles, and, once the ventricles are filled, they contract and propel the blood into the systemic and pulmonary circuits.

Cardiac muscle cells, especially those of the atria and the interventricular septum, manufacture and store a hormone known as **atrial natriuretic peptide**. Cardiac muscle cells of the ventricles also manufacture and store a hormone known as **B-type natriuretic peptide**. Both hormones have similar functions, in that they decrease blood volume, thereby reducing blood pressure.

Arteries

Arteries, by definition, conduct blood away from the heart; they are classified into three categories: elastic (also known as conducting or large), muscular (also known as distributing or medium), and arterioles (Table 9-1; also see Fig. 9-1).

Elastic Arteries

Elastic arteries, such as the aorta, receive blood directly from the heart and consequently are the largest of the arteries. Because they arise directly from the heart, they are subject to cyclic changes of blood pressure, high as the ventricles pump blood into their lumina and low between the emptying of these ventricles. To compensate for these intermittent pressure alterations, an abundance of elastic fibers is located in the tunica media of these vessels. These elastic fibers not only provide structural stability and permit distention of the elastic arteries but also assist in the maintenance of blood pressure in between heartbeats by recoiling the artery back to its

CLINICAL CONSIDERATIONS 9-1

Valve Defects and Rheumatic Fever

Children who have had rheumatic fever may develop **valve defects**. These valve defects may be related to improper closing (**incompetency**) or narrowed opening (**stenosis**). Fortunately, most of these defects can be repaired surgically. **Rheumatic fever**, a frequent sequela of **group A ß-hemolytic streptococcal pharyngitis**, is an inflammatory response to the bacterial insult. Although many body organs may be affected, most patients recover; however, in some cases, the heart bears permanent injury. In developed countries, where the streptococcal infection is aggressively treated by antibiotics, the occurrence of rheumatic fever is much less than in developing nations. In affected children, usually between age 5 and 15 years, symptoms such as painful, swollen joints, skin rash, chest pain, fever, and small nodules deep to the skin appear a few weeks after the resolution of an untreated strep throat infection. The symptoms disappear in less than a month; however, a number of years later, a small percentage of these children develop damaged **mitral valves** (left AV valve).

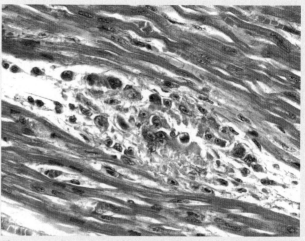

The myocardium of a decedent who died from acute rheumatic fever displays the presence of Aschoff bodies, composed of plasma cells, lymphocytes, macrophages, and multinucleated giant Aschoff cells. (Reprinted with permission from Mills SE, et al., eds. *Sternberg's Diagnostic Surgical Pathology*, 6th ed. Philadelphia: Wolters Kluwer, 2015. p. 1319, Figure 29-23.)

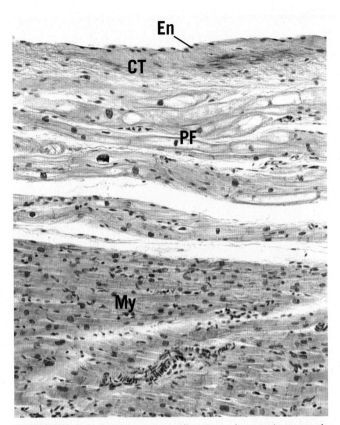

FIGURE 9-3. This low-magnification photomicrograph of the heart displays the simple squamous **endothelial lining** (En) of the ventricle, the subendothelial **connective tissue** (CT), and the well-defined **Purkinje fibers** (PF), branches of the conducting system of the heart. Observe the thick **myocardium** (My). ×135.

original size and propelling the excess blood within. The tunica adventitia of these vessels is much thinner than one would expect; however, it is well supplied with vasa vasorum. Because the elastic laminae of the fenestrated membranes have numerous openings, the nutrients

delivered by the vasa vasorum have good access to the tunica media.

Muscular Arteries

Muscular arteries comprise most of the named arteries of the body and supply blood to various organs. Their tunica media is composed mostly of many layers of smooth muscle cells. Both elastic and muscular arteries are supplied by **vasa vasorum** (Fig. 9-4; also see Fig. 9-1) and nerve fibers.

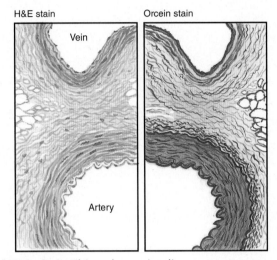

FIGURE 9-4. This schematic diagram compares the walls of an artery and the corresponding vein using H&E and Orcein stains. Arteries have a more muscular wall, thus a much thicker tunica media than the veins, and they have a greater amount of elastic tissue. Conversely, the tunicae adventitia of veins are much thicker than those of the arteries. The outermost layer is the **tunica adventitia**, composed of fibroelastic connective tissue, whose vessels, the **vasa vasorum**, penetrate the outer regions of the tunica media, supplying its cells with nutrients.

Table 9-1	Characteristics of Types of Arteries		
Artery	**Tunica Intima**	**Tunica Media**	**Tunica adventitia**
Elastic arteries (conducting) (e.g., aorta, pulmonary trunk)	Endothelium (containing Weibel–Palade bodies), basal lamina, subendothelial layer, incomplete internal elastic lamina	Layers of smooth muscle cells interspersed with 40–70 fenestrated elastic membranes, thin incomplete external elastic lamina, vasa vasorum	Thin layer of fibroelastic CT, limited vasa vasorum, lymphatic vessels, nerve fibers
Muscular arteries (distributing) (e.g., carotid and femoral arteries)	Endothelium (containing Weibel–Palade bodies), basal lamina, subendothelial layer, thick internal elastic lamina	~40 layers of smooth muscle cells, thick external elastic lamina, relatively little additional elastic tissue	Thin layer of fibroelastic CT, limited vasa vasorum, lymphatic vessels, nerve fibers
Arterioles	Endothelium (containing Weibel–Palade bodies), basal lamina, subendothelial layer, internal elastic lamina mostly replaced by elastic fibers	1–2 layers of smooth muscle cells	Ill-defined sheath of loose connective tissue, nerve fibers
Metarterioles	Endothelium and basal lamina	Precapillary sphincter formed by smooth muscle cells	Sparse loose connective tissue

CLINICAL CONSIDERATIONS 9-2

Aneurysm

A damaged vessel wall may, over time, become weakened and begin to enlarge and form a bulging defect known as an **aneurysm**. This condition occurs most often in elastic arteries such as the aorta and renal artery. If undetected or left untreated, it may rupture without warning and cause internal bleeding with fatal consequences. Surgical repair is possible, depending on the health of the individual.

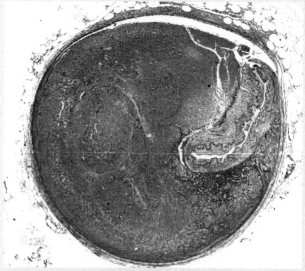

This is a photomicrograph of an aneurysm of the renal artery. The blood escaping from the lumen dissected the vessel wall and pooled between the tunica media and the tunica adventitia. (Reprinted with permission from Mills SE, et al., eds. *Sternberg's Diagnostic Surgical Pathology*, 6th ed. Philadelphia: Wolters Kluwer, 2015. p. 1356, Figure 30-6.)

CLINICAL CONSIDERATIONS 9-3

Atherosclerosis

Atherosclerosis, the deposition of plaque within the walls of large- and medium-sized arteries, results in stenosis and reduced blood flow within that vessel. If this condition involves the coronary arteries, the decreased blood flow to the myocardium causes coronary heart disease. The consequences of this disease may be angina pectoris, myocardial infarct, chronic ischemic cardiopathy, or sudden death.

Arterioles

Arterioles are the smallest arteries and are responsible for regulating blood pressure. Their tunica intima is composed of endothelium with a negligible amount of subendothelial connective tissue. Their tunica media is composed of a few layers of smooth muscle cells, but in small arterioles, it is reduced to a single smooth muscle cell layer. The tunica adventitia is also slight with the occasional presence of fibroblasts. Arterioles usually provide smaller branches known as metarterioles.

CLINICAL CONSIDERATIONS 9-4

Raynaud's Disease

Raynaud's disease is an idiopathic condition in which the arterioles of the fingers and toes go into sudden spasms lasting minutes to hours, cutting off blood supply to the digits, resulting in cyanosis and loss of sensation. This condition, affecting mostly younger women, is believed to be caused by exposure to cold and the patient's emotional state. Other causes include atherosclerosis, scleroderma, injury, and reaction to certain medications.

CLINICAL CONSIDERATIONS 9-5

Stroke

Stroke is a condition in which blood flow to a part of the brain is interrupted because of a blockage of blood vessels or hemorrhage of blood vessels. The lack of blood causes anoxia of the affected region with consequent death of the neurons of that region, resulting in weakness, paralysis, sensory loss, or the inability to speak. If stroke victims can reach a health facility equipped with dealing with the problem, and, depending on the extent of the injury, they can be rehabilitated to recover some or all of the lost function.

Metarterioles are the terminal ends of the arterioles, and they are characterized by the presence of incomplete rings of smooth muscle cells (**precapillary sphincters**) that encircle the origins of the capillaries (Figs. 9-5 and 9-6). Metarterioles form the arterial (proximal) end of a **central channel**, and they are responsible for delivering blood into the capillary bed. The venous (distal) end of the central channel, known as a **thoroughfare channel**, is responsible for draining blood from the capillary bed and delivering it into venules. Contraction of precapillary sphincters of the metarteriole shunts the blood into the **thoroughfare channel** and from there into the venule; this way, the blood bypasses the capillary bed (see Fig. 9-5).

Arteriovenous anastomoses (shunts) are direct connections between arteries and venules, and they also function in having blood bypass the capillary bed. These shunts function in **thermoregulation** and blood pressure control by opening (when precapillary sphincters close) to bypass the capillary beds in the skin, thereby conserving heat; then by closing (when precapillary sphincters open) to channel blood into capillary beds, thereby dissipating heat through the skin.

Capillaries

Capillaries are very small vessels that consist of a single layer of endothelial cells surrounded by a basal lamina and occasional **pericytes**, but these vessels possess no smooth muscle cells; therefore, they do not exhibit vasomotor activities. Capillaries exhibit **selective permeability** and they, along with venules, are responsible for the exchange of gases, metabolites, and other substances between the bloodstream and the tissues of the body. Capillaries are composed of highly attenuated **endothelial cells** that form narrow vascular channels 8 to 10 μm in diameter and are usually less than 1 mm long. There are three types of capillaries: continuous, fenestrated, and sinusoidal (Fig. 9-7 and Table 9-2):

- **Continuous capillaries** lack fenestrae, display only occasional pinocytotic vesicles, and possess a continuous basal lamina. They are present in regions such as peripheral nerve fibers, skeletal muscle, lungs, and thymus. The continuous nature of the endothelial cytoplasm ensures a highly controlled and regulated exchange of materials between the capillary and the extracapillary environments.

- **Fenestrated capillaries** are penetrated by relatively large diaphragm-covered pores called fenestrae. The

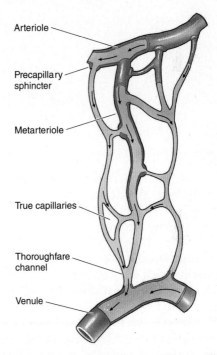

FIGURE 9-5. Schematic illustration of controlling blood flow through a capillary bed. Some capillary beds, such as those of the skin, are designed such that they may be bypassed under certain circumstances. One method whereby blood flow may be controlled is the use of **central channels** that convey blood from an arteriole to a venule. The proximal half of the central channel is a **metarteriole**, a vessel with an incomplete smooth muscle coat. Flow of blood into each capillary that arises from the metarteriole is controlled by a smooth muscle cell, the **precapillary sphincter**. The distal half of the central channel is the **thoroughfare channel**, which possesses no smooth muscle cells and accepts blood from the capillary bed. If the capillary bed is to be bypassed, the precapillary sphincters contract, preventing blood flow into the capillary bed, and the blood goes directly into the venule.

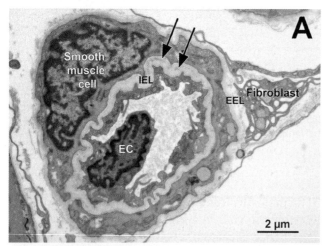

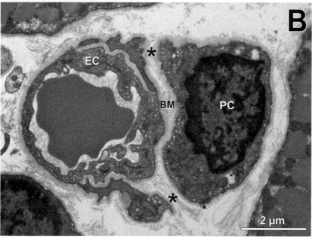

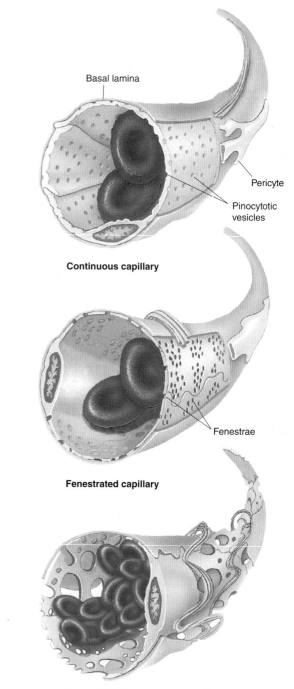

Basal lamina

Pericyte

Pinocytotic
vesicles

Continuous capillary

Fenestrae

Fenestrated capillary

Sinusoidal (Discontinuous) capillary

FIGURE 9-6. A. Transmission electron micrograph of a metarteriole from skeletal muscle. Note the single smooth muscle cell with its **external elastic lamina** (EEL) separating it from the connective tissue elements, including a fibroblast. The external lamina of the smooth muscle cell fuses with the basal lamina of the **endothelial cell** (EC) of the metarteriole and is known as the internal elastic lamina (IEL). Observe the slender elastic fibers in the internal elastic lamina (*arrows*). **B.** Observe that the **endothelial cell** (EC) of the capillary is surrounded by a **basal lamina** (BM), which fuses (*asterisks*) with the basal lamina of the **pericyte** (PC). (Courtesy of Dr. Oliver Baum.)

FIGURE 9-7. Schematic illustration of the three types of capillaries, continuous, fenestrated, and sinusoidal (discontinuous). Capillaries consist of a simple squamous epithelium rolled into a narrow cylinder 8 to 10 μm in diameter. **Continuous (somatic) capillaries** have no fenestrae: material transverses the endothelial cell in either direction via pinocytotic vesicles. **Fenestrated (visceral) capillaries** are characterized by the presence of perforations, **fenestrae**, 60 to 80 μm in diameter, which may or may not be bridged by a diaphragm. **Sinusoidal capillaries** have a large lumen (30 to 40 μm) in diameter, possess numerous fenestrae, have discontinuous basal lamina, and lack pinocytotic vesicles. Frequently, adjacent endothelial cells of sinusoidal capillaries incompletely overlap one another.

diaphragm can be seen in transmission electron micrograph as an electron-dense glycocalyx bridging the fenestrae. These cells also possess pinocytotic vesicles and are enveloped by a continuous basal lamina. The fenestrate allow rapid exchange of larger molecules, such as proenzymes, hormones, and large carbohydrate moieties between the capillary and the extracapillary environments. Fenestrated capillaries are located in endocrine glands, pancreas, and lamina propria of the intestines, and they also constitute the glomeruli of the kidneys, although their fenestrae are not covered by a diaphragm.

Table 9-2	Characteristics of Types of Capillaries		
Characteristics	**Continuous Capillaries**	**Fenestrated Capillaries**	**Sinusoidal Capillaries**
Location	CT, muscle, neural tissue; modified in brain tissue	Endocrine glands, pancreas, intestines	Bone marrow, spleen, liver, lymph nodes, certain endocrine glands
Diameter	Smallest diameter	Intermediate diameter	Largest diameter
Endothelium	Forms tight junctions at marginal fold with itself or adjacent cells	Forms tight junctions at marginal fold with itself or adjacent cells	Frequently, the endothelium and basal lamina are discontinuous.
Fenestrae (pores through the endothelial cells)	Not present	Present	Present in addition to gaps

- **Sinusoidal capillaries** (also known as **sinusoids, discontinuous capillaries**) are much larger than their fenestrated or continuous counterparts. They are enveloped by a discontinuous basal lamina, and their endothelial cells do not possess pinocytotic vesicles. The intercellular junctions of their endothelial cells display gaps, thus permitting leakage of material, including cells, into and out of these vessels. Frequently, macrophages are associated with sinusoidal capillaries. Sinusoidal capillaries are located in the liver, spleen, lymph nodes, bone marrow, and suprarenal cortex.

Capillary Permeability

Capillary permeability is dependent not only on the endothelial cells comprising the capillary but also on the physicochemical characteristics, such as size, charge, and shape, of the traversing substance. Some molecules, such as H_2O, diffuse through, whereas others are actively transported by carrier proteins across the endothelial cell plasma membrane. Other molecules move through fenestrae or through gaps in the intercellular junctions. Certain pharmacologic agents, such as **bradykinin** and **histamine**, have the ability to alter capillary permeability. Leukocytes leave the bloodstream by passing through intercellular junctions of the endothelial cells (**diapedesis**) to enter the extracellular spaces of tissues and organs.

Endothelial Cell Functions

Endothelial cells function in the formation of a selectively permeable membrane, vasoconstriction, vasodilation, initiation of coagulation, facilitation of transepithelial migration of inflammatory cells, angiogenesis, synthesis of growth factors, converting angiotensin I to angiotensin II by angiotensin-converting enzyme that is present on the luminal aspect of the endothelial cell plasmalemma, binding lipoprotein lipase, and oxidation of lipoproteins.

Vasoconstriction is due not only to the action of sympathetic nerve fibers that act on the smooth muscles of the tunica media but also to the pharmacologic agent **endothelin 1**, produced and released by endothelial cells

of blood vessels. Additionally, **antidiuretic hormone (ADH, vasopressin)** released by the posterior pituitary functions in vasoconstriction.

Vasodilation is accomplished by parasympathetic nerve fibers in an indirect fashion. Instead of acting on smooth muscle cells, acetylcholine, released by the nerve end-foot, is bound to receptors on the endothelial cells, inducing them to release **nitric oxide (NO)**, previously known as endothelial-derived releasing factor (EDRF). Nitric oxide acts on the cyclic guanosine monophosphate (cGMP) system of the smooth muscle cells, causing their relaxation. Additionally, endothelial cells can produce **prostacyclins**, pharmacologic agents that induce the cAMP second messenger pathway in smooth muscle cells, effecting their relaxation.

In case blood clotting is necessary, endothelial cells stop producing inhibitors of coagulation and instead release **tissue factor** (also known as **thromboplastin**), an agent that facilitates entry into the common pathway of **blood coagulation**, and **von Willebrand factor**, which activates and facilitates the adhesion of platelets to the exposed laminin and collagens and induces them to release ADP and thrombospondin, which encourages platelets to adhere to one another.

When inflammatory cells must leave the bloodstream to enter the connective tissue spaces, endothelial cells express on their luminal plasma membranes **E-selectins**. These signaling molecules are recognized by carbohydrate ligands on the surface of the inflammatory cells, triggering their **epithelial transmigration**.

Angiogenesis occurs in adult tissues in response to repair of damaged vessels, establishment of new vessels in repairing injuries, formation of new vessels after menstruation, formation of the corpus luteum, as well as in response to tumor formation. New vessels arise from existing vessels due to the interactions of various signaling molecules, such as angiopoietins 1 and 2, with specific receptors on endothelial cells that induce mitotic activity in preexisting endothelial cells and recruit smooth muscle cells to form the tunica media of the developing vessels.

CLINICAL CONSIDERATION 9-6

Von Willebrand Disease

Von Willebrand disease is a genetic disorder in which the individual is either incapable of producing a normal quantity of von Willebrand factor or the factor that they produce is deficient. Most individuals have a mild form of the condition that is not life-threatening. These individuals have problems with the process of blood clotting and display symptoms such as bruising easily, longer bleeding time, excessive bleeding from tooth extraction, excessive menstrual bleeding, and bloody mucous membranes.

Endothelial cells also **synthesize growth factors** such as various colony-stimulating factors, which induce cells of blood lineage to undergo mitosis and produce various blood cells. They also manufacture growth inhibitors, such as transforming growth factor-β.

Additionally, as indicated above, endothelial cells convert angiotensin I to angiotensin II, a powerful smooth muscle contractant and inducer of aldosterone release by the suprarenal cortex.

Endothelial cells also oxidize high-cholesterol-containing low-density lipoproteins and very low-density lipoproteins, so that the oxidized by-product can be phagocytosed by macrophages.

These cells also secrete several types of collagen and laminin.

Lipoprotein lipase, the enzyme in endothelial cells, cleaves triglycerides in the blood into glycerol and fatty acids so that these can leave the blood and enter the fat cells of adipose tissue.

Veins

Veins are low-pressure vessels that conduct blood away from body tissues and back to the heart (see Figs. 9-1 and 9-3). Generally, the diameters of veins are larger than those of corresponding arteries; however, veins are thinner walled because they do not bear high blood pressures. Veins also possess three concentric, more or less definite layers: **tunica intima**, **tunica media**, and **tunica adventitia**. Furthermore, veins have fewer layers of smooth muscle cells in their tunica media than do arteries. Finally, many veins possess valves that act to prevent regurgitation of blood. Because the lumina of veins are much larger than those of their companion arteries, veins contain at least twice the amount of blood as the arteries. The three categories of veins are **venules**, **medium**, and **large veins** (Table 9-3):

- The smallest of the **veins**, **venules**, and especially **postcapillary venules**, are also responsible for the exchange of materials.
  - Postcapillary venules have **pericytes** instead of a tunica media and their walls are more permeable than those of venules and even of capillaries.
  - **Vasodilator substances**, such as **serotonin** and **histamine**, appear to act on small venules, causing them to become "leaky" by increasing the intercellular distances between the membranes of contiguous endothelial cells.
  - Most such intercellular gaps occur in postcapillary venules rather than in capillaries.
  - Leukocytes preferentially leave the vascular system at the postcapillary venules to enter the connective tissue spaces via **diapedesis**.
- **Medium veins** receive blood from most of the body, including the upper and lower extremities. They also possess three layers.
  - The tunica intima frequently forms valves, especially in the lower extremities, to counteract the gravitational forces and avert the backflow of blood.

Table 9-3	Characteristics of Types of Veins		
Type of Vein	**Tunica Intima**	**Tunica Media**	**Tunica Adventitia**
Large veins	Endothelium, basal lamina, subendothelial CT, some veins possess valves	Connective tissue and a few layers of smooth muscle cells	Thickest layer with bundles of smooth muscle cells oriented longitudinally within dense irregular CT. Vasa vasorum are present.
Medium	Endothelium, basal lamina, subendothelial CT, some veins possess valves	Reticular and elastic fibers and some smooth muscle cells	Layers of dense irregular CT with vasa vasorum
Venules	Endothelium, basal lamina (pericytes are associated with some postcapillary venules)	Some connective tissue, along with a few smooth muscle cells	Some collagen fiber bundles and a few fibroblasts

- The tunica media is slender and houses only a loosely organized network of smooth muscle cells interspersed with fibroblasts and type I collagen fibers.
- The tunica adventitia is the thickest of the three layers consisting mostly of elastic fibers and type I collagen bundles arranged parallel to the longitudinal axis of the vein. Occasional smooth muscle cells are also present in the adventitia.
- **Large veins**, such as the venae cavae, pulmonary, and renal veins, are greater than 1 cm in diameter.
  - As the venae cavae and pulmonary veins approach the heart, they exhibit the presence of cardiac muscle cells in their adventitia.
  - Most of the large veins (except for those in the lower extremities) possess few smooth muscle cells in their tunica media; instead, more smooth muscle cells are located in their tunica adventitia.
- The tunica intima of large veins are rich in elastic fibers and fibroblasts.
- The walls of these large veins are supplied by slender vessels derived from the vasa vasorum located in their adventitia.

Lymph Vascular System

Excess extracellular fluid, which does not enter the venous return system at the level of the capillary bed or venule, gains entry into **lymphatic capillaries**, blindly ending thin vessels of the lymph vascular system. After passing through chains of lymph nodes and larger lymph vessels, the fluid known as lymph enters the blood vascular system at the root of the neck.

PLATE 9-1A   Elastic Artery

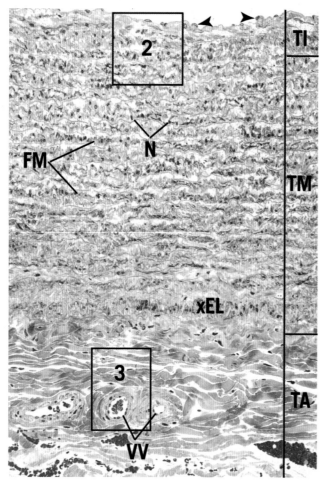

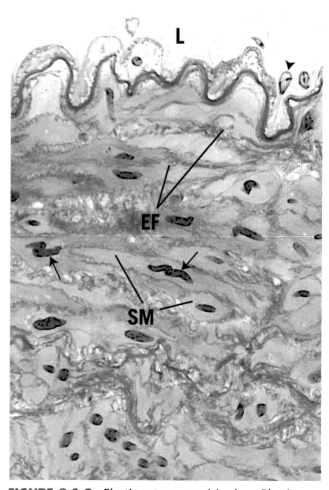

FIGURE 9-1-1. Elastic artery. l.s. Aorta. Monkey. Plastic section. ×132.

FIGURE 9-1-2. Elastic artery. x.s. Monkey. Plastic section. ×540.

This low-magnification photomicrograph displays almost the entire thickness of the wall of the aorta, the largest artery of the body. The **tunica intima** (TI) is lined by a simple squamous epithelium whose nuclei (*arrowheads*) bulge into the lumen of the vessel. The lines, which appear pale at this magnification, are elastic fibers and laminae, whereas the nuclei belong to smooth muscle cells and connective tissue cells. The internal elastic lamina is not readily identifiable because the tunicae intima and the media are rich in elastic fibers. The **tunica media** (TM) is composed of smooth muscle cells whose **nuclei** (N) are evident. These smooth muscle cells lie in the spaces between the concentrically layered **fenestrated membranes** (FM), composed of elastic connective tissue. The **external elastic lamina** (xEL) is that portion of the media that adjoins the adventitia. The outermost coat of the aorta, the **tunica adventitia** (TA), is composed of collagenous and elastic fibers interspersed with connective tissue cells and blood vessels, the **vasa vasorum** (VV). Regions similar to the *boxed areas* are presented in Figures 9-1-2 and 9-1-3.

This is a higher magnification of a region of the tunica intima, similar to the *boxed area* of Figure 9-1-1. The endothelial lining of the blood vessel presents **nuclei** (*arrowhead*), which bulge into the **lumen** (L). The numerous **elastic fibers** (EF) form an incomplete elastic lamina. Note that the interstices of the tunica intima house many **smooth muscle cells** (SM), whose nuclei are corkscrew-shaped (*arrows*), indicative of muscle contraction. Although most of the cellular elements are smooth muscle cells, it has been suggested that fibroblasts and macrophages may also be present; however, it is believed that the elastic fibers and the amorphous intercellular substances are synthesized by the smooth muscle cells.

KEY					
EF	elastic fibers	**SM**	smooth muscle cells	**TM**	tunica media
FM	fenestrated membranes	**TA**	tunica adventitia	**VV**	vasa vasorum
L	lumen	**TI**	tunica intima	**xEL**	external elastic lamina
N	nuclei				

PLATE 9-1B Elastic Artery

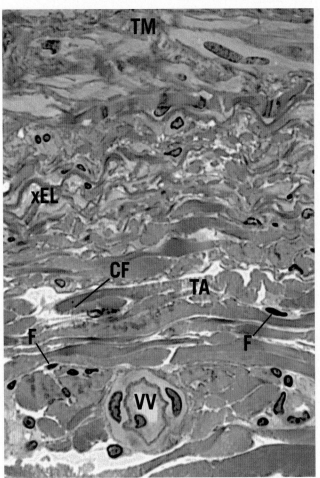

FIGURE 9-1-3. Elastic artery. x.s. Monkey. Plastic section. ×540.

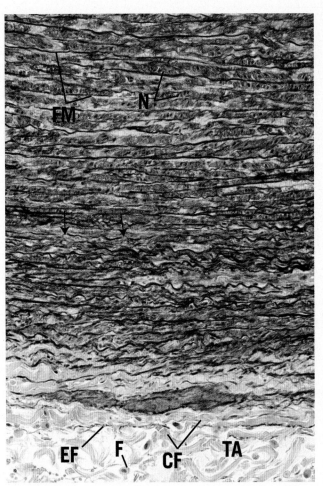

FIGURE 9-1-4. Elastic artery. x.s. Human. Elastic stain. Paraffin section. ×132.

This is a higher magnification of the tunica adventitia similar to the *boxed region* of Figure 9-1-1. The outermost region of the **tunica media** (TM) is demarcated by the **external elastic lamina** (xEL). The **tunica adventitia** (TA) is composed of thick bundles of **collagen fibers** (CF) interspersed with elastic fibers. Observe the nuclei of **fibroblasts** (F) located in the interstitial spaces among the collagen fiber bundles. Because the vessel wall is very thick, nutrients diffusing from the lumen cannot serve the entire vessel; therefore, the adventitia is supplied by small vessels known as **vasa vasorum** (VV). Vasa vasorum provide circulation not only for the tunica adventitia but also for the outer portion of the tunica media. Moreover, lymphatic vessels (not observed here) are also present in the adventitia.

The use of a special stain to demonstrate the presence of concentric elastic sheets, known as **fenestrated membranes** (FM), displays the highly elastic quality of the aorta. The number of fenestrated membranes, as well as the thickness of each membrane, increases with age so that the adult will possess almost twice as many of these structures as an infant. These membranes are called fenestrated because they possess spaces (*arrows*) through which nutrients and waste materials diffuse. The interstices between the fenestrated membranes are occupied by smooth muscle cells, whose **nuclei** (N) are evident, as well as amorphous intercellular materials, collagen, and fine elastic fibers. The **tunica adventitia** (TA) is composed mostly of **collagenous fiber bundles** (CF) and some **elastic fibers** (EF). Numerous **fibroblasts** (F) and other connective tissue cells occupy the adventitia.

KEY					
CF	collagen fiber	**FM**	fenestrated membrane	**TM**	tunica media
EF	elastic fiber	**N**	nucleus	**VV**	vasa vasorum
F	fibroblast	**TA**	tunica adventitia	**xEL**	external elastic lamina

PLATE 9-2A   Muscular Artery, Vein

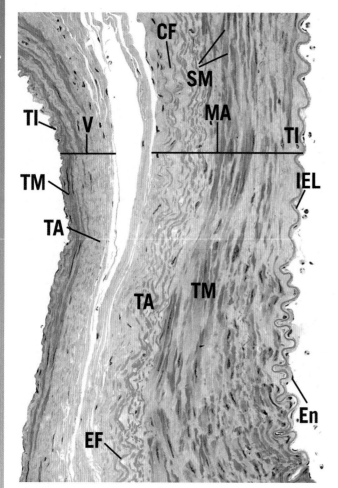

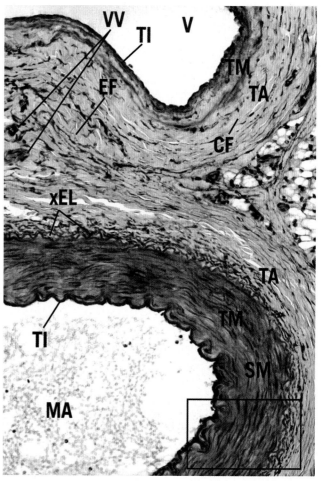

FIGURE 9-2-1. Artery and vein. x.s. Monkey. Plastic section. ×132.

FIGURE 9-2-2. Artery and vein. x.s. Elastic stain. Paraffin section. ×132.

This low-magnification photomicrograph presents a **muscular artery** (MA) and corresponding **vein** (V). Observe that the wall of the artery is much thicker than that of the vein and contains considerably more muscle fibers. The three concentric tunicae of the artery are evident. The **tunica intima** (TI), with its **endothelial layer** (En) and **internal elastic lamina** (IEL), is readily apparent. The thick **tunica media** (TM) is identified by the circularly or spirally displayed **smooth muscle cells** (SM) that are embedded in an elastic type of intercellular material. These elastic fibers, as well as the external elastic lamina—the outermost layer of the tunica media—are not easily apparent with hematoxylin and eosin stain. The **tunica adventitia** (TA), almost as thick as the media, contains no smooth muscle cells. It is composed chiefly of **collagen** (CF) and **elastic** (EF) fibers as well as fibroblasts and other connective tissue cells. The wall of the companion vein presents the same three tunicae: **intima** (TI), **media** (TM), and **adventitia** (TA); however, all three (but especially the media) are reduced in thickness.

The elastic stain used in this transverse section of a **muscular artery** (MA) and corresponding **vein** (V) clearly demonstrates the differences between arteries and veins. The **tunica intima** (TI) of the artery stains dark due to the thick internal elastic lamina, whereas that of the vein does not stain nearly as intensely. The thick **tunica media** (TM) of the artery is composed of numerous layers of circularly or spirally disposed **smooth muscle cells** (SM) with many elastic fibers ramifying through this tunic. The **tunica media** (TM) of the vein has only a few smooth muscle cell layers with little intervening elastic fibers. The **external elastic lamina** (xEL) of the artery is much better developed than that of the vein. Finally, the **tunica adventitia** (TA) constitutes the bulk of the wall of the vein and is composed of **collagenous** (CF) and **elastic** (EF) fibers. The **tunica adventitia** (TA) of the artery is also thick, but it comprises only about half the thickness of its wall. It is also composed of collagenous and elastic fibers. Both vessels possess their own **vasa vasorum** (VV) in their tunicae adventitia. A region similar to the *boxed area* is presented at higher magnification in Figure 9-2-3.

KEY							
CF	collagen fiber		**MA**	muscular artery		**TM**	tunica media
EF	elastic fiber		**SM**	smooth muscle cell		**V**	vein
En	endothelial layer		**TA**	tunica adventitia		**VV**	vasa vasorum
IEL	internal elastic lamina		**TI**	tunica intima			

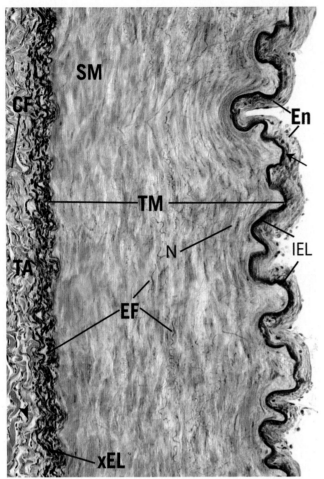

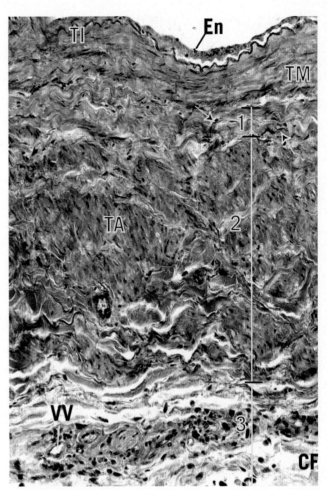

FIGURE 9-2-3. Artery. x.s. Elastic stain. Paraffin section. ×270.

FIGURE 9-2-4. Large vein. Vena cava. x.s. Human. Paraffin section. ×270.

This photomicrograph is a higher magnification of a region similar to the *boxed area* of Figure 9-2-2. The **endothelium** (En), subendothelial connective tissue (*arrow*), and the highly contracted **internal elastic lamina** (IEL) are readily evident. These three structures constitute the tunica intima of the muscular artery. The **tunica media** (TM) is very thick and consists of many layers of spirally or circularly disposed **smooth muscle cells** (SM), whose **nuclei** (N) are readily identifiable with this stain. Numerous **elastic fibers** (EF) ramify through the intercellular spaces between smooth muscle cells. The **external elastic lamina** (xEL), which comprises the outermost layer of the tunica media, is seen to advantage in this preparation. Finally, note the **collagenous** (CF) and **elastic** (EF) fibers of the **tunica adventitia** (TA), as well as the nuclei (*arrowhead*) of the various connective tissue cells.

Large veins, as the inferior vena cava in this photomicrograph, are very different from the medium-sized veins of Figures 9-2-1 and 9-2-2. The **tunica intima** (TI) is composed of **endothelium** (EN) and some subendothelial connective tissue, whereas the **tunica media** (TM) is greatly reduced in thickness and contains only occasional smooth muscle cells. The bulk of the wall of the vena cava is composed of the greatly thickened **tunica adventitia** (TA), consisting of three concentric regions. The innermost layer (1) displays thick collagen bundles (*arrows*) arrayed in a spiral configuration, which permits it to become elongated or shortened, with respiratory excursion of the diaphragm. The middle layer (2) presents smooth muscle (or cardiac muscle) cells, longitudinally disposed. The outer layer (3) is characterized by thick bundles of **collagen fibers** (CF) interspersed with elastic fibers. This region contains **vasa vasorum** (VV) that supply nourishment to the wall of the vena cava.

KEY					
EF	elastic fiber	SM	smooth muscle cell	TM	tunica media
En	endothelial layer	TA	tunica adventitia	VV	vasa vasorum
IEL	internal elastic lamina	TI	tunica intima	xEL	external elastic lamina
N	nucleus				

PLATE 9-3A   Arterioles and Venules

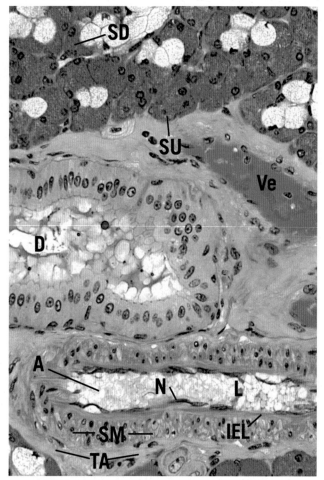

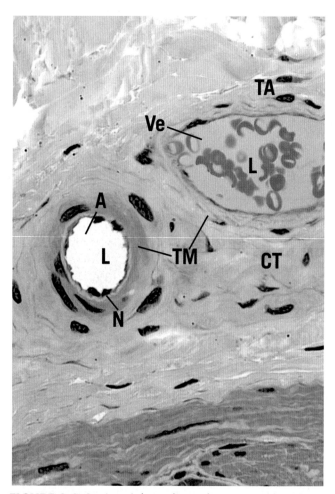

FIGURE 9-3-1. Arteriole and venule. l.s. Monkey. Plastic section. ×270.

FIGURE 9-3-2. Arteriole and venule. x.s. Monkey. Plastic section. ×540.

This longitudinal section of a large **arteriole** (A) and companion **venule** (Ve) from the connective tissue septum of a monkey submandibular gland displays a **duct** (D) of the gland between the two vessels. Observe that the thickness of the arteriole wall approximates the diameter of the **lumen** (L). The endothelial cell **nuclei** (N) are readily evident in both vessels, as are the **smooth muscle cells** (SM) of the tunica media. The arteriole also presents an **internal elastic lamina** (IEL) between the tunica media and the endothelial cells. The **tunica adventitia** (TA) of the arteriole displays nuclei of fibroblasts, whereas those of the venule merge imperceptibly with the surrounding connective tissue. Glandular acini are evident in this field as are **serous units** (SU) and **serous demilunes** (SD).

This small **arteriole** (A) and its companion **venule** (Ve) are from the submucosa of the fundic region of a monkey stomach. Observe the obvious difference between the diameters of the **lumina** (L) of the two vessels as well as the thickness of their walls. Due to the greater muscularity of the **tunica media** (TM) of the arteriole, the **nuclei** (N) of its endothelial cells bulge into its round lumen. The **tunica media** (TM) of the venule is much reduced, whereas the **tunica adventitia** (TA) is well developed and composed of **collagenous connective tissue** (CT) interspersed with elastic fibers (not evident in this hematoxylin and eosin section).

KEY					
A	arteriole	**L**	lumen	**SU**	serous unit
CT	connective tissue	**N**	nucleus	**TA**	tunica adventitia
D	duct	**SD**	serous demilune	**TM**	tunica media
IEL	internal elastic lamina	**SM**	smooth muscle cell	**Ve**	venule

PLATE 9-3B Capillaries and Lymph Vessels

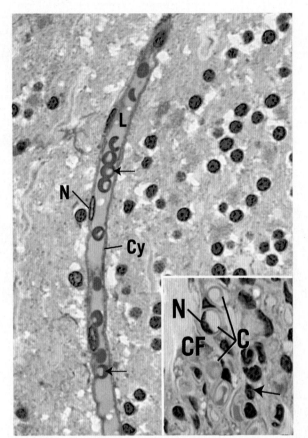

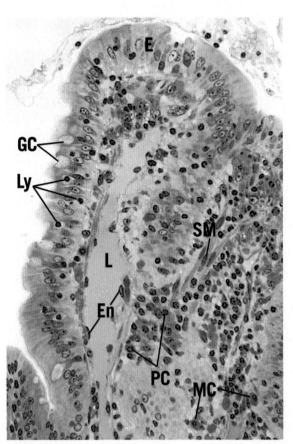

FIGURE 9-3-3. Capillary. l.s. Monkey. Plastic section. ×540.

FIGURE 9-3-4. Lymphatic vessel. l.s. Monkey. Plastic section. ×270.

In this photomicrograph of the monkey cerebellum, the molecular layer displays longitudinal sections of a capillary. Note that the endothelial cell **nuclei** (N) are occasionally in the field of view. The **cytoplasm** (Cy) of the highly attenuated endothelial cells is visible as thin, dark lines, bordering the **lumina** (L) of the capillary. Red blood cells (*arrows*) are noted to be distorted as they pass through the narrow lumina of the vessel. *Inset.* **Capillary**. **x.s. Monkey**. **Plastic section**. ×540. The connective tissue represented in this photomicrograph displays bundles of **collagen fibers** (CF), nuclei of connective tissue cells (*arrow*), and a cross section of a **capillary** (C), whose endothelial cell **nucleus** (N) is clearly evident.

This photomicrograph presents a villus from monkey duodenum. Note the simple columnar **epithelium** (E) interspersed with occasional **goblet cells** (GC). The connective tissue lamina propria displays numerous **plasma cells** (PC), **mast cells** (MC), **lymphocytes** (Ly), and **smooth muscle fibers** (SM). The longitudinal section of the **lumen** (L) lined with **endothelium** (En) is a lacteal, blindly ending lymphatic channel. Because lymph vessels do not transport red blood cells, the lacteal appears to be empty, but in fact, it contains lymph. After a fatty meal, lacteals contain chylomicrons. Observe that the wall of the lacteal is very flimsy in relation to the diameter of the vessel.

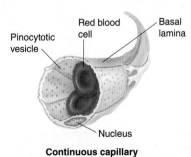

Continuous capillary

KEY					
C	Capillary	En	endothelium	MC	mast cell
CF	collagen fiber	GC	goblet cells	N	nucleus
Cy	cytoplasm	L	lumen	PC	plasma cells
E	epithelium	Ly	lymphocytes	SM	smooth muscle cell

PLATE 9-4A   Heart: Endocardium and Myocardium

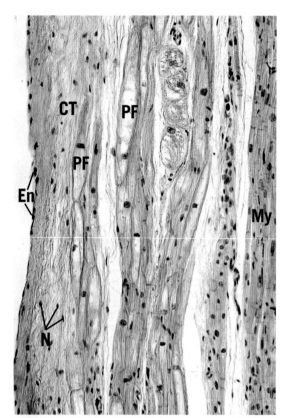

FIGURE 9-4-1. Endocardium. Human. Paraffin section. ×132.

The endocardium, the innermost layer of the heart, is lined by a simple squamous epithelium that is continuous with the endothelial lining of the various blood vessels entering or exiting the heart. The endocardium is composed of three layers, the innermost of which consists of the **endothelium** (En) and the subendothelial **connective tissue** (CT), whose collagenous fibers and connective tissue cell **nuclei** (N) are readily evident. The middle layer of the endocardium, although composed of dense collagenous and elastic fibers and some smooth muscle cells, is occupied in this photomicrograph by branches of the conducting system of the heart, the **Purkinje fibers** (PF). The third layer of the endocardium borders the thick **myocardium** (My) and is composed of looser connective tissue elements housing blood vessels, occasional adipocytes, and additional connective tissue cells.

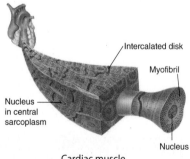

Intercalated disk

Myofibril

Nucleus in central sarcoplasm

Nucleus

Cardiac muscle

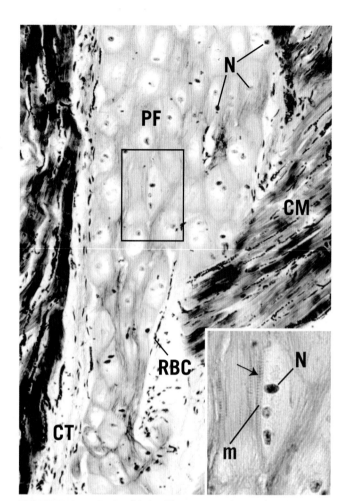

FIGURE 9-4-2. Purkinje fibers. Iron hematoxylin. Paraffin section. ×132.

The stain utilized in preparing this section of the ventricular myocardium intensely stains **red blood cells** (RBC) and **cardiac muscle cells** (CM). Therefore, the thick bundle of **Purkinje fibers** (PF) is shown to advantage because of its less dense staining quality. The **connective tissue** (CT) surrounding these fibers is highly vascularized, as evidenced by the red blood cell–filled capillaries. Purkinje fibers are composed of individual cells, each with a centrally placed single **nucleus** (N). These fibers form numerous gap junctions with each other and with cardiac muscle cells. The *boxed area* is presented at a higher magnification in the inset. *Inset.* **Purkinje fibers. Iron hematoxylin. Paraffin section.** ×270. Individual cells of Purkinje fibers are much larger than cardiac muscle cells. However, the presence of peripherally displaced **myofibrils** (m) displaying A and I bands (*arrow*) clearly demonstrates that they are modified cardiac muscle cells. The **nucleus** (N) is surrounded by a clear area, housing glycogen and mitochondria.

KEY					
CM	cardiac muscle cell	**m**	myofibril	**PF**	Purkinje fiber
CT	connective tissue	**My**	myocardium	**RBC**	red blood cell
En	endothelium	**N**	nuclei		

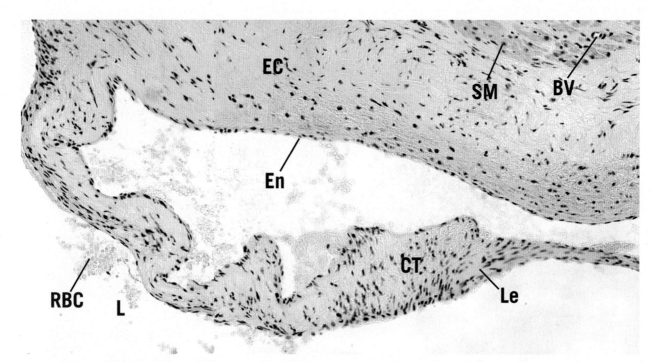

FIGURE 9-4-3. Heart valve. l.s. Paraffin section. ×132.

This figure is a montage, displaying a **valve leaflet** (Le) as well as the **endocardium** (EC) of the heart. The leaflet is in the **lumen** (L) of the ventricle, as evidenced by the numerous trapped **red blood cells** (RBC). The **endothelial** (En) lining of the endocardium is continuous with the endothelial lining of the leaflet. The three layers of the endocardium are clearly evident, as are the occasional **smooth muscle cells** (SM) and **blood vessels** (BV). The core of the leaflet is composed of dense collagenous and elastic **connective tissue** (CT), housing numerous cells whose nuclei are readily observed. Because the core of these leaflets is devoid of blood vessels, the connective tissue cells receive their nutrients directly from the blood in the lumen of the heart via simple diffusion. The connective tissue core of the leaflet is continuous with the skeleton of the heart, which forms a fibrous ring around the opening of the valves.

KEY					
BV	blood vessel	**En**	endothelium	**RBC**	red blood cell
CT	connective tissue	**L**	lumen	**SM**	smooth muscle cell
EC	endocardium	**Le**	valve leaflet		

PLATE 9-5 Capillary, Transmission Electron Microscopy

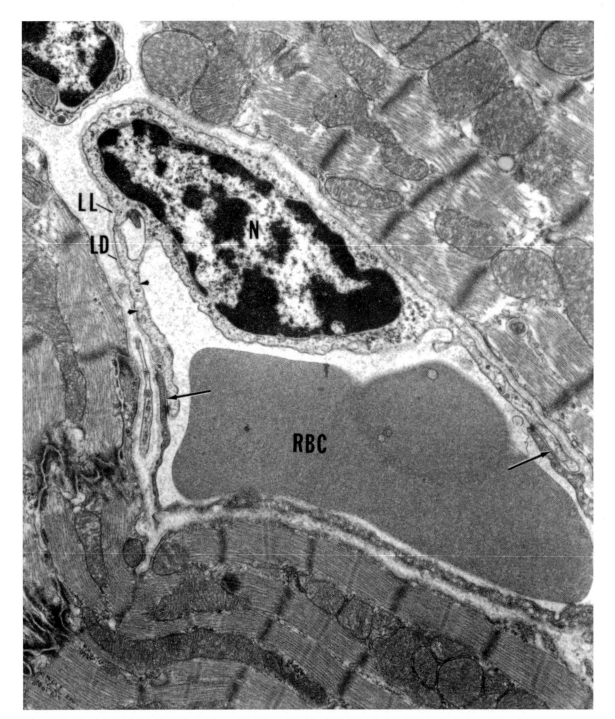

FIGURE 9-5-1. Continuous capillary. x.s. Cardiac muscle. Mouse. Electron microscopy. ×29,330.

This electron micrograph of a continuous capillary in cross section was taken from mouse heart tissue. Observe that the section passes through the **nucleus** (N) of one of the endothelial cells constituting the wall of the vessel and that the lumen contains **red blood cells** (RBC). Note that the endothelial cells are highly attenuated and that they form tight junctions (*arrows*) with each other. *Arrowheads* point to pinocytotic vesicles that traverse the endothelial cell. The **lamina densa** (LD) and **lamina lucida** (LL) of the basal lamina are clearly evident.

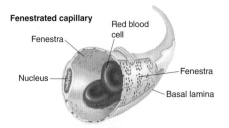

PLATE 9-6 Freeze Etch, Fenestrated Capillary, Electron Microscopy

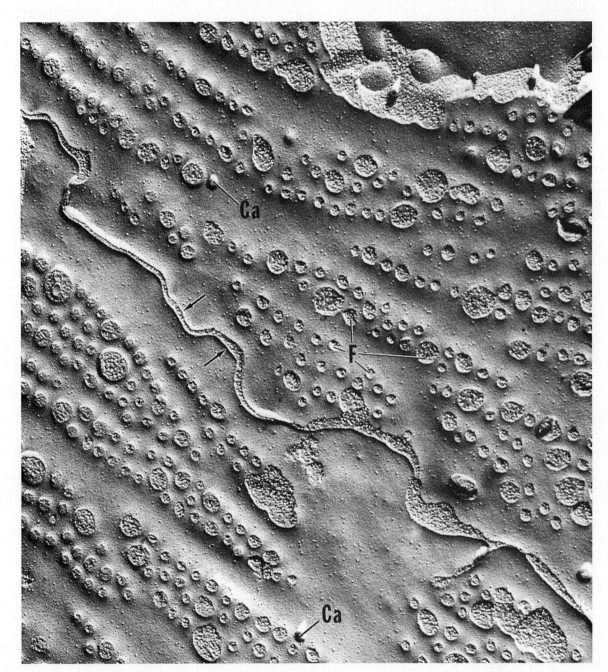

FIGURE 9-6-1. Fenestrated capillary. Hamster. Electron microscopy. Freeze fracture. ×205,200.

This electron micrograph is a representative example of fenestrated capillaries from the hamster adrenal cortex, as revealed by the freeze-fracture replica technique. The parallel lines (*arrows*) running diagonally across the field represent the line of junction between two endothelial cells, which are presented in a surface view. Note that the numerous **fenestrae** (F), whose diameters range from 57 to 166 nm, are arranged in tracts, with the regions between tracts nonfenestrated. Occasional **caveolae** (Ca) are also present. (Reprinted from Ryan US, et al. Fenestrated endothelium of the adrenal gland: freeze-fracture studies. *Tissue Cell* 1975;7(1):181–190. Copyright © 1975 Elsevier, With permission.)

Selected Review of Histologic Images

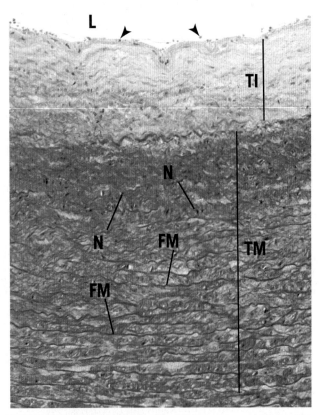

REVIEW FIGURE 9-1-1. Elastic artery. x.s. Aorta. Human. Elastic stain. Paraffin section. ×132.

This low-magnification image of a transverse section of the aorta displays the tunica intima and part of the tunica media. Note that the **tunica intima** (TI) is relatively thick, and the **lumen** (L) of the vessel is lined by a **simple squamous epithelium** (*arrowheads*) known as the endothelium. The **tunica media** (TM) is very thick and is separated from the tunica intima by the internal elastic lamina (not labeled in this photomicrograph). The **fenestrated membranes** (FM) and **nuclei** (N) of the smooth muscle cells are clearly evident.

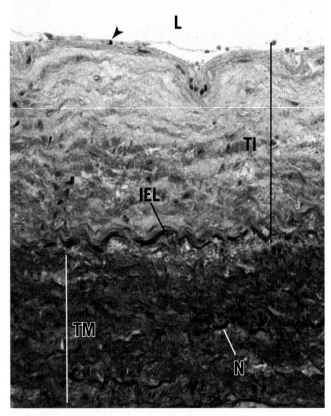

REVIEW FIGURE 9-1-2. Elastic artery. x.s. Aorta. Human. Elastic stain. Paraffin section. ×270.

This image is a higher magnification of the tunica intima and part of the tunica media of Review Figure 9-1-1. Observe that the **lumen** (L) of the aorta is lined by endothelium, composed of a **simple squamous epithelium** (*arrowhead*). The deepest portion of the **tunica intima** (TI) is the **internal elastic lamina** (IEL) that adjoins the **tunica media** (TM). Note the **nuclei** (N) of the smooth muscle cells of the tunica media.

KEY					
FM	fenestrated membranes	**L**	lumen	**TI**	tunica intima
IEL	internal elastic lamina	**N**	nucleus	**TM**	tunica media

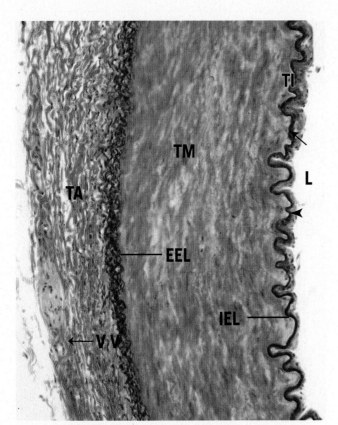

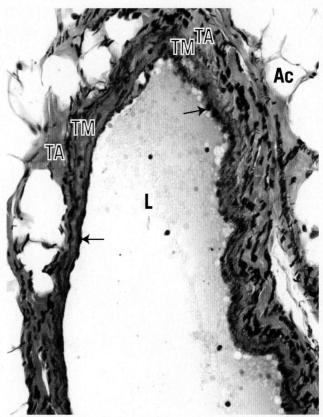

REVIEW FIGURE 9-1-3. Muscular artery. x.s. Human. Elastic stain. Paraffin section. ×132.

The **endothelium** (*arrowhead*), **subendothelial connective tissue** (*arrow*), and the **internal elastic lamina** (IEL) compose the **tunica intima** (TI). Observe the thick smooth muscle layer and the well-defined **external elastic lamina** (EEL) of this muscular artery, which form the **tunica media** (TM). The collagenous connective tissue **tunica adventitia** (TA) houses the **vasa vasorum** (VV).

REVIEW FIGURE 9-1-4. Medium-sized vein. x.s. Human. Paraffin section. ×270.

The cross section of this medium-sized vein displays the **lumen** (L) partly filled with blood. The **nuclei** (*arrows*) of the endothelial cells lining the vein bulge into the lumen. The smooth muscle cells of the **tunica media** (TM) stain much darker than the collagen fibers of the **tunica adventitia** (TA). As usual, the vein is surrounded by **adipose cells** (Ac) of the adipose tissue.

KEY					
Ac	adipose cells	**L**	lumen	**TM**	tunica media
EEL	external elastic lamina	**TA**	tunica adventitia	**VV**	vasa vasorum
IEL	internal elastic lamina	**TI**	tunica intima		

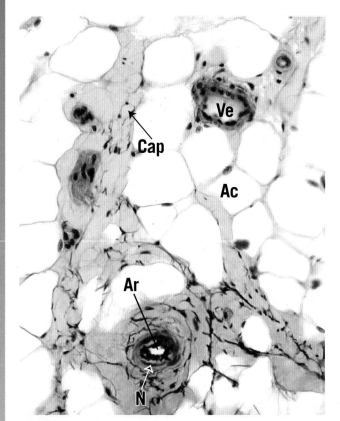

REVIEW FIGURE 9-2-1. Arteriole and venule. x.s. Human. Elastic stain. Paraffin section. ×270.

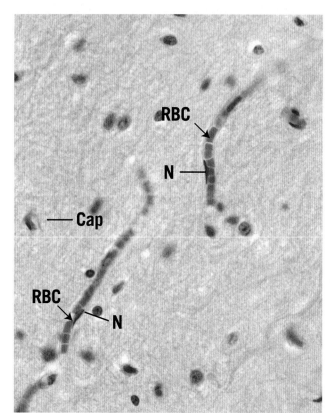

REVIEW FIGURE 9-2-2. Capillary. Cerebellum. Human. Paraffin section. ×540.

Arterioles (Ar) and **venules** (Ve) are small vessels that are usually surrounded by **adipose tissue** (Ac). Note that the tunica intima of the arteriole has smooth muscle cells whose **nuclei** (N) are clearly evident. The connective tissue of the tunica adventitia stains lighter than the smooth muscle layer of the tunica media. The venule has a much larger lumen than does the arteriole and its wall is much thinner than that of the arteriole. Note the **capillary** (Cap) in the upper half of the field.

This is a section of the molecular layer of the cerebellum displaying the presence of numerous **capillaries** (Cap) in cross section and longitudinal section. Note the presence of numerous **red blood cells** (RBC) as well as the endothelial cell **nuclei** (N) of these narrow vessels. Observe that the erythrocytes are the same width as the lumen of the capillary.

KEY					
Ac	adipose tissue	**Cap**	capillary	**RBC**	red blood cell
Ar	arterioles	**N**	nucleus	**Ve**	venules

Summary of Histologic Organization

I. Elastic Artery (Conducting Artery)

Among these are the **aorta**, **common carotid**, and **subclavian arteries**.

A. Tunica Intima

Lined by short, polygonal **endothelial cells**. The **subendothelial connective tissue** is fibroelastic and houses some longitudinally disposed smooth muscle cells. **Internal elastic lamina** is not clearly defined.

B. Tunica Media

Characterized by numerous **fenestrated membranes** (spiral to concentric sheets of fenestrated elastic membranes). Enmeshed among the elastic material are circularly disposed **smooth muscle cells** and associated **collagenous**, **reticular**, and **elastic fibers**.

C. Tunica Adventitia

Thin, **collagenous connective tissue** containing some **elastic fibers** and a few longitudinally oriented **smooth muscle cells**. **Vasa vasorum** (vessels of vessels) are also present.

II. Muscular Artery (Distributing Artery)

Among these are the named arteries, except the elastic arteries.

A. Tunica Intima

These are lined by polygonal-shaped, flattened **endothelial cells** that bulge into the lumen during vasoconstriction. The **subendothelial connective tissue** houses fine **collagenous fibers** and few longitudinally disposed **smooth muscle cells**. The **internal elastic lamina**, clearly evident, is frequently split into two membranes.

B. Tunica Media

Characterized by many layers of circularly disposed **smooth muscle cells**, with some **elastic**, **reticular**, and collagenous fibers among the muscle cells. The **external elastic lamina** is well defined.

C. Tunica Adventitia

Usually a very thick **collagenous** and **elastic tissue**, with some longitudinally oriented **smooth muscle fibers**. **Vasa vasorum** are also present.

III. Arterioles

These are arterial vessels whose diameter is less than 100 μm.

A. Tunica Intima

Endothelium and a variable amount of **subendothelial connective tissue** are always present. The **internal elastic lamina** is present in larger arterioles but absent in smaller arterioles.

B. Tunica Media

The spirally arranged **smooth muscle fibers** may be up to three layers thick. An **external elastic lamina** is present in larger arterioles but absent in smaller arterioles.

C. Tunica Adventitia

This is composed of **collagenous** and **elastic connective tissues**, whose thickness approaches that of the tunica media.

IV. Capillaries

Most **capillaries** in cross section appear as thin, circular profiles 8 to 10 μm in diameter. Occasionally, a fortuitous section will display an **endothelial cell nucleus**, a red blood cell, or, very infrequently, a white blood cell. Frequently, capillaries will be collapsed and not evident with the light microscope. **Pericytes** are usually associated with capillaries.

V. Venules

Venules possess much larger lumina and thinner walls than corresponding arterioles.

A. Tunica Intima

Endothelium lies on a very thin **subendothelial connective tissue** layer, which increases with the size of the vessel. **Pericytes** are frequently associated with smaller venules.

B. Tunica Media

Absent in smaller venules, whereas in larger venules one or two layers of **smooth muscle cells** may be observed.

C. Tunica Adventitia

Consists of **collagenous connective tissue** with **fibroblasts** and some **elastic fibers**.

VI. Medium-Sized Veins

A. Tunica Intima

The **endothelium** and a scant amount of **subendothelial connective tissue** are always present. Occasionally, a thin **internal elastic lamina** is observed. **Valves** may be evident.

B. Tunica Media

Much thinner than that of the corresponding artery but does possess a few layers of **smooth muscle cells**. Occasionally, some of the muscle fibers, instead of being circularly disposed, are longitudinally disposed. Bundles of **collagen fibers** interspersed with a few **elastic fibers** are also present.

C. Tunica Adventitia

Composed of **collagen** and some **elastic fibers**, which constitute the bulk of the vessel wall. Occasionally, longitudinally oriented **smooth muscle cells** may be present. **Vasa vasorum** are noted to penetrate even the **tunica media**.

VII. Large Veins

A. Tunica Intima

Same as that of medium-sized veins but displays thicker **subendothelial connective tissue**. Some large veins have well-defined **valves**.

B. Tunica Media

Not very well defined, although it may present some **smooth muscle cells** interspersed among **collagenous** and **elastic fibers**.

C. Tunica Adventitia

Thickest of the three layers and accounts for most of the vessel wall. May contain longitudinally oriented **smooth muscle fiber bundles** among the thick layers of **collagen** and **elastic fibers**. **Vasa vasorum** are commonly present.

VIII. Heart

An extremely thick, muscular organ composed of three layers: **endocardium**, **myocardium**, and **epicardium**. The presence of **cardiac muscle** is characteristic of this organ. Additional structural parameters may include **Purkinje fibers**, thick **valves**, **atrioventricular** and **sinoatrial nodes**, as well as the **chordae tendineae** and the thick, connective tissue **cardiac skeleton**.

IX. Lymphatic Vessels

Lymphatic vessels are either collapsed and therefore not discernible or are filled with lymph. In the latter case, they present the appearance of a clear, endothelium-lined space resembling a blood vessel. However, the lumina contain no **red blood cells**, though **lymphocytes** may be present. The **endothelium** may display **valves**.

Chapter Review Questions

9-1. The idiopathic condition, known as Raynaud's disease, is characterized by which of the following?

A. Spasms of the small veins of the thighs

B. Relaxation of the arterioles of the toes

C. Spasms of the arterioles of the fingers

D. Relaxation of the small veins of the thighs

E. Relaxation of the arterioles of the fingers

9-2. The myocardium of a patient who died of rheumatic fever presents with Aschoff bodies. These structures are composed of which of the following cells?

A. Macrophages

B. Neutrophils

C. Eosinophils

D. Basophils

E. Mast cells

9-3. B-type natriuretic peptide is a hormone manufactured by which of the following cells?

A. Smooth muscle cells of the vena cava

B. Smooth muscle cells of the aorta

C. Purkinje fibers

D. Cardiac muscle cells of the atria

E. Cardiac muscle cells of the ventricle

9-4. Continuous capillaries are present in which of the following?

A. Endocrine glands

B. Intestines

C. Muscle

D. Spleen

E. Lymph nodes

9-5. Weibel–Palade bodies, located in endothelial cells of blood vessels contain which of the following substances?

A. Vasopressin

B. E-selectin

C. Tissue factor

D. Factor VIII

E. Laminin

CHAPTER

10

LYMPHOID (IMMUNE) SYSTEM

CHAPTER OUTLINE

The **lymphoid (immune) system** forms the basis of the immune defense of the body and is organized into **diffuse lymphoid tissue**, **lymphoid follicles** (mucosa-associated lymphoid tissue [MALT]), and **capsulated lymphatic organs** (lymph nodes, tonsils, spleen, and thymus). The lymphocytes and **macrophages** are the principal cells of, and are responsible for, the proper functioning of the immune system (Fig. 10-1). Although morphologically identical, small lymphocytes may be functionally categorized into three groups: null cells, B lymphocytes (B cells), and T lymphocytes (T cells); macrophages are also of various types. *These cells are merely introduced here; they are discussed in more detail later in this chapter.*

- **Null cells** are composed of two categories of cells, namely stem cells and natural killer (NK) cells.
  - **Stem cells** are undifferentiated cells that give rise to the various cellular elements of blood, whereas **NK cells** are cytotoxic cells that are responsible for the destruction of certain categories of foreign cells; they resemble cytotoxic T cells (CTLs), but they are immunocompetent without having to enter the thymus to receive "instruction" on how to become mature killer cells.

- **B lymphocytes (B cells)**, which "learn" to become immunocompetent cells in the bone marrow are responsible for the **humoral immune response**. They have the capability of transforming into plasma cells.
  - **Plasma cells** possess the ability to manufacture humoral **antibodies**, which once released, bind to and thus inactivate the specific **antigen**. Additionally, the attachment of antibodies to antigens may enhance phagocytosis (by opsonization) or precipitate complement activation, resulting in chemotaxis of neutrophils and even lysis of the invader.

- **T lymphocytes (T cells)**, which are potentiated in the thymus, do not produce antibodies; instead, they function in the **cell-mediated immune response**, in which they search out, identify, and kill foreign or virally transformed cells. T lymphocytes, activated by the presence of an antigen, release **cytokines**, substances that, in turn, activate macrophages, attract them to the site of antigenic invasion, and enhance their phagocytic capabilities. Frequently, T lymphocytes also assist B lymphocytes in the performance of their functions. The various types of T cells are discussed later in this chapter.

- **Macrophages** can identify, bind to, and destroy cells that have antibodies, complement proteins, and unusual carbohydrates attached to them. Macrophages are also known as **antigen-presenting cells (APCs)** because they can present epitopes to both B and T lymphocytes. Moreover, they release signaling molecules to facilitate the immunologic defense of the body.

General Plan of the Immune System

The body protects itself against invading pathogens in three ways: (1) by the establishment of a physical barrier in the form of an epithelium that completely covers (epidermis of the skin) and lines (mucosa of the respiratory, digestive, urogenital systems and conjunctivae of the eyes) the body, thus isolating it from the external milieu; (2) by activating the **secondary defense system**, that is the **innate (nonspecific) immune system**; and (3) by triggering a response from the tertiary defense system, that is the adaptive (specific) immune system.

- The physical barrier is the primary defense, but it can be damaged (e.g., a splinter in the skin) permitting the ingress of pathogens into the subepithelial connective tissue activating the secondary and tertiary defense systems to perform their protective roles.

- The innate immune system is an evolutionarily older system than its adaptive counterpart. It possesses no immunologic memory but acts rapidly in response to the presence of specific molecules common to most pathogens, known as **pathogen-associated molecular patterns (PAMPs)**. Therefore, the innate immune system is nonspecific in that it is not designed to combat a single, particular antigen. The components of the innate immune system that recognize these PAMPs are listed in Table 10-1 and one of their components, the toll-like receptors, are presented in Table 10-2. The innate immune system possesses **innate B cells** that can manufacture **polyreactive antibodies (natural antibodies)** even in utero. Unlike antibodies of the adaptive immune system, polyreactive antibodies are not very specific in that they can bind to a number of antigens and they can form only weak bonds. Another component of the innate immune system is composed of a series of blood-borne proteins, known as **complement**. These proteins recognize bacteria in the bloodstream; they assemble on the bacterial surface forming a **membrane attack complex (MAC)** that damages the bacterial cell and making it a target for phagocytosis.

- The **adaptive immune system** is *specific* in that it has four primary characteristics: **immunologic memory**, **immunologic specificity**, **immunologic diversity**, and the **ability to differentiate between self and non-self**. Additionally, the adaptive immune system

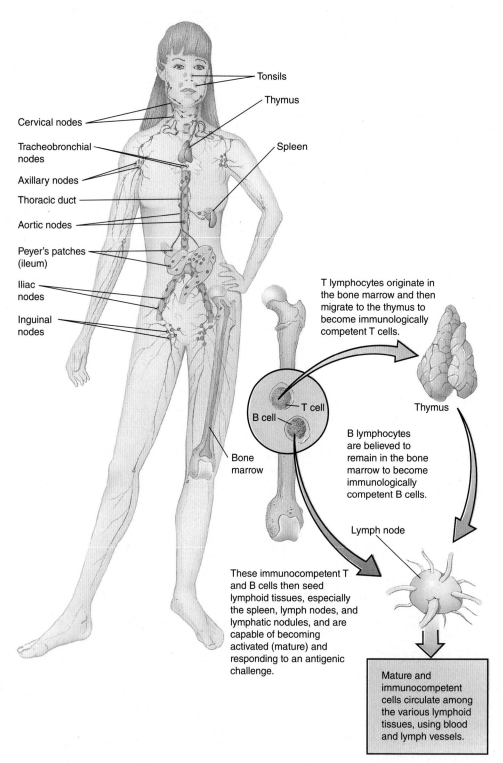

FIGURE 10-1. Schematic representation of the components of the lymphoid (immune) system. Lymphoid tissue consists of several encapsulated organs, lymph nodes, tonsils, thymus, and spleen as well as diffuse lymphoid tissue, composed of loose conglomerates of the lymphoid cells: B lymphocytes, T lymphocytes, plasma cells, macrophages, and antigen-presenting cells (APCs). Frequently, these lymphoid cells are collected as lymphatic nodules that appear as they are needed, although they are always present in the gut (gut-associated lymphoid tissue [GALT] and Peyer's patches), in the bronchial tubes (bronchus-associated lymphoid tissue [BALT]), and certain mucosae (mucosa-associated lymphoid tissue [MALT]).

CLINICAL CONSIDERATIONS 10-1

Polyreactive Antibodies

It has been demonstrated that polyreactive antibodies have an affinity to bind to apoptotic cells, whereas other antibodies do not bind to such cells. It was also noted that certain signal molecules were also attracted to the apoptotic cells with bound polyreactive antibodies, and this complex encouraged macrophages to phagocytose these apoptotic cells.

Table 10-1	Components of the Innate Immune System
Component	**Function**
Complement	This series of blood-associated macromolecules combines in a predetermined order to form a membrane attack complex on the plasmalemmae of intravascular pathogens.
Toll-like receptors (TLR)	TLRs are a family of 15 or more integral proteins located on the plasmalemmae of dendritic cells, macrophages, and mast cells as well as in endosomal membranes. TLRs recognize extracellular pathogens as well as intracellular ligands formed because of cell injury and initiate responses to combat them. TLRs activate not only cells of the innate immune system but also those of the adaptive immune system. See Table 10-2 for some of their functions.
Mast cells	See Chapter 4
Eosinophils	See Chapter 6
Neutrophils	See Chapter 6
Macrophages	Macrophages phagocytose foreign substances, breaking them down to epitopes (antigenic determinants). They present these epitopes on their cell surface in conjunction with major histocompatibility complex (MHC) molecules and other membrane-associated markers.
Natural killer (NK) cells	NK cells kill virally altered cells and tumor cells in a nonspecific and non–MHC-restricted manner. These cells become activated by the Fc portions of those antibodies that are bound to cell surface epitopes and thus kill these decorated cells by a procedure known as antibody-dependent cell-mediated cytotoxicity (ADCC).

Table 10-2	Toll-Like Receptors	
Location	**Receptor Pair**	**Function**
Extracellular and intracellular	TLR1–TLR2	Binds to parasite proteins and bacterial lipoproteins
	TLR2–TLR2	Binds to bacterial wall peptidoglycans
	TLR2–TLR6	In gram-positive bacteria, binds to lipoteichoic acid; in fungi, it binds to zymosan
	TLR4–TLR4	In gram-negative bacteria, binds to lipopolysaccharides (lipoglycans) of the outer membranes
	TLR5–?*	Binds to the protein flagellin (principal constituent of bacterial flagella)
	TLR11–?*	Host recognition of *Toxoplasmosis gondii*
Intracellular only	TLR3–?*	Binds to double-stranded RNA of viruses
	TLR7–?*	Binds to single-stranded RNA of viruses
	TLR8–?*	Binds to single-stranded RNA of viruses
	TLR9–?*	Binds to viral and bacterial DNA
Unknown	TLR10–?*	Unknown
	TLR12–?*	Unknown
	TLR13–?*	Unknown
	TLR15–?*	Unknown

*Currently, TLR partner is unknown.
TLR, toll-like receptor.

establishes a relatively small number of identical cells, known as a **clone**, that are effective against a particular antigen. If required, the body can increase the number of cells of a particular clone, a process known as **clonal expansion**.

The adaptive immune system relies on the interactions of its primary cell components, lymphocytes, and APCs, which act in concert to:

- Initiate a cell-mediated immune response against microorganism, foreign cells, and virally altered cells or
- Initiate a humoral immune response by the release of **antibodies** against antigens.

Antibodies

Antibodies (immunoglobulins) are glycoproteins produced by plasma cells, and they form the principal armamentarium of the **humoral immune response**. These glycoproteins bind to those antigens for which they are specific, forming antibody–antigen complexes. Each antibody is composed of two heavy chains and two light chains and possesses a **constant region (Fc fragment** [c refers to its being able to crystallize easily]) and a **variable region (Fab fragment** [ab refers to antigen binding]). The constant regions are the same for all antibodies of the same class (isotype), whereas the variable regions are identical only in antibodies against a specific antigen. There are **five classes (isotypes)** of immunoglobulins: IgA, IgD, IgE, IgG, and IgM (Table 10-3). The heavy chains of these isotypes differ from one another in their amino acid composition. Most **antigens** (a contraction for **anti**body **gen**erators) are large molecules and have numerous antigenic regions, known as **epitopes**, where each epitope can have a specific antibody generated against it. The variable region recognizes and attaches to the epitope, and the constant region is available to be recognized by certain cells of the adaptive immune system.

Table 10-3	Immunoglobulin Isotypes and Their Characteristics		
Class	**Cytokines***	**Binding to Cells**	**Biologic Characteristics**
IgA Secretory immunoglobulin	TGF-β	Forms temporary attachment to epithelial cells as it is being secreted	IgA is secreted as a dimer, which is protected by its secretory component, into saliva, tears, bile, gut lumen, nasal discharge, and milk (providing passive immunity for infants), and it provides protection against pathogens and invading antigens.
IgD Reaginic antibody		B-cell plasmalemma	The presence of IgD on B-cell plasma membranes permits them to recognize antigens and initiate an immune response by inducing B cells to differentiate into plasma cells.
IgE Reaginic antibody	IL-4 and IL-5	Plasmalemmae of mast cells and basophils	When antigens bind to IgE antibodies attached to mast cells and basophil plasma membranes, the binding prompts the release of pharmacologic agents from these cells initiating the immediate hypersensitivity response.
IgG Serum immunoglobulin	IFN-γ, IL-4, and IL-6	Neutrophils and macrophages	IgG is a serum antibody that crosses the placental barrier protecting the fetus (passive immunity). In the bloodstream, IgG binds to antigenic sites on invading microorganisms, opsonizing these pathogens so that neutrophils and macrophages can phagocytose them. NK cells are activated by IgG, thereby initiating ADCC.
IgM First to be formed in immune response		Although a pentamer, monomeric form binds to B cells	The pentameric form activates the complement system.

ADCC, antibody-dependent cell-mediated cytotoxicity; IFN, interferon; IL, interleukin; NK, natural killer; TGF-β=Transforming growth factor-β
*Cytokines responsible for switching to this isotype.

CLINICAL CONSIDERATIONS 10-2

Monoclonal Antibodies

Monoclonal antibodies are manufactured by clones of an antigen-specific plasma cell so that the antibodies produced are identical and bind to identical epitopes; therefore, they are monovalent antibodies. By convention, pharmaceutical companies that manufacture large amounts of these monoclonal antibodies developed the nomenclature so that the name ends with "mab," thus the pharmaceutical agent can be recognized as a monoclonal antibody. Many of these monoclonal antibodies target specific molecules to disrupt their functions to assist patients with autoimmune diseases, induce apoptotic responses and immune responses against cancer cells, and fight hepatitis C as well as certain other conditions.

Immune Response

The immune system relies on the interactions of its primary cell components, lymphocytes, and APCs, to effect an immune response. These responses are meticulously controlled and directed, but a complete description of the mechanisms of their actions is beyond the purposes of this book. Therefore, only the salient features of the mechanisms of the immune process will be described, readers interested in a more thorough description should consult a textbook of immunology.

Cells of the Adaptive and Innate Immune Systems

B Lymphocytes

B lymphocytes (B cells) are formed and become immunocompetent in the bone marrow where **pre-B cells** are transformed into **transitional B cells**, which develop into **mature B cells** in the spleen. Mature B cells establish clones whose members seed various lymphoid organs and, if necessary, can respond to initiate a **humoral immune response**. As B cells achieve immunocompetency, they synthesize IgM or IgD and place them on their cell membrane (as **surface immunoglobulins [SIGs]**) in such a fashion that the epitope-binding sites are located in the extracellular space and the Fc moiety of the SIGs is embedded in the plasmalemma in association with two pairs of integral proteins, **Igα** and **Igβ**. Every SIG of a particular B cell targets identical epitopes.

When a newly formed B cell binds to its epitope, the integral proteins Igα and Igβ transduce the information and the mature B cell becomes activated. Although there are several different B-cell populations, they will not be discussed in this text. For more information about B cells, the reader is encouraged to consult one of the many immunology textbooks.

B cells display **CD40 molecules** (cluster of differentiation 40 molecules) on their cell membranes, which allow these cells to communicate with a particular population of T helper cells (T_H2 cells).

Additionally, B cells display class II MHC molecules on their cell membranes with which they can present **epitopes** to T_H2 cells during an immune response (Fig. 10-2). As they present the **MHC II–epitope complex** to the T_H2 cell, that cell releases the following cytokines:

- Interleukin (IL)-10 that inhibits T_H1 cells from undergoing mitosis,
- IL-4 and IL-6 that induces the activation, proliferation, and differentiation of B cells into **plasma cells** and **B memory cells**, and
- IL-5 that not only induces B cells to proliferate but also instructs the B cells to manufacture the explicit type of immunoglobulins (known as **isotype switching**) that are required to battle the specific pathogen that triggered the immune reaction.

The T-cell receptor (TCR) and CD4 molecules of the T_H2 cell recognize the B cell's MHC II–epitope complex. Additionally, binding of the B cell's CD40 molecule to the T_H2 cell's CD40 receptor induces the B cell to proliferate and the T_H2 cell to release IL-4, IL-5, and IL-6.

IL-4, IL-5, and IL-6 induce the activation of B cells and their differentiation into B memory cells and plasma cells.

Plasma cells do not possess SIGs but synthesize and release an enormous number of identical copies of the same antibody that is specific against only a particular epitope (although it may cross-react with very similar epitopes). They release their antibodies into the connective tissues from which the antibodies are distributed via the blood or lymph vascular system, thus the term "humoral response."

B memory cells are long-lived, circulating cells that are added to and increase the number of cells of the original clone. Similarly, it is this increase in the size of the clone that is responsible for the **anamnestic response** against a subsequent encounter with the same antigen. Antibodies, once released, bind to a specific antigen. In some instances, binding inactivates the antigen, whereas in others the attachment of antibodies to antigens may enhance phagocytosis (**opsonization**) or activate the

CLINICAL CONSIDERATIONS 10-3

Major Histocompatibility Complex Molecules

It should be noted that most nucleated cells possess **major histocompatibility complex (MHC) I molecules (class I MHC molecules)** on the extracellular aspect of their plasmalemma. APCs also possess **MHC II molecules (class II MHC molecules)** on the extracellular aspect of their plasmalemma. All MHC I molecules are identical for a particular individual but differ from those of other individuals (except for identical twins), and that is also true for all MHC II molecules. Therefore, MHC I and MHC II molecules identify "self." MHC molecules bind to epitopes to form an MHC–epitope complex, which APCs can present to T helper cells. In humans, some authors use the term HLA molecules (for human leukocyte antigens).

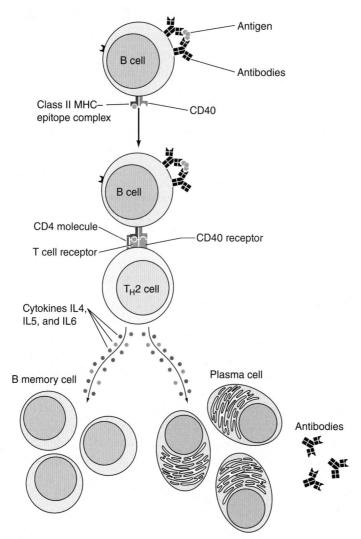

FIGURE 10-2. Schematic illustration of the interaction between B cells and T$_H$2 cells. Antigen-dependent cross-linking of the surface antibodies activates the B cell, which places the epitope–MHC II complex on the external aspect of its plasmalemma.

complement cascade, resulting in chemotaxis of neutrophils and, frequently, lysis of the invader.

T Lymphocytes

T-lymphocyte precursors are immunoincompetent until they enter the cortex of the thymus.

Here, under the influence of the cortical environment, they express their **T-cell receptors** and **cluster of differentiation markers** (CD2, CD3, CD4, CD8, and CD28) and, after numerous programmed alterations, become immunocompetent. Once immunocompetent, the T cells enter the medulla of the thymus or, are killed in the thymic medulla if they are committed against the self. In the medulla, they will lose either their CD4 or their CD8 markers and thus develop into **CD8$^+$** or **CD4$^+$ cells**, respectively. These cells enter the blood vessels of the thymic medulla to become members of the circulating population of lymphocytes.

There are several categories of T cells that are responsible not only for the **cell-mediated immune response** but also for inducing the **humoral-mediated response** of B cells (Fig. 10-2) to **thymic-dependent antigens** (i.e., antigens that require the involvement of T cells). T cells have characteristic integral membrane proteins on their cell surfaces, which assist them in executing their functions. One of these integral proteins is the TCR that is analogous to the SIGs of B cells. A TCR can recognize that particular epitope to which the cell is genetically programmed to respond; however, T cells can recognize only those epitopes that are bound to MHC molecules present on the surface of APCs. Thus, T cells are said to be **MHC restricted**. It should be stressed that although TCRs are analogous to immunoglobulins, they are always bound to the T-cell plasma membrane and are not secreted. T cells, instead of acting at a distance, always perform their functions by contacting other cells; therefore, they are responsible for the cell-mediated immune response. Once a T lymphocyte becomes activated by contacting an APC bearing the proper signals, it releases cytokines, substances that activate cytotoxic T cells (CTLs), causing their proliferation and their ability to kill virally transformed or foreign cells (Fig. 10-3).

There are three general categories of T cells: naive T cells, memory T cells, and effector T cells.

- **Naive T cells** are immunologically competent. They possess CD45RA molecules on their plasma membrane, but they have to become activated before they can perform their functions as T cells. Activation involves the interaction of the naive T cell's TCR–CD3 complex with the MHC–epitope complex of APCs as well as the interaction of the T cell's CD28 molecule with the APC's B7 molecule. The activated naive T cell enters the cell cycle and forms memory T cells and effector T cells.

- **Memory T cells**, the progeny of activated T cells, are long-lived, circulating cells that exhibit CD45RA molecules on their cell membranes. They undergo mitosis, thereby increasing the number of cells of the original clone permitting a more rapid and a more vigorous secondary response (anamnestic response) against another encounter with the same antigen.

There are two types of memory T cells: those that possess CR7 molecules (CR7$^+$) on their cell membranes (**central memory T cells [TCMs]**) and those that do not have CR7 molecules (CR7$^-$) on their plasmalemma (**effector T memory cells [TEMs]**). TCMs express IL-12 receptors on their cell membranes and reside in the lymph node **paracortex** (T-cell–rich zone of the lymph node). When TCMs contact the proper APC, the APC releases IL-12, which binds to the IL-12 receptor of the TCM, causing it to transform itself into a TEM. The newly formed TEMs travel to the region of inflammation and undergo a rapid course of cell divisions to form **effector T cells**.

- **Effector T cells** are immunocompetent descendants of TEM cells that have the ability to initiate an immune response. There are three categories of effector T cells: T helper cells (T$_H$ cells), cytotoxic T lymphocytes (CTLs, T killer cells), and regulatory T cells (T reg cells). An additional type of T cells is known as natural T killer cells.
  - **T helper cells** are all CD4$^+$ cells. Collectively, T helper cells are responsible for: producing and releasing various interleukins that initiate a cell-mediated immune response against intracellular pathogens, parasites, and virally altered cells; inducing B cell proliferation and differentiation into plasma cells; and recruiting neutrophils to the site of immune response.

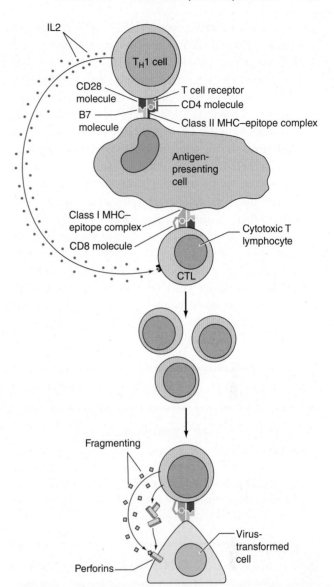

FIGURE 10-3. Schematic diagram illustrating the interactions between antigen-presenting cells (APCs) and T$_H$1 cells and APCs with CTLs. The T-cell receptor (TCR) and CD4 molecule of the T$_H$1 cell bind to the epitope and the MHC II of the APC, respectively. The binding induces the APC to express B7 molecules on its plasmalemma, which then binds to the CD28 molecule of the T$_H$1 cell, inducing that cell to release IL-2.

The same APC expresses the MHC I–epitope complex, which is recognized by the CD28 molecule and the TCR of the cytotoxic T lymphocyte (CTL). Additionally, the CD28 molecule of the CTL binds with the B7 molecule on the APC plasmalemma. These interactions induce the expression of IL-2 receptors on the CTL plasma membrane. Binding of IL-2 (released by the T$_H$1 cell) to the IL-2 receptors of the CTL induces that cell to proliferate.

The plasmalemma of virally transformed cells expresses an MHC I–epitope complex, which is recognized by the CD28 molecule and TCR of the newly formed CTLs. The binding of the CTL induces these cells to secrete perforins and fragmentins. The former assembled to form pores in the plasma membrane of the transformed cell, and fragmentin drives the transformed cell into apoptosis.

- **Cytotoxic T lymphocytes** are CD8⁺ cells that also express TCRs and CD3 on their cell membranes. Upon contacting the proper class I MHC–epitope complex displayed by APCs and having been activated by IL-2, they enter the cell cycle to form CTLs. These newly formed cells kill foreign and virally transformed self-cells by secreting **perforins** and **fragmentins** and by expressing CD95L (**death ligand**) on their plasmalemma, which activates CD95 (**death receptor**) on the target cell's plasma membrane that drives the target cell into apoptosis (see Fig. 10-3).
- **Regulatory T cells** (**T Reg cells**) are CD4⁺ cells that function in the suppression of the immune response by binding to APCs or effector T cells and by releasing cytokines that inhibit T helper cells.
- **Natural T killer cells** (not to be confused with NK cells discussed below) are similar to NK cells in that they act in a rapid fashion, but they have to enter the cortex of the thymus to become immunocompetent. They are quite unusual because their TCRs have the ability to recognize **lipid antigens** that are complexed to CD1 molecules on the APC's surface.

Natural Killer Cells

Natural killer cells (**NK cells**) are members of the **null cell** division of lymphocytes. NK cells do not have the cell surface determinants typical of T or B cells, and they are immunocompetent as soon as they are formed in the bone marrow. These cells kill virally altered cells, non-self-cells, and tumor cells in a nonspecific manner. NK cells are not MHC restricted, do not have to enter the thymus to be competent killer cells, and they recognize, bind to, and become activated by the Fc portions of those antibodies that are bound to cell surface epitopes of foreign, tumor, or virally altered cells. Once activated, NK cells release perforins and fragmentins to kill these decorated cells by a procedure

CLINICAL CONSIDERATIONS 10-4

Wiskott–Aldrich Syndrome

Wiskott–Aldrich syndrome is an immunodeficiency disorder occurring only in boys and is characterized by eczema (dermatitis), lowered platelet count, and lymphocytopenia (abnormally low levels of lymphocytes, both B- and T-cell populations). The immunosuppressed state of these children leads to recurring bacterial infections, hemorrhage, and death at an early age. Most children who survive the first decade of life are stricken with leukemia or lymphoma.

CLINICAL CONSIDERATIONS 10-5

Hodgkin's Disease

Hodgkin's disease is a neoplastic transformation of lymphocytes that is prevalent mostly in young males. Its clinical signs are asymptomatic initially because the swelling of the liver, spleen, and lymph nodes is not accompanied by pain. Other manifestations include the loss of weight, elevated temperature, diminished appetite, and generalized weakness. Histopathologic characteristics include the presence of Reed–Sternberg cells, easily recognizable by their large size, and the presence of two large, pale, oval nuclei in each cell.

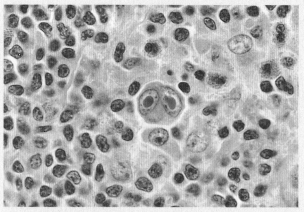

This photomicrograph is from the lymph node of a patient with Hodgkin's lymphoma displaying the characteristic binucleate Reed–Sternberg cell in the center of the field. Note the distinguishing eosinophilic nuclei that resemble nuclear inclusions. (Reprinted with permission from Mills SE, et al., eds. *Sternberg's Diagnostic Surgical Pathology*, 6th ed. Philadelphia: Wolters Kluwer, 2015. p. 770, Figure 17-21.)

known as **antibody-dependent cell-mediated cytotox-icity (ADCC)**. Perforins assemble as pores within the plasmalemma of these foreign, tumor, or virally altered cells, whereas fragmentins drive these cells into apoptosis. NK cells also possess integral proteins known as **killer activating receptors** that have an affinity to specific proteins on the cell membranes of nucleated cells. To protect self-cells from this response, NK cells also possess additional transmembrane proteins, known as **killer-inhibitor receptors**, that avoid the killing of healthy self-cells by recognizing MHC I molecules on the plasmalemmae of these cells.

Antigen-Presenting Cells and Macrophages

APCs, macrophages, and B lymphocytes possess both class I and class II MHC molecules, whereas all other nucleated cells possess only MHC I molecules.

An APC phagocytoses and degrades the antigen into epitopes, small highly antigenic peptides 7 to 11 amino acids long. Each epitope is attached to a class II MHC molecule, and this complex is placed on the external aspect of its cell membrane (Fig. 10-4). The MHC II–epitope complex is recognized by the **T cell receptor (TCR)** in conjunction with the CD4 molecule of the T helper cells. Because the epitope must be complexed with a class II MHC molecule for the T cell to recognize it, the process is known as MHC II restriction.

APCs and, specifically, macrophages produce and release a variety of cytokines that modulate the immune response. These include IL-1, which stimulates T helper cells and self-activated macrophages as well as prostaglandin E_2 that attenuates some immune responses. Cytokines, such as **interferon-γ**, released by other lymphoid cells, as well as by macrophages, enhance the phagocytic and cytolytic avidity of macrophages.

Diffuse Lymphoid Tissue

Diffuse lymphoid tissue occurs throughout the body, mostly in the loose connective tissue of the lamina propria deep to wet epithelial membranes. Lamina propria and wet lining epithelium are collectively referred to as mucosa. This loose connective tissue of the mucosa is infiltrated by lymphoid cells, namely lymphocytes, plasma cells, macrophages, and reticular cells, hence the name **mucosa-associated lymphoid tissue (MALT)**. MALT is particularly evident in the lamina propria of the respiratory tract and of the digestive tract, where they are known as **bronchus-associated lymphoid tissue (BALT)** and **gut-associated lymphoid tissue (GALT)**, respectively (see Chapter 15 for more information about GALT). It may be noted that the lymphoid cells are not arranged in any particular pattern but are scattered in an apparently haphazard manner.

Lymphoid Follicles (Lymphoid Nodules)

Lymphoid follicles or **nodules** are transitory dense cellular aggregates, composed mostly of lymphocytes. Lymphoid nodules may be **primary** or **secondary**.

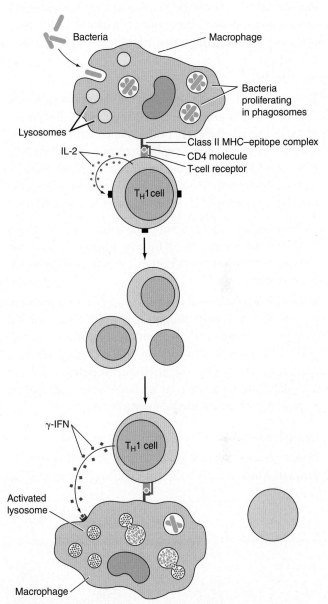

FIGURE 10-4. Schematic diagram illustrating the interaction between T_H1 cells and macrophages. Bacteria-infected macrophages bear MHC II–epitope complexes on their plasmalemma that, if recognized by the CD4 molecule and TCR of T_H1 cells, activates these cells, causing them to release IL-2 and to express IL-2 receptors on their plasma membrane. Binding of IL-2 to IL-2 receptors induces proliferation of the T_H1 cells.

The TCR and CD4 molecules of the newly formed T_H1 cells recognize and bind to the MHC II–epitope complexes of bacteria-infected macrophages. The binding causes activation of these T_H1 cells so that they release interferon-γ, a cytokine that encourages the macrophages to destroy their endocytosed bacteria.

The primary nodules are composed mostly of homogenously dense lymphocyte aggregates. The secondary lymphoid nodules are more active, therefore contain a lighter-staining **germinal center** and a darker, peripherally located **corona** or **mantle zone**. The germinal centers are sites of lymphocyte proliferation, whereas the corona is composed mostly of newly formed B lymphocytes that are migrating away from the germinal center.

Lymphoid Organs

The **lymphoid organs** function in the expansion and "training" of immune cells as well as providing the proper milieu in which these cells can organize an immune response. Histologically, lymphoid organs are typically a mixture of diffuse lymphoid tissue and lymphoid follicles surrounded by a complete or incomplete capsule. There are two classes of lymphoid organs, primary and secondary.

- Bone marrow and thymus constitute the **primary lymphoid organs** of the human adult; it is here that lymphocytes are formed and develop into immunocompetent cells.

- Lymph nodes, tonsils, spleen, and bone marrow (as well as MALT, even though it is a diffuse lymphoid tissue) constitute the **secondary lymphoid organs** of the human adult; it is here that a proper milieu is established so that the immunocompetent cells can collaborate to launch an immune response against pathogens that invaded the organism.

Lymph Nodes

Lymph nodes are ovoid- to kidney-shaped structures through which lymph is filtered (Fig. 10-5). They possess a **convex surface**, which receives afferent lymph vessels, and a **hilum**, where efferent lymph vessels leave, draining lymph from the organ, and both afferent and efferent blood vessels enter and exit.

Lymphocytes enter lymph nodes via the **afferent lymph vessels** and also by way of **arterioles**. Arterioles penetrate the lymph node at the hilum, using connective tissue trabeculae they travel to the paracortex where they deliver their blood into **high endothelial vessels (postcapillary venules)** that function in permitting T cells and B cells to leave the circulatory system, enter the parenchyma of the lymph node, and following specific chemotactic chemokines for each, migrate to their respective locations; T cells to the paracortex and B cells to lymphoid nodules.

Each lymph node has a dense irregular connective tissue **capsule**. **Septa**, derived from the capsule, partition the cortex into incomplete compartments (see Fig. 10-6). Attached to the septa and the internal aspect of the capsule is a network of reticular connective tissue that acts as a framework for housing reticular cells as well as numerous free and migratory cells, mostly lymphocytes, APCs, and macrophages, that reside in the organ. The cortex of the lymph node houses lymphoid nodules, composed mainly of B lymphocytes, APCs (such as follicular dendritic cells), macrophages, and reticular cells as well as the capsular and cortical lymphatic sinuses. Between the cortex and the medulla is the paracortex, populated by T lymphocytes, APCs (such as dendritic cells), and macrophages. The medulla consists of medullary cords and medullary sinuses. The medullary cords are composed mainly of T cells, B cells, follicular dendritic cells, and plasma cells that arise in the cortex and paracortex and

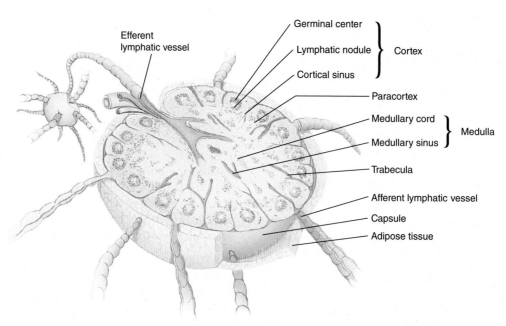

FIGURE 10-5. Schematic diagram of a lymph node. Lymph nodes function in T and B cell formation as well as in the cleaning of lymph.

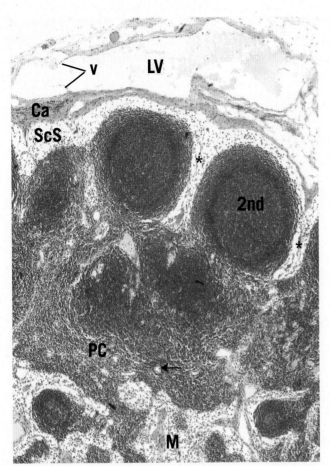

FIGURE 10-6. A low magnification of the convex region of a human lymph node. Note the **capsule** (Ca) and an afferent **lymph vessel** (LV) with its **valves** (v) bringing lymph into the **subcapsular sinus** (ScS). Observe the secondary lymphatic nodules (2nd), the paratrabecular sinuses (*asterisks*), and the **paracortex** (PC) with its high endothelial vessels (*arrow*), and a small region of the **medulla** (M). ×56.

migrate into the medulla. The medullary sinuses are continuous with the capsular and cortical sinuses. T cells and B cells enter the medullary sinuses and leave the lymph node via efferent lymph vessels.

Additional cell components of lymph nodes are macrophages, APCs, and some granulocytes. Aside from functioning in the maintenance and production of immunocompetent B and T cells and destroying those fugitive T cells that managed to leave the thymus even though they are programmed to recognize and attack

"self-antigens," lymph nodes also filter lymph. Lymph enters the node via afferent lymph vessels on the convex aspect, then flows through the subcapsular sinuses, radial/paratrabecular sinuses through the cortex and paracortex, then through the medullary sinuses before leaving the lymph node via efferent lymph vessel at the hilum. The filtering procedure is facilitated by the elongated processes of reticular cells that span the sinuses of the lymph node thereby disturbing and retarding lymph flow, providing more time for the resident macrophages to phagocytose antigens and other debris.

Tonsils

Tonsils are collections of diffuse lymphoid tissue and lymphoid follicles partially encapsulated by dense irregular connective tissue and situated at the entrances to the oral pharynx and the nasal pharynx. **Pharyngeal, lingual,** and **two palatine tonsils** form the **tonsillar ring (Waldeyer's ring)** at the major oronasal entryway. Plasma cells of the tonsils produce antibodies against the numerous antigens and microorganisms that abound in their vicinity. The palatine tonsils also produce T lymphocytes. Due to their location and their histologic anatomy, some authors consider them to be members of GALT, whereas other authors suggest that they are lymphoid organs.

Spleen

The **spleen** is the largest lymphoid organ of the body that functions in filtering blood, eliminating pathogens and senescent erythrocytes, facilitating the formation of effector T and B lymphocytes, and providing a locale for plasma cells to manufacture antibodies. Unlike lymph nodes, the spleen is not divided into cortical and medullary regions nor is it supplied by afferent lymphatic vessels. Blood vessels enter and leave the spleen at its hilum and travel within the parenchyma via trabeculae derived from its connective tissue capsule (Fig. 10-7).

The substance of the spleen is subdivided into white and red pulps. **White pulp** is composed of lymphoid tissue, which is organized either as **periarterial lymphatic sheaths (PALS)** composed of T lymphocytes or as lymphoid nodules consisting of B lymphocytes (Fig. 10-8). **Red pulp** consists of **pulp (splenic) cords (of Billroth)** interposed between a spongy network of sinusoids lined by unusually elongated endothelial cells, called stave

CLINICAL CONSIDERATIONS 10-6

Lymph Nodes During Infection

In a healthy patient with a normal amount of adipose tissue, the lymph nodes are small, soft structures that cannot be palpated easily. However, during an infection, the regional lymph nodes become enlarged and hard to the touch because of the large number of lymphocytes that are being formed within the node.

CLINICAL CONSIDERATIONS 10-7

Burkitt's Lymphoma

Burkitt's lymphoma is a very rapidly growing non-Hodgkin's lymphoma that has its origins in B cells. It is relatively rare in the United States but is more common in Central Africa, where it affects young males infected with the Epstein-Barr virus. It is also prevalent in people afflicted with human immunodeficiency virus. The lymphoma cells proliferate quickly and spread to lymph nodes and the small intestine. In more severe cases, the lymphoma cells can invade the central nervous system, bone marrow, and blood. If untreated, the disease is fatal, but treatment, especially in the early stages of the disease, has a very good prognosis.

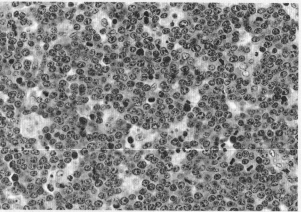

This photomicrograph is from a lymph node of a patient with Burkitt's lymphoma. Note the presence of several mitotic figures in the field. The image resembles a "starry sky" owing to the presence of an abundance of tingible-body macrophages. (Reprinted with permission from Mills SE, et al., eds. *Sternberg's Diagnostic Surgical Pathology*, 6th ed. Philadelphia: Wolters Kluwer, 2015. p. 789, Figure 17-48.)

CLINICAL CONSIDERATIONS 10-8

Tonsillitis

Tonsillitis is one of the most common complaints in children and even in young adults that affects the palatine, but also frequently, the pharyngeal tonsils. A number of viruses, such as rhinoviruses, adenoviruses, parainfluenza, and influenza viruses can cause tonsillitis, but usually they do not pose serious problems. However, the bacterium *Streptococcus pyogenes* is a culprit that can cause serious suppurative and nonsuppurative aftereffects. In some cases, suppuration may lead to peritonsillar abscesses that may dissect into the mediastinum or even into the cranial cavity leading to life-threatening results.

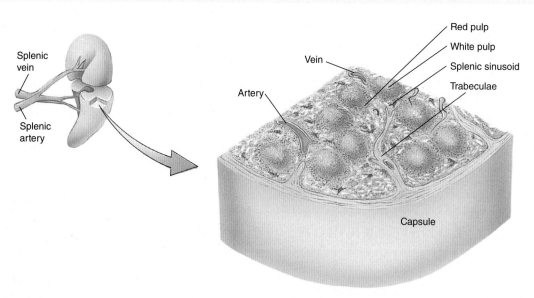

FIGURE 10-7. Schematic illustration of the microscopic morphology of the spleen. The spleen cleanses the blood, eliminates defunct red blood cells (RBCs), and forms T and B cells. In some animals (but not humans), the spleen stores RBCs.

cells, displaying large intercellular spaces, supported by a thick, discontinuous, hoop-like basement membrane. Healthy erythrocytes can pass through the gaps in between stave cells; however, damaged or old erythrocytes cannot pass through, thus getting trapped in the spleen for destruction by the macrophages. Reticular cells and reticular fibers associated with these sinusoids extend into the pulp cords to provide structural support to the cell population that consists of macrophages, plasma cells, and extravasated blood cells.

The red and white pulps are separated from one another by the **marginal zone**, composed of a group of small sinusoids, macrophages, T and B cells, APCs, and plasma cells (Fig. 10-9). Capillaries arising from the central arteries deliver their blood to sinusoids of the marginal zone with its avidly phagocytic macrophages. APCs of the marginal zone monitor this blood for the presence of antigens and foreign substances.

Understanding its vascular supply is key to comprehending the organization of the spleen.

- The splenic artery entering at the hilum is distributed to the interior of the organ via trabeculae as trabecular arteries. This vessel leaves the trabecula and enters the splenic parenchyma, where it becomes surrounded by the PALS (and occasional lymphoid nodules) and is known as the central artery (central arteriole).

- Central arteries lose their PALS as they enter the red pulp, and they subdivide into numerous small, straight vessels known as penicillar arteries, which possess three regions:
  - pulp arterioles,
  - sheathed arterioles, and
  - terminal arterial capillaries.

- Whether these terminal arterial capillaries drain directly into the sinusoids (closed circulation) or terminate as open-ended vessels in the pulp cords (open circulation) has not been determined conclusively; however, in humans, the open circulation is believed to predominate.

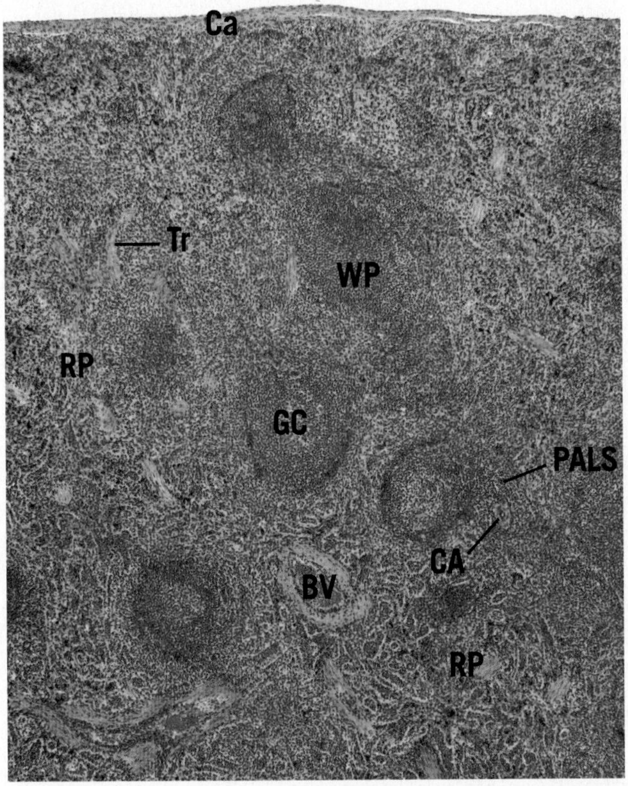

FIGURE 10-8. This very low-magnification photomicrograph of the human spleen displays its connective tissue **capsule** (Ca), the **trabeculae** (Tr) derived from the capsule ferrying **blood vessels** (BV), as well as the **red pulp** (RP) and **white pulp** (WP). Note that the white pulp is composed of **periarterial lymphatic sheaths** (PALS) with their centrally placed **central arteriole** (CA) and the frequent lymphoid nodules, some with **germinal centers** (GC) inserted into the PALS.

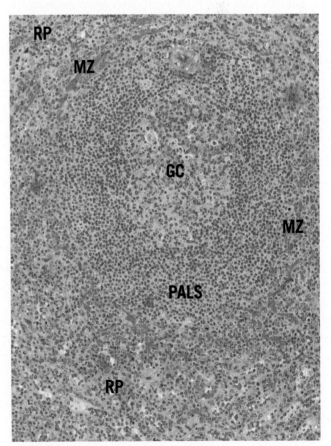

FIGURE 10-9. This low-magnification photomicrograph of the monkey spleen displays the **red pulp** (RP) as well as the white pulp, composed of the **periarterial lymphoid sheath** (PALS) and a lymphoid nodule with its **germinal center** (GC). Observe that the white pulp is separated from the red pulp by the **marginal zone** (MZ) that has a rich vascular supply composed of small sinuses.

- During this passage of RBCs from the splenic cords into the sinusoids, damaged and aging erythrocytes are eliminated.

- Sinusoids are drained by pulp veins, which lead to trabecular veins and eventually join the splenic vein.

Thymus

The **thymus** is a bilobed, encapsulated lymphoid organ located in the anterosuperior mediastinum, overlying the great vessels of the heart. The thymus attains its greatest proportionate size shortly after birth, but after puberty, it begins to **involute** and becomes infiltrated by adipose tissue; however, even in the adult, the thymus retains its ability to form a reduced number of T lymphocytes. The slender connective tissue capsule of the thymus sends septa deep into the lobes of the organ, incompletely subdividing them into lobules, and ferrying blood vessels into its substance (Fig. 10-10).

CLINICAL CONSIDERATIONS 10-9

Peripheral T-Cell Lymphoma in the Spleen

A relatively rare disease, **peripheral T-cell lymphomas in the spleen** are derived from T cells and T-cell precursors that proliferate and invade various organs, including the skin and the spleen. When the spleen is affected, the cells are large and aggressive with clear cytoplasms. They congregate in the vicinity of the PALS. The prognosis of patients with peripheral T-cell lymphomas depends on whether the invading cells express the protein anaplastic lymphoma kinase (ALK). Patients whose cells express ALK respond to treatment much better than patients whose cells do not express this protein.

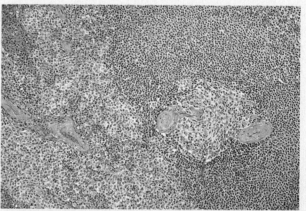

This photomicrograph is of the spleen of a patient with peripheral T-cell lymphoma. The large, clear cells that surround the PALS and the B cell–rich germinal center appear unaffected. (Reprinted with permission from Mills SE, et al., eds. *Sternberg's Diagnostic Surgical Pathology*, 6th ed. Philadelphia: Wolters Kluwer, 2015. p. 829, Figure 18-20A.)

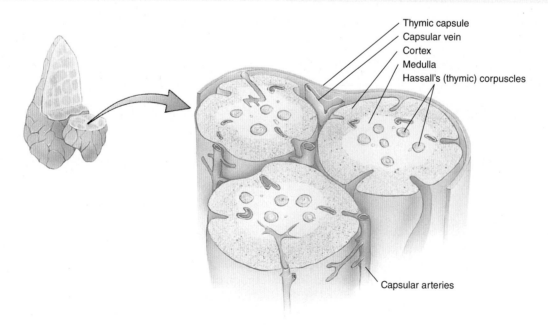

Thymic capsule
Capsular vein
Cortex
Medulla
Hassall's (thymic) corpuscles

Capsular arteries

FIGURE 10-10. Schematic diagram of the histology of an adult thymus. The thymus is responsible for the maturation of T cells. T helper cells play a pivotal role in the development and maintenance of the immune response. They interact with antigen-presenting cells and release cytokines, resulting in the generation of plasma cells for the humoral and T killer (cytotoxic) cells for the cell-mediated response.

Unlike lymph nodes and the spleen, the thymus possesses no lymphoid nodules; instead, its lobules are divided into an outer darker-staining cortex, composed of epithelial reticular cells, macrophages, and small T lymphocytes (thymocytes), and an inner lighter-staining medulla consisting of large T lymphocytes, epithelial reticular cells, and **thymic (Hassall's) corpuscles** (Table 10-4 and Fig. 10-11). The endoderm-derived epithelial reticular cells are different from the reticular cells of other lymphoid organs in that they provide many important structural and functional support to the thymus. Unlike in most organs, the medullae of neighboring lobules often tend to merge.

The principal functions of this primary lymphoid organ are the formation, potentiation, and, when necessary, the destruction of T lymphocytes, which the thymus accomplishes in the following manner.

- Immunoincompetent (immature) T-lymphocyte precursors enter the corticomedullary junction of the thymus, where they become known as thymocytes, migrate to the outer cortex where they are activated by cytokines released by epithelial reticular cells to express certain T-cell markers.

- The markers that thymocytes express do not include CD4, CD8, or the CD3–TCR complex and, because of that, they are known as **double-negative thymocytes**.

- These double-negative thymocytes migrate into the inner cortex, express pre-TCRs that trigger their propagation.

- The progeny of the pre-TCR-bearing thymocytes express both CD4 and CD8 molecules as well as a limited number of CD3–TCR molecules and are known as **double-positive thymocytes**.

- Cortical epithelial reticular cells assess if double-positive thymocytes are able to recognize **self-MHC–self-epitope complexes**.

- About 90% of double-positive thymocytes are unable to recognize these complexes, and they undergo apoptosis.

- The remaining 10% of these double-positive thymocytes that do recognize the self-MHC–self-epitope complexes mature, express many more TCRs, and lose either CD8 or CD4 molecules from their cell surface.

- Thymocytes that express many TCRs and either CD4 or CD8 molecules are known as **single-positive thymocytes**, which pass through the corticomedullary border to enter the medulla.

- Dendritic cells and epithelial reticular cells of the medulla assess the abilities of single-positive thymocytes to initiate an immune response against the self.

Table 10-4	Thymic Epithelial Reticular Cells	
Cell Type	**Location**	**Function**
Type I	Cortex	Surrounds blood vessels and isolates cortex from capsule and septa thus aiding in the formation of the blood–thymus barrier
Type II	Midcortex	Forms a boundary around and present MHC I, MHC II, and self-antigen molecules to thymocytes
Type III	Corticomedullary junction	Present MHC I, MHC II, and self-antigen molecules to thymocytes
Type IV	Corticomedullary junction	Isolates type III epithelial reticular cells from the medulla
Type V	Medulla	Forms the cellular scaffolding of the medulla
Type VI	Medulla	Forms Hassall's corpuscles; releases the cytokine thymic stromal lymphopoietin responsible for T reg cell formation

MHC, major histocompatibility complex.

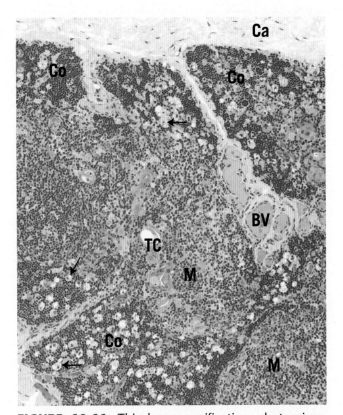

FIGURE 10-11. This low-magnification photomicrograph of an adult human thymus displays the **capsule** (Ca), darker **cortex** (Co), and the lighter-staining **medulla** (M). Note the rich **vascular supply** (BV) of the thymus as well as the **thymic (Hassall's) corpuscles** (TC) in the medulla. The numerous lightly staining circular profiles in the cortex represent mostly type II epithelial reticular cells (*arrows*). ×132.

- Single-positive thymocytes that can initiate an immune response against the self undergo apoptosis (**clonal deletion**) due to the effect of thymic stromal lymphopoietin, released by epithelial reticular cells of Hassall's corpuscles.
  - The signaling molecule, thymic stromal lymphopoietin, may also function in facilitating regulatory T cell formation.
- Single-positive thymocytes that are unable to attack the self are released from the thymus as **naive T lymphocytes**.
- These naive T cells migrate to the secondary lymphoid organs to set up clones of T cells.

Blood vessels travel in the connective tissue septa, which they exit at the corticomedullary junction, where they provide capillary loops to the cortex. The capillaries that enter the cortex are the continuous type and are surrounded by epithelial reticular cells that isolate them from the cortical lymphocytes, thus establishing a **blood–thymus barrier**, providing an antigen-free environment for the potentiation of the immunocompetent T lymphocytes. The blood vessels of the medulla are not unusual and present no blood–thymus barrier. The thymus is drained by venules in the medulla, which also receives blood from the cortical capillaries. Epithelial reticular cells form a specialized barrier between the cortex and medulla to prevent medullary material from gaining access to the cortex.

CLINICAL CONSIDERATIONS 10-10

DiGeorge's Syndrome

DiGeorge's syndrome is a congenital disorder in which the thymus fails to develop, and the patient is unable to produce T lymphocytes. These patients cannot mount a cell-mediated immune response, and some of their humorally mediated responses are also disabled or curtailed. Most individuals with this syndrome die in early childhood as a result of uncontrollable infections.

CLINICAL CONSIDERATIONS 10-11

Thymoma

Thymomas, 80% of which are benign tumors of the thymus, are most frequently located in the anterosuperior mediastinum. These dense, grayish tumors can be as large as 5 to 6 inches in length and are subdivided into segments by connective tissue septa derived from their dense irregular connective tissue capsule. Their most common cells are lymphocytes and proliferating spindle-shaped epithelial cells that may resemble abnormal Hassall's corpuscles. Interestingly, ~15% of myasthenia gravis patients exhibit thymomas.

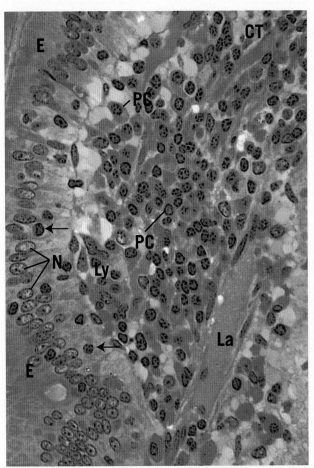

FIGURE 10-1-1. Lymphatic infiltration. Monkey. Plastic section. ×540.

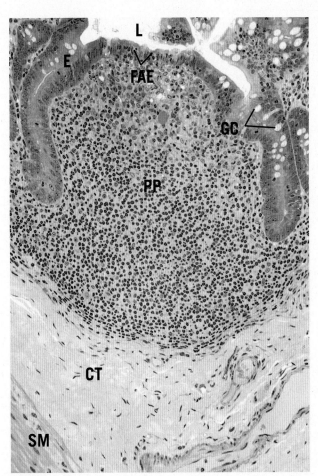

FIGURE 10-1-2. Lymphatic nodule. Monkey. Plastic section. ×132.

The **connective tissue** (CT) of the lamina propria deep to wet epithelia is usually infiltrated by loosely aggregated **lymphocytes** (Ly) and **plasma cells** (PC), as is exemplified by this photomicrograph of the monkey duodenum. Observe that the simple columnar **epithelium** (E) contains not only the **nuclei** (N) of epithelial cells but also dark dense nuclei of lymphocytes (*arrows*), some of which are in the process of migrating from the lamina propria (connective tissue) into the lumen of the duodenum. Note also the presence of a **lacteal** (La), a blindly ending lymphatic channel containing lymph. These vessels may be recognized by the absence of red blood cells.

The gut-associated lymphatic nodule in this photomicrograph is part of a cluster of nodules known as **Peyer's patches** (PP) and is taken from the monkey ileum. The **lumen** (L) of the small intestine is lined by a simple columnar **epithelium** (E) with numerous **goblet cells** (GC). However, note that the epithelium is modified over the lymphoid tissue into a **follicle-associated epithelium** (FAE), which is composed of shorter, specialized M cells, lymphocyte infiltrates, and no goblet cells. Observe that this particular lymphatic nodule presents no germinal center but is composed of several cell types, as recognized by nuclei of various sizes and densities. These will be described in Figures 10-1-3 and 10-1-4. Although this lymphatic nodule is unencapsulated, the **connective tissue** (CT) between the **smooth muscle** (SM) and the lymphatic nodule is free of infiltrate.

KEY					
CT	connective tissue	GC	goblet cell	N	nucleus
E	epithelium	L	lumen	PC	plasma cell
FAE	follicle-associated epithelium	La	lacteal	PP	Peyer's patch
		Ly	small lymphocyte	SM	smooth muscle

PLATE 10-1B Lymphoid Nodules

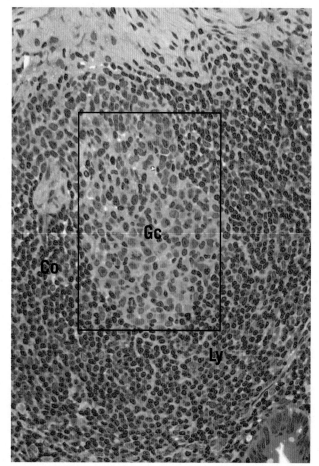

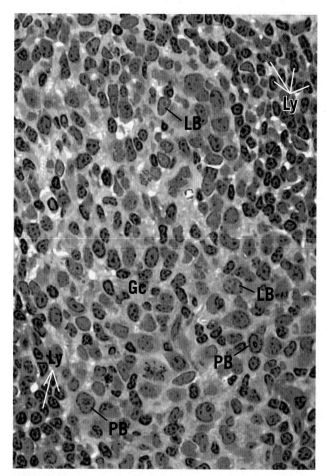

FIGURE 10-1-3. Lymphoid nodule. Monkey. Plastic section. ×270.

This is a higher magnification of a lymphoid nodule from Peyer's patches in the monkey ileum. Note that the lighter-staining **germinal center** (Gc) is sur-rounded by the **corona** (Co) of darker-staining cells possessing only a limited amount of cytoplasm around a dense nucleus. These cells are small **lymphocytes** (Ly). Germinal centers form in response to an antigenic challenge and are composed of lymphoblasts and plas-mablasts, whose nuclei stain much lighter than those of small lymphocytes. The *boxed area* is presented at a higher magnification in Figure 10-1-4.

FIGURE 10-1-4. Lymphoid nodule. Monkey. Plastic section. ×540.

This is a higher magnification of the *boxed area* of Fig-ure 10-1-3. Observe the small **lymphocytes** (Ly) at the periphery of the **germinal center** (Gc). The activity of this center is evidenced by the presence of mitotic figures as well as the **lymphoblasts** (LB) and **plas-mablasts** (PB). The germinal center is the site of pro-duction of small lymphocytes that then migrate to the periphery of the lymphoid nodule to form the corona.

KEY					
Co	corona	**LB**	lymphoblast	**PB**	plasmablast
Gc	germinal center	**Ly**	small lymphocyte		

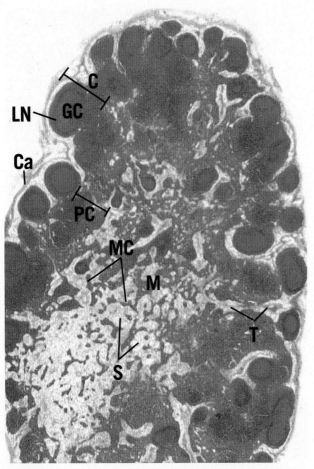

FIGURE 10-2-1. Lymph node. Paraffin section. ×14.

Lymph nodes are kidney-shaped structures possessing a convex and a concave (hilus) surface. They are invested by a connective tissue **capsule** (Ca) that sends **trabeculae** (T) into the substance of the node, subdividing it into incomplete compartments. The compartmentalization is particularly evident in the **cortex** (C), the peripheral aspect of the lymph node. The lighter-staining central region is the **medulla** (M), whereas the zone between the medulla and cortex is the **paracortex** (PC). Observe that the cortex displays numerous **lymphoid nodules** (LN), many with **germinal centers** (GC). This is the region of B lymphocytes, whereas the paracortex is particularly rich in T lymphocytes. Note that the medulla is composed of medullary **sinuses** (S), **trabeculae** (T) of connective tissue conducting blood vessels, and **medullary cords** (MC). The medullary cords are composed of lymphocytes, macrophages, and plasma cells. Lymph enters the lymph node through the afferent lymph vessels on the convex surface, and as it percolates through cortex, paracortex, and medullary sinuses, foreign substances are removed from it by phagocytic activity of macrophages.

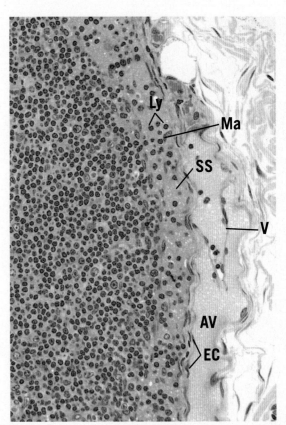

FIGURE 10-2-2. Lymph node. Monkey. Plastic section. ×270.

Afferent lymphatic vessels (AV) enter the lymph node at its convex surface. These vessels bear **valves** (V) that regulate the direction of flow. Lymph enters the **subcapsular sinus** (SS), which contains numerous **macrophages** (Ma), **lymphocytes** (Ly), and antigen presenting cells. These sinuses are lined by **endothelial cells** (EC), which also cover the fine collagen fibers that frequently span the sinus to create turbulence in lymph flow. Lymph from the subcapsular sinus enters the cortical sinus, then moves into the medullary sinus. Here, lymphocytes also migrate into the sinus, leaving the lymph node via the efferent lymph vessels eventually to enter the general circulation.

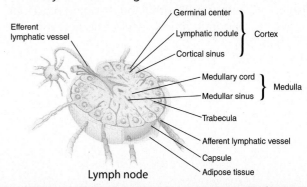

KEY					
AV	afferent lymphatic vessel	**LN**	lymphatic nodule	**PC**	paracortex
C	cortex	**Ly**	small lymphocyte	**S**	sinusoid
Ca	capsule	**M**	medulla	**SS**	subcapsular sinus
EC	endothelial cell	**Ma**	macrophage	**T**	trabeculae
GC	germinal center	**MC**	medullary cord	**V**	valve

PLATE 10-2B Lymph Node

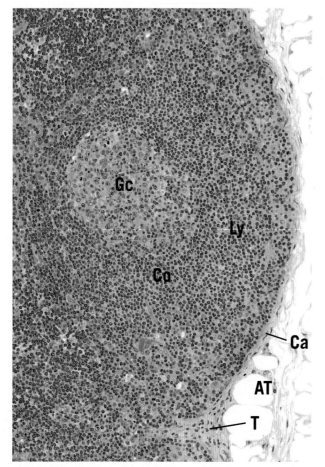

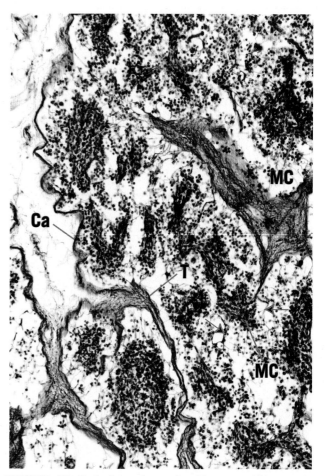

FIGURE 10-2-3. Lymph node. Monkey. Plastic section. ×132.

The cortex of the lymph node is composed of numerous lymphoid nodules, one of which is presented in this photomicrograph. Observe that the lymph node is usually surrounded by **adipose tissue** (AT). The thin connective tissue **capsule** (Ca) sends **trabeculae** (T) into the substance of the lymph node. Observe that the lymphatic nodule possesses a dark-staining **corona** (Co), composed mainly of small **lymphocytes** (Ly), whose heterochromatic nuclei are responsible for their staining characteristics. The **germinal center** (Gc) displays numerous cells with lightly staining nuclei, belonging to dendritic reticular cells, plasmablasts, and lymphoblasts.

FIGURE 10-2-4. Lymph node. Human. Silver stain. Paraffin section. ×132.

The hilus of the human lymph node displays the dense irregular connective tissue **capsule** (Ca), which sends numerous **trabeculae** (T) into the substance of the lymph node. Observe that the region of the hilus is devoid of lymphoid nodules but is particularly rich in **medullary cords** (MC). Note that the basic framework of these medullary cords, as well as of the lymph node, is composed of thin reticular fibers (*arrows*), which are connected to the collagen fiber bundles of the trabeculae and capsule.

KEY					
AT	adipose tissue	**GC**	germinal center	**MC**	medullary cord
Ca	capsule	**Ly**	small lymphocyte	**T**	trabeculae
Co	corona				

PLATE 10-3A   Lymph Node

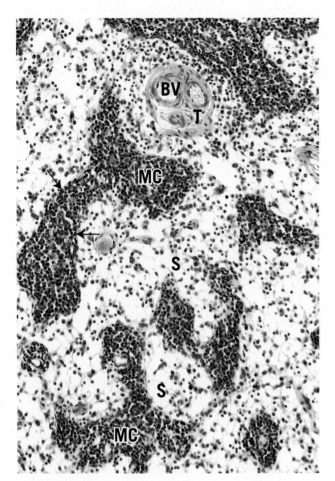

FIGURE 10-3-1. Lymph node. Paraffin section. ×132.

The medulla of the lymph node consists of numerous endothelially lined **sinuses** (S), which receive lymph from the cortical sinuses. Surrounding the medullary sinuses are many **medullary cords** (MC), composed of macrophages, small lymphocytes, and plasma cells, whose nuclei (*arrows*) stain intensely. Both T and B lymphocytes are found in medullary cords because they are in the process of migrating from the paracortex and cortex, respectively. Some of these lymphocytes will leave the lymph node using the medullary sinuses and efferent lymphatic vessels at the hilus. The medulla also displays connective tissue **trabeculae** (T) housing **blood vessels** (BV), which enter the lymph node at the hilus.

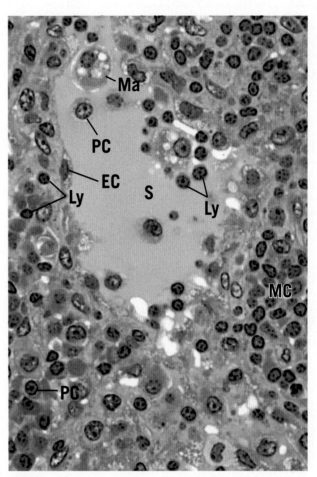

FIGURE 10-3-2. Lymph node. Monkey. Plastic section. ×540.

This photomicrograph is a high magnification of a medullary **sinus** (S) and surrounding **medullary cords** (MC) of a lymph node medulla. Note that the medullary cords are composed of macrophages, **plasma cells** (PC), and small **lymphocytes** (Ly). The sinuses are lined by **endothelial cells** (EC), which do not form a continuous lining. The lumen contains lymph, small **lymphocytes** (Ly), and **macrophages** (Ma). These cells are actively phagocytosing particulate matter as is evidenced by their vacuolated appearance.

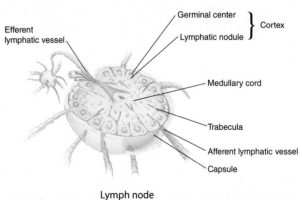

Lymph node

KEY							
BV	blood vessel		**Ma**	macrophage		**S**	sinusoid
EC	endothelial cell		**MC**	medullary cord		**T**	trabeculae
Ly	lymphocyte		**PC**	plasma cell			

PLATE 10-3B   Tonsils

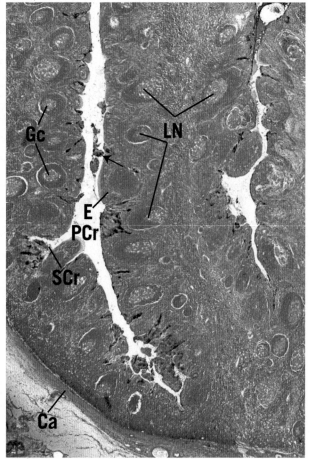

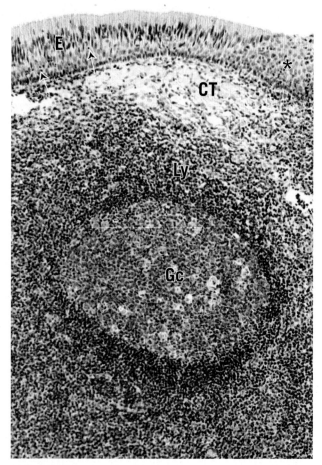

FIGURE 10-3-3. Palatine tonsil. Human. Paraffin section. ×14.

The palatine tonsil is an aggregate of **lymphatic nodules** (LN), many of which possess **germinal centers** (Gc). The palatine tonsil is covered by a stratified squamous nonkeratinized **epithelium** (E) that lines the deep **primary crypts** (PCr) that invaginate deeply into the substance of the tonsil. Frequently, **secondary crypts** (SCr) are evident, also lined by the same type of epithelium. The deep surface of the palatine tonsil is covered by a thickened connective tissue **capsule** (Ca). The crypts frequently contain debris (*arrow*) that consists of decomposing food particles as well as lymphocytes that migrate from the lymphatic nodules through the epithelium to enter the crypts.

FIGURE 10-3-4. Pharyngeal tonsil. Human. Paraffin section. ×132.

The pharyngeal tonsil, located in the nasopharynx, is an aggregate of lymphatic nodules, often displaying **germinal centers** (Gc). The **epithelial lining** (E) is pseudostratified ciliated columnar with occasional patches of stratified squamous nonkeratinized epithelium (*asterisk*). The lymphatic nodules are located in a loose, collagenous **connective tissue** (CT) that is infiltrated by small **lymphocytes** (Ly). Note that lymphocytes migrate through the epithelium (*arrows*) to gain access to the nasopharynx.

KEY					
Ca	capsule	**GC**	germinal center	**PCr**	primary crypt
CT	connective tissue	**LN**	lymphatic nodule	**SCr**	secondary crypt
E	epithelium	**Ly**	lymphocyte		

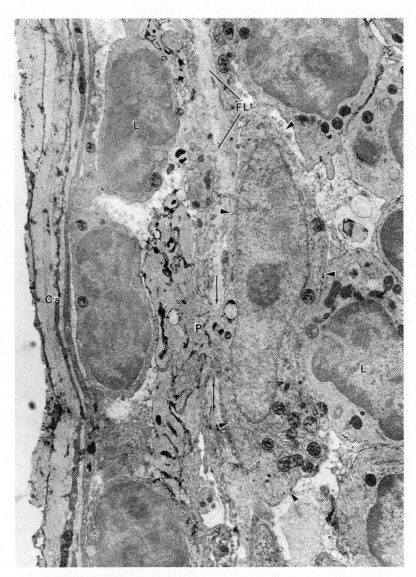

FIGURE 10-4-1. Lymph node. Mouse. Electron microscopy. ×8,608.

This electron micrograph of a mouse popliteal lymph node presents the **capsule** (Ca) and the subcapsular sinus. The sinus is occupied by three **lymphocytes**, one of which is labeled (L), as well as the **process** (P) of an antigen presenting cell, whose cell body (*arrowheads*) and nucleus are in the cortex, deep to the sinus. The process enters the lumen of the subcapsular sinus via a pore (*arrows*) in its **floor** (FL). It is believed that antigen presenting cells trap antigens at the site of antigenic invasion and transport them to lymphoid nodules of lymph nodes, where they mature to become dendritic reticular cells. (Reprinted with permission from Szakal AK, et al. Transport of immune complexes from the subcapsular sinus to lymph node follicles on the surface of nonphagocytic cells, including cells with dendritic morphology. *J Immunol* 1983;131(4):1714–1727. Copyright © 1983 by American Association of Immunologists.)

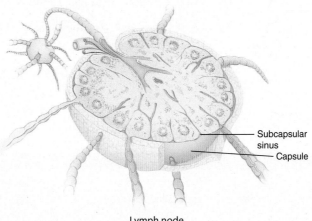

Subcapsular sinus

Capsule

Lymph node

PLATE 10-5A Thymus

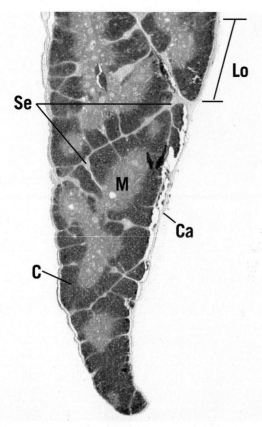

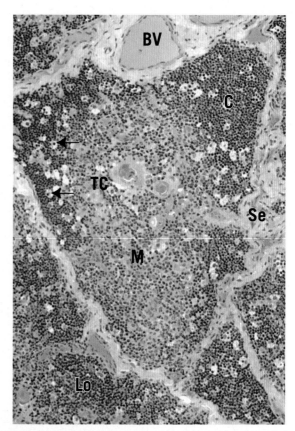

FIGURE 10-5-1. Thymus. Human infant. Paraffin section. ×14.

The thymus of an infant is a well-developed organ that displays its many characteristics to advantage. This photomicrograph presents a part of one lobe. It is invested by a thin connective tissue **capsule** (Ca) that incompletely subdivides the thymus into **lobules** (Lo) by connective tissue **septa** (Se). Each lobule possesses a darker-staining peripheral **cortex** (C) and a lighter-staining **medulla** (M). The medulla of one lobule, however, is continuous with that of other lobules. The connective tissue capsule and septa convey blood vessels into the medulla of the thymus. Shortly after puberty, the thymus begins to involute, and the connective tissue septa become infiltrated with adipocytes.

FIGURE 10-5-2. Thymus. Monkey. Plastic section. ×132.

The lobule of the thymus presented in this photomicrograph appears to be surrounded completely by connective tissue **septa** (Se); however, in a three-dimensional reconstruction, it would be seen that this lobule is continuous with surrounding **lobules** (Lo). Observe the numerous **blood vessels** (BV) in the septa, as well as the darker-staining **cortex** (C) and the lighter-staining **medulla** (M). The light patches of the cortex probably present epithelial reticular cells and macrophages (*arrows*), whereas the darker-staining structures are nuclei of the T-lymphocyte series. The medulla contains the characteristic **thymic corpuscles** (TC) as well as blood vessels, macrophages, and epithelial reticular cells.

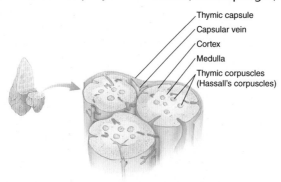

Thymic capsule
Capsular vein
Cortex
Medulla
Thymic corpuscles
(Hassall's corpuscles)

Thymus

KEY					
BV	blood vessel	**Lo**	lobule	**Se**	septum
C	cortex	**M**	medulla	**TC**	thymic corpuscle
Ca	capsule				

PLATE 10-5B   Thymus

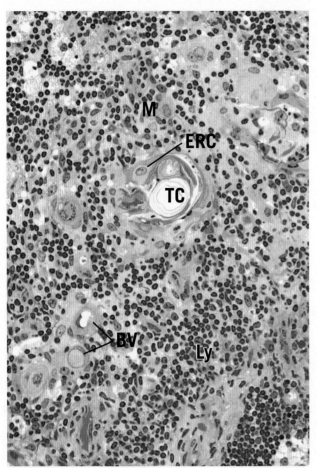

FIGURE 10-5-3. Thymus. Monkey. Plastic section. ×270.

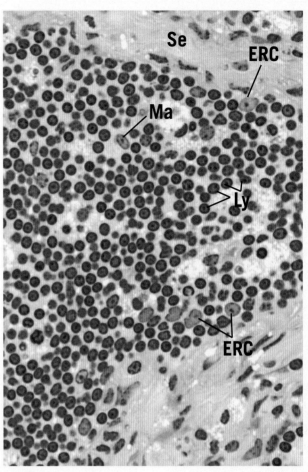

FIGURE 10-5-4. Thymus. Monkey. Plastic section. ×540.

The center of this photomicrograph is occupied by the **medulla** (M) of the thymus, presenting a large **thymic (Hassall's) corpuscle** (TC), composed of concentrically arranged **epithelial reticular cells** (ERC). Thymic corpuscles manufacture the cytokine thymic stromal lymphopoietin that is involved in T reg cell generation. The thymic medulla houses numerous **blood vessels** (BV), macrophages, **lymphocytes** (Ly), and occasional plasma cells.

The cortex of the thymus is bounded externally by collagenous connective tissue **septa** (Se). The substance of the cortex is separated from the septa by a border of **epithelial reticular cells** (ERC), recognizable by their pale nuclei. Additional epithelial reticular cells form a cellular reticulum, in whose interstices **lymphocytes** (Ly) develop into mature T lymphocytes. Numerous **macrophages** (Ma) are also evident in the cortex. These cells phagocytose lymphocytes destroyed in the thymus.

KEY					
BV	blood vessel	**M**	medulla	**Se**	septum
ERC	epithelial reticular cell	**Ma**	macrophage	**TC**	thymic corpuscle
Ly	lymphocyte				

PLATE 10-6A Spleen

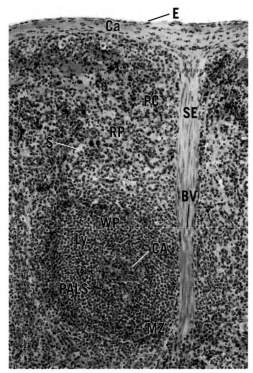

FIGURE 10-6-1. Spleen. Human. Paraffin section. ×132.

The spleen, the largest lymphoid organ, possesses a thick collagenous connective tissue **capsule** (Ca). Because it lies within the abdominal cavity, it is surrounded by a simple squamous **epithelium** (E) or mesothelium. Connective tissue **septa** (SE), derived from the capsule, penetrate the substance of the spleen, conveying **blood vessels** (BV) into the interior of the organ. The spleen is not subdivided into cortex and medulla; instead, it is composed of **white pulp** (WP) and **red pulp** (RP). White pulp is arranged as a cylindrical sheath of **lymphocytes** (Ly) surrounding a blood vessel known as the **central artery** (CA), whereas red pulp consists of **sinusoids** (S) meandering through a cellular tissue known as **pulp cords** (PC). The white pulp of the spleen is found in two different arrangements. The one represented in this photomicrograph is known as a **periarterial lymphatic sheath** (PALS) composed mostly of T lymphocytes. The zone of lymphocytes at the junction of the PALS and the red pulp is known as the **marginal zone** (MZ).

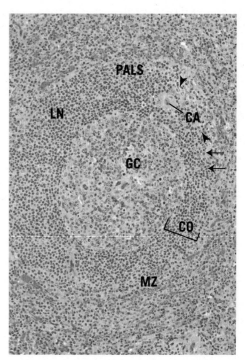

FIGURE 10-6-2. Spleen. Monkey. Plastic section. ×132.

Lying within the **periarterial lymphatic sheaths** (PALS) of the spleen, a second arrangement of white pulp may be noted, namely **lymphatic nodules** (LN) bearing a **germinal center** (Gc). Lymphatic nodules frequently occur at the branching of the **central artery** (CA). Nodules are populated mostly by B lymphocytes (*arrows*), which account for the dark staining of the **corona** (CO). The germinal center is the site of active production of B lymphocytes during an antigenic challenge. The **marginal zone** (MZ), also present around lymphatic nodules, is the region where lymphocytes leave the small capillaries and first enter the connective tissue spaces of the spleen. From here, T lymphocytes migrate to the periarterial lymphatic sheaths, whereas B lymphocytes seek out lymphatic nodules. Both the marginal zone and the white pulp house numerous macrophages as well as antigen-presenting cells (*arrowheads*) in addition to lymphocytes.

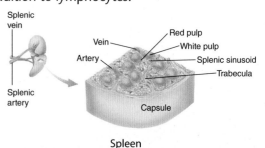

Spleen

KEY							
BV	blood vessel	**GC**	germinal center	**PC**	pulp cord
Ca	capsule	**LN**	lymphatic nodule	**RP**	red pulp
CA	central artery	**Ly**	lymphocyte	**S**	sinusoid
CO	corona	**MZ**	marginal zone	**SE**	septum
E	epithelium	**PALS**	periarterial lymphatic sheath	**WP**	white pulp

PLATE 10-6B Spleen

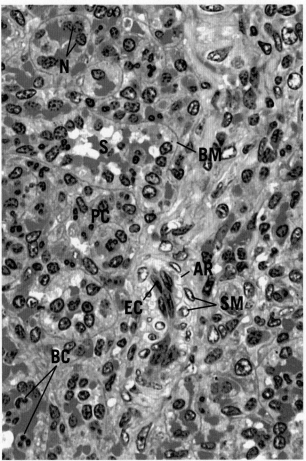

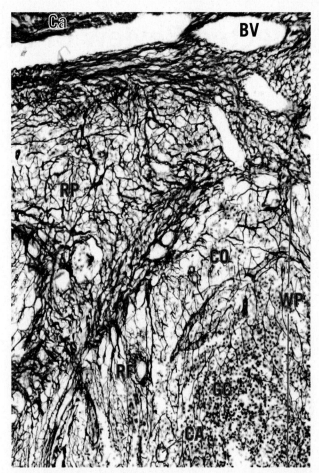

FIGURE 10-6-3. Spleen. Monkey. Plastic section. ×540.

The red pulp of the spleen, presented in this photomicrograph, is composed of splenic **sinusoids** (S) and **pulp cords** (PC). The splenic sinusoids are lined by a discontinuous type of epithelium comprised of stave cells and surrounded by an unusual arrangement of **basement membrane** (BM) that encircles the sinusoids in a discontinuous fashion. Sinusoids contain numerous **blood cells** (BC). **Nuclei** (N) of the stave cells bulge into the lumen. The regions between sinusoids are occupied by pulp cords, housing various cells of the blood, macrophages, reticular cells, and plasma cells. The vascular supply of the red pulp is derived from penicillar arteries, which give rise to **arterioles** (AR) whose **endothelial cells** (EC) and **smooth muscle** (SM) cells are evident in the center of this field.

FIGURE 10-6-4. Spleen. Human. Silver stain. Paraffin section. ×132.

The connective tissue framework of the spleen is demonstrated by the use of silver stain, which precipitates around reticular fibers. The **capsule** (Ca) of the spleen is pierced by **blood vessels** (BV) that enter the substance of the organ via **trabeculae** (T). The **white pulp** (WP) and **red pulp** (RP) are evident. In fact, the lymphatic nodule presents a well-defined **germinal center** (GC) as well as a **corona** (CO). The **central artery** (CA) is also evident in this preparation. **Reticular fibers** (RF), which form an extensive network throughout the substance of the spleen, are attached to the capsule and the trabeculae.

KEY					
AR	arteriole	**CO**	corona	**RF**	reticular fiber
BC	blood cell	**EC**	endothelial cell	**RP**	red pulp
BM	basement membrane	**GC**	germinal center	**S**	sinusoid
BV	blood vessel	**N**	nucleus	**SM**	smooth muscle
Ca	capsule	**PC**	pulp cord	**WP**	white pulp
CA	central artery				

Selected Review of Histologic Images

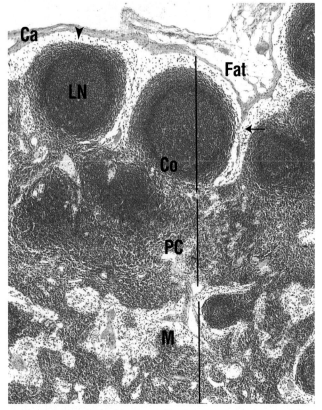

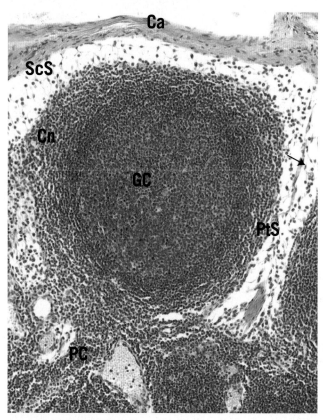

REVIEW FIGURE 10-1-1. Lymph node. Human adult. Paraffin section. ×56.

This low-magnification photomicrograph of a human lymph node demonstrates that it is surrounded by **adipose tissue** (Fat). The **capsule** (Ca) of the lymph node is composed of dense irregular collagenous connective tissue. Note the subcapsular (*arrowhead*) and the paratrabecular sinuses (*arrow*) as well as the **lymphoid nodules** (LN) in the **cortex** (Co). The **paracortex** (PC) is the T-cell–rich area located between the cortex and the **medulla** (M).

REVIEW FIGURE 10-1-2. Lymph node. Human adult. Paraffin section. ×132.

This is a higher-magnification photomicrograph of the cortex of the lymph node in Review Figure 10-1-1. Note the **capsule** (Ca), **subcapsular sinus** (ScS), and the paratrabecular sinus (PtS). The B cell–rich **corona** (Cn) and **germinal center** (GC) of the lymphoid nodule are well defined. The **paracortex** (PC) is the T-cell–rich area just below the lymphoid nodule.

KEY							
Ca	capsule	**GC**	germinal center	**PC**	paracortex
Co	cortex	**M**	medulla	**PtS**	paratrabecular sinus
Cn	corona	**LN**	lymphoid nodule	**ScS**	subcapsular sinus
Fat	adipose tissue				

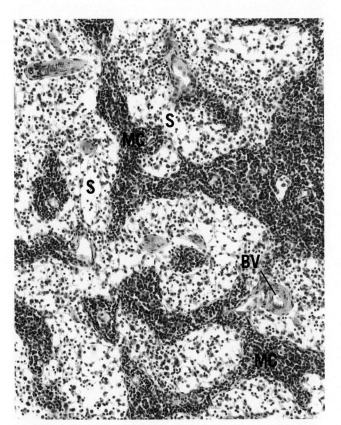

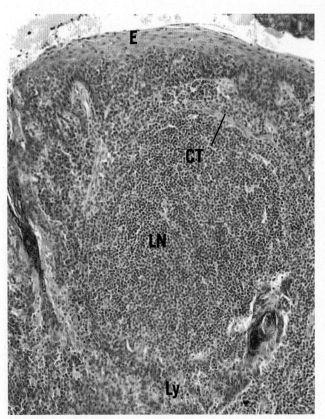

REVIEW FIGURE 10-1-3. Lymph node medulla. Human adult. Paraffin section. ×132.

This is a higher-magnification photomicrograph of the medulla of the lymph node in Review Figure 10-1-1. Note that the **medullary cords** (MC) are interspersed with the medullary **sinuses** (S). Trabeculae house **blood vessels** (BV) in the medulla.

REVIEW FIGURE 10-1-4. Palatine tonsil. Human. Paraffin section. ×132.

The palatine tonsils, located on either side of the base of the tongue, are composed of **lymphoid nodules** (LN), many with germinal centers. Each tonsil is covered by a stratified squamous **epithelium** (E). **Connective tissue trabeculae** (CT) arise from the capsule at the base of the tonsil carrying blood vessels into its substance. The numerous dark dots are the nuclei of **lymphocytes** (Ly).

KEY					
BV	blood vessel	**E**	stratified squamous	**LN**	lymphoid nodule
CT	connective tissue		epithelium	**Ly**	lymphocyte
	trabecula	**MC**	medullary cord	**S**	medullary sinus

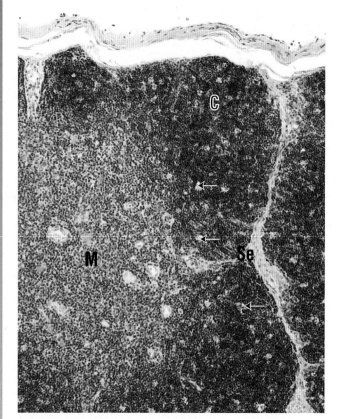

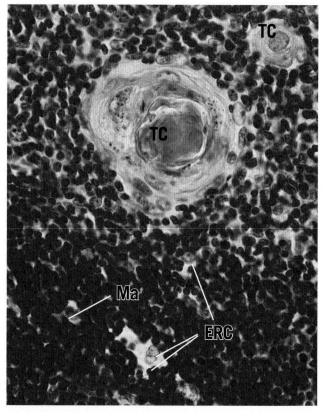

REVIEW FIGURE 10-2-1. Thymus. Human adult. Paraffin section. ×270.

This is a photomicrograph of three adjoining lobules of a human adult thymus. Note that **septa** (Se) arise from the connective tissue **capsule** (Ca) and separate the thymic lobe into lobules. The separation of the two lobules on the left-hand side is evident by the connective tissue septum at the "Se" label marker. The darker **cortex** (Co) is occupied by large numbers of thymocytes (T cells in various stages of development) as well as by numerous macrophages and epithelial reticular cells (*arrows*). The **medulla** (M) is lighter-staining than the cortex, and it is evident that the medullae of the two adjacent lobules are continuous with each other.

REVIEW FIGURE 10-2-2. Thymus medulla. Human adult. Paraffin section. ×540.

This is a photomicrograph of the human thymic adult medulla. Note the presence of **thymic corpuscles** (TC) as well as the presence of **macrophages** (Ma) and **epithelial reticular cells** (ERC). At this magnification, the two cells are easily distinguishable from each other because the epithelial reticular cells possess lighter-staining nucleoli with finer chromatin material than that of the macrophage.

KEY					
Ca	capsule	**M**	medulla	**Se**	septum
Co	cortex	**Ma**	macrophage	**TC**	thymic corpuscle
ERC	epithelial reticular cell				

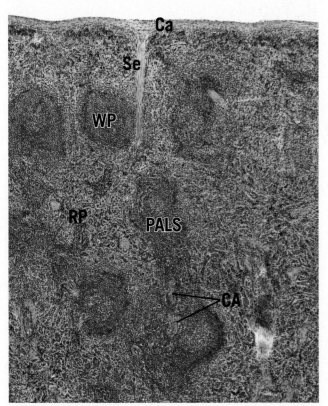

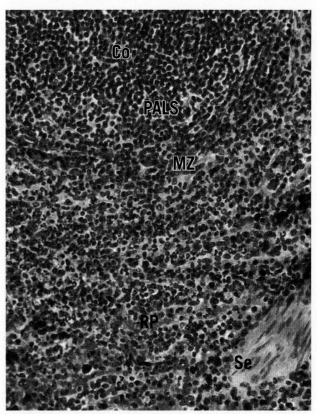

REVIEW FIGURE 10-2-3. Spleen. Human. Paraffin section. ×56.

This low-magnification photomicrograph of the human spleen displays its dense irregular collagenous connective tissue **capsule** (Ca) covered by a simple squamous epithelium, the peritoneum. **Septa** (Se) arising from the capsule convey blood vessels, arterial vessels into and venous vessels out of the spleen. Instead of the cortex and medulla, the spleen is subdivided into **white pulp** (WP) composed mostly of lymphocytes and **red pulp** (RP) composed mostly of venous sinusoids. The boundary between the red and white pulps is known as the marginal zone. The white pulp is organized into lymphoid nodules (mostly B cells) and **periarterial lymphatic sheath** (PALS), composed mostly of T cells. The center of the PALS is occupied by a **central arteriole** (CA).

REVIEW FIGURE 10-2-4. Spleen. Human. Paraffin section. ×270.

This photomicrograph is a higher magnification of a lymphoid nodule similar to the lymphoid nodule of Review Figure 10-2-3. Note that the **corona** (Co) of the lymphoid nodule is surrounded by the **periarterial lymphatic sheath** (PALS), which, in turn, is surrounded by the **marginal zone** (MZ). The **red pulp** (RP) and a piece of the **septum** (Se) are also identified.

KEY					
Ca	capsule	**MZ**	marginal zone	**RP**	red pulp
CA	central arteriole	**PALS**	periarterial lymphatic	**Se**	septum
Co	corona		sheath	**WP**	white pulp

Summary of Histologic Organization

Lymphoid tissue consists of diffuse and dense lymphoid tissue. The principal cell of lymphoid tissue is the lymphocyte, of which there are three categories: B lymphocytes, T lymphocytes, and null cells. Additionally, macrophages, reticular cells, plasma cells, dendritic cells, and APCs perform important functions in lymphoid tissue.

I. Lymph Node

A. Capsule

The capsule, usually surrounded by adipose tissue, is composed of dense irregular collagenous connective tissue containing some elastic fibers and smooth muscle. Afferent lymphatic vessels enter the convex aspect; efferent lymphatics and blood vessels pierce the hilum.

B. Cortex

Lymphoid nodules are composed of a dark corona (mostly B lymphocytes) and lighter-staining germinal centers, housing activated B lymphoblasts, macrophages, and follicular dendritic cells. Connective tissue trabeculae subdivide the cortex into incomplete compartments. Subcapsular and cortical sinuses display lymphocytes, reticular cells, and macrophages.

C. Paracortex

The paracortex is the region between the cortex and medulla, composed of T lymphocytes and dendritic cells. Postcapillary venules, with their characteristic cuboidal endothelium, are also present.

D. Medulla

The medulla displays connective tissue trabeculae, medullary cords (composed of macrophages, plasma cells, and lymphocytes), and medullary sinuses lined by discontinuous endothelial cells. Sinusoids contain lymphocytes, plasma cells, and macrophages. The region of the hilum is evident as a result of the thickened capsule and lack of lymphatic nodules.

E. Reticular Fibers

With the use of special stains, an extensive network of reticular fibers may be demonstrated to constitute the framework of lymph nodes.

II. Tonsils

A. Palatine Tonsils

1. Epithelium

Covered by stratified squamous nonkeratinized epithelium that extends into the tonsillar crypts. Lymphocytes may migrate through the epithelium.

2. Lymphoid Nodules

Surround crypts and frequently display germinal centers.

3. Capsule

Dense irregular collagenous connective tissue capsule separates the tonsil from the underlying pharyngeal wall musculature. Septa, derived from the capsule, extend into the tonsil.

B. Pharyngeal Tonsils

1. Epithelium

For the most part, pseudostratified ciliated columnar epithelium (infiltrated by lymphocytes) covers the free surface, as well as the folds that resemble crypts.

2. Lymphoid Nodules

Most lymphoid nodules display germinal centers.

3. Capsule

The thin capsule, situated deep to the tonsil, provides septa for the tonsil.

4. Glands

Ducts of the seromucous glands may be seen beneath the capsule, piercing the tonsil to open onto the epithelially covered surface.

C. Lingual Tonsils

1. Epithelium

Stratified squamous nonkeratinized epithelium covers the tonsil and extends into the shallow crypts.

2. Lymphoid

Most lymphoid nodules present germinal centers.

3. Capsule

The capsule is thin, not clearly defined.

4. Glands

Seromucous glands opening into the base of crypts may be seen.

III. Spleen

A. Capsule

The capsule, composed of dense irregular collagenous connective tissue thickest at the hilum, possesses some elastic fibers and smooth muscle cells. It is covered by mesothelium but is not surrounded by adipose tissue. Trabeculae, bearing blood vessels, extend from the capsule into the substance of the spleen.

B. White Pulp

White pulp is composed of PALS and lymphoid nodules with germinal centers. Both PALS (housing T lymphocytes) and lymphoid nodules (housing B lymphocytes) surround the acentrically located central artery, a distinguishing characteristic of the spleen.

C. Marginal Zone

A looser accumulation of lymphocytes, macrophages, and plasma cells is located between white and red pulps. It is supplied by capillary loops derived from the central artery.

D. Red Pulp

Red pulp is composed of pulp cords and sinusoids. Pulp cords are composed of delicate reticular fibers, stellate-shaped reticular cells, plasma cells, macrophages, and cells of the circulating blood. Sinusoids are lined by elongated discontinuous endothelial cells called stave cells which are surrounded by thickened hoop-like basement membrane in association with reticular fibers. The various regions of penicilli are evident in the red pulp. These are pulp arterioles, sheathed arterioles, and terminal arterial capillaries. Convincing evidence to determine whether circulation in the red pulp is open or closed is not available.

E. Reticular Fibers

With the use of special stains, an extensive network of reticular fibers may be demonstrated to constitute the framework of the spleen.

IV. Thymus

A. Capsule

The thin capsule is composed of dense irregular collagenous connective tissue (with some elastic fibers) that extends interlobular trabeculae that incompletely subdivide the thymus into lobules.

B. Cortex

The cortex has no lymphoid nodules or plasma cells. It is composed of lightly staining epithelial reticular cells, macrophages, and densely packed, darkly staining, small T lymphocytes (thymocytes) in various stages of development responsible for the dark appearance of the cortex. Epithelial reticular cells also surround capillaries, the only blood vessels present in the cortex.

C. Medulla

The medulla, which stains much lighter than the cortex, is continuous from lobule to lobule. It contains plasma cells, lymphocytes, macrophages, and epithelial reticular cells. Moreover, thymic (Hassall's) corpuscles, concentrically arranged epithelial reticular cells, are characteristic features of the thymic medulla.

D. Involution

The thymus begins to involute after puberty. The cortex becomes less dense because its population of lymphocytes and epithelial reticular cells is, to some extent, replaced by fat. In the medulla, thymic corpuscles increase in number and size.

E. Reticular Fibers and Sinusoids

The thymus possesses neither reticular fibers nor sinusoids.

Chapter Review Questions

10-1. The lymph node of a patient with Hodgkin's disease is characterized by which of the following?

A. Proliferation of monocytes

B. Presence of Reed–Sternberg cells

C. Hypertrophy of the kidneys

D. Atrophy of the spleen

E. Unusual weight gain

10-2. A physician received the biopsy report of one of their patients indicating the presence of tingible-body macrophages. What is the most probable diagnosis?

A. Leukemia

B. Thymoma

C. Acute tonsillitis

D. Burkitt's lymphoma

E. DiGeorge's syndrome

10-3. Antibody-dependent cell-mediated cytotoxicity is a procedure that is related to which of the following cells?

A. B memory cells

B. Natural T killer cells

C. Cytotoxic T cells

D. Plasma cells

E. Natural killer cells

10-4. Which of the following conditions is characterized by the patient's inability to form T lymphocytes?

A. DiGeorge's syndrome

B. Burkitt's lymphoma

C. Wiskott–Aldrich syndrome

D. Hodgkin's disease

E. Thymoma

10-5. Lipid antigens that are complexed to CD-1 molecules are recognized by which of the following cells?

A. Natural killer cells

B. B cells

C. Antigen-presenting cells

D. Natural T killer cells

ENDOCRINE SYSTEM

The endocrine system, in cooperation with the nervous system, orchestrates homeostasis by influencing, coordinating, and integrating the physiologic functions of the body. It consists of several organs (glands), isolated groups of cells within certain organs, and individual cells scattered among parenchymal cells of the body. The individual endocrine cells and structures such as pancreatic islets (islets of Langerhans), interstitial cells of Leydig, ovarian structures, and diffuse neuroendocrine cells (DNES) are discussed in organ-specific chapters.

The **endocrine glands** to be discussed here are the:

- pituitary,
- thyroid,
- parathyroid,
- suprarenal (adrenal) glands, and
- pineal body.

All these glands produce **hormones**, low-molecular-weight molecules, that they secrete into the connective tissue spaces where they enter a rich network of fenestrated capillaries to be disseminated by the vascular system throughout the body.

- If these hormones act on the same cells that produce them, then they are called **autocrine hormones**.

- If these hormones act on target cells in their immediate vicinity, then they are known as **paracrine hormones**.

- If these hormones enter blood vessels to be transported to their target cells, then they are referred to as **endocrine hormones** (identified as just **hormones** in this chapter).

The current chapter details hormones (Tables 11-1 and 11-2), whereas other chapters (on nervous tissue and the respiratory and digestive systems) discuss autocrine and paracrine hormones.

Pituitary Gland

The **pituitary gland (hypophysis)** is a small ovoid organ attached to the hypothalamus of the brain by a thin stalk called the infundibulum. It sits in a bony depression called sella turcica of the sphenoid bone and is covered by the dura mater on its superior surface. This small but important organ develops from two separate embryonic origins; therefore, it is subdivided into two parts, the **adenohypophysis (anterior pituitary)** and **neurohypophysis (posterior pituitary)**. Together, the two subunits of the pituitary secrete numerous hormones that regulate other endocrine organs (**pituitary-dependent endocrine glands**) and many other aspects of bodily functions (Fig. 11-1).

Table 11-1	Pituitary Gland Hormones			
Region	**Hormone Produced or Stored**	**Releasing Hormone**	**Inhibiting Hormone**	**Principal Functions**
Anterior pituitary	Somatotropin (growth hormone [GH])	SRH	Somatostatin	Generally increases cellular metabolism; stimulates the liver to release insulin-like growth factors I and II, resulting in cartilage proliferation and long bone growth
	Prolactin	PRH	PIF	Stimulates mammary gland development during pregnancy and production of milk after parturition
	Adrenocorticotropic hormone (ACTH, corticotropin)	CRH		Induces the zona fasciculata to synthesize and secrete cortisol and corticosterone and cells of the zona reticularis to synthesize and release androgens
	Follicle-stimulating hormone (FSH)	GnRH and leptin	Inhibin (in males)	Promotes secondary and Graafian follicle development as well as estrogen secretion in females; stimulates Sertoli cells to produce androgen-binding protein in males
	Luteinizing hormone (LH) in females	GnRH		Promotes ovulation, corpus luteum formation, secretion of estrogen and progesterone in females
	Luteinizing hormone (LH) in males			Promotes secretion of testosterone by Leydig cells in men
	TSH (thyrotropin)	TRH		Stimulates secretion and release of triiodothyronine and thyroxine by thyroid follicular cells
Posterior pituitary	Oxytocin			Stimulates uterine smooth muscle contraction during parturition. Stimulates contractions of mammary gland myoepithelial cells during suckling
	Vasopressin (antidiuretic hormone [ADH])			Elevates blood pressure by inducing vascular smooth muscle contraction; causes water resorption in collecting tubules of the kidney

CRH, corticotropin-releasing hormone; GnRH, gonadotropin-releasing hormone; PIH, prolactin-inhibiting hormone; PRH, prolactin-releasing hormone; SRH, somatotropin-releasing hormone; TRH, thyrotropin-releasing hormone.

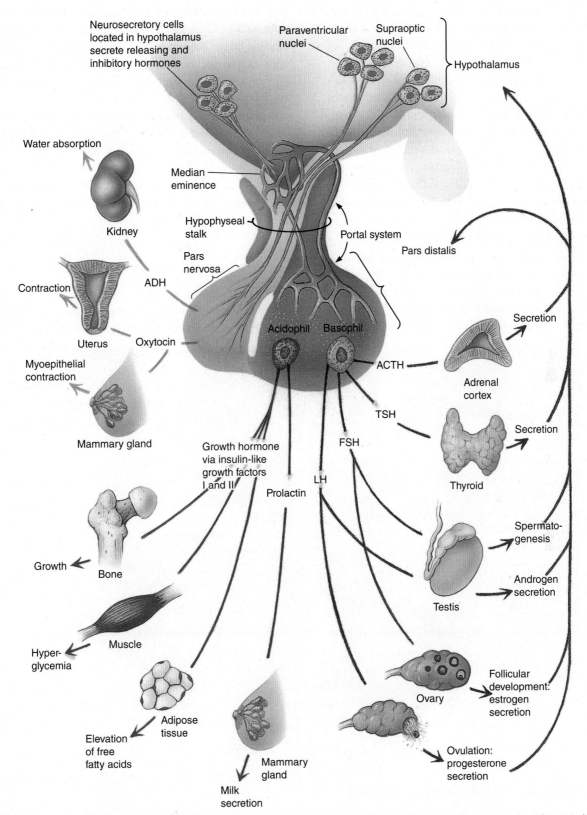

FIGURE 11-1. Pituitary gland and its hormones. ACTH, adrenocorticotropic hormone; ADH, antidiuretic hormone; FSH, follicle-stimulating hormone; LH, luteinizing hormone; TSH, thyroid-stimulating hormone.

- **Adenohypophysis** derives from the oral ectodermal epithelium lining the roof of the oral cavity. Adenohypophysis forms initially as an epithelial thickening that grows into the mesenchymal connective tissue, forming an epithelium-lined pouch called Rathke's pouch. As the Rathke's pouch grows bigger and moves closer to the developing neurohypophysis, the connecting stalk between the oral cavity and the Rathke's pouch degenerates, leaving behind a group of epithelial cells that elaborate and differentiate into adenohypophysis. Adenohypophysis is subdivided into three regions, **pars anterior (pars distalis)**, **pars tuberalis**, and **pars intermedia** (Fig. 11-2).

- **Neurohypophysis** derives from the downgrowth of neuroectoderm from the floor of the diencephalon, the precursor of the median eminence of the hypothalamus. Certain neurons whose cell bodies are located in the hypothalamus, grow their axons into the neurohypophysis and transfer the hormones, manufactured in their cell bodies, through the axons and store them within their dilated axon terminals, known as **Herring bodies (HB)**. Therefore, the neurohypophysis, physically connected to the median eminence of the hypothalamus by a thin stalk of neural tissue, is subdivided into two regions of neural tissue origin, the **infundibulum (infundibular stalk)** and the **pars nervosa**. The nonmyelinated axons of the neuron cell bodies that are located in the **paraventricular** and **supraoptic nuclei** of the **hypothalamus** constitute the infundibulum, whereas the axon terminals and supporting glial cells, known as **pituicytes**, compose the pars nervosa (see Figs. 11-1 and 11-2).

Vascular Supply of the Pituitary Gland

The pituitary gland receives its **blood supply** from the right and left **superior hypophyseal arteries**, serving the median eminence, pars tuberalis, and the infundibulum,

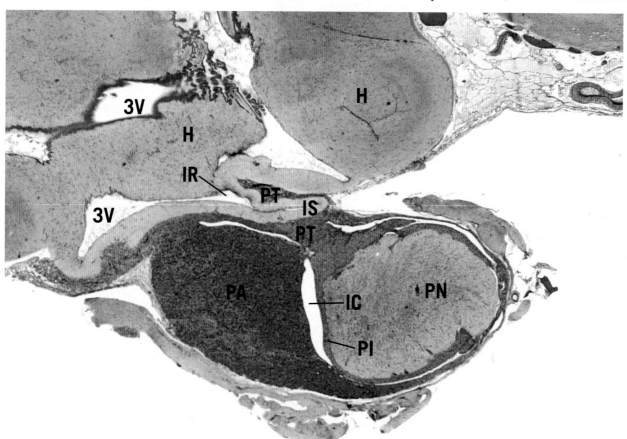

FIGURE 11-2. Pituitary gland. Paraffin section. ×19.

This survey photomicrograph of the pituitary gland demonstrates the relationship of the gland to the **hypothalamus** (H), from which it is suspended by the infundibulum. The infundibulum is composed of a neural portion, the **infundibular stem** (IS) and the surrounding **pars tuberalis** (PT). Note that the **third ventricle** (3V) of the brain is continuous with the **infundibular recess** (IR). The largest portion of the pituitary is the **pars anterior** (PA), which is glandular and secretes numerous hormones. The neural component of the pituitary gland is the **pars nervosa** (PN), which does not manufacture its hormones but stores and releases them. Even at this magnification, its resemblance to the brain tissue and to the substance of the infundibular stalk is readily evident. Between the pars anterior and pars nervosa is the **pars intermedia** (PI), which frequently presents an **intraglandular cleft** (IC), a remnant of Rathke's pouch.

demonstrating that there is not only a neural but also a vascular connection between the median eminence and the pituitary gland. Additionally, branches from the right and left **inferior hypophyseal arteries** provide blood supply to the pars nervosa.

The two superior hypophyseal arteries give rise to the **hypothalamic–hypophyseal portal system** which is comprised of two fenestrated capillary beds that are connected to each other by a set of portal veins (see Fig. 11-1).

- Superior hypophyseal arteries give rise to the **primary capillary plexus** located in the median eminence; these capillaries receive **releasing hormones** produced by the hypothalamic neurons.

- **Hypophyseal portal veins** drain the primary capillary plexus and deliver the blood containing these releasing hormones into the **secondary capillary plexus**.

- The secondary capillary plexus is located in the pars anterior, where these releasing hormones regulate the hormone secretion of the parenchymal cells.

- The hormones released by the cells of adenohypophysis are carried away by the blood from the secondary capillary plexus for systemic distribution.

It should be noted that blood also flows in the opposing direction, that is, from the pituitary into the median eminence, thereby ensuring that communication occurs seamlessly in both directions. Moreover, the hypothalamus receives information from the entire body as well as from other regions of the brain, permitting it to perform its function in regulating homeostasis.

Pars Anterior (Pars Distalis)

The **pars anterior (pars distalis)** is composed of numerous parenchymal cells arranged in thick cords, with the secondary capillary plexus, comprising **fenestrated capillaries**, richly vascularizing the intervening regions. The parenchymal cells are classified into two main categories: those whose granules readily take up stain, **chromophils**; and those cells that do not possess a strong affinity for stains, **chromophobes** (Fig. 11-3).

- **Chromophils** are of two types, **acidophils** and **basophils**. Although considerable controversy surrounds the classification of these cells vis-à-vis their function, probably, at least six of the seven hormones manufactured by the pars anterior are made by separate cells (Figs. 11-4 and 11-5; also see Table 11-1).

- It is believed that two types of acidophils produce **somatotropin (growth hormone [GH])** and **prolactin.**

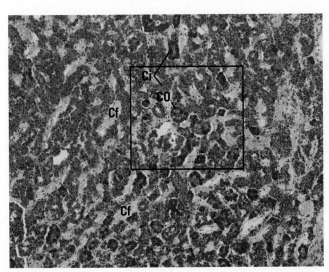

FIGURE 11-3. Pituitary gland. Pars anterior. Paraffin section. ×100.

The pars anterior is composed of large cords of cells that branch and anastomose with each other. These cords are surrounded by an extensive **fenestrated capillary** (Cf) network. The parenchymal cells of the anterior pituitary are divided into two groups: **chromophils** (Ci) and **chromophobes** (CO). With hematoxylin and eosin, the distinction between chromophils and chromophobes is obvious. The former stain blue or pink, whereas the latter stain poorly. The *boxed area* is presented at a higher magnification in Figure 11-4.

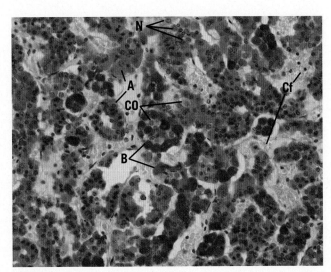

FIGURE 11-4. Pituitary gland. Pars anterior. Paraffin section. ×256.

This is a higher magnification of the *boxed area* of Figure 11-3. Note that the **chromophobes** (CO) do not take up the stain well, and only their **nuclei** (N) are demonstrable. These cells are small; therefore, chromophobes are easily recognizable because their nuclei appear to be clumped together. Chromophils may be classified into two categories by their affinity to histologic dyes: blue-staining **basophils** (B) and pink-colored **acidophils** (A). The distinction between these two cell types in sections stained with hematoxylin and eosin is not as apparent as with some other stains. Note also the presence of **fenestrated capillaries** (Cf).

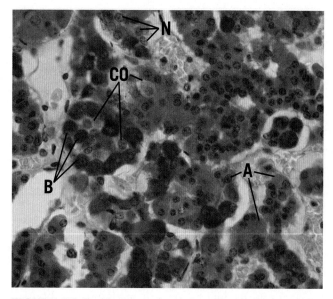

FIGURE 11-5. Pituitary gland. Paraffin section. ×400.

In this hematoxylin and eosin stain, **acidophils** (A) stain pink to red and are slightly smaller in size than the **basophils** (B), which stain bluish to purple. **Chromophobe**s (CO) are readily recognizable; because their cytoplasms do not take up stain, they present as pale cells with centrally placed nuclei. Cords of chromophobes display clusters of **nuclei** (N) crowded together.

- Various populations of basophils produce the remaining five hormones **thyrotropin (thyroid-stimulating hormone [TSH])**, **follicle-stimulating hormone (FSH)**, **luteinizing hormone (LH)**, **adrenocorticotropin (ACTH)**, and **melanocyte-stimulating hormone (MSH)**.
- **Chromophobes** are believed to be acidophils and basophils that have released their granules.

An additional group of parenchymal cells are the nonsecretory **folliculostellate cells** whose function is not completely understood. The long processes of these cells create gap junctions with each other, a characteristic that implies that they communicate with one another and perhaps aid in the regulation of chromophil function. It is also possible that they act as phagocytes or as regenerative cells to replace defunct acidophils and/or basophils.

Control of Anterior Pituitary Hormone Release

The axons whose cell bodies are located in the paraventricular and arcuate nuclei of the hypothalamus terminate at the median eminence containing the primary capillary bed.

- These axons store the regulatory hormones of the chromophils (see Table 11-1):
  - **somatotropin-releasing hormone (SRH)** stimulating acidophils to release somatotropin (GH)

- **prolactin-releasing hormone (PRH)** stimulating acidophils to release prolactin
- **corticotropin-releasing hormone (CRH)** stimulating basophils to release ACTH
- **thyrotropin-releasing hormone (TRH)** stimulating basophils to release TSH
- **gonadotropin-releasing hormone (GnRH)** stimulating basophils to release FSH and LH
- **inhibin** inhibiting basophils from releasing FSH
- **prolactin-inhibiting factor (PIF)** inhibiting acidophils from releasing prolactin
- **somatostatin** inhibiting acidophils from releasing SRH

- The hormones are released by these axons into the primary capillary plexus and are conveyed to the secondary capillary plexus by the hypophyseal portal veins.
- The hormones then activate (or inhibit) the **basophils** and **acidophils** of the pars anterior, causing them to release or prevent them from releasing their hormones (see Table 11-1).

An additional control is the mechanism of negative feedback so that the presence of specific plasma levels of the pituitary hormones prevents the chromophils from releasing additional quantities of their hormones (see Fig. 11-1).

Pars Intermedia

The **pars intermedia** is not well developed in humans (Fig. 11-6). It is believed that the basophil cell population of this region produces **proopiomelanocortin**. This large protein is cleaved within the basophil into **lipotropic hormone (LPH)** and **adrenocorticotropic hormone (ACTH)**. Other enzymes within these cells can convert ACTH into **melanotropic hormone (MSH)** and LPH into β-**endorphin**.

Pars Tuberalis

The pars tuberalis forms a partial coat around the infundibular stalk (see Fig. 11-2). It may house basophils that may manufacture both LH and FSH.

Pars Nervosa and Infundibular Stalk

The **pars nervosa** is a neural tissue comprised of unmyelinated axons, axon terminals, and **pituicytes**, cells believed to be neuroglial in nature (Fig. 11-7; also see Fig. 11-6).

- The unmyelinated axons originate from the cell bodies located in the **supraoptic** and **paraventricular nuclei** of the hypothalamus, where hormones **oxytocin** and **antidiuretic hormone (ADH, vasopressin)** are

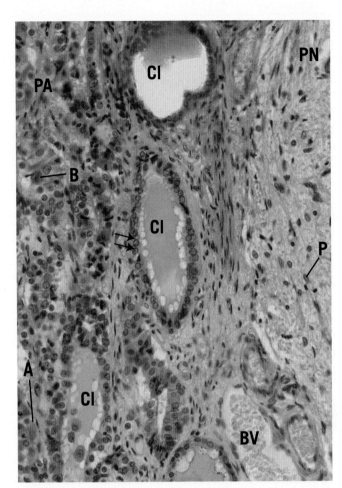

FIGURE 11-6. Pituitary gland. Pars intermedia. Human. Paraffin section. ×280.

The pars intermedia of the pituitary gland is situated between the **pars anterior** (PA) and the **pars nervosa** (PN). It is characterized by **basophils** (B), which are smaller than those of the pars anterior. Additionally, the pars intermedia contains **colloid** (Cl)-filled follicles, lined by pale, small, low cuboidal shaped cells (*arrows*). A few **acidophils** (A) are present, but they are not as numerous here. Note that some of the basophils extend into the pars nervosa. Numerous **blood vessels** (BV) and **pituicytes** (P) are evident in this area of the pars nervosa.

synthesized, respectively. The axons from these nuclei form the **hypothalamo-hypophyseal tract** as they emerge from the median eminence and enter the pars nervosa. The hormones produced and packaged into vesicles in the cell body are transported by the kinesins along the microtubules within the axons.

- The hormones are then stored in the dilated axon terminals referred to as **Herring bodies**, within the pars nervosa (Fig. 11-8; also see Fig. 11-7).

- *Oxytocin* is a powerful smooth muscle constrictor that affects the muscular wall of the uterus during parturition (birth process) and also the myoepithelial cells of the mammary glands to eject milk as the baby is feeding. Oxytocin is also known to play a role in the feeling of love and pair-bonding.

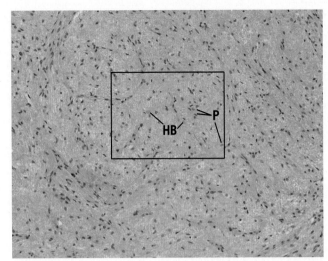

FIGURE 11-7. Pituitary gland. Pars nervosa. Paraffin section. ×132.

The pars nervosa of the pituitary gland is composed of elongated cells with long processes known as **pituicytes** (P), which are thought to be neuroglial in nature. These cells, which possess more or less oval nuclei, appear to support numerous unmyelinated nerve fibers of the hypothalamo-hypophyseal tract. These nerve fibers cannot be distinguished from the cytoplasm of pituicytes in a hematoxylin and eosin-stained preparation. Neurosecretory materials pass along these nerve fibers and are stored in expanded regions, known as **Herring bodies** (HB), at the termination of the fibers. Note that the pars nervosa resembles neural tissue. The *boxed area* is presented at a higher magnification in Figure 11-8.

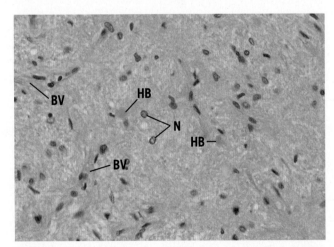

FIGURE 11-8. Pituitary gland. Pars nervosa. Paraffin section. ×400.

This photomicrograph is a higher magnification of the *boxed area* of Figure 11-7. Note the numerous more or less oval **nuclei** (N) of the pituicytes, some of whose processes (*arrows*) are clearly evident at this magnification. The unmyelinated nerve fibers and processes of pituicytes constitute the cellular network of the pars nervosa. The expanded terminal regions of the nerve fibers, which house neurosecretions, are known as **Herring bodies** (HB). Also observe the presence of **blood vessels** (BV) in the pars nervosa.

- *Antidiuretic hormone (ADH, vasopressin)* influences the cells in the collecting tubules of the kidney to increase aquaporin expression in the cell membrane, prompting water reabsorption, thereby concentrating the urine.

- The release of these neurosecretory hormones (neurosecretions) is mediated by nerve impulses and occurs at the interface between the axon terminals and the fenestrated capillaries. When the axon is ready to *release its secretory products*, the pituicytes withdraw their processes and permit the secretory product clear access to the capillaries.

Thyroid Gland

The **thyroid gland** consists of right and left lobes that are interconnected by a narrow isthmus across the thyroid cartilage and upper trachea (Fig. 11-9; also see Table 11-2). It is enveloped by a connective tissue capsule whose septa penetrate the substance of the gland, forming not only its supporting framework but also a conduit for its rich vascular supply.

Thyroid Hormone

Thyroid hormones are unusual among the amino acid derivative and nonsteroid-based hormones, in that they directly enter the nucleus, where they bind with **receptor molecules**. The hormone–receptor complexes control the activities of **operators** and/or **promoters**, resulting in mRNA transcription. The newly formed mRNAs enter the cytoplasm, where they are translated into proteins that elevate the cell's metabolic activity.

Synthesis of Thyroid Hormone

The process of thyroid hormone synthesis relies on the availability of **dietary iodine**, which is converted to **iodide (I^-)** by cells of the alimentary canal and released into the bloodstream. Iodide is preferentially transported into the thyroid follicular cells via sodium/iodide

Gland	Hormone	Stimulating Hormone	Principal Functions
Thyroid gland	Thyroxine (T_4) and triiodothyronine (T_3)	Thyroid-stimulating hormone (TSH)	Promotes gene transcription and stimulates carbohydrate and fat metabolism. Increases basal metabolism, growth rates, endocrine gland secretion, heart rate, and respiration. Decreases cholesterol, phospholipid, and triglyceride levels, and lowers body weight
	Calcitonin (thyrocalcitonin)		Lowers blood calcium levels by suppressing osteoclastic activity
Parathyroid gland	Parathyroid hormone (PTH)		Increases blood calcium levels
Suprarenal (adrenal) gland			
Cortex			
Zona glomerulosa	Mineralocorticoids (aldosterone and deoxycorticosterone)	Angiotensin II and Adrenocorticotropic hormone (ACTH)	Stimulates distal convoluted tubules of the kidney to resorb sodium and excrete potassium
Zona fasciculata	Glucocorticoids (cortisol and corticosterone)	ACTH	Controls carbohydrate, lipid, and protein metabolism. Stimulates gluconeogenesis. Reduces inflammation and suppresses the immune system
Zona reticularis	Androgens (dehydroepiandrosterone and androstenedione)	ACTH	No significant effect in a healthy individual
Medulla	Catecholamines (epinephrine and norepinephrine)	Preganglionic sympathetic and splanchnic nerves	Epinephrine—increases blood pressure and heart rate; promotes glucose release by the liver Norepinephrine—elevates blood pressure via vasoconstriction
Pineal body (pineal gland)	Melatonin	Norepinephrine	Influences the individual's diurnal rhythm and inhibits Follicle-stimulating hormone (FSH) release, thus regulating the reproductive cycle in animals that reproduce only at a specific time of the year

Table 11-2   Hormones of the Thyroid, Parathyroid, Adrenal, and Pineal Glands

CLINICAL CONSIDERATIONS 11-1

Disorders of the Pituitary Gland

Diabetes Insipidus The symptom of diabetes insipidus is polyurea (excessive urination) and polydipsia (excessive drinking and thirst) caused by reduction or lack of antidiuretic hormone (ADH, vasopressin). This condition may occur from tumors, injury, or trauma involving paraventricular nuclei or the infundibulum. The lack of ADH causes the inability to absorb water from the collecting ducts in the kidney, thereby excreting diluted urine in large volume, which in turn triggers dehydration and unquenchable thirst.

Galactorrhea is a condition in which a male produces breast milk or a woman who is not breastfeeding produces breast milk. In men, it is often accompanied by impotence, headache, and loss of peripheral vision and in women by hot flashes, vaginal dryness, and an abnormal menstrual cycle. This rather uncommon condition is usually a result of prolactinoma, a tumor of prolactin-producing cells of the pituitary gland. The condition is usually treated by drug intervention or surgery, or both.

Postpartum pituitary infarct is a condition caused by the pregnancy-induced enlargement of the pituitary gland and its concomitant increase in its vascularity. The high vascularity of the pituitary increases the chances of a vascular accident, such as hemorrhage, which results in the partial destruction of the pituitary gland. The condition may be severe enough to produce Sheehan's syndrome, which is recognized by the lack of milk production, the loss of pubic and axillary hair, and fatigue.

Pituitary somatotrope adenoma is one of the pituitary adenomas, benign tumors, that are more common in adults than in children. Somatotrope adenomas involve proliferation of acidophils that produce an excess of GH, which in children result in **gigantism**, whereas in adults, it results in **acromegaly**. These acidophils grow slowly and usually do not grow outside the sella turcica. Individuals afflicted with untreated acromegaly frequently suffer from complications that increase their chance of succumbing to cardiovascular, cerebrovascular, and respiratory problems. These individuals also present with hypertension.

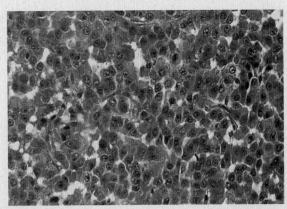

This is a photomicrograph from the pituitary gland of a patient with pituitary somatotrope adenoma. Note that the adenoma cells are arranged in ribbons and cords. (Reprinted with permission from Strayer DS, et al., eds. Rubin's Pathology. *Clinicopathologic Foundations of Medicine*, 7th ed. Philadelphia: Wolters Kluwer, 2014. Figure 27-7.)

---

transporters, located at the basal cell membrane, against a concentration gradient (an energy-requiring mechanism). The iodide then leaves the follicular cell at the apical cell membrane via **pendrin**, an iodide/chloride transporter. As the iodide enters the colloid, two processes occur at the colloid–cell interphase: **thyroglobulin**, a protein manufactured on the rough endoplasmic reticulum (rER) and modified and packaged in the Golgi apparatus, also enters the colloid along with **thyroid peroxidase**, an enzyme that oxidizes and thereby activates iodide. Either one or two activated iodides attach to tyrosine residues of thyroglobulin, forming **monoiodinate tyrosine (MIT)** or **diiodinated tyrosine (DIT)**, respectively. One MIT and one DIT can combine to form **triiodothyronine (T_3)** or two DITs can combine to form **thyroxine (T_4)**, and the iodinated thyroglobulin is stored in the colloid. Interestingly, T_4 concentration in the colloid is almost 10 times greater than the concentration of T_3.

Release of Thyroid Hormone

Thyroid-stimulating hormone (TSH) released by the basophils of the anterior pituitary binds to **TSH receptors** on the follicular cell's basal membrane inducing the production and activation of cAMP that, in turn, activates protein kinase A resulting in the release of the thyroid hormones **triiodothyronine** and **thyroxine**. The binding of TSH also induces the follicular cells to increase in height, becoming columnar cells that form finger-like extension, known as **filopodia**, at the colloidal interface. These filopodia encircle small volumes of the colloid, form endocytic vesicles, and transfer them into the cytoplasm. The endocytic vesicles fuse with endosomes, and within these organelles, enzymes liberate the iodinated tyrosines from the thyroglobulins and release them as MITs, DITs, T_3s, and T_4s. MITs and DITs are deiodinated by the enzyme **iodotyrosine**

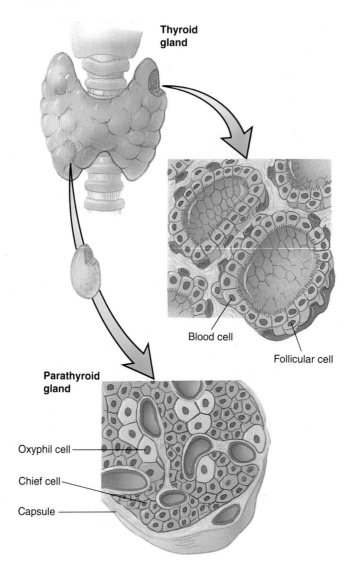

Thyroid gland

Blood cell

Follicular cell

Parathyroid gland

Oxyphil cell

Chief cell

Capsule

FIGURE 11-9. Thyroid and parathyroid glands.

The parenchymal cells of the thyroid gland are arranged in numerous follicles, composed of a **simple cuboidal epithelium** lining a central **colloid-filled lumen** (Figs. 11-10 and 11-11). The colloid, secreted and resorbed by the **follicular cells**, is composed of **thyroglobulin** the **thyroid hormone** that is bound to a large protein. Thyroid hormone is essential for regulating basal metabolism and for influencing growth rate and mental processes and generally stimulates endocrine gland functioning. An additional secretory cell type, **parafollicular cells (clear cells, C cells)**, a member of the **DNES** family of cells, is present in the thyroid. Most of these cells are found in between the follicles, but occasionally, they are found interspersed among the follicular cells as well. Parafollicular cells manufacture the hormone **calcitonin**, which is released directly into the connective tissue in the immediate vicinity of capillaries. Calcitonin helps to decrease calcium concentrations in the blood by inhibiting bone resorption by osteoclasts (i.e., when blood calcium levels are high, calcitonin is released).

dehalogenase, and the amino acid and iodine remain in the cytosol as entities that are independent of each other. The thyroid hormones T_3 and T_4 are released into the connective tissue of the thyroid and enter the perifollicular capillary network where they bind to various thyroid hormone carrier proteins to be delivered to their target cells. The hormone is transported into the target cell cytoplasm and from there enters the nucleus to bind to **nuclear thyroid hormone–receptor protein** to trigger transcription of various genes. It should be

mentioned that although the concentration and half-life of T_3 are much less than that of T_4, T_3 is a lot more potent than T_4.

Parathyroid Glands

The **parathyroid glands**, usually four in number, are embedded in the fascial sheath of the posterior aspect of the thyroid gland (see Fig. 11-9). They possess slender connective tissue capsules from which septa are derived to

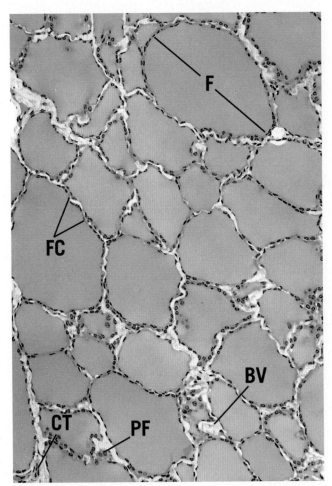

FIGURE 11-10. Thyroid gland. Monkey. Plastic section. ×132.

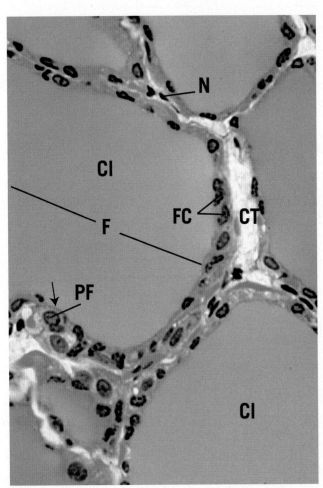

FIGURE 11-11. Thyroid gland. Monkey. Plastic section. ×540.

The capsule of the thyroid gland sends septa of connective tissue into the substance of the gland, subdividing it into incomplete lobules. This photomicrograph presents part of a lobule displaying many **follicles** (F) of varied sizes. Each follicle is surrounded by slender **connective tissue** (CT), which supports the follicles and brings **blood vessels** (BV) in close approximation. The follicles are composed of **follicular cells** (FC), whose low cuboidal morphology indicates that the cells are not producing secretory product. During the active secretory cycle, these cells become taller in morphology. In addition to the follicular cells, another parenchymal cell type is found in the thyroid gland. These cells do not border the colloid, are located on the periphery of the follicles, and are known as **parafollicular cells** (PF) or C cells. They are large and possess centrally placed round nuclei, and their cytoplasm appears paler.

The thyroid **follicle** (F) presented in this photomicrograph is surrounded by several other follicles and intervening **connective tissue** (CT). **Nuclei** (N) in the connective tissue may belong either to endothelial cells or to connective tissue cells. Because most capillaries are collapsed in excised thyroid tissue, it is often difficult to identify endothelial cells with any degree of certainty. The **follicular cells** (FC) are flattened, indicating that these cells are not actively secreting thyroglobulin. Note that the follicles are filled with a **colloid** (Cl) material. Observe the presence of a **parafollicular cell** (PF), which may be distinguished from the surrounding cells by its pale cytoplasm (*arrow*) and larger nucleus.

penetrate the glands and convey a vascular supply to the interior. In the adult, two types of parenchymal cells are present in the parathyroid glands: numerous small **chief cells** and a smaller number of large **acidophilic cells**, the **oxyphils** (Fig. 11-12 and Fig. 11-13). Fatty infiltration

of the glands is common in older individuals. Although there is no known function of oxyphils, some suggest that they may be a nonsecretory phase of the chief cells.

Chief cells produce **parathyroid hormone (PTH)**, the most important, "minute-to-minute," regulator of calcium in the body. If the blood calcium levels drop below normal, G protein binds calcium-sensing receptors on the chief cells, known as **transmembrane calcium receptors (CaSR)**. If there is enough Ca^{2+} present in the blood, then the CaSR has calcium complexed with it and

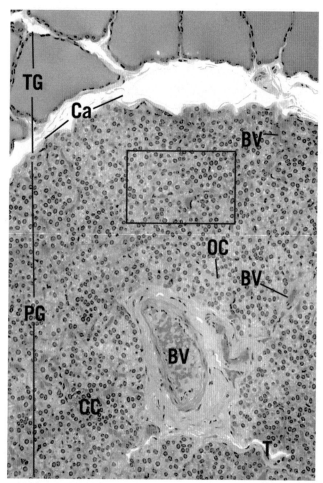

FIGURE 11-12. Thyroid and parathyroid glands. Monkey. Plastic section. ×132.

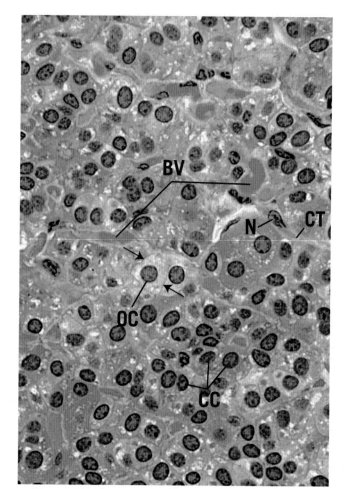

FIGURE 11-13. Parathyroid gland. Monkey. Plastic section. ×540.

Although the **parathyroid** (PG) and **thyroid glands** (TG) are separated by their respective **capsules** (Ca), they are extremely close to each other. The capsule of the parathyroid gland sends **trabeculae** (T) of connective tissue carrying **blood vessels** (BV) into the substance of the gland. The parenchyma of the gland consists of two types of cells, namely, **chief cells** (CC), also known as principal cells, and **oxyphil cells** (OC). Chief cells are more numerous and possess darker-staining cytoplasm. Oxyphil cells stain lighter and are usually larger than chief cells, and their cell membranes are evident. A region similar to the *boxed area* is presented at a higher magnification in Figure 11-13.

This photomicrograph is a region similar to the *boxed area* of Figure 11-12. The **chief cells** (CC) of the parathyroid gland form small cords surrounded by slender **connective tissue** (CT) elements and **blood vessels** (BV). The **nuclei** (N) of connective tissue cells may be easily recognized because of their elongated appearance. **Oxyphil cells** (OC) possess a paler cytoplasm, and frequently, the cell membranes are evident (*arrows*). The glands of older individuals may become infiltrated by adipocytes.

the cell is inhibited from releasing PTH. If the blood calcium level is below normal, then calcium ions are not available to bind to CaSR, and it activates the G proteins to cause these cells to release PTH. Parathyroid hormone helps control serum calcium levels by (1) acting directly on osteoblasts prompting them to release osteoclast stimulating hormone which in turn increases osteoclastic activity, (2) reducing calcium loss through the kidneys, and (3) promoting the production of vitamin D (**calcitriol**) by the proximal tubule cells of the kidneys because calcitriol is essential for calcium absorption in the intestines.

CLINICAL CONSIDERATIONS 11-2

Disorders of the Thyroid Gland

Graves disease is caused by the binding of autoimmune IgG antibodies to TSH receptors, thus stimulating increased thyroid hormone production (**hyperthyroidism**). Clinically, the thyroid gland becomes enlarged, and there is evidence of exophthalmic goiter (protrusion of the eyeballs).

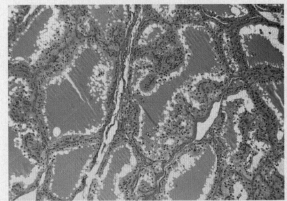

This photomicrograph is from the thyroid gland of a patient with Graves disease. Note that the follicular cells are high columnar hyperplastic cells enclosing pinkish colloid that is scalloped along its periphery. (Reprinted with permission from Strayer DS, et al., eds. *Rubin's Pathology. Clinicopathologic Foundations of Medicine*, 7th ed. Philadelphia: Wolters Kluwer, 2014. Figure 27-24.)

CLINICAL CONSIDERATIONS 11-3

Disorders of the Parathyroid Gland

Hyperparathyroidism may be caused by the presence of a benign tumor causing the excess production of PTH.

The high levels of circulating PTH cause increased bone resorption, resulting in a greatly elevated blood calcium level. The excess calcium may become deposited in arterial walls and in the kidneys, creating kidney stones.

Suprarenal Glands

The **suprarenal glands** (adrenal glands) are positioned just above the kidneys and are invested by a thin connective tissue capsule (Figs. 11-14 to 11-16; also see Fig. 11-3). The glands are derived from two different embryonic origins, namely, **mesodermal epithelium**, which gives rise to the **cortex**, and **neural crest** derived from neuroectoderm, from which the **medulla** originates. The rich vascular supply of the gland is conveyed to the interior in connective tissue elements derived from the capsule.

Cortex

The **cortex** is subdivided into three concentric regions or zones that secrete specific hormones (Fig. 11-17; also see Table 11-2 and Fig. 11-16). Control of these hormonal secretions is mostly regulated by ACTH from the pituitary gland.

- The outermost region, just beneath the capsule, is the **zona glomerulosa**, where the cells are arranged in arches and spherical clusters with numerous capillaries surrounding them (Fig. 11-18; also see Fig. 11-17).

  - Cells of the zona glomerulosa secrete **aldosterone**, a mineralocorticoid that acts on cells of the distal convoluted tubules of the kidney to modulate water and electrolyte balance.

- The second region, the **zona fasciculata**, is the most extensive. Its parenchymal cells, usually known as **spongiocytes**, are arranged in long cords, with numerous capillaries between the cords (see Figs. 11-17 and 11-18).

  - The spongiocytes secrete **cortisol** and **corticosterone**, steroid-based hormones that have been extracted at processing, which accounts for lack of staining with hematoxylin and eosin (H&E), resulting in the spongy appearance of the zona fasciculata cells.

  - These glucocorticoids regulate carbohydrate metabolism, facilitate the catabolism of fats and proteins, exhibit anti-inflammatory activity, and suppress the immune response.

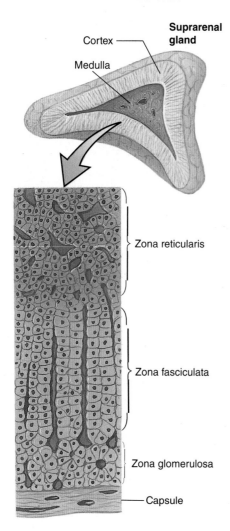

FIGURE 11-14. Diagram of the suprarenal gland and the three layers of the cortex.

- The innermost region of the cortex, the **zona reticularis**, is arranged in anastomosing cords of cells with a rich intervening capillary network (see Figs. 11-17 and 11-18).

  - Zona reticularis cells secrete weak **androgens** (dehydroepiandrosterone [DHEA]) that promote the development of masculine characteristics.

At the junction of the zona fasciculata with the zona glomerulosa, there are regenerative cells, known as **progenitor cells**, that can enter the cell cycle to form new cells to replace defunct parenchymal cells of the suprarenal cortex.

Medulla

Parenchymal cells of the **medulla**, derived from the neural crest, are disposed in irregularly arranged short cords surrounded by capillary networks (Fig. 11-19). They contain numerous granules that stain intensely when the freshly cut tissue is exposed to chromium salts. This is referred to as the chromaffin reaction; therefore, the cells are called **chromaffin cells**.

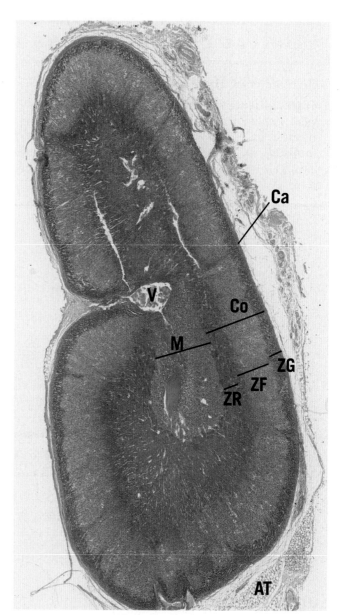

FIGURE 11-15. Suprarenal gland. Paraffin section. ×12.

The suprarenal gland, usually embedded in **adipose tissue** (AT), is invested by a collagenous connective tissue **capsule** (Ca) that provides thin connective tissue elements that carry blood vessels and nerves into the substance of the gland. The **cortex** (Co) of the suprarenal gland completely surrounds the flattened **medulla** (M) in the center. The cortex is divided into three concentric regions: the outermost **zona glomerulosa** (ZG), middle **zona fasciculata** (ZF), and the innermost **zona reticularis** (ZR). The medulla, which is always bounded by the zona reticularis, possesses several large **veins** (V), which are always accompanied by a considerable amount of connective tissue.

There are two populations of **chromaffin cells** that secrete the two hormones (see Table 11-2) of the suprarenal medulla, mainly:

- **epinephrine** (adrenaline) or
- **norepinephrine** (noradrenaline).

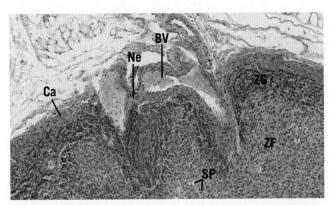

FIGURE 11-16. Suprarenal gland. Cortex. Monkey. Plastic section. ×136.

The collagenous connective tissue **capsule** (Ca) of the suprarenal gland is surrounded by adipose tissue through which **blood vessels** (BV) and **nerves** (Ne) reach the gland. The parenchymal cells of the cortex, immediately deep to the capsule, are arranged in an irregular array, forming the more or less oval to round clusters or arch-like cords of the **zona glomerulosa** (ZG). The cells of the **zona fasciculata** (ZF) form long, straight columns of cords oriented radially, each being one to two cells in width. These cells are larger than those of the zona glomerulosa. They present a vacuolated appearance owing to the numerous lipid droplets that were extracted during processing and are often referred to as **spongiocytes** (Sp). The interstitium is richly vascularized by **blood vessels** (BV).

The secretion of these two catecholamines is directly regulated by preganglionic axon fibers of the sympathetic nervous system that synapse with the chromaffin cells. For this reason, chromaffin cells are considered as the modified postganglionic sympathetic neurons (Fig. 11-20). Catecholamine release occurs in physical and psychological stress. Moreover, scattered, large **postganglionic sympathetic ganglion cells** in the medulla act on smooth muscle cells of the medullary veins, thus controlling blood flow in the cortex.

Pineal Gland

The **pineal gland (pineal body, epiphysis)** is a projection of the roof of the diencephalon (Fig. 11-21). The connective tissue covering of the pineal gland is the pia mater, which sends trabeculae and septa into the substance of the pineal gland, subdividing it into incomplete lobules. Blood vessels along with postganglionic sympathetic nerve fibers from the superior cervical ganglia travel in these connective tissue elements. As the nerve fibers enter the pineal gland, they lose their myelin sheath. The parenchyma of the pineal gland is composed of **pinealocytes** and **neuroglial cells** (Figs. 11-22 and 11-23).

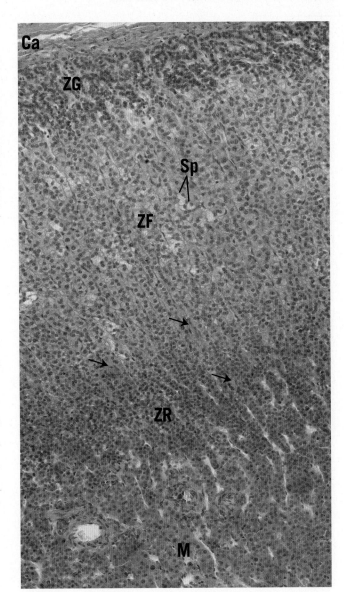

FIGURE 11-17. Suprarenal gland. Paraffin section. ×136.

Deep to the **capsule** (Ca), is the thin layer of **zona glomerulosa** (ZG). composed of small cells forming arches and clusters. The columnar arrangement of the cords of the **zona fasciculata** (ZF) is readily evident by viewing the architecture of the blood vessels indicated by the *arrows*. The cells in the deeper region of the zona fasciculata are smaller and appear denser than the more superficially located **spongiocytes** (Sp). Cells of the **zona reticularis** (ZR) are arranged in irregular, anastomosing cords whose interstices contain wide capillaries. The cords of the zona reticularis merge almost imperceptibly with those of the zona fasciculata. This is a relatively narrow region of the cortex. The **medulla** (M) is clearly evident because its cells are much larger than those of the zona reticularis.

• The pinealocytes form gap junctions with each other and manufacture, and immediately release, **melatonin** with the assistance of the rate-limiting enzyme **arylalkylamine *N*-acetyltransferase (AANAT).**

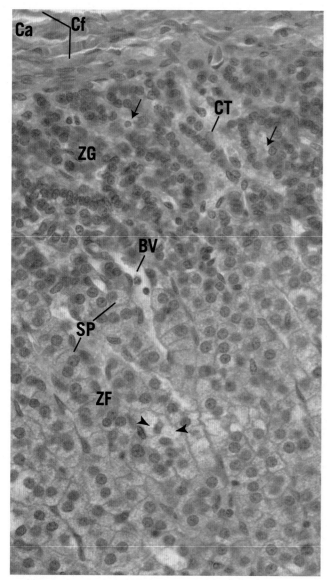

FIGURE 11-18. Suprarenal gland. Paraffin section. ×400.

The **capsule** (Ca) of the suprarenal gland displays its **collagen fibers** (Cf) and the **nuclei** (N) of the fibroblasts. The **zona glomerulosa** (ZG), which occupies the upper part of the photomicrograph, displays relatively small cells with few vacuoles (*arrows*). The lower part of the photomicrograph demonstrates the **zona fasciculata** (ZF), whose cells are larger and display a more vacuolated (*arrowheads*) appearance. Note the presence of **connective tissue** (CT) elements and **blood vessels** (BV) in the interstitium between cords of parenchymal cells.

- Neuroglial cells do not appear to have any secretory functions, but they lend support to pinealocytes.

- Interestingly, melatonin is manufactured only at night because the activity of AANAT is repressed in daylight. The pineal body receives indirect input from special

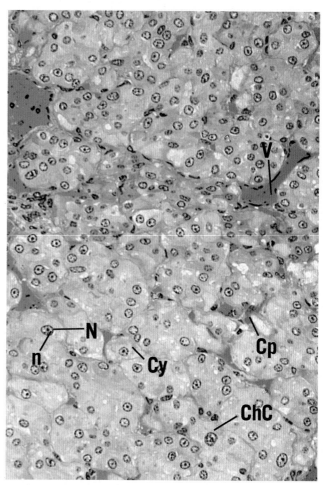

FIGURE 11-19. Suprarenal gland. Medulla. Monkey. Plastic section. ×270.

The cells of the adrenal medulla, often referred to as **chromaffin cells** (ChC), are arranged in round to ovoid clusters or in irregularly arranged short cords. The cells are large and more or less round to polyhedral in shape with a pale **cytoplasm** (Cy) and vesicular-appearing **nucleus** (N), displaying a single, large **nucleolus** (n). The interstitium presents large **veins** (V) and an extensive **capillary** (Cp) network. Large ganglion cells are occasionally noted.

ganglion cells of the **retina**, which allows the pineal gland to differentiate between day and night and, in that manner, assists in the establishment of the circadian rhythm. Melatonin is used in some instances to treat jet lag and in regulating emotional responses related to shortened daylight during winter, a condition called seasonal affective disorder (SAD).

- The intercellular spaces of the pineal body contain calcified granular material known as **brain sand (corpora arenacea)**, whose significance, if any, is not known.

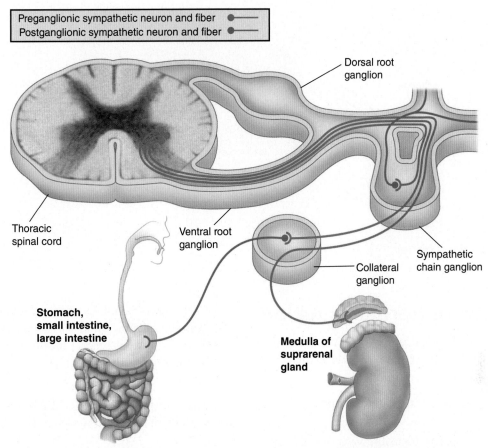

Preganglionic sympathetic neuron and fiber ●——
Postganglionic sympathetic neuron and fiber ●——

Dorsal root ganglion

Thoracic spinal cord

Ventral root ganglion

Sympathetic chain ganglion

Collateral ganglion

Stomach, small intestine, large intestine

Medulla of suprarenal gland

FIGURE 11-20. Sympathetic innervation of the viscera and the medulla and suprarenal gland.

CLINICAL CONSIDERATIONS 11-4

Disorders of the Suprarenal Gland

Addison's disease is an autoimmune disease, although it may also be the aftermath of tuberculosis. It is characterized by decreased production of adrenocortical hormones owing to the destruction of the suprarenal cortex, and without the administration of steroid treatment, it may have fatal consequences.

Type 2 polyglandular syndrome, a hereditary disorder, affects the thyroid and suprarenal glands in such a fashion that they are underactive (although the thyroid may become overactive). Frequently, patients with this disorder also develop diabetes.

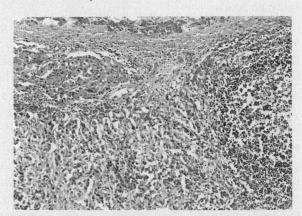

This photomicrograph of the adrenal gland of a patient with Addison's disease displays cortical fibrosis and inflammation as well as a mass of atrophic cortical cells. (Reprinted with permission from Strayer DS, et al., eds. *Rubin's Pathology: Clinicopathologic Foundations of Medicine,* 7th ed. Philadelphia: Wolters Kluwer, 2014. Figure 27-32.)

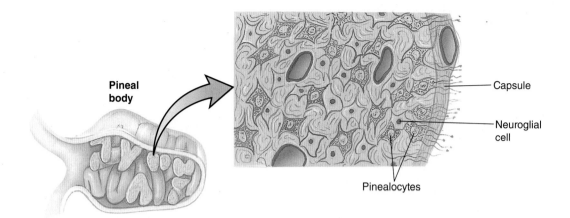

FIGURE 11-21. Pineal gland.

Mechanism of Hormonal Action

Hormones may be classified according to various criteria including lipid solubility. Lipid-insoluble (nonsteroid-based) hormones are derived from:

- amino acids (melatonin, catecholamines, thyroid hormones),
- small polypeptides (oxytocin and vasopressin), and
- proteins (glucagon, insulin, anterior pituitary proteins, and PTH).

Whereas lipid-soluble (steroid-based) hormones are derived from fatty acids or steroids (aldosterone, cortisol, estrogen, progesterone, and testosterone).

Regardless of the type of hormones, all are released by specific **releasing cells** and are designed for their specific **target cells**. Because the hormones discussed in this chapter travel through the bloodstream, they can come in contact with a plethora of cells, but they affect only those cells that express **receptors** designed for a particular hormone. These receptors may be embedded on the target cell plasma membrane (**cell-surface receptors**), they may be in the cytosol (**intracytoplasmic receptors**), or they may be within the nucleus (**intranuclear receptors**) of the target cell. When the hormone binds to its receptor, the target cell responds either by actively performing a specific task or by becoming inhibited from performing a particular task.

- Hormones that bind to a receptor inside the nucleus or a hormone–receptor complex formed in the cytosol enter the nucleus, attach to the DNA of the cell, and activate its **transcription**.
- Hormones that bind to **cell-surface receptors**, **catalytic receptors**, or **G protein complexes** cause the intracytoplasmic moiety of the receptor to initiate the activation of **regulatory molecules/ions**, such as

cAMP, cGMP, members of the **inositol family**, or the release of **calcium ions**. These regulatory molecules/ions are known as second messengers. It is these second messengers that induce the required response by the target cell.

Because of the specificity of the reaction, only a minute quantity of the hormone is required.

Nonsteroid-Based Hormones and Amino Acid Derivatives

Nonsteroid-based endocrine hormones and amino acid derivatives bind to **receptors** (some are G protein-linked, and some are catalytic) located on the target cell membrane, activate them, and thus initiate a sequence of intracellular reactions. These may act by altering the state of an **ion channel** (opening or closing) or by activating (or inhibiting) an **enzyme** or group of enzymes associated with the cytoplasmic aspect of the cell membrane.

Opening or closing an ion channel will permit the particular ion to traverse or inhibit the particular ion from traversing the cell membrane, thus altering the membrane potential. Neurotransmitters and **catecholamines** act on ion channels. The binding of most hormones to their receptor will have only a single effect, which is the activation of **adenylate cyclase**. This enzyme functions in the transformation of ATP to **cyclic adenosine monophosphate** (cAMP), the major **second messenger** of the cell. cAMP then activates a specific sequence of enzymes that are necessary to accomplish the desired result. There are a few hormones that activate a similar compound, **cyclic guanosine monophosphate** (cGMP), which functions comparably. Some hormones facilitate the opening of **calcium channels**; calcium enters the cell, and three or four calcium ions bind to the protein **calmodulin**,

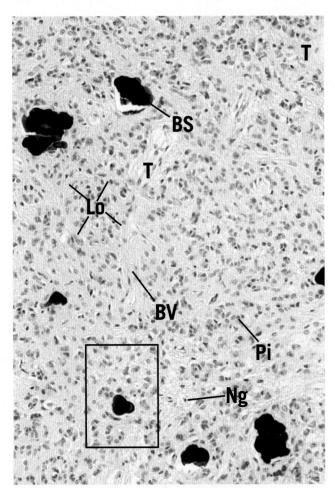

FIGURE 11-22. Pineal gland. Human. Paraffin section. ×132.

The pineal gland is covered by a capsule of connective tissue derived from the pia mater. From this capsule, connective tissue **trabeculae** (T) enter the substance of the pineal gland, subdividing it into numerous incomplete **lobules** (Lo). Nerves and **blood vessels** (BV) travel in the trabeculae to be distributed throughout the pineal gland, providing it with a rich vascular supply. In addition to endothelial and connective tissue cells, two other types of cells are present in the pineal gland, namely, the parenchymal cells, known as **pinealocytes** (Pi), and **neuroglial supporting cells** (Ng). A characteristic feature of the pineal gland is the deposit of calcified material known as corpora arenacea or **brain sand** (BS). The *boxed area* is presented at a higher magnification in Figure 11-23.

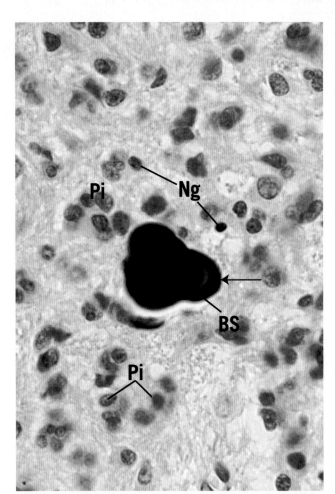

FIGURE 11-23. Pineal body. Human. Paraffin section. ×540.

This photomicrograph is a higher magnification of the *boxed area* of Figure 11-22. With the use of hematoxylin and eosin stain, only the nuclei of the two cell types are clearly evident. The larger, paler, more numerous nuclei belong to the **pinealocytes** (Pi). The smaller, denser nuclei are those of the **neuroglial cells** (Ng). The pale background is composed of the long, intertwining processes of these two cell types. The center of the photomicrograph is occupied by **brain sand** (BS). Observe that these concretions increase in size by apposition of layers on the surface of the calcified material, as may be noted at the *arrow*.

altering its conformation. The altered calmodulin is a **second messenger** that activates a sequence of enzymes, causing a specific response.

Steroid-Based Hormones

Steroid-based endocrine hormones diffuse into the target cell through the plasma membrane and, once inside the cell, bind to a **receptor molecule**. The receptor molecule–hormone complex enters the nucleus, seeks out a specific region of the DNA molecule, and initiates the synthesis of mRNA. The newly formed mRNA codes for the formation of specific enzymes that will accomplish the desired result. The presence of most hormones also elicits a vascularly mediated negative feedback response, in that subsequent to a desired response, the further production and/or release of that particular hormone is inhibited.

Selected Review of Histologic Images

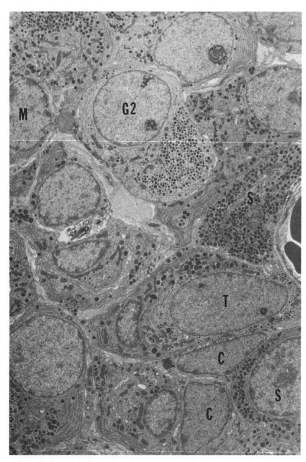

REVIEW FIGURE 11-1-1. Pituitary gland. Pars anterior. Electron microscopy. ×4,950.

Although considerable controversy surrounds the precise fine structural identification of the cells of the pars anterior, it is reasonably certain that the several cell types presented in this electron micrograph are acidophils, basophils, and chromophobes, as observed by light microscopy. The acidophils are **somatotropes** (S) and **mammotropes** (M), whereas only two types of basophils are included in this electron micrograph, namely, **type II gonadotropes** (G2) and **thyrotropes** (T). The **chromophobes** (C) may be recognized by the absence of secretory granules in their cytoplasm. (From Poole MC, et al. Cellular distribution within the rat adenohypophysis: a morphometric study. *Anat Rec* 1982;204(1):45–53. Copyright © 1982 Wiley-Liss, Inc. Reprinted by permission of John Wiley & Sons, Inc.)

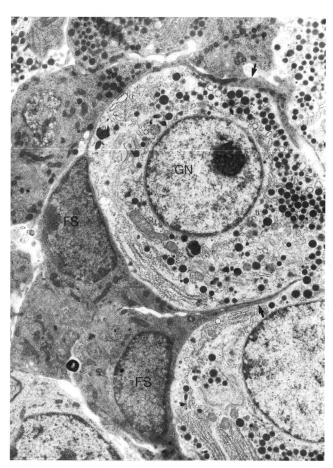

REVIEW FIGURE 11-1-2. Pituitary gland. Rat. Electron microscopy. ×8,936.

The pars distalis of the rat pituitary houses various cell types, two of which are represented here. The granule-containing **gonadotrophs** (GN) are surrounded by nongranular **folliculostellate cells** (FS), whose processes are demarcated by *arrows*. The functions of folliculostellate cells are in question, although some believe them to be supportive, phagocytic, regenerative, or secretory in nature. (Reprinted by permission from Springer: Stokreef JC, et al. A possible phagocytic role for folliculo-stellate cells of anterior pituitary following estrogen withdrawal from primed male rats. *Cell Tissue Res* 1986;243(2):255–261. Copyright © 1986 Springer Nature.)

KEY					
C	chromophobes	**GN**	gonadotrophs	**S**	somatotropes
FS	folliculostellate cells	**M**	mammotropes	**T**	thyrotropes
G2	type II gonadotropes				

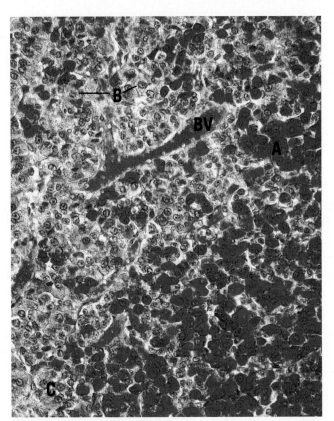

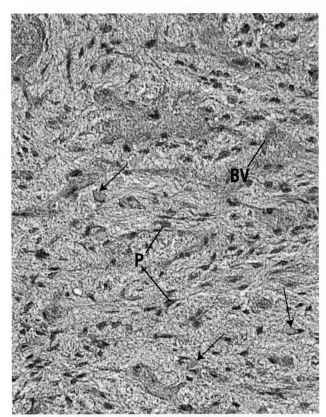

REVIEW FIGURE 11-1-3. Pituitary gland. Pars anterior. Human. Paraffin section. Masson stain. ×270.

REVIEW FIGURE 11-1-4. Pituitary gland. Pars nervosa. Human. Paraffin section. Masson stain. ×270.

The pars anterior of the pituitary gland is derived from the epithelium of the pharyngeal roof and is composed of parenchymal cells arranged in thick cords. These cords of cells are surrounded by a rich **vascular tissue** (BV) whose blood carries their secretions to their target cells. Three types of parenchymal cells are visible with this stain: those whose granules stain red, known as **acidophils** (A); those whose granules stain blue, known as **basophils** (B); and those whose cytoplasm is limited and is devoid of granules, known as **chromophobes** (C). Because chromophobes have very little cytoplasm, the nuclei of the cells are very closely clustered, making them easy to recognize.

The pars nervosa of the pituitary gland is derived from the hypothalamus and is composed of axons of neurons located in the paraventricular and supraoptic nuclei of the hypothalamus. The axons display expanded regions both along their length and at their termini, and these swellings, known as **Herring bodies** (*arrows*), house vasopressin or oxytocin, depending on the origin of the axon. They release their hormones into the connective tissue surrounding **blood vessels** (BV). **Pituicytes** (P), neuroglia-like cells, envelop these axons, providing physical and metabolic support.

KEY					
A	acidophils	BV	blood vessels	P	pituicytes
B	basophils	C	chromophobes		

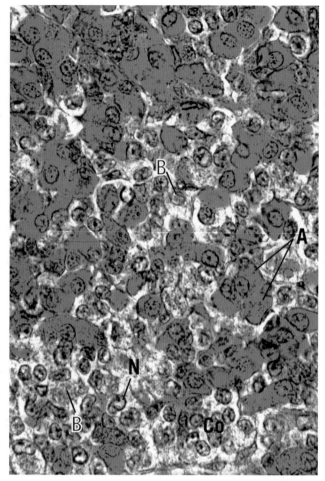

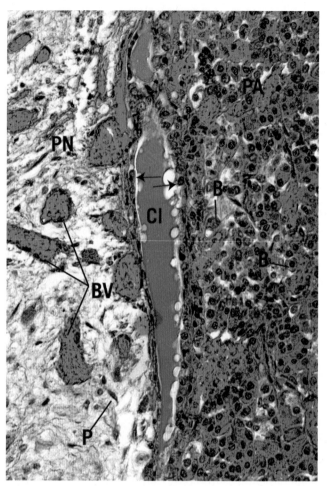

REVIEW FIGURE 11-2-1. Pituitary gland. Paraffin section. ×540.

REVIEW FIGURE 11-2-2. Pituitary gland. Pars intermedia. Human. Paraffin section. ×270.

It is somewhat difficult to discriminate between the **acidophils** (A) and **basophils** (B) of the pituitary gland stained with hematoxylin and eosin. Even at high magnification, such as in this photomicrograph, only slight differences are noted. Acidophils stain pinkish and are slightly smaller in size than the basophils, which stain pale blue. In a black and white photomicrograph, basophils appear darker than acidophils. **Chromophobes** (Co) are readily recognizable because their cytoplasm is small and does not take up stain. Moreover, cords of chromophobes present clusters of **nuclei** (N) crowded together.

The pars intermedia of the pituitary gland is situated between the **pars anterior** (PA) and the **pars nervosa** (PN). It is characterized by **basophils** (B), which are smaller than those of the pars anterior. Additionally, the pars intermedia contains **colloid** (Cl)-filled follicles, lined by pale, small, low cuboidal shaped cells (*arrows*). Note that some of the basophils extend into the pars nervosa. Numerous **blood vessels** (BV) and **pituicytes** (P) are evident in this area of the pars nervosa.

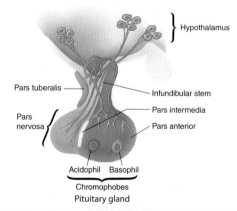

KEY

A	acidophils	Cl	colloid	P	pituicytes
B	basophils	Co	chromophobes	PA	pars anterior
BV	blood vessels	N	nucleus	PN	pars nervosa

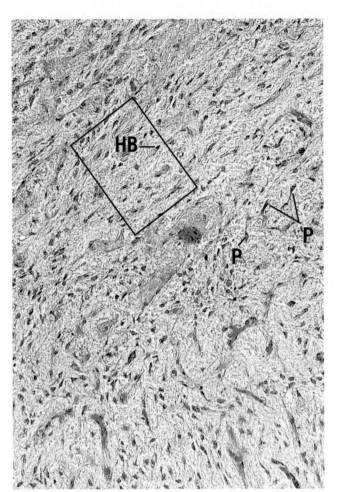

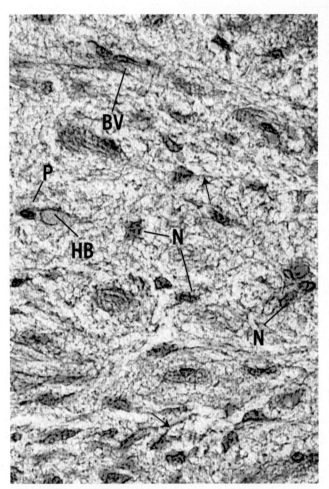

REVIEW FIGURE 11-2-3. Pituitary gland. Pars nervosa. Paraffin section. ×132.

REVIEW FIGURE 11-2-4. Pituitary gland. Pars nervosa. Paraffin section. ×540.

The pars nervosa of the pituitary gland is composed of elongated cells with long processes known as **pituicytes** (P), which are thought to be neuroglial in nature. These cells, which possess more or less oval nuclei, appear to support numerous unmyelinated nerve fibers traveling from the hypothalamus via the hypothalamo-hypophyseal tract. These nerve fibers cannot be distinguished from the cytoplasm of pituicytes in a hematoxylin and eosin-stained preparation. Neurosecretory materials pass along these nerve fibers and are stored in expanded regions at the termination of the fibers, which are then referred to as **Herring bodies** (HB). Note that the pars nervosa resembles neural tissue. The *boxed area* is presented at a higher magnification in Review Figure 11-2-4.

This photomicrograph is a higher magnification of the *boxed area* of Review Figure 11-2-3. Note the numerous more or less oval **nuclei** (N) of the pituicytes, some of whose processes (*arrows*) are clearly evident at this magnification. The unmyelinated nerve fibers and processes of pituicytes make up the cellular network of the pars nervosa. The expanded terminal regions of the nerve fibers, which house neurosecretions, are known as **Herring bodies** (HB). Also observe the presence of **blood vessels** (BV) in the pars nervosa.

KEY					
BV	blood vessels	**N**	nucleus	**P**	pituicytes
HB	Herring bodies				

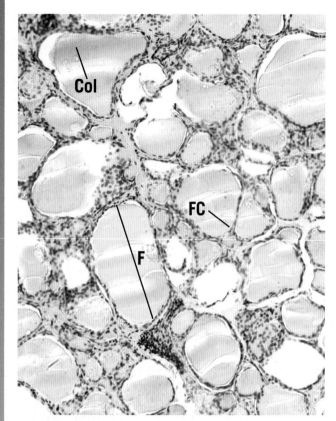

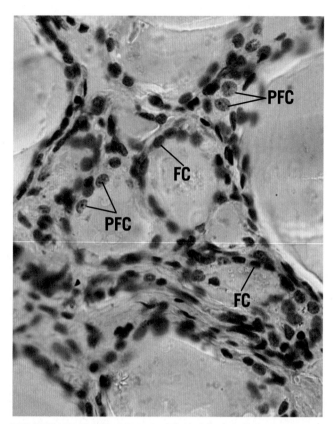

REVIEW FIGURE 11-3-1. Thyroid gland. Human. Paraffin section. ×132.

This is a paraffin section of the human thyroid that is similar to the plastic section of the monkey thyroid depicted in Review Figure 11-1-3. The low cuboidal **follicular cells** (FC) form the **follicles** (F) that are filled with **colloid** (Col).

REVIEW FIGURE 11-3-2. Thyroid gland. Human. Paraffin section. ×540.

This is a higher magnification of a region similar to Review Figure 11-3-1. The low cuboidal **follicular cells** (FC) are clearly evident as are the **parafollicular cells** (PFC) whose clear cytoplasm is responsible for their additional name, that is, "clear cells." Note also that the nuclei of the follicular cells are dark, whereas the nuclei of the parafollicular cells are stained much lighter.

KEY					
Col	colloid	**FC**	follicular cell	**PFC**	parafollicular cell
F	follicle				

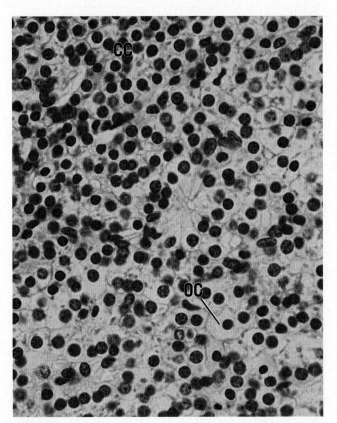

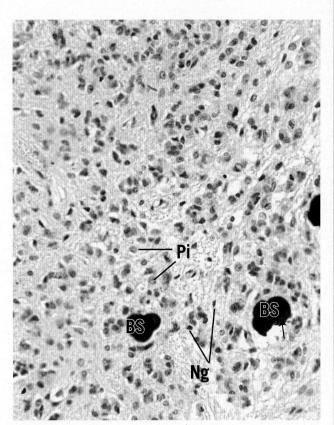

REVIEW FIGURE 11-3-3. Parathyroid gland. Human. Paraffin section. ×540.

Note that the smaller **chief cells** (CC) are crowded together, whereas the **oxyphil cells** (OC) that are equally as crowded together appear to be more loosely arranged owing to their larger cytoplasm.

REVIEW FIGURE 11-3-4. Pineal gland. Human. Paraffin section. ×270.

Note that two types of cells present in the pineal gland, the **pinealocytes** (Pi), whose nuclei are larger and lighter staining than those of the **neuroglia** (Ng). **Brain sand** (BS) occupies some of the intercellular spaces of the pineal gland.

KEY					
BS	brain sand	**Ng**	neuroglial cell	**Pi**	pinealocyte
CC	chief cells	**OC**	oxyphil cells		

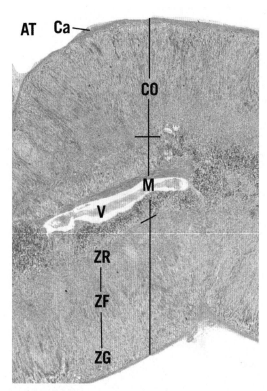

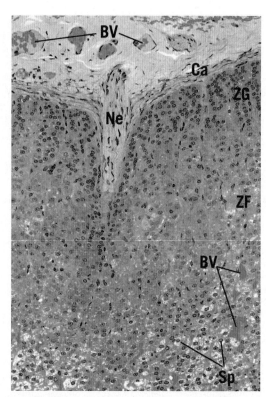

REVIEW FIGURE 11-4-1. Suprarenal gland. Paraffin section. ×14.

The suprarenal gland, usually embedded in **adipose tissue** (AT), is invested by a collagenous connective tissue **capsule** (Ca) that provides thin connective tissue elements that carry blood vessels and nerves into the substance of the gland. Because the **cortex** (Co) of the suprarenal gland completely surrounds the flattened **medulla** (M), it appears duplicated in any section that completely transects the gland. The cortex is divided into three concentric regions: the outermost **zona glomerulosa** (ZG), middle **zona fasciculata** (ZF), and the innermost **zona reticularis** (ZR). The medulla, which is always bounded by the zona reticularis, possesses several large **veins** (V), which are always accompanied by a considerable amount of connective tissue.

REVIEW FIGURE 11-4-2. Suprarenal gland. Cortex. Monkey. Plastic section. ×132.

The collagenous connective tissue **capsule** (Ca) of the suprarenal gland is surrounded by adipose tissue through which **blood vessels** (BV) and **nerves** (Ne) reach the gland. The parenchymal cells of the cortex, immediately deep to the capsule, are arranged in an irregular array, forming the more or less oval to round clusters or arch-like cords of the **zona glomerulosa** (ZG). The cells of the **zona fasciculata** (ZF) form long, straight columns of cords oriented radially, each being one to two cells in width. These cells are larger than those of the zona glomerulosa. They present a vacuolated appearance owing to the numerous lipid droplets that were extracted during processing and are often referred to as **spongiocytes** (Sp). The interstitium is richly vascularized by **blood vessels** (BV).

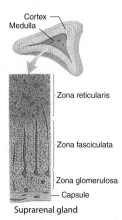

Suprarenal gland

KEY					
AT	adipose tissue	M	medulla	ZF	zona fasciculata
BV	blood vessels	Ne	nerves	ZG	zona glomerulosa
Ca	capsule	Sp	spongiocytes	ZR	zona reticularis
Co	Cortex	V	vein		

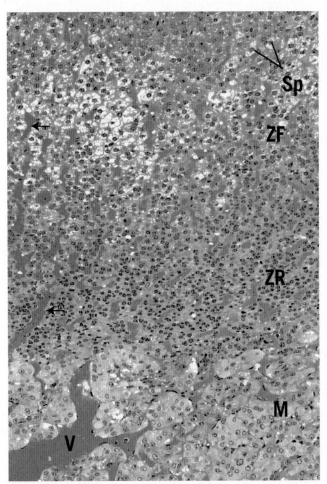

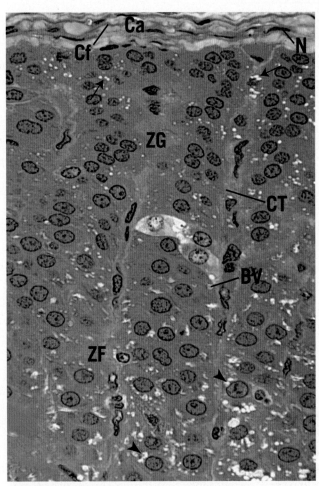

REVIEW FIGURE 11-4-3. Suprarenal gland. Monkey. Plastic section. ×132.

REVIEW FIGURE 11-4-4. Suprarenal gland. Monkey. Plastic section. ×540.

The columnar arrangement of the cords of the **zona fasciculata** (ZF) is readily evident by viewing the architecture of the blood vessels indicated by the *arrows*. The cells in the deeper region of the zona fasciculata are smaller and appear denser than the more superficially located **spongiocytes** (Sp). Cells of the **zona reticularis** (ZR) are arranged in irregular, anastomosing cords whose interstices contain wide capillaries. The cords of the zona reticularis merge almost imperceptibly with those of the zona fasciculata. This is a relatively narrow region of the cortex. The **medulla** (M) is clearly evident because its cells are much larger than those of the zona reticularis. Moreover, numerous large **veins** (V) are characteristic of the medulla.

The **capsule** (Ca) of the suprarenal gland displays its **collagen fibers** (Cf) and the **nuclei** (N) of the fibroblasts. The **zona glomerulosa** (ZG), which occupies the upper part of the photomicrograph, displays relatively small cells with few vacuoles (*arrows*). The lower part of the photomicrograph demonstrates the **zona fasciculata** (ZF), whose cells are larger and display a more vacuolated (*arrowheads*) appearance. Note the presence of **connective tissue** (CT) elements and **blood vessels** (BV) in the interstitium between cords of parenchymal cells.

KEY					
BV	blood vessels	**M**	medulla	**ZF**	zona fasciculata
Ca	capsule	**N**	nuclei	**ZG**	zona glomerulosa
Cf	collagen fibers	**Sp**	spongiocytes	**ZR**	zona reticularis
CT	connective tissue	**V**	veins		

REVIEW PLATE 11-5A

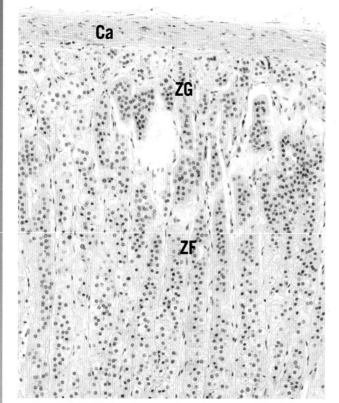

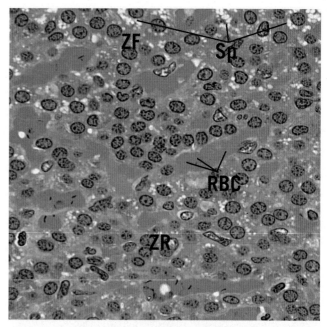

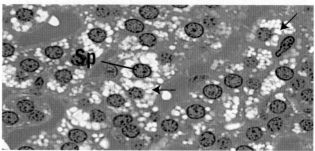

REVIEW FIGURE 11-5-1. Suprarenal gland. Cortex. Human. Paraffin section. ×132.

Observe the collagenous connective tissue **capsule** (Ca) that invests the **zona glomerulosa** (ZG) of the suprarenal cortex. Note that the cells of the zona glomerulosa are arranged in a spherical configuration, whereas the cells of the **zona fasciculata** (ZF) are arranged in vertical columns.

REVIEW FIGURE 11-5-2. Suprarenal gland. Cortex. Monkey. Plastic section. ×540.

The upper part of this photomicrograph presents the border between the **zona fasciculata** (ZF) and the **zona reticularis** (ZR). Note that the **spongiocytes** (Sp) of the fasciculata are larger and more vacuolated than the cells of the reticularis. The parenchymal cells of the zona reticularis are arranged in haphazardly anastomosing cords. The interstitium of both regions houses large capillaries containing **red blood cells** (RBC). *Inset.* **Zona fasciculata. Monkey. Plastic section.** ×540. The **spongiocytes** (Sp) of the zona fasciculata are of two different sizes. Those positioned more superficially in the cortex, as in this *inset*, are larger and more vacuolated (*arrows*) than spongiocytes close to the zona reticularis.

KEY					
Ca	capsule	**Sp**	spongiocytes	**ZG**	zona glomerulosa
RBC	red blood cells	**ZF**	zona fasciculata	**ZR**	zona reticularis

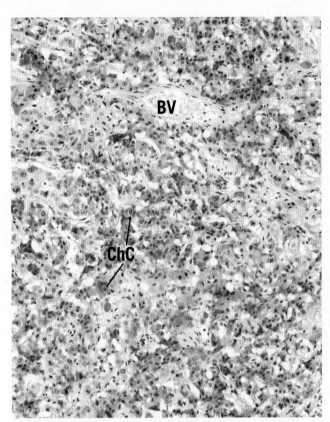

REVIEW FIGURE 11-5-3. Suprarenal gland. Medulla. Human. Paraffin section. ×132.

This is the medulla of the suprarenal gland displaying its rich **vascular supply** (BV) as well as the numerous clusters of **chromaffin cells** (ChC) that populate the medulla.

Summary of Histologic Organization

Endocrine glands are characterized by the absence of ducts and the presence of a rich vascular network. The parenchymal cells of endocrine glands are usually arranged in short **cords**, **follicles**, or **clusters**, although other arrangements are also common.

I. Pituitary Gland

The pituitary gland is invested by a connective tissue capsule. The gland is embryonically and histologically divided into two parts, adenohypophysis and neurohypophysis, each further subdivided into smaller structural and functional regions.

A. Adenohypophysis (Anterior Pituitary)

Derived from oral ectodermal epithelium which differentiates into two categories of cells based on staining patterns with H&E.

1. Chromophils

i. *Acidophils*

Stain pink to red with H&E. They are more densely present in the center of the pars anterior (pars distalis).

ii. *Basophils*

Stain darker in bluish to purple hues with H&E. They are more frequently found at the periphery of the pars anterior (pars distalis), pars intermedia, and pars tuberalis.

2. Chromophobes

Chromophobes are smaller cells whose cytoplasm is not granular and pale staining owing to little affinity for stain. They may be recognized as clusters of nuclei throughout the adenohypophysis.

3. Three Subdivisions of Adenohypophysis

i. *Pars Anterior (Pars Distalis)*

The bulk of the adenohypophysis, comprising of chromophils and chromophobes.

ii. *Pars Intermedia*

The **pars intermedia** is rudimentary in humans, and it is positioned between the pars anterior and pars nervosa. Small basophils are present, as well as **colloid-filled follicles**.

iii. *Pars Tuberalis*

The **pars tuberalis** extends around the infundibulum and is composed of mostly basophils arranged in cords. Small colloid-filled **follicles** may be present.

B. Neurohypophysis (Posterior Pituitary)

Neurohypophysis derives from the downgrowth of the hypothalamus; therefore, it is comprised of neural tissue.

1. Two Subdivisions of Neurohypophysis

i. *Infundibulum (Infundibular Stalk)*

Infundibulum is comprised of the unmyelinated axons extending from the neuron cell bodies in the paraventricular and supraoptic nuclei in the hypothalamus. This collection of unmyelinated axons is known as the hypothalamic–hypophyseal tract. Vasopressin and oxytocin synthesized in the cell bodies are transported into the axon terminals in the pars nervosa.

ii. *Pars Nervosa*

The expanded axon terminals of the hypothalamic–hypophyseal tract, located in the pars nervosa, are known as **Herring bodies**, and they contain vasopressin and oxytocin. Numerous nuclei in the pars nervosa belong to the **pituicytes** which perform neuroglial functions such as supporting the unmyelinated axon fibers.

II. Thyroid Gland

A. Capsule

The **capsule** of the thyroid gland consists of a thin **collagenous dense irregular connective tissue** from which **septa** extend into the substance of the gland, subdividing it into lobules.

B. Parenchymal Cells

The **parenchymal cells** of the thyroid gland form **colloid**-filled **follicles**. These parenchymal cells are of two types:

- **follicular cells** (simple cuboidal epithelium) which synthesize thyroid hormones and
- **parafollicular cells** (clear cells) located at the periphery of the follicles which produce calcitonin.

C. Connective Tissue

Slender connective tissue elements support a rich vascular supply.

III. Parathyroid Gland

A. Capsule

The gland is invested by a slender collagenous dense irregular connective tissue **capsule** from which **septa** arise to penetrate the substance of the gland.

B. Parenchymal Cells

1. Chief Cells

Chief cells are numerous, small cells with large nuclei that form cords and produce PTH.

2. Oxyphils

Oxyphils are larger, acidophilic, and much fewer in number than chief cells with unclear functions.

C. Connective Tissue

Collagenous connective tissue **septa** as well as slender **reticular fibers** support a rich vascular supply. **Fatty infiltration** is common in older individuals.

IV. Suprarenal (Adrenal) Gland

The **suprarenal gland** is invested by a collagenous denser irregular connective tissue **capsule**. The gland is subdivided into a **cortex** and a **medulla**.

A. Cortex

The **cortex** derives from the mesodermal epithelium and is divided into three concentric zones:

1. Zona Glomerulosa

The **zona glomerulosa** is immediately deep into the capsule. It consists of cuboidal cells, arranged in arches and spherical clusters, which release aldosterone.

2. Zona Fasciculata

The thickest zone of the cortex is the **zona fasciculata**. The more or less cuboidal cells (**spongiocytes**) are arranged in long, parallel cords. **Spongiocytes** appear highly vacuolated owing to extraction of the steroid-based hormone cortisol during tissue processing. Spongiocytes in the deepest region are smaller and much less vacuolated.

3. Zona Reticularis

The innermost zone of the cortex is the **zona reticularis**. It is composed of small, darker cells arranged in irregularly anastomosing cords secreting weak androgen DHEA. The intervening capillaries are enlarged.

B. Medulla

The **medulla** derives from the neural crest and is composed of large, granule-containing **chromaffin cells** arranged in short cords. In response to presynaptic sympathetic neuron firing, chromaffin cells release epinephrine and norepinephrine. Additionally, large autonomic ganglion cells are present. A characteristic of the medulla is the presence of large veins.

V. Pineal Gland

A. Capsule

The **capsule**, derived from **pia mater**, is thin collagenous connective tissue. **Septa** derived from the capsule divide the pineal body into incomplete lobules.

B. Parenchymal Cells

1. Pinealocytes

Pinealocytes produce melatonin and are recognized by the large size of their nuclei.

2. Neuroglial Cells

Neuroglial cells possess smaller, denser nuclei than the pinealocytes.

C. Brain Sand (Corpora Arenacea)

Brain sand or **corpora arenacea** are characteristic of the pineal body and are calcified accretions in the intercellular spaces. Currently, there are no known functions of these concretions.

Chapter Review Questions

Case scenario for questions 11-1 to 11-4: A 28-year-old male patient who is a professional boxer presents to his primary physician with chief concerns of dizziness, irritability, and "unquenchable" thirst persisting the past 2 days, despite consuming over a gallon of water daily. The patient reports that 2 days ago, he was knocked out during a sparring session from an accidental headbutt to his forehead. Physical exam revealed a bruise on the forehead, tachycardia, and tachypnea.

11-1. **What is the most likely diagnosis?**

    A. Addison's disease

    B. Diabetes insipidus

    C. Graves disease

    D. Hyperparathyroidism

    E. Somatotrope adenoma

11-2. **Which cells are injured in this case?**

    A. Parathyroid oxyphils

    B. Pinealocytes

    C. Pituitary acidophils

    D. Pituitary basophils

    E. Supraoptic nucleus neurons

11-3. **Target cells in which structures are receiving significantly reduced hormonal signals in this patient?**

    A. Collecting tubule cells

    B. Cells of the paraventricular nuclei

    C. Thyroid follicular cells

    D. Spongiocytes

11-4. **Which structure is impaired in this patient?**

    A. Adrenal medulla

    B. Infundibulum

    C. Pars distalis

    D. Thyroid gland

    E. Zona reticularis

11-5. **Patients with high blood calcium levels and exogenous calcifications should be examined for adenoma of which organ?**

    A. Adrenal cortex

    B. Anterior pituitary

    C. Parathyroid

    D. Pineal gland

    E. Posterior pituitary

INTEGUMENT

The integument, the largest and heaviest organ of the body, is composed of skin and its various derivatives, including sebaceous glands, sweat glands, hair, and nails. The skin covers the entire body and is continuous with the mucous membranes at the lips, at the anus, in the nose, at the leading edges of the eyelids, and at the external orifices of the urogenital system. Some of the many functions of skin include protection against physical, chemical, and biologic assaults; providing a waterproof barrier; absorbing ultraviolet radiation for both vitamin D synthesis and protection; excretion (i.e., sweat) and thermoregulation; monitoring the external milieu via its various nerve endings; and immunologic defense of the body.

Skin

Skin is composed of two layers of different tissue types. The superficial layer is the **epidermis**, composed of **keratinized stratified squamous epithelium**, and the deep layer is the **dermis**. The dermis is divided into two sublayers, the thin layer of **papillary dermis** comprised of **loose connective tissue**, positioned just deep to the epidermis, and the remainder of the deeper layer, the **reticular dermis**, composed of **dense irregular connective tissue** (Fig. 12-1).

- The epidermis and dermis interdigitate with each other by way of **epidermal ridges (epidermal pegs)** and **dermal ridges (dermal papillae)**, which form an undulating interface between the two tissue types, separated by a basement membrane. The interdigitation increases the surface area available for strong adhesion between the epidermis and dermis via numerous hemidesmosomes.

  - Frequently, a dermal ridge is subdivided into two secondary dermal ridges with an intervening interpapillary peg from the epidermis.

- The interdigitation creates the ridges on the epidermis of the fingertip surfaces that imprint as fingerprints.

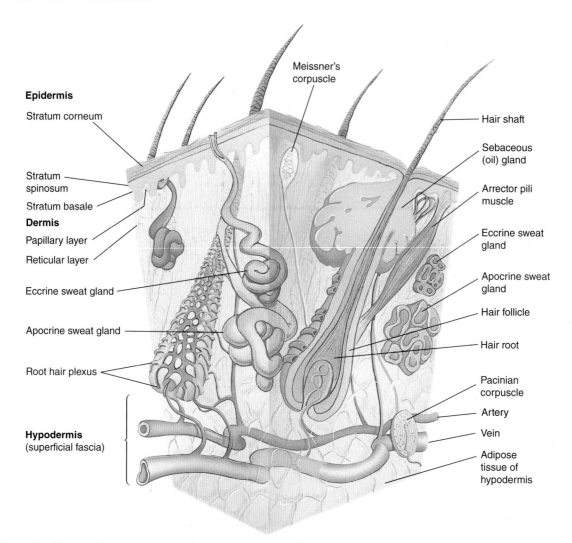

FIGURE 12-1. Skin and its appendages, hair, sweat glands (both eccrine and apocrine), sebaceous glands, arrector pili muscles, and nails, are known as the integument. Skin is composed of the epidermis and dermis and may be thick or thin, depending on the thickness of its epidermis. Skin is richly vascularized and contains various sensory cells and structures.

Interposed between the skin and deeper structures is a fascial sheath known as the hypodermis (superficial fascia), which is *not* a part of the skin. Skin can be classified as **thick skin**, as on the sole of the foot and the palm of the hand, or **thin skin (glabrous skin)** as over the remainder of the body (Table 12-1). Thick skin is characterized by the thickness of the epidermis of about 0.5 mm, prominent epidermal and dermal ridges, numerous sweat glands, and lack of hair follicles and sebaceous glands (Fig. 12-2A). Thin skin is characterized by a thinner epidermis of about 0.1 to 0.15 mm, numerous sweat glands, hair follicles, and sebaceous glands (Fig. 12-2B). Observed under a microscope, five distinct histologic layers within the keratinized stratified squamous epithelium comprise the epidermis of the thick skin, whereas only four layers are distinguishable in thin skin.

Epidermis

The epidermis is composed of four cell types, keratinocytes, melanocytes, Langerhans cells, and Merkel cells. Approximately 95% of the cells of the epidermis are keratinocytes, and their morphology is responsible for the characteristics of the five layers of the epidermis.

• The deepest layer, the **stratum basale**, is a single layer of cuboidal to columnar-shaped keratinocytes (Fig. 12-3A; also see Fig. 12-2B). Distributed within this layer are melanocytes and Merkel cells that produce skin pigments and perform fine sensory functions, respectively. The keratinocytes of this layer are responsible not only for forming strong adhesions between the epidermis and the dermis via hemidesmosomes but also for epidermal renewal and maintenance, via

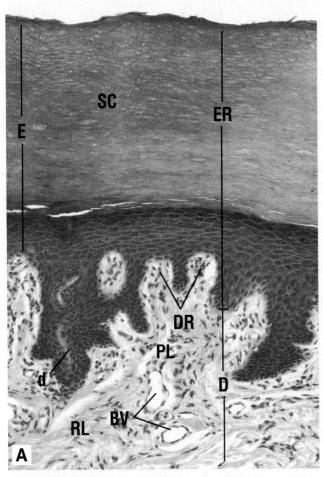

FIGURE 12-2A. Thick skin. Paraffin section. ×132.

Skin is composed of the superficial **epidermis** (E) and the deeper **dermis** (D). The interface of the two tissues is demarcated by **epidermal ridges** (ER) and **dermal ridges** (DR) (dermal papillae). Between successive epidermal ridges are the interpapillary pegs, which divide each dermal ridge into secondary dermal ridges. Note that in thick skin, the keratinized layer, **stratum corneum** (SC), is highly developed. Observe also that the **duct** (d) of the sweat gland pierces the base of an epidermal ridge. The dermis of the skin is subdivided into two regions, a **papillary layer** (PL), comprising loose connective tissue of the dermal ridges, and the deeper, dense irregular connective tissue of the **reticular layer** (RL). **Blood vessels** (BV) from the reticular layer enter the dermal ridges.

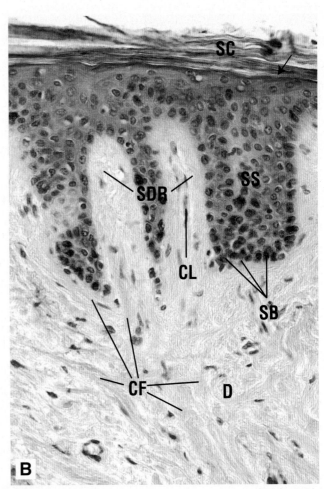

FIGURE 12-2B. Thin skin. Human. Paraffin section. ×270.

Compared to thick skin, the epidermis of thin skin is much thinner composed of only four of the layers found in thick skin. The **stratum basale** (SB) is present as a single layer of cuboidal to columnar cells. Most of the epidermis is composed of the prickle cells of the **stratum spinosum** (SS) and scattered cells of the stratum granulosum (*arrow*) and **stratum corneum** (SC) are especially thin, whereas stratum lucidum is absent. The papillary layer of the **dermis** (D) is richly vascularized by **capillary loops** (CL), which penetrate the **secondary dermal ridges** (SDR). Observe that the **collagen fiber** (CF) bundles of the dermis become coarser as the distance from the epidermis increases.

mitosis (usually at night). Furthermore, the keratinocytes manufacture and start accumulating bundles of **keratin** intermediate filaments known as **tonofilaments**. The daughter cells of keratinocyte mitosis are pushed surfaceward, giving rise to the layer just superficial to the stratum basale.

• **Stratum spinosum** is the thickest layer of the epidermis and is composed of several layers of polyhedral **keratinocytes** (also called **prickle cells**) characterized by the appearance of numerous cell processes on their periphery that make the cells seem prickly (see

Figs. 12-3A,B). As the cells shrink during tissue processing, their processes become accentuated, highlighting the desmosome-induced adherence of the cell–cell junctions (intercellular bridges) among neighboring prickle cells. The strong desmosomes, along with the tonofilaments that anchor the desmosomal plagues remain intact. Prickle cells also undergo mitotic activity (usually at night) and contribute to the renewal and maintenance of the epidermis. Furthermore, the prickle cells continue to manufacture keratin that becomes surrounded by a material

Table 12-1 Characteristics of Thick and Thin Skin

Cellular Strata (*Superficial to deepest*)	Thick Skin	Thin Skin
Epidermis	Is a stratified squamous keratinized epithelium derived from ectoderm. Cells of the epidermis consist of four cell types: keratinocytes, melanocytes, Langerhans cells, and Merkel cells.	
Stratum corneum (*cornified cell layer*)	Composed of several layers of dead, anucleate, flattened keratinocytes (squames) that are continuously sloughed from the surface. As many as 50 layers of keratinocytes are located in the thickest skin (e.g., sole of the foot).	Only about five or so layers of keratinocytes (squames) comprise this layer in the thinnest skin (e.g., eyelids).
Stratum lucidum (*clear cell layer*)	Poorly stained, thin keratinocytes filled with keratin compose this thin, well-defined layer. Organelles and nuclei are absent.	Layer is absent, but individual cells of the layer are probably present.
Stratum granulosum (*granular cell layer*)	Only three to five layers thick with flattening nucleated keratinocytes with a normal complement of organelles as well as keratohyalin and membrane-coating granules	Layer is attenuated.
Stratum spinosum (*prickle cell layer*)	This thickest living cell layer is composed of mitotically active and maturing polygonal keratinocytes (prickle cells) that interdigitate with one another via projections (intercellular bridges) that are attached to each other by desmosomes. The cytoplasm is rich in tonofilaments, organelles, and membrane-coating granules. Langerhans cells are present in this layer.	This stratum is the same as in thick skin, but the number of layers is reduced.
Stratum basale (*stratum germinativum*)	This deepest stratum is composed of a single layer of mitotically active tall cuboidal keratinocytes that are in contact with the basal lamina. Keratinocytes of the more superficial strata originate from this layer and eventually migrate to the surface where they are sloughed. Melanocytes and Merkel cells are also present in this layer.	This layer is the same in thin skin as well as in thick skin.
Dermis	Located deep into the epidermis, and separated from it by a basement membrane, the dermis is derived from mesoderm and is composed mostly of connective tissue. It contains capillaries, nerves, sensory organs, hair follicles, sweat and sebaceous glands, and arrector pili muscles. It is divided into two layers: a superficial papillary layer and a deeper reticular layer.	
Papillary layer	Is comprised of loose connective tissue containing capillary loops, and terminals of mechanoreceptors. These dermal papillae interdigitate with the epidermal ridges of the epidermis. These interdigitations are pronounced in thick skin.	The papillary layer is comprised of the same loose connective tissue as in thick skin. However, its volume is much reduced. The depth of the dermal/epidermal interdigitations is also greatly reduced.
Reticular layer	Is composed of dense irregular connective tissue containing the usual array of connective tissue elements, including cells, blood, and lymphatic vessels. Sweat glands and cutaneous nerves are also present, and their branches extend into the papillary layer and the epidermis.	Same as in thick skin with the addition of sebaceous glands and hair follicles along with their arrector pili muscles

known as **keratohyalin** whose principal components are the histidine and cystine-rich proteins **filaggrin** and **trichohyalin**. Additionally, prickle cells form **membrane-coating granules** (**Odland bodies, lamellar bodies**), whose lipid-rich content is composed of ceramides, phospholipids, and glycosphingolipids. Intermixed among the cells of the stratum spinosum are Langerhans cells, resident macrophages of the skin that also function as antigen-presenting cells. Cytoplasmic extensions of melanocytes extend into the extracellular spaces of the stratum spinosum and here, they transfer melanosomes to the resident keratinocytes.

- **Stratum granulosum** is a thin layer of keratinocytes, which continue to accumulate **keratohyalin granules** until they eventually overfill the cells, destroying their nuclei and organelles (Fig. 12-3B). These cells also continue to manufacture membrane-coating lipid-rich granules that contribute to forming a moisture barrier. Cells of the stratum granulosum contact each other via desmosomes and, in their superficial layers, also form claudin-containing **occluding junctions** with each other as well as with cells of the stratum lucidum (or, in the absence of the stratum lucidum, with the cells of the stratum corneum). Cells in the superficial layers of the stratum granulosum release the contents of their membrane-coating granules into the extracellular space. These keratinocytes undergo apoptosis, contain neither organelles nor a nucleus, and are moved to the next superficial layer of the epidermis.

- The fourth epidermal layer, the **stratum lucidum**, is present only in the thick skin, and usually appears as a relatively thin and translucent region, interposed between stratum granulosum and stratum corneum (see Fig. 12-3B). The dead keratinocytes of the stratum lucidum have no nuclei or organelles

but contain tonofibrils (densely packed keratin filaments) and eleidin, a transformation product of keratohyalin.

- The superficial-most layer is the **stratum corneum**, composed of preferentially arranged stacks of hulls of dead keratinocytes (now called **squames**) still filled with keratin. The superficial layers of the stratum corneum are desquamated at the same rate as they are being replaced by the mitotic activity of the stratum basale and stratum spinosum (see Fig. 12-3B).

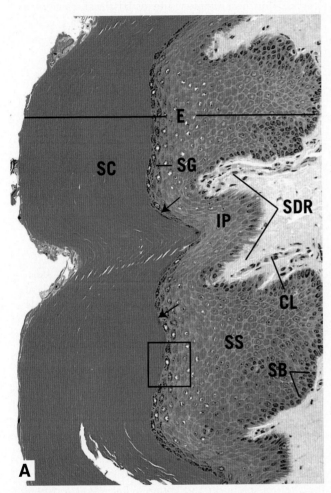

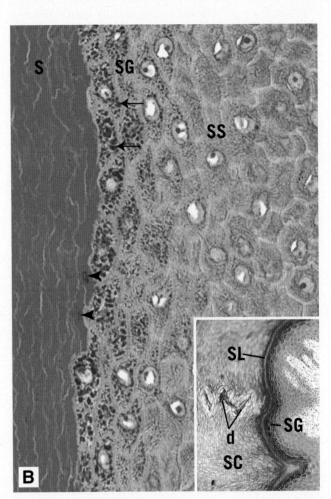

FIGURE 12-3A. Thick skin. Monkey. Plastic section. ×132.

The five layers of the **epidermis** (E) are clearly delineated in this plastic section. Observe that the squames of the **stratum corneum** (SC) appear to lie directly on the **stratum granulosum** (SG), whose cells contain keratohyalin granules. The thickest layer of living cells in the epidermis is the **stratum spinosum** (SS), whereas the **stratum basale** (SB) is only a single cell layer thick. The stratum lucidum is not evident, although a few transitional cells (*arrows*) may be identified. Note that the **secondary dermal ridges** (SDR), on either side of the **interpapillary peg** (IP), present **capillary loops** (CL). A region similar to the *boxed area* is presented in Figure 12-3B at higher magnification.

FIGURE 12-3B. Thick skin. Monkey. Plastic section. ×540.

This is a higher magnification of a region similar to the *boxed area* of Figure 12-3A. Observe that as the cells of the **stratum spinosum** (SS) are being pushed surfaceward, they become somewhat flattened. As the cells reach the **stratum granulosum** (SG), they accumulate keratohyalin granules (*arrows*), which increase in number as the cells progress through this layer. Occasional transitional cells (*arrowheads*) of the poorly defined stratum lucidum may be observed, as well as the **squames** (S) of the **stratum corneum** (SC). *Inset.* **Thick skin. Paraffin section**. ×132. This photomicrograph displays the **stratum lucidum** (SL) to advantage. This layer is between the **stratum granulosum** (SG) and **stratum corneum** (SC). Observe the **duct** (d) of a sweat gland.

CLINICAL CONSIDERATIONS 12-1

Psoriasis Vulgaris

Psoriasis vulgaris is a commonly occurring condition characterized by reddish patchy lesions on the skin with grayish sheen, located especially around the joints, the sacral region, the navel, and the scalp. This condition is produced by increased proliferation of keratinocytes and an acceleration of the cell cycle, resulting in an accumulation of cells in the stratum corneum but with an absence of a stratum granulosum and, frequently, the presence of lymphocytic infiltrates in the papillary layer. The condition is cyclic and is of unknown etiology.

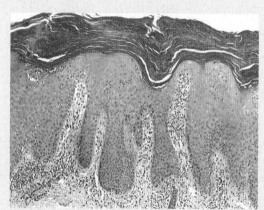

This photomicrograph is of a patient suffering from psoriasis vulgaris. Note that the stratum spinosum and stratum corneum are thickened and that the stratum granulosum is absent. The papillary layer of the dermis displays an infiltration by lymphocytes. (Reprinted with permission from Mills SE, et al., eds. *Sternberg's Diagnostic Surgical Pathology*, 6th ed. Philadelphia: Wolters Kluwer, 2015. p. 7, Figure 1-5.)

Warts

Warts are benign epidermal growths on the skin caused by papilloma viral infection of the keratinocytes. Warts are common in young children, in young adults, and in immunosuppressed patients.

Basal and Squamous Cell Carcinoma

Basal cell carcinoma is the most common malignancy of the skin. It develops in the stratum basale from the accumulation of mutations caused by ultraviolet radiation. The foremost type of basal cell carcinoma is the **nodulocystic type** where small hyperchromatic cells form spherical nodules that are separated from the surrounding connective tissue elements of the dermis by narrow spaces. The most frequent site of basal cell carcinoma is on the nose, occurring as papules or nodules, which eventually craters. Surgery is usually 90% effective with no recurrence.

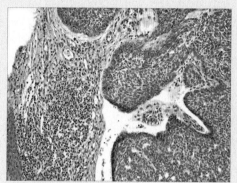

This photomicrograph is of a patient with basal cell carcinoma. Note that the lesion is composed of dark, dense basal cells that form rounded nodules that are separated from the dermal connective tissue by narrowed spaces. (Reprinted with permission from Mills SE, et al., eds. *Sternberg's Diagnostic Surgical Pathology*, 6th ed. Philadelphia: Wolters Kluwer, 2015. p. 53, Figure 2-31.)

Squamous cell carcinoma, the second most frequent skin malignancy, is more invasive and metastatic than basal cell carcinoma. Its probable etiology is environmental factors, such as ultraviolet radiation and x-irradiation, as well as a variety of chemical carcinogens, including arsenic. The carcinoma originates in cells of the stratum spinosum and appears clinically as a hyperkeratotic, scaly plaque with a deep invasion of underlying tissues, often accompanied by bleeding. Surgery is the treatment of choice.

Recent investigations indicate that keratinocytes produce immunogenic molecules and are probably active in the immune process. Evidence also shows that these cells are capable of producing several interleukins, colony-stimulating factors, interferons, tumor necrosis factors, as well as platelet- and fibroblast-stimulating growth factors.

Nonkeratinocytes of the Epidermis

There are three types of nonkeratinocytes in the epidermis: melanocytes, Langerhans cells, and Merkel cells (Table 12-2).

Melanocytes

Melanocytes, derived from neural crest cells, are the second most populous cell type in the epidermis. They are interspersed among the keratinocytes of the stratum basale and are also present in hair follicles and the dermis (Figs. 12-4A,B). Although the main cell bodies of the melanocytes reside in the stratum basale, they extend long thin cytoplasmic processes into the extracellular spaces between keratinocytes of the stratum spinosum. Melanocytes are responsible for synthesizing pigments called **melanin**. There are two types of melanin:

Table 12-2	Nonkeratinocytes of the Epidermis			
Nonepithelial Cells	**Origin**	**Location**	**Features**	**Function**
Melanocytes	Derived from neural crest	Migrate into stratum basale during embryonic development; some remain undifferentiated even in adulthood (reserved to maintain melanocyte population). Do not form desmosomal contact with keratinocytes, but some may form hemidesmosomes with basal lamina	Melanocytes extend long processes (dendrites) into the stratum spinosum. Melanosomes containing melanin are manufactured within their cytoplasm and are transferred to the distal ends of the dendrites for melanin donation to the associated keratinocytes (epidermal–melanin unit). Melanocytes comprise ~3% of the epidermal cell population in all individuals regardless of skin color.	Melanocytes manufacture melanin pigment. Melanosomes located in the cytoplasm are activated to produce melanin (eumelanin in dark hair and pheomelanin in red and blond hair). Once melanosomes are filled with melanin, they travel up the dendrites and are released into the extracellular space. Keratinocytes of the strata basale and spinosum phagocytose these melanin-laden melanosomes. The melanosomes migrate to the supranuclear region of the keratinocyte and form a protective umbrella, shielding the nucleus (and its chromosomes) from the ultraviolet rays of the sun. Soon the melanosomes are destroyed by keratinocyte lysosomes. UV rays increase melanin production, its darkening, and its endocytosis. Light-skinned individuals produce fewer melanosomes, which congregate around the nucleus, whereas in dark-skinned individuals, melanosomes are produced in larger quantity and size, and are dispersed throughout the cytoplasm. Melanosome destruction is also slower in darker skin.
Langerhans cells	Derived from bone marrow	Mostly located in the stratum spinosum	Because they possess long processes, they are known as dendritic cells. Nucleus possesses many indentations. Cytoplasm contains Birbeck granules, elongated vesicles exhibiting a ballooned-out terminus. They do not form desmosomal contact with keratinocytes.	Langerhans cells are antigen-presenting cells. These cells possess surface markers and receptors as well as langerin, a transmembrane protein associated with Birbeck granules. Some of these elements facilitate an immune response against the organism responsible for leprosy. Additionally, Langerhans cells phagocytose antigens that enter the epidermis and migrate to lymph vessels located in the dermis and from there into the paracortex of a lymph node to present these antigens to T cells, thereby activating a delayed-type hypersensitivity response.
Merkel cells	Probably derived from neural crest	Interspersed with keratinocytes of the stratum basale; they are most abundant in the fingertips	Merkel cells form complexes, known as Merkel disks, with terminals of afferent nerves.	Merkel cells function as mechanoreceptors (touch receptors). There is some evidence that they may also function as neurosecretory cells.

- **eumelanin**, a dark brown-to-black pigment composed of polymers of **hydroxyindole** and

- **pheomelanin**, a red-to-rust-colored compound composed of **cysteinyl dopa** polymers.

The former is present in individuals with dark hair, and the latter is found in individuals with red and blond hair. Both types of melanin are derived from the amino acid **tyrosine**, which is transported into specialized **tyrosinase**-containing vesicles derived from the trans-Golgi network, known as melanosomes. Within these oval (1.0 by 0.5 μm) melanosomes, tyrosinase, through a series of steps, converts tyrosine into **melanin**. Although the activation of tyrosinase is owing to the presence of **UV light** (ultraviolet), the process requires the presence of the protein **microphthalmia-associated transcription factor** whose expression is dependent on the **melanocyte-stimulating hormone**, produced by basophils of the pituitary gland.

Once produced, the **melanosomes** are transported into the distal ends of the melanocyte processes extending into the stratum spinosum. Here, in the process called **melanosome transfer**, either the melanocyte releases its tip filled with melanosomes or the melanocyte tip releases melanosomes into the extracellular space. The keratinocytes endocytose the released materials and store them in the supranuclear region, thereby protecting the nucleus (and its chromosomes) from exposure to ultraviolet rays and subsequent damage. Within a few days, lysosomes of the prickle cells attack and destroy the transferred melanosomes. Ultraviolet rays not only increase the rates of darkening of melanin and endocytosis

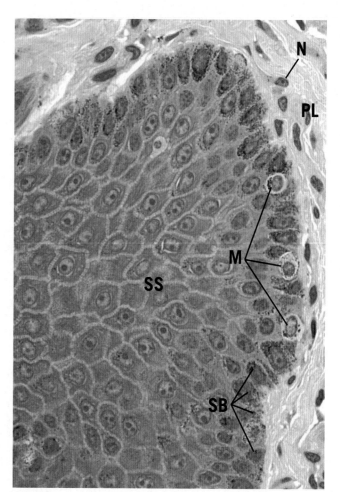

FIGURE 12-4B. Thick skin. Monkey. Plastic section. ×540.

The basal compartment of the epidermis is highlighted in this photomicrograph, along with the interface between the dermis and the **stratum basale** (SB). Observe that in stratum basale, keratinocytes are cuboidal to columnar, and contain numerous brown melanosomes in their cytoplasm. Interspersed among the keratinocytes within this layer are occasional cuboidal cells with clear cytoplasm, most of which are **melanocytes** (M). Merkel cells can also appear as clear cells; however, they are not as numerous. Keratinocytes of the **stratum spinosum** (SS) are polyhedral in shape, possessing numerous intercellular bridges, which interdigitate with those of other cells, accounting for their spiny appearance. The **papillary layer** (PL) of the dermis displays **nuclei** (N) of the various connective tissue cells.

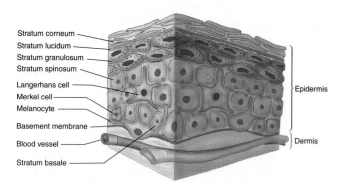

FIGURE 12-4A. The epidermis is composed of histologically distinct layers of keratinocytes (strata basale, spinosum, granulosum, lucidum, and corneum) in the thick skin, and all but the stratum lucidum in the thin skin. Interspersed within the epidermis are three additional cell types, melanocytes, Merkel cells, and Langerhans cells. Note the relative positions and cellular extensions of the melanocytes and of the Langerhans cells.

of melanosomes but also enhance tyrosinase activity and, thus, melanin production.

A group of keratinocytes receiving melanosomes from a single melanocyte is called the **epidermal–melanin unit**. The epidermal–melanin units tend to be smaller (fewer keratinocytes supplied with melanosomes by a single melanocyte) around the genitals and axilla, which

CLINICAL CONSIDERATIONS 12-2

Vitiligo

A condition in which the skin has patches of white areas caused by the lack of pigmentation is known as **vitiligo**. The melanocytes of the affected region are destroyed in an autoimmune response. The condition may appear suddenly after a physical injury or as a consequence of sunburn. If the area affected has hair, as the hair grows, it will be white. Although there are no physical consequences to vitiligo, there may be psychological sequelae.

Melanoma

Malignant melanoma may be a life-threatening malignancy. It develops in the epidermis where melanocytes become mitotically active and form a dysplastic nevus. It may then enter a **radial growth phase** where individual melanocytes invade the dermis, then enter the **vertical growth phase** where they begin to form tumors in the dermis, and eventually become a full-fledged, **metastatic melanoma** whose cells eventually enter the lymphatic and circulatory system to metastasize to other organ systems.

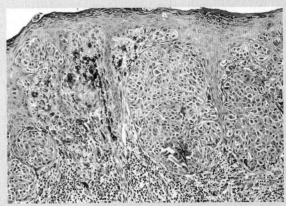

This photomicrograph is of a patient suffering from malignant melanoma. Note that the melanocytes, some still producing melanosomes, are invading the dermis in large numbers, indicating that the melanoma is in the vertical growth phase. (Reprinted with permission from Mills SE, et al., eds. *Sternberg's Diagnostic Surgical Pathology*, 6th ed. Philadelphia: Wolters Kluwer, 2015. p. 102, Figure 3-34.)

accounts for relatively darker pigmentation of these areas in most individuals. However, the skin color differences among different races result from the amount of melanin synthesis and melanosome distribution within keratinocytes rather than the total number of melanocytes or the size of the epidermal–melanin unit which is similar in all humans. In dark-skinned individuals, abundant melanosomes are produced and dispersed throughout the keratinocyte cytoplasm, whereas in light-skinned individuals fewer melanosomes are produced and stored around the keratinocyte nucleus.

Langerhans Cells

Langerhans cells (also known as **dendritic cells** because of their long processes), derived from bone marrow and located mostly in the stratum spinosum, function as antigen-presenting cells in immune responses (see Fig. 12-4A). Langerhans cells do not make desmosomal contact with the keratinocytes of the stratum spinosum. They express **CD1a** surface marker and major histocompatibility complex **(MHC) I, MHC II, Fc receptors for IgG, C3b receptors**, and the transmembrane protein **langerin**. Langerin and CD1a facilitate the immune defense against *Mycobacterium leprae*, the microorganism responsible for **leprosy**. Langerhans cells **phagocytose antigens** entering the epidermis, including nonprotein antigens. When they phagocytose an antigen, these cells

migrate into a lymph vessel of the dermis to enter the paracortex of a nearby lymph node. Here, the Langerhans cells present their antigens to T cells to activate a **delayed-type hypersensitivity response**.

Merkel Cells

Merkel cells are interspersed among the keratinocytes of the stratum basale and most abundant in the fingertips (see Fig. 12-4A). Afferent nerve terminals approximate these cells, forming **Merkel cell–neurite complexes** that are believed to function as **mechanoreceptors** (touch receptors). There is some evidence that Merkel cells originate from the neural crest and may have a neurosecretory function.

Thin skin differs from thick skin in that it has only three or four strata. Stratum lucidum is always absent in thin skin, whereas strata corneum, granulosum, and spinosum are greatly reduced in size. In fact, frequently only an incomplete layer of stratum granulosum is present.

Dermis

The **dermis** of the skin, deep to the epidermis, is derived from the mesoderm. It is composed of two types of connective tissues that form two ill-defined sublayers of the dermis:

- The **papillary layer** is a thin superficial region of the dermis that forms the primary and secondary dermal papillae or ridges that interdigitate with the epidermal ridges (and interpapillary pegs) of the epidermis. This layer is composed of loose connective tissue, rich with capillary network and immune cells that provide nutrient and host-defense support to the avascular epidermis.

- The **reticular layer** is a much thicker and deeper layer of the dermis composed of dense irregular connective tissue, rich with type I collagen fibers and elastic fibers that provide strength and elasticity to the skin and also assist in securing the skin to the underlying **hypodermis (superficial fascia)**.

Sensory Structures in the Dermis

In addition to the Merkel cells in the epidermis, there are several sensory structures in the dermis responsible for detecting variable forms and strengths of stimuli applied to the skin:

- **Meissner's corpuscles** reside in the **dermal ridges** (as well as secondary dermal ridges) of the papillary dermis and display encapsulated nerve endings (Fig. 12-5). Meissner's corpuscles detect fine touch and low-frequency vibrations.

- **Ruffini's corpuscles** reside in the superficial aspect of the reticular dermis and detect pressure and low vibrations and continue to register sustained change, such as stretching, in the skin.

- **Krause's end bulbs** are encapsulated sensory receptors believed to be present in the dermis of limited regions of the body detecting temperature (cold) as well as pressure and vibration.

- **Pacinian corpuscles** reside in the deep aspect of the reticular dermis or even deeper in the hypodermis.

Pacinian corpuscles are quite large, up to 1 mm in diameter, owing to elaborate layers of glial cells and connective tissue surrounding the nerve ending in the center (Fig. 12-6). This design allows for quick detection of pressure and vibration, and adaptation of sensation to prevent the prolonged changes to the skin does not continuously register as a stimulus.

Derivatives of Skin

Derivatives of the skin include hair follicles, sebaceous glands, sweat glands, and nails (Fig. 12-7). These structures develop from the down growth of epidermal cells into the dermis and hypodermis, while maintaining their connection to the epidermis, therefore the outside.

- **Hair follicles** produce **hair**. Each hair is composed of a root contained within a hair follicle and a shaft composed of cornified cells (Figs. 12-8A,B and 12-9; also see Fig. 12-7). The hair follicle is continuous with strata basale and spinosum of the epidermis, which form the external root sheath and the internal root sheath, respectively (see Fig. 12-8A). The deepest end of the hair follicle is dilated into a hair bulb whose invagination houses the highly vascularized dermal papilla. Melanocytes, present in the region of the hair bulb that adjoins the dermal papilla, provide pigments to the growing hair.

- **Sebaceous glands** are simple branched acinar exocrine glands associated with each hair follicle, releasing oily **sebum** into the neck of the hair follicle via holocrine secretion (Fig. 12-10; also see Fig. 12-9).

- **Arrector pili muscle** is a small bundle of smooth muscle cells that attach to the hair follicle and, cradling the sebaceous gland, inserts into the epidermis (see Figs. 12-8A, 12-9, and 12-10). Contraction of the arrector pili muscles raises the hair, and in the process,

CLINICAL CONSIDERATIONS 12-3

Pruritus and Erythema Multiforme

The sensation of **itching (pruritus)** is accompanied by an instinctive, almost irrepressible urge to scratch. There are many different causes of itching, some as simple as a fly walking on one's skin and moving the hair follicles or as serious as debilitating systemic conditions such as kidney failure or liver disease. If the itching is accompanied by a rash, then the probable cause is not the kidney or the liver. Parasitic infestations (mites, scabies, etc.), insect bites, plant toxins (such as poison oak and poison ivy), and drug allergies are usually accompanied by a rash and require medical intervention. If the itching is long term,

the patient should seek the assistance of a physician. Pregnancy and cold, dry weather may also be contributing factors to itching.

Patches of elevated red skin, frequently resembling a target, displaying symmetrical distribution over the face and extremities, that occurs periodically, indicate the disorder **erythema multiforme**. It is most frequently caused by herpes simplex infection. The condition is not usually accompanied by itching, although painful lesions (blisters) on the lips and buccal cavity are common occurrences. Usually, the condition resolves itself, but in more severe cases, medical intervention is indicated.

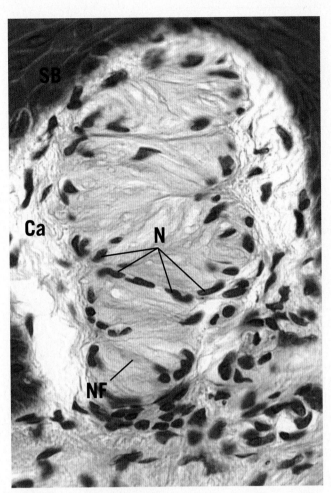

FIGURE 12-5. Meissner's corpuscle. Paraffin section. ×540.

Meissner's corpuscles are oval, encapsulated mechanoreceptors lying in dermal ridges just deep to the **stratum basale** (SB). They are especially prominent in the genital areas, lips, fingertips, and soles of the feet. A connective tissue **capsule** (Ca) envelops the corpuscle. The **nuclei** (N) within the corpuscle belong to flattened (probably modified) Schwann cells, which are arranged horizontally in this structure. The afferent **nerve fiber** (NF) pierces the base of the Meissner's corpuscle, branches, and follows a tortuous course within the corpuscle.

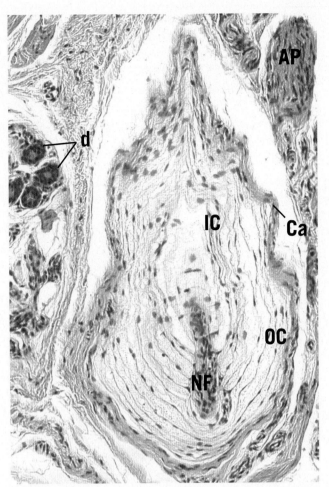

FIGURE 12-6. Pacinian corpuscle. Paraffin section. ×132.

Pacinian corpuscles, located in the dermis and hypodermis, are mechanoreceptors. They have an **inner core** (IC) and an **outer core** (OC) as well as a surrounding **capsule** (Ca). The inner core invests the afferent **nerve fiber** (NF), which loses its myelin sheath soon after entering the corpuscle. The core cells are modified Schwann cells, whereas the components of the capsule are continuous with the endoneurium of the afferent nerve fiber. Pacinian corpuscles are readily recognizable in the section because they resemble the cut surface of an onion. Observe the presence of an **arrector pili muscle** (AP) and profiles of **ducts** (d) of a sweat gland in the vicinity of, but not associated with, the Pacinian corpuscle.

also creates small dimples and raised areas in the skin, commonly known as goosebumps. Because **thick skin** is devoid of hair follicles and hair, it is also called **glabrous skin**, whereas **thin skin** has hair follicles.

- **Eccrine sweat glands** do not develop in association with hair follicles. These are simple, coiled, tubular exocrine glands whose secretory units produce sweat, which is delivered to the surface of the skin by long ducts (Fig. 12-11; also see Fig. 12-9).

  - **Myoepithelial cells** surround the secretory portion of these glands.

- **Apocrine sweat glands** are also simple, coiled tubular exocrine glands, but these are much larger than

eccrine sweat glands, and they are associated with and drain into hair follicles of the axilla (armpit), areola of the mammary gland, and of the anus and genitals. Apocrine sweat glands become active at puberty and secrete viscous fluids which epidermal microbiome metabolize and produce distinct odor.

- **Nails** are cornified structures on the distal phalanx of each finger or toe. The nail is composed of the broad nail plate and the tapered nail root embedded within the distal phalanx (Figs. 12-12A,B; also see Fig. 12-7).

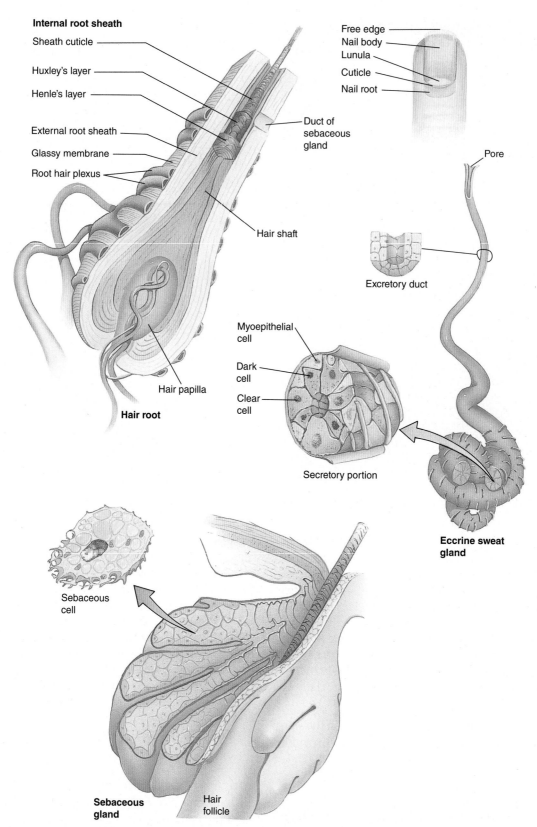

FIGURE 12-7. Derivatives of the skin. Secretory components of **eccrine sweat glands** consist of simple cuboidal epithelium composed of **dark cells**, **clear cells**, and **myoepithelial cells**. The **ducts** of these glands are composed of a stratified cuboidal (two layers of cuboidal cells) epithelium. **Sebaceous glands** are branched acinar holocrine glands whose short ducts empty into a hair follicle into the space created by the disappearance of the internal root sheath.

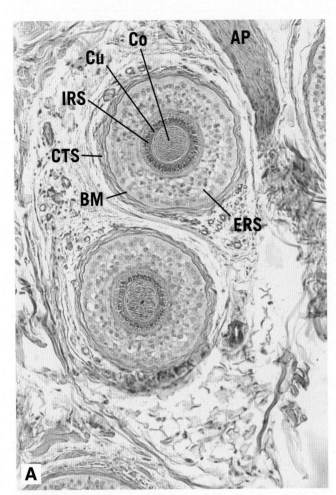

A

FIGURE 12-8A. Hair follicle. x.s. Human. Paraffin section. ×132.

Many of the layers comprising the growing hair follicle may be observed in these cross sections. The entire structure is surrounded by a **connective tissue sheath** (CTS), which is separated from the epithelial-derived components by a specialized **basement membrane** (BM), the inner glassy membrane. The clear polyhedral cells compose the **external root sheath** (ERS), which surrounds the **internal root sheath** (IRS), whose cells become keratinized. At the neck of the hair follicle, where the ducts of the sebaceous glands enter, the internal root sheath disintegrates, providing a lumen into which sebum and apocrine sweat are discharged. The **cuticle** (Cu) and **cortex** (Co) constitute the highly keratinized components of the hair, whereas the medulla is not visible at this magnification. Note the presence of **arrector pili muscle** (AP).

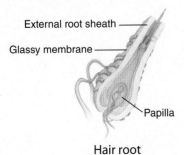

External root sheath

Glassy membrane

Papilla

Hair root

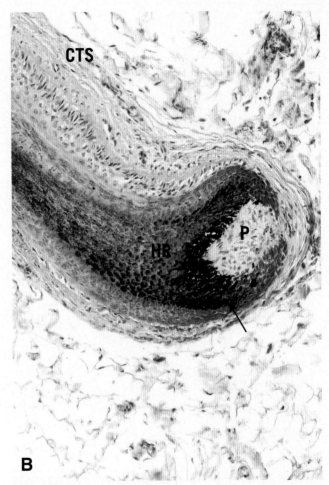

B

FIGURE 12-8B. Hair follicle. l.s. Human. Paraffin section. ×132.

The terminal expansion of the hair follicle, known as the bulb, is composed of a connective tissue, **papilla** (P), enveloped by epithelium-derived cells of the **hair root** (HR). The mitotic activity responsible for the growth of hair occurs in the matrix, from which several concentric sheaths of epithelial cells emerge to be surrounded by a **connective tissue sheath** (CTS). The color of hair is owing to the intracellular pigment that accounts for the dark appearance of some cells (*arrow*).

These horny plates lie on a nail bed and are bounded laterally by nail walls.

- The **nail matrix**, situated deep to the nail root, is equivalent to the strata basale and spinosum of epidermis and continues to supply cornified cells at the nail root, thus allowing the nail to grow (see Figs. 12-12A,B).
- **Nail bed** lies deep to the nail plate and attaches the nail plate to the underlying connective tissue (see Figs. 12-12A,B).
- **Cuticle** (**eponychium**) is equivalent to the stratum corneum of the epidermis and lies over the **lunula**, an opaque, crescent-shaped area of the nail plate (see Fig. 12-12A).

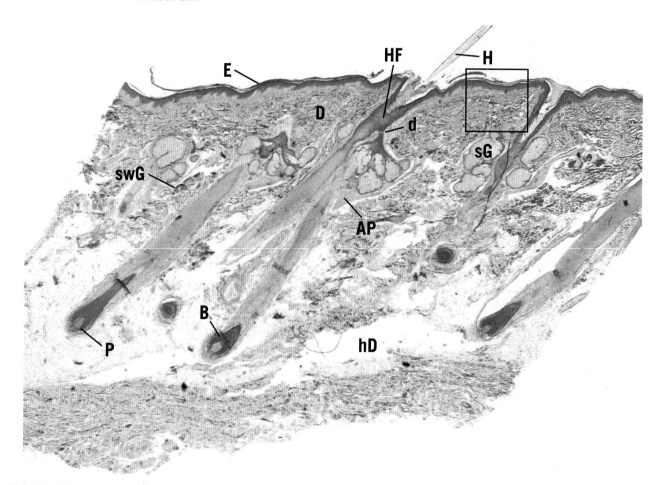

FIGURE 12-9. Thin skin. Human. Paraffin section. ×19.

Thin skin is composed of a very slender layer of **epidermis** (E) and the underlying **dermis** (D). Although thick skin has no hair follicles and sebaceous glands associated with it, most thin skin is richly endowed with both. Observe the **hair** (H) and the **hair follicles** (HF), whose expanded **bulb** (B) presents the connective tissue **papilla** (P). Much of the follicle is embedded beneath the skin in the superficial fascia, the fatty connective tissue layer known as the **hypodermis** (hD), which is not a part of the integument. **Sebaceous glands** (sG) secrete their sebum into short **ducts** (d), which empty into the lumen of the hair follicle. Smooth muscle bundles, **arrector pili muscle** (AP), cradle these glands, in passing from the hair follicle to the papillary layer of the dermis. **Sweat glands** (swG) are also present in the reticular layer of the dermis.

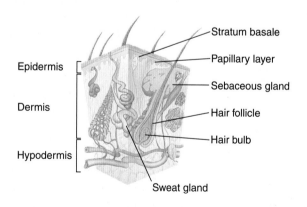

- The **hyponychium** is also equivalent to the stratum corneum of the epidermis and is located beneath the free edge of the nail plate (see Fig. 12-12B).

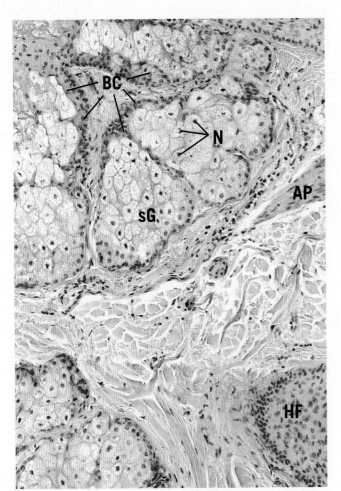

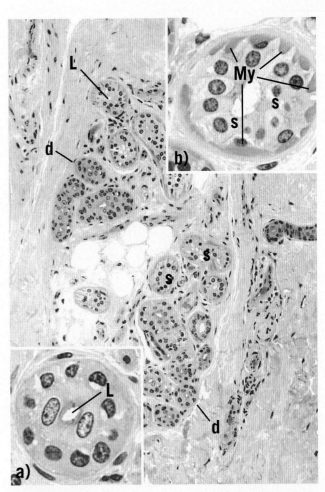

FIGURE 12-10. Sebaceous gland. Human. Paraffin section. ×132.

FIGURE 12-11. Eccrine sweat gland. Monkey. Plastic section. ×132.

Sebaceous glands (sG) are branched, acinar holocrine glands, which produce oily sebum. The secretion of these glands is delivered into the lumen of a **hair follicle** (HF), with which sebaceous glands are associated. **Basal cells** (BC), located at the periphery of the gland, undergo mitotic activity to replenish the dead cells, which, in holocrine glands, become the secretory product. Note that as these cells accumulate sebum in their cytoplasm, they degenerate, as evidenced by the gradual pyknosis of their **nuclei** (N). Observe the **arrector pili muscle** (AP), which cradles the sebaceous glands.

The simple, coiled, tubular exocrine gland is divided into two compartments: a **secretory portion** (s) and a **duct** (d). The secretory portion of the gland consists of a simple cuboidal epithelium, composed of larger and clear staining secretory cells. Intercellular canaliculi are noted between clear cells, which are smaller than the **lumen** (L) of the gland. **Ducts** (d) may be recognized by the darker staining stratified cuboidal epithelium owing to smaller and darker staining cells. *Insets a and b*. **Duct and secretory unit**. **Monkey**. **Plastic section**. ×540. The duct is recognized by the **lumen** (L) surrounded by two layers of small and darker staining cuboidal cells. **Secretory cells** (s) of the eccrine sweat gland are surrounded by darker staining **myoepithelial cells** (My).

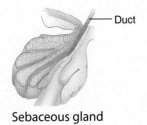

Sebaceous gland

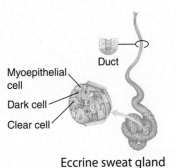

Eccrine sweat gland

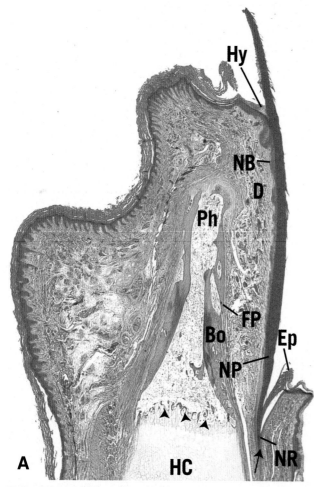

FIGURE 12-12A. Fingernail. l.s. Paraffin section. ×14.

The nail is a highly keratinized structure that is located on the dorsal surface of the distal **phalanx** (Ph) of each finger and toe. The horny **nail plate** (NP) extends deep into the dermis, forming the **nail root** (NR). The epidermis of the distal phalanx forms a continuous fold, resulting in the **eponychium** (Ep), or cuticle, the **nail bed** (NB) underlying the nail plate, and the **hyponychium** (Hy). The epithelium (*arrow*) surrounding the nail root is the nail matrix responsible for the continuous elongation of the nail. The **dermis** (D) between the nail bed and the **bone** (Bo) of the distal phalanx is tightly secured to the **fibrous periosteum** (FP). Note that this is a developing finger, as evidenced by the presence of **hyaline cartilage** (HC) and endochondral osteogenesis (*arrowheads*).

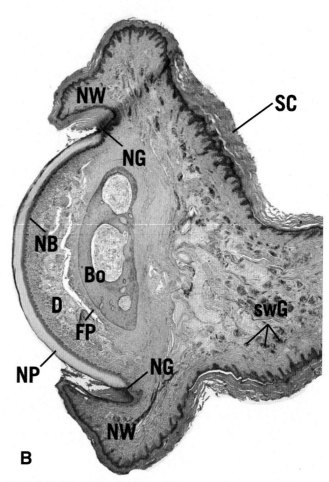

FIGURE 12-12B. Fingernail. x.s. Paraffin section. ×14.

The **nail plate** (NP) in this cross section presents a convex appearance. On either side, it is bordered by a **nail wall** (NW), and the groove it occupies is referred to as the lateral **nail groove** (NG). The **nail bed** (NB) is analogous to four layers of the epidermis, whereas the nail plate represents the stratum corneum. The **dermis** (D), deep to the nail bed, is firmly attached to the **fibrous periosteum** (FP) of the **bone** (Bo) of the terminal phalanx. Observe that the fingertip is covered by thick skin whose **stratum corneum** (SC) is extremely well developed. The small, darkly staining structures in the dermis are **sweat glands** (swG).

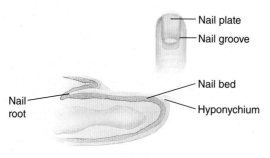

Fingernail

Selected Review of Histologic Images

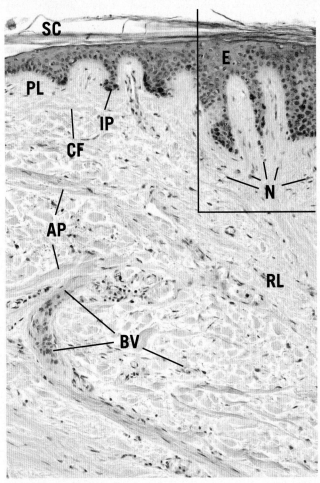

REVIEW FIGURE 12-1-1. Thin skin. Human. Paraffin section. ×132.

Observe that the **epidermis** (E) is much thinner than that of thick skin and that the **stratum corneum** (SC) is significantly reduced. The epidermal ridges and **interpapillary pegs** (IP) are well represented in this photomicrograph. Note that the **papillary layer** (PL) of the dermis is composed of much finer bundles of **collagen fibers** (CF) than those of the dense irregular connective tissue of the **reticular layer** (RL). The dermis is quite vascular, as evidenced by the large number of **blood vessels** (BV) whose cross-sectional profiles are readily observed. The numerous **nuclei** (N) of the various connective tissue cells attest to the cellularity of the dermis. Note also the presence of the **arrector pili muscle** (AP), whose contraction elevates the hair and is responsible for the appearance of "goosebumps."

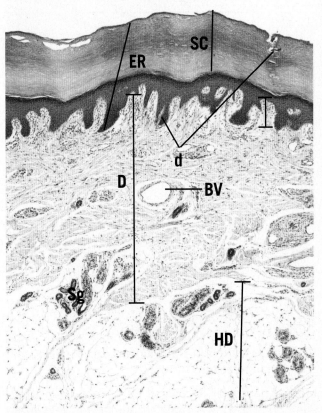

REVIEW FIGURE 12-1-2. Thick skin. Human. Paraffin section. ×56.

This low-magnification photomicrograph of the skin of the human palm displays a much thicker epidermis with clearly visible **stratum corneum** (SC) even at this magnification. The **ducts** (d) of the sweat glands as they penetrate the epidermis are also readily observed. Observe the interdigitating **epidermal ridges** (ER) and the **dermis** (D) and the **deep hypodermis** (HD). The dermis is quite **vascular** (BV), but the epidermis is always avascular. **Sweat glands** (Sg) span both the dermis and the hypodermis.

KEY					
AP	arrector pili muscle	**E**	epidermis	**PL**	papillary layer
BV	blood vessels	**ER**	epidermal ridges	**RL**	reticular layer
CF	collagen fibers	**HD**	deep hypodermis	**SC**	stratum corneum
d	ducts	**IP**	interpapillary pegs	**Sg**	sweat glands
D	dermis	**N**	nuclei		

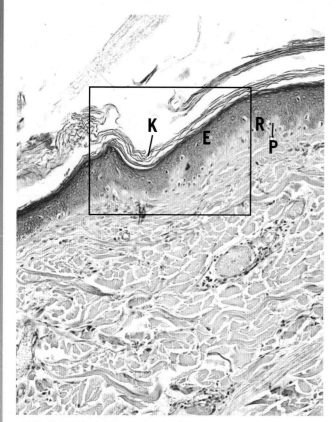

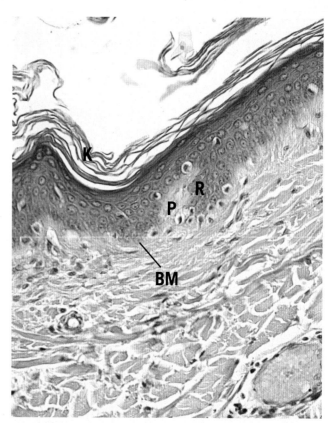

REVIEW FIGURE 12-1-3. Human glabrous skin (thin skin). Paraffin section. ×132.

REVIEW FIGURE 12-1-4. Human glabrous skin (thin skin). Paraffin section. ×270.

Most of the body is covered by glabrous skin (hairy skin), composed of a stratified, squamous, keratinized epithelium and an underlying connective tissue component known as the dermis. Note that the **keratin layer** (K) of the **epithelium** (E) of glabrous skin is relatively thin when compared to the thick skin of the palm of the hand and the sole of the foot. The rete apparatus, composed of **epithelial ridges** (R) and **dermal ridges** (P), is well developed but not as extensive as that of thick skin. The *boxed area* appears at higher magnification in Review Figure 12-1-4.

This higher magnification of the boxed area of the glabrous skin of the previous photomicrograph displays the **keratin** (K) sloughing off the free surface of the stratified squamous keratinized epithelium. Note that a **basement membrane** (BM) separates the epidermis from the dermis. Also observe the rete apparatus as evident from the presence of **epithelial ridges** (R) that interdigitate with **dermal ridges** (P) of the dermis.

KEY					
BM	basement membrane	**K**	keratin layer	**R**	epithelial ridges
E	epithelium	**P**	dermal ridges		

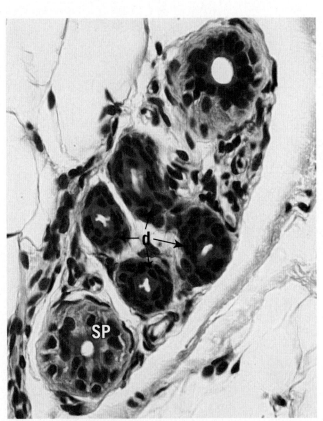

REVIEW FIGURE 12-1-5. Eccrine sweat gland. Human glabrous skin (thin skin). Paraffin section. ×540.

Eccrine sweat glands are simple coiled tubular exocrine glands, producing a watery solution. The **secretory portion** (SP) of the gland is composed of a simple cuboidal epithelium with two cell types, a lightly staining cell that makes up most of the secretory portion and a darker staining cell that usually cannot be distinguished with the light microscope. Surrounding the secretory portion are myoepithelial cells, which, with their numerous branching processes, encircle the secretory tubule and assist in expressing the fluid into the ducts. The **ducts** (d) are composed of a stratified cuboidal epithelium, whose cells are smaller than those of the secretory unit. In histologic sections, therefore, the ducts are darker than the secretory units.

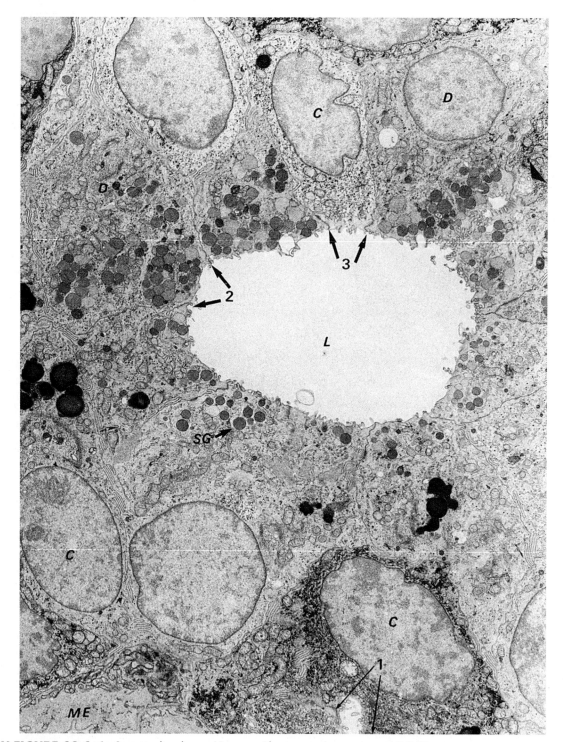

REVIEW FIGURE 12-1-6. Sweat gland. x.s. Human. Electron microscopy. ×5,040.

Tight junctions (*arrows*) occur at three locations in the secretory coil of human sweat glands: (1) between **clear cells** (C) separating the lumen of the intercellular canaliculus (*arrowhead*) and the basolateral intercellular space; (2) between two **dark cells** (D) separating the main lumen and the lateral intercellular space; and (3) between a clear cell and a dark cell, separating the main **lumen** (L) and intercellular space. Note the presence of **secretory granules** (SG) and **myoepithelial cell** (ME). (From Briggman JV, et al. Structure of the tight junctions of the human eccrine sweat gland. *Am J Anat* 1981;162(4):357–368. Copyright © 1981 Wiley-Liss, Inc. Reprinted by permission of John Wiley & Sons, Inc.)

KEY					
C	clear cells	**L**	lumen	**SG**	secretory granules
d	ducts	**ME**	myoepithelial cell	**Sp**	secretory portion
D	dark cells				

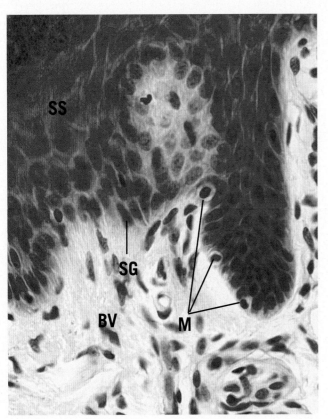

REVIEW FIGURE 12-1-7. Thick skin. Human. Paraffin section. ×270.

The interface between the epidermis and the dermis presents the **stratum spinosum** (SS) and stratum basale also known as **stratum germinativum** (SG) of the epidermis. Observe the rich **vascular supply** (BV), mostly capillaries of the papillary region of the dermis and the numerous **melanocytes** (M) located in the stratum basale.

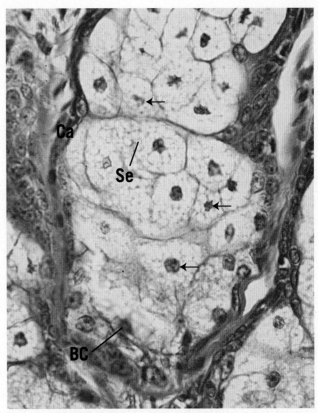

REVIEW FIGURE 12-1-8. Sebaceous gland. Human glabrous skin (thin skin). Paraffin section. ×540.

This photomicrograph is a high magnification of a sebaceous gland displaying the regenerative **basal cells** (BC) that are responsible for the maintenance of the gland by providing new cells that replace the sebum-forming cells of the gland lie pressed against the **capsule** (Ca) of the gland. **Sebum** (Se) collects in vesicles that fuse as the cell degenerates, and the entire dead cell is expressed as the secretory product of this holocrine gland. Observe that as the cell degenerates, its nucleus becomes more and more pyknotic (*arrows*).

KEY					
Ca	capsule	**M**	melanocytes	**SG**	stratum germinativum
BC	basal cells	**Se**	sebum	**SS**	stratum spinosum
BV	vascular supply				

Summary of Histologic Organization

I. Skin

A. Epidermis

The **epidermis** constitutes the superficial, keratinized, stratified squamous epithelium of the skin. It is composed of four cell types: **keratinocytes**, **melanocytes**, **Langerhans cells**, and **Merkel cells**. The keratinocytes are arranged in five layers, and the remaining three cell types are interspersed among them. The five layers of the epidermis are as follows:

1. Stratum Basale

A single layer of cuboidal to columnar cells abutting the **basement membrane**, forming abundant hemidesmosomes. This is a layer of cell division. It also contains **melanocytes** and **Merkel cells**.

2. Stratum Spinosum

Composed of many layers of polyhedral **prickle cells** bearing **intercellular bridges**. Mitotic activity is also present. It also contains **Langerhans cells** and processes of **melanocytes**.

3. Stratum Granulosum

Keratinocytes in this layer are flattened and contain **keratohyalin granules**. Lamellar granules in the intercellular space contribute to the moisture barrier. This layer is attenuated in thin skin.

4. Stratum Lucidum

A thin, translucent layer of flattened, dead keratinocytes containing **eleidin** is observable in thick, but not in thin, skin.

5. Stratum Corneum

Composed of dead keratinocytes called **squames** packed with **keratin** are continuously desquamated at the superficial surface.

B. Dermis

The **dermis** is a **connective tissue** deep to the epidermis and is subdivided into two layers: papillary and reticular.

1. Papillary Layer

Composed of loose connective tissue and forms the **dermal ridges** (dermal papillae) and **secondary dermal ridges** which interdigitate with the **epidermal ridges** (and **interpapillary pegs**) of the epidermis. Dermal ridges house **capillary loops** and **Meissner's corpuscles**.

2. Reticular Layer

The **reticular layer** of skin is composed of dense irregular connective tissue. It supports a **vascular plexus** and interdigitates with the underlying **hypodermis**. Frequently, it houses **hair follicles**, **sebaceous glands**, and **sweat glands**. **Krause's end bulbs** and **Pacinian corpuscles** may also be present.

II. Appendages

A. Hair

Hair is an **epidermal** downgrowth embedded into dermis or hypodermis. It has a free **shaft** surrounded by several layers of cylindrical sheaths of cells. The terminal end of the hair follicle is expanded as the **hair bulb**, consisting of the connective tissue core **dermal papilla** and the **hair root**. The concentric layers of the follicle from the outside to the center are:

1. Connective Tissue Sheath

2. Glassy Membrane

A modified basement membrane.

3. External Root Sheath

Composed of a few layers of polyhedral cells, it is continuous with the epidermis.

4. Internal Root Sheath

Composed of up to three layers of cuboidal cells, which stop at the neck of the follicle, where sebaceous gland ducts open into the hair follicle, forming a **lumen** into which the sebum is delivered.

5. Cuticle of the Hair

Composed of highly keratinized cells that overlap each other.

6. Cortex

The bulk of the hair composed of highly keratinized cells.

7. Medulla

Present only in thick hair and is the thin core of the hair whose cells contain soft keratin.

B. Sebaceous Glands

Sebaceous glands are in the form of **saccules** associated with hair follicles. They are **simple branched acinar glands** that produce and secrete an oily **sebum** via **holocrine** mode. Secretions are delivered into the neck of the hair follicle via short, wide **ducts**. **Basal cells** are regenerative cells of sebaceous glands, located at the periphery of the **saccule**.

C. Arrector Pili Muscle

Arrector pili muscles are bundles of smooth muscle cells extending from the **hair follicle** to the **papillary layer** of the dermis. They cradle the **sebaceous gland**. Contractions of these muscle fibers elevate the hair, forming "goosebumps," release heat, and assist in the delivery of sebum from the gland into its duct.

D. Sweat Glands

1. Sweat Glands

Simple coiled tubular exocrine glands whose **secretory portion** is composed of a simple cuboidal epithelium. **Dark cells** and **light cells** are present with **intercellular canaliculi** between cells. **Myoepithelial cells** surround the secretory portion.

2. Ducts

Are composed of a stratified cuboidal (two-cell-thick) epithelium. Smaller cells with scant cytoplasm comprise the ducts; therefore, ducts stain darker owing to nuclear crowding compared to secretory portion. Ducts pierce the base of the epidermal ridges to deliver sweat to the outside.

E. Nail

The hard **nail plate** sits on the **nail bed**. It is bordered laterally by the **nail wall**, the base of which forms the **lateral nail groove**. The **eponychium** (cuticle) is above the proximal nail plate. The **hyponychium** is located below the free, distal end of the nail plate. The proximal most aspect of the nail plate, embedded in the epidermal fold is the **nail root**, which lies above the **matrix**, the area responsible for the growth of the nail.

Chapter Review Questions

Clinical vignette for questions 12-1–12-3: The parents of a 2-month-old infant complain to the pediatrician that their baby has constant rashes and blisters around the joints and that the baby is always fussy. The pediatrician observes several clear fluid-filled papules concentrated in the folds of the skin and around the diaper line. Microscopic observation of the biopsied papules reveals that the epidermis has separated from the dermis.

12-1. Structural integrity of which of the following may be weakened?

A. Gap junctions

B. Hemidesmosomes

C. Keratohyalin granules

D. Tight junctions

12-2. Which layer of the skin is adversely affected?

A. Hypodermis

B. Reticular dermis

C. Stratum basale

D. Stratum granulosum

E. Stratum corneum

12-3. Which protein is adversely affected?

A. Collagen

B. Fibrillin

C. Integrin

D. Keratin

12-4. Microscopic observation of a metastatic tumor mass biopsied from the liver reveal some of the tumor cells containing numerous brown pigments in the cytoplasm. Immunohistochemistry using an antibody against which protein is likely to stain the tumor cells?

A. Integrin

B. Keratohyalin

C. Tonofilament

D. Tyrosinase

12-5. Which structure of the skin is responsible for sensing heavy pressure or vibration applied to the skin?

A. Merkel cells

B. Meissner's corpuscles

C. Pacinian corpuscle

D. Ruffini's corpuscle

RESPIRATORY SYSTEM

CHAPTER OUTLINE

The respiratory system functions in exchanging carbon dioxide for oxygen, which will then be distributed to all body tissues. The process of **respiration** is a four-part endeavor, only two of which, **breathing (ventilation)** and the exchange of oxygen for carbon dioxide, known as **external respiration**, occur within the respiratory system. The third and fourth components, the **transport of gases** by the bloodstream and the exchange of carbon dioxide for oxygen that occurs at the cellular level, known as **internal respiration**, occur outside the respiratory system. To accomplish the exchange of oxygen for carbon dioxide, that is, external respiration, air must be brought to that portion of the respiratory system where the exchange of gases can occur.

This process of inspiration requires energy, in that it depends on the contraction of the **diaphragm** and elevation of the **ribs**, increasing the size of the **thoracic cavity**. Because the **visceral pleura** adheres to the lungs and is separated from the **parietal pleura** by the pleural cavity, that cavity is also enlarged, reducing the pressure within it. Because the pressure in the enlarged pleural cavities is less than the atmospheric pressure in the lungs, air enters the lungs, and they as well as their **elastic fiber** networks become stretched, and the volume of the pleural cavity is reduced.

The process of expiration does not require energy because it is dependent on **relaxation** of the muscles responsible for inspiration as well as on relaxation of the stretched **elastic fibers** of the expanded lungs, which return to their **resting length**. As the muscles relax, the volume of the thoracic cage decreases, increasing the pressure inside the lung, which exceeds atmospheric pressure. The additional force of the elastic fibers returning to their resting length drives air out of the lungs.

Anatomically and histologically, the respiratory system is subdivided into a **conducting portion**, conduits that transport air between the atmosphere and the sites of gas exchange in the lungs, and a **respiratory portion** in which gas exchange between air and blood occurs. Some of the larger conduits of the conducting portion are extrapulmonary (anatomically positioned external to the lungs) whereas its smaller components are intrapulmonary. The respiratory portions, however, are completely intrapulmonary. The lumina of the larger conduits are supported by bone and/or cartilage to remain patent, and the luminal diameters of most conduits can be modified by the presence of smooth muscle cells along their length.

Conducting Portion of the Respiratory System

The extrapulmonary region of the conducting portion consists of the nasal cavities, pharynx, larynx, trachea, and primary bronchi. The intrapulmonary region consists of a series of branching conduits of decreasing diameter, from intrapulmonary bronchi to the smaller branches called bronchioles to the distal-most terminal bronchioles (Fig. 13-1 and Table 13-1). The lumina of the larger conducting portions, from nasal cavities to the bronchi, are lined by the ciliated pseudostratified columnar epithelium, also known as the **respiratory epithelium**, that is separated from the underlying fibroelastic connective tissue, the lamina propria, by a basement membrane. Additionally, these larger conduits are supported by a skeleton composed of bone and/or cartilage that assists in the maintenance of a patent lumen. The lining epithelia of the bronchioles transition from ciliated simple columnar epithelium to simple cuboidal epithelium with decreasing luminal diameter. Although bronchiolar walls do not possess cartilage, the surrounding fibroelastic connective tissues help support the patency of the lumina. The luminal diameter throughout the conducting portion of the respiratory system is controlled by smooth muscle cells.

Respiratory Epithelium

The respiratory epithelium of the larger conduits of the conducting portion is composed of various cell types, namely, goblet cells, ciliated cells, basal cells, brush cells, serous cells, and diffuse neuroendocrine system (DNES) cells (Figs. 13-2 and 13-3).

- **Goblet cells** constitute about 30% of the epithelial cells. Goblet cells are unicellular exocrine glands that produce **mucinogen**, a mucous substance (heavily glycosylated protein) that is released onto the wet epithelial surface where it becomes hydrated to form **mucin**. Once particular substances in the tracheal lumen are intermixed with mucin, that viscous material becomes known as **mucus**.

- **Ciliated cells** also compose about 30% of the cell population. They are tall, ciliated cells whose cilia sweep the mucus toward the larynx.

- **Basal cells** also constitute approximately 30% of the epithelial cell population. They are regenerative cells that function in replacing the epithelial lining of the trachea.

- **Brush cells** form only 3% of the cell population of the respiratory epithelium. They possess small mucinogen-containing granules in their cytoplasm and long microvilli that reach into the lumen of the trachea. Brush cells may have neurosensory functions, or they may be defunct goblet cells that released their mucinogen.

- **Serous cells** are tall, columnar cells whose cytoplasm houses small vesicles containing a serous secretion whose function is not understood. Serous cells form 3% of the epithelial cell population.

- **DNES cells** constitute 3% to 4% of the epithelial cell population, and they synthesize and store polypeptide hormones in small granules localized in their subnuclear basal cytoplasms. When released into the underlying lamina propria, these hormones may act locally (paracrine hormones) or at a distance (hormones) to regulate respiratory functions. Nerve fibers often contact many of these DNES cells, to form structures, known as **pulmonary neuroepithelial bodies**, that by monitoring local hypoxic conditions can alert the brain's respiratory center to increase respiration.

Extrapulmonary Region

The mucosa of the extrapulmonary region of the conducting portion modifies the inspired air by humidifying, cleansing, and adjusting its temperature. This **mucosa** is composed of

- **pseudostratified ciliated columnar epithelium** (respiratory epithelium) with numerous **goblet cells** and

- an underlying connective tissue sheath of lamina propria that is well endowed with **seromucous glands**.

Nasal Cavity

The nasal cavity is divided into right and left cavities by a thin nasal septum, and each cavity has three curved, shelf-like protrusions from the lateral wall designed to increase the surface area of the nasal cavity and to create turbulence in the inspired air stream. Therefore, mucosa of the nasal cavity is composed of the respiratory epithelium and underlying lamina propria with rich vasculature and seromucous glands, suited for filtration and modulation of the temperature and humidity of the inspired air (Fig. 13-4).

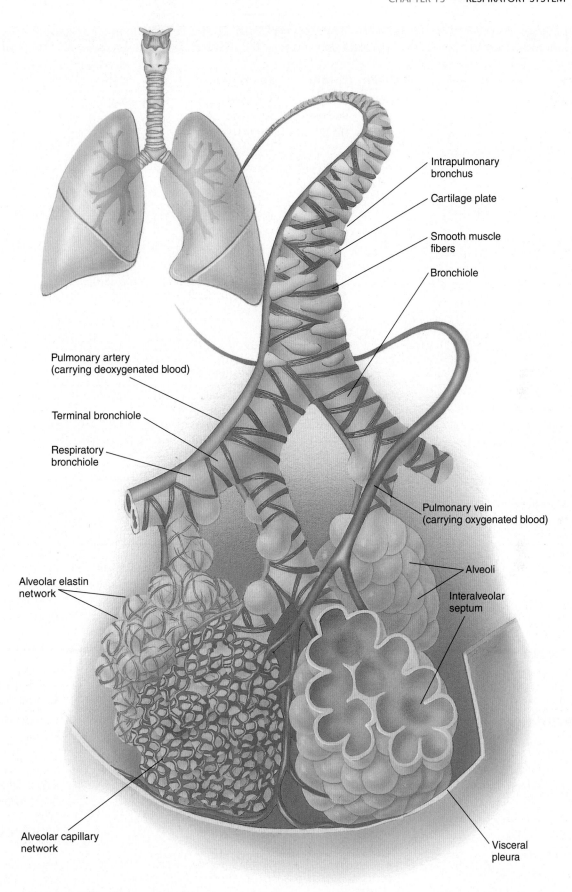

FIGURE 13-1. Respiratory system overview.

Table 13-1 Summary Table of Respiratory System

Division	Region	Skeleton	Glands	Epithelium	Cilia	Goblet Cells	Special Features
Nasal cavity	Vestibule	Hyaline cartilage	Sebaceous and sweat glands	Stratified squamous keratinized and nonkeratinized	No	No	Vibrissae
	Respiratory	Bone and hyaline cartilage	Seromucous	Pseudostratified ciliated columnar	Yes	Yes	Large venous plexus
	Olfactory	Nasal conchae (bone)	Bowman's glands	Pseudostratified ciliated columnar	Yes	No	Basal cells, sustentacular cells, olfactory cells, nerve fibers
Pharynx	Nasal	Muscle	Seromucous glands	Pseudostratified ciliated columnar	Yes	Yes	Pharyngeal tonsil, eustachian tube
	Oral	Muscle	Seromucous glands	Stratified squamous nonkeratinized	No	No	Palatine tonsils
Larynx		Hyaline and elastic cartilage	Mucous and seromucous glands	Stratified squamous nonkeratinized and pseudostratified ciliated columnar	Yes	Yes	Vocal cords, epiglottis, some taste buds
Trachea and extrapulmonary (primary bronchi)		C-rings of hyaline cartilage	Mucous and seromucous glands	Pseudostratified ciliated columnar	Yes	Yes	Trachealis muscle, elastic lamina
Intrapulmonary conducting	Secondary bronchi	Plates of hyaline cartilage	Seromucous glands	Pseudostratified ciliated columnar	Yes	Yes	Two helical-oriented ribbons of smooth muscle
	Bronchioles	Smooth muscle	None	Simple columnar to simple cuboidal	Yes	Only in larger bronchioles	Club cells
	Terminal bronchiole	Smooth muscle	None	Simple cuboidal	Some	None	Less than 0.5 mm in diameter, club cells
Respiratory	Respiratory bronchiole	Some smooth muscle	None	Simple cuboidal and simple squamous	Some	None	Outpocketings of alveoli
	Alveolar duct	None	None	Simple squamous	None	None	Outpocketings of alveoli, type I pneumocytes, type II pneumocytes, dust cells
	Alveolus	None	None	Simple squamous	None	None	Type I pneumocytes, type II pneumocytes, dust cells

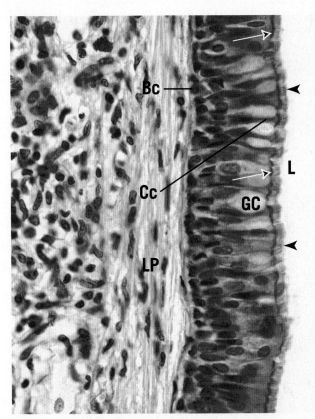

FIGURE 13-2. Respiratory epithelium. Monkey trachea l.s. Paraffin section. ×540.

The cilia (*arrowheads*) of the respiratory epithelium, pseudostratified ciliated columnar epithelium, are evident as they project into the **lumen** (L). Three of the cell types composing this epithelium can be recognized, the short **basal cells** (Bc), the large **goblet cells** (GC) with their expanded theca, and the narrow, tall **ciliated cells** (Cc). Observe the **terminal bars** (*white arrows*) at the apical regions of the tall cells. The **lamina propria** (LP) is separated from the epithelium by the basement membrane.

In the superior aspect of the nasal cavity, the mucosa is modified to function in olfaction and is referred to as the **olfactory mucosa** (Fig. 13-5A,B). Unlike the respiratory mucosa of the rest of the nasal cavity, the ciliated pseudostratified columnar olfactory epithelium is composed mostly of **olfactory cells** that perceive the sensory stimuli and interspersed **supporting cells** and **basal cells**. Supporting cells do not possess any sensory function, but they manufacture a yellowish brown pigment that is responsible for the coloration of the olfactory mucosa; additionally, they insulate and support the olfactory cells. Basal cells are small, dark cells that lie on the basement membrane and, probably, are regenerative in function. The glands in the lamina propria, known as **Bowman's glands**, produce a thin serous secretion that dissolves odoriferous substances. Axons of the olfactory cells are collected into small nerve bundles that pass through

the cribriform plate of the ethmoid bone and form the first cranial nerve, the olfactory nerve. Thus, it should be noted that the cell bodies of the olfactory nerve (cranial nerve I) are located in a rather vulnerable place, in the surface epithelium lining the nasal cavity.

Mechanism of Olfaction

The olfactory cells of the olfactory epithelium are bipolar neurons whose receptor ends are modified **cilia** that extend into the overlying mucus and whose axons go through the cribriform plate at the roof of the nasal cavity to enter the floor of the cranial cavity to synapse with cells of the olfactory bulb.

- **Odorant-binding proteins** (integral membrane proteins that are **odorant receptors**) embedded within the plasma membrane of the cilia are sensitive to molecules of specific odor groups, where each of these molecules is known as an **odorant**.

- When odorants bind to a threshold number of their corresponding odorant receptors, the opening of the ion channels results in **depolarization** of the cell membrane and generation of **action potentials**.

- The action potentials are transmitted to the **olfactory bulbs**, dilated distal ends of the olfactory nerve where approximately 2,000 olfactory cells, each reacting to the same (or similar) odorants, form synapses with a group of interneurons called **mitral cells**.

- A single odorant may bind to a number of olfactory cells that in turn may form synapses with mitral cells. This permits the discernment of various odors that resemble each other (such as the odor of oranges and grapefruits).

- The axons of the mitral cells form the **olfactory tract**, which transmits signals to the amygdala of the brainstem, and from there, the information is delivered to the olfactory cortex. It is now believed that humans have the ability to discern as many as 1 trillion different scents.

Larynx and Trachea

The **larynx**, a region of the conducting portion, is designed for the passage of air into and out of the lower respiratory tract, phonation and to prevent food, liquid, and foreign objects from entering its lumen. It is composed of three paired and three unpaired cartilages, numerous extrinsic and intrinsic muscles, and several ligaments. The actions of these muscles on the cartilages and ligaments modulate the tension and positioning of the vocal folds, thus permitting variations in the pitch of the sound being produced (Fig. 13-6).

The largest two unpaired cartilages of the larynx are composed of the hyaline cartilage which functions in structural support and maintenance of patent lumen.

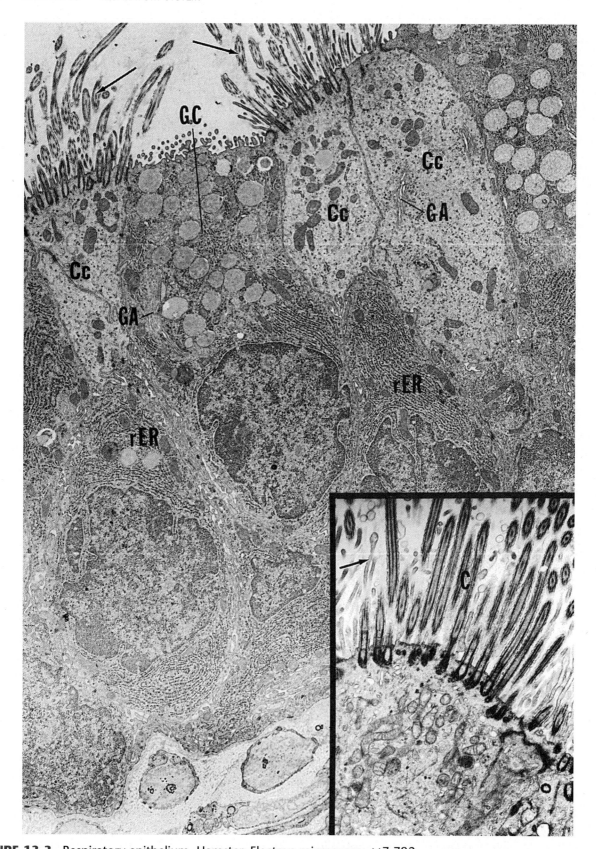

FIGURE 13-3. Respiratory epithelium. Hamster. Electron microscopy. ×7,782.

The tracheal epithelium of the hamster presents mucinogen-producing **goblet cells** (GC) as well as ciliated **columnar cells** (Cc), whose cilia (*arrows*) project into the lumen. Note that both cell types are well endowed with **Golgi apparatus** (GA), whereas goblet cells are particularly rich in **rough endoplasmic reticulum** (rER). (Courtesy of Dr. E. McDowell.) *Inset.* **Bronchus. Human. Electron microscopy.** ×7,782. The apical region of a ciliated epithelial cell presents both **cilia** (C) with apparent axonemes and microvilli (*arrow*). (Courtesy of Dr. E. McDowell.)

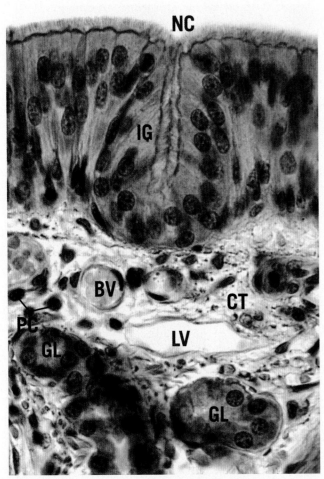

FIGURE 13-4. Nasal Cavity. Human. Paraffin section. ×540.

The epithelium of the nasal cavity occasionally displays small, **intraepithelial glands** (IG). Note that these structures are clearly demarcated from the surrounding epithelium. The secretory product is released into the space that is continuous with the **nasal cavity** (NC). The subepithelial **connective tissue** (CT) of the lamina propria is richly supplied with **blood vessels** (BV) and **lymph vessels** (LV). Observe the **plasma cells** (PC), characteristic of the subepithelial connective tissue of the respiratory system, which also displays the presence of **glands** (GL).

The third unpaired cartilage, the **epiglottis**, however, has an elastic cartilage core and functions as a regulatory flap that folds over the laryngeal inlet to prevent food or liquid from entering the respiratory tract (Fig. 13-7). The lingual aspect and the tip of the epiglottis exposed to the pharyngeal space are lined by the nonkeratinized stratified squamous epithelium. The laryngeal aspect of the epiglottis that does not frequently contact food or liquid is lined by the respiratory epithelium. Respiratory epithelium lines the rest of the luminal mucosa in the larynx except for the **vocal folds**, where nonkeratinized stratified squamous epithelium once again protects these

structures against the frequent vibration required in vocalization (see Fig. 13-6).

The trachea is a long, flexible tube supported by 15 to 20 horseshoe-shaped **hyaline cartilage**, called **C-rings** along its length, whose open ends, bridged by smooth muscle fibers (trachealis muscle), face toward the back of the body (Figs. 13-8A,B). The rigidity of the C-rings ensures the trachea can withstand pressure changes and remain patent during inhalation and exhalation, and the incompleteness of the C-rings accommodates boluses to pass down the esophagus. The **perichondria** of succeeding C-rings are connected to each other, thereby permitting the ability of the trachea to stretch during inhalation.

The tracheal wall is composed of the respiratory epithelium and loose connective tissue of the lamina propria, the dense connective tissue of the submucosa layer which also contains seromucous glands and blends with the perichondrium of the C-ring, and the adventitia that adheres to that of the esophagus posteriorly (Fig. 13-9). The distal end of the trachea branches into the two primary bronchi that lead to the right and the left lungs.

Intrapulmonary Region

The intrapulmonary region of the conducting respiratory portion is composed of branches of the primary bronchi which travel within the lung parenchyma (Figs. 13-10 and 13-11). These **intrapulmonary bronchi** include distal ends of the right and left primary bronchi each of which branches into secondary bronchi. Each secondary bronchus leads into each lung lobe and further branches into tertiary bronchi, which conduct air into the bronchopulmonary segments. The intrapulmonary bronchial walls are supported by irregular plates of hyaline cartilage which progressively become smaller as the bronchi continue to branch into smaller and distal divisions. Respiratory epithelium continues to line the lumen of the intrapulmonary bronchi. The lamina propria between the epithelium and the cartilage layers contains seromucous glands and mucosa-associated lymphoid follicles which are also called bronchus-associated lymphoid tissue (BALT).

Each distal intrapulmonary bronchus gives rise to several **bronchioles**, tubes of decreasing diameters and wall thickness that do not possess a cartilaginous supporting skeleton. The lining epithelium of the bronchioles transition from a ciliated simple columnar epithelium with a few interspersed goblet cells in the larger bronchioles to a simple cuboidal epithelium in the smaller bronchioles (Fig. 13-12). As the lining epithelium transitions to a thinner type, the goblet cells are replaced by **club cells** (formerly known as **Clara cells**). These club cells manufacture **club cell secretory protein** believed to protect the epithelial lining as well as a **surfactant-like substance**

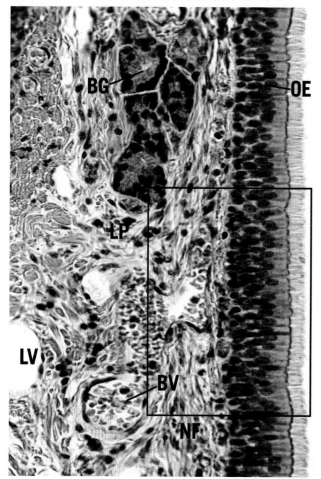

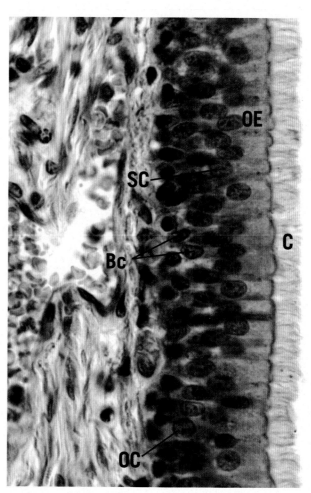

FIGURE 13-5A. Olfactory mucosa. Human. Paraffin section. ×270.

FIGURE 13-5B. Olfactory epithelium. Human. Paraffin section. ×540.

The olfactory mucosa of the nasal cavity is composed of a thick **olfactory epithelium** (OE) and a **lamina propria** (LP) richly endowed with **blood vessels** (BV), **lymph vessels** (LV), and **nerve fibers** (NF) frequently collected into bundles. The lamina propria also contains **Bowman's glands** (BG), which produce a watery secretion that is delivered onto the ciliated surface by short ducts. The *boxed area* is presented at higher magnification in Figure 13-5B.

This is a higher magnification of the *boxed area* of Figure 13-5. The **epithelium** (OE) is pseudostratified ciliated columnar, whose **cilia** (C) are particularly evident. Although hematoxylin and eosin–stained tissue does not permit clear identification of the various cell types, the positions of the nuclei facilitate tentative identification. **Basal cells** (Bc) are short, and their nuclei are near the basement membrane. **Olfactory cell** (OC) nuclei are centrally located, whereas nuclei of **supporting cells** (SC) are positioned near the apex of the cell.

that helps prevent these flimsy conduits from collapsing by reducing surface tension. The distal-most region of the conducting portion of the respiratory system is composed of **terminal bronchioles** whose mucosa is further decreased in thickness and complexity (Fig. 13-13).

The patency of the bronchiolar airways whose walls do not possess cartilaginous support is maintained by elastic fibers that radiate from their periphery and intermingle with elastic fibers emanating from nearby structures. During inspiration, these elastic fibers become stretched, thereby keeping open the bronchiolar lumina.

Respiratory Portion of the Respiratory System

The respiratory portion of the respiratory system begins with **respiratory bronchioles** that branch from the terminal bronchiole (Figs. 13-14 through 13-16; also see Table 13-1). Respiratory bronchioles are histologically similar to terminal bronchioles except for the alveoli, the thin-walled outpocketings, which protrude out of the respiratory bronchiolar wall and permit gaseous exchange.

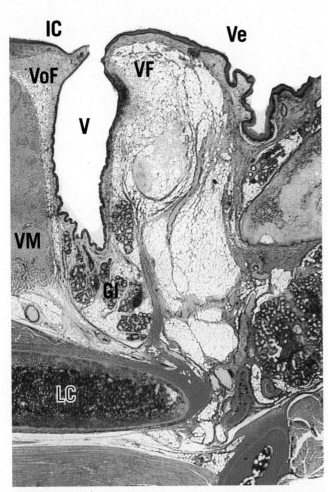

FIGURE 13-6. Larynx. l.s. Human. Paraffin section. ×14.

The right half of the larynx, at the level of the **ventricle** (V), is presented in this survey photomicrograph. The ventricle is bounded superiorly by the **ventricular folds** (false vocal cords) (VF) and inferiorly by the **vocal folds** (VoF). The space above the ventricular fold is the beginning of the **vestibule** (Ve) and that below the vocal fold is the beginning of the **infraglottic cavity** (IC). The **vocalis muscle** (VM) regulates the vocal ligament present in the vocal fold. Acini of mucous and seromucous **glands** (Gl) are scattered throughout the connective tissue of the lamina propria. The **laryngeal cartilages** (LC) are also shown to advantage.

Respiratory bronchioles lead to alveolar ducts, each of which ends in an expanded region, known as an **atrium**, that leads to several **alveolar sacs**, with each alveolar sac being composed of a number of alveoli (see Figs. 13-14 through 13-16). The epithelium of alveolar sacs and alveoli is composed of two types of cells:

- highly attenuated **type I pneumocytes**, which form much of the lining of the alveolus and alveolar sac, and

- **type II pneumocytes**, cells that manufacture **surfactant**, a phospholipid compound that forms a film

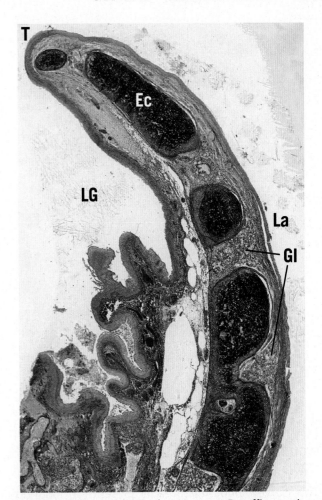

FIGURE 13-7. Epiglottis. l.s. Human. Paraffin section. ×8.

The sagittal section of the epiglottis reveals an **elastic cartilage** (Ec) core responsible for the maintenance of the leaf-like shape that can fold over the laryngeal inlet during swallowing. The **lingual** (LG) side and the **tip** (T) of the epiglottis are covered by the nonkeratinized stratified squamous epithelium, whereas the **laryngeal aspect** (La) is covered with respiratory epithelium. Numerous seromucous **glands** (Gl), particularly more on the laryngeal aspect, are also evident in the lamina propria.

over the watery fluid coating the type I pneumocytes to reduce surface tension.

Associated with the respiratory portion of the lungs is an extremely rich capillary network, supplied by the pulmonary and bronchial arteries and drained by the pulmonary veins (see Fig. 13-14).

- The capillaries invest each alveolus, and their highly attenuated continuous endothelial cells closely approximate the type I pneumocytes.

- In fact, in many areas, the basal laminae of the type I pneumocytes and endothelial cells fuse into a single

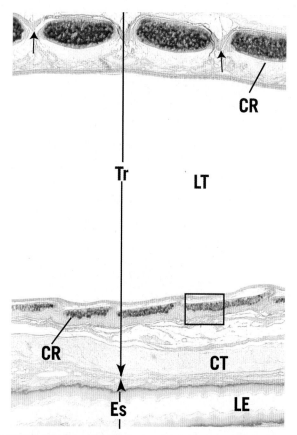

FIGURE 13-8A. Trachea. l.s. Monkey. Paraffin section. ×20.

This survey photomicrograph presents a longitudinal section of the **trachea** (Tr) and **esophagus** (Es). Observe that the **lumen** (LT) of the trachea is patent because of the presence of discontinuous cartilaginous **C-rings** (CR) in its wall. The C-rings of the trachea are thicker anteriorly than posteriorly and are separated from each other by thick, fibrous connective tissue (*arrows*) that is continuous with the perichondrium of the C-rings. The adventitia of the trachea adheres to the esophagus via a loose type of **connective tissue** (CT), which frequently contains adipose tissue. Note that the **lumen** (LE) of the esophagus is normally collapsed. A region similar to the *boxed area* is presented at higher magnification in Figure 13-10. *Inset.* **Trachea.** This illustration demonstrates the trachea extending from the larynx down to its branching point. The regularly spaced C-rings along the length provide allow the trachea to be flexible while maintaining the lumen patent. The openings of the C-rings allow for the expansion of the adjacent esophagus during the passage of the bolus.

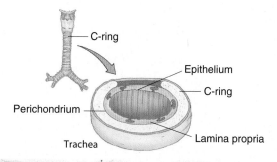

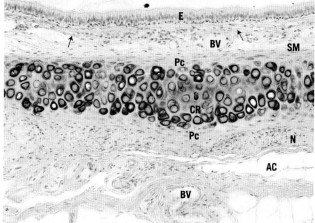

FIGURE 13-8B. Trachea. l.s. Monkey. Paraffin section. ×200.

This photomicrograph is a higher magnification of a region similar to the *boxed area* of Figure 13-8A. The respiratory, ciliated pseudostratified columnar **epithelium** (E) lies on a basement membrane that separates it from the underlying lamina propria. The outer extent of the lamina propria is demarcated by an elastic lamina (*arrows*), deep to which is the **submucosa** (SM), containing a rich **vascular supply** (BV). The **C-ring** (CR), with its attendant **perichondrium** (Pc), constitutes the most substantive layer of the tracheal wall. The adventitia of the trachea, which some consider to include the C-ring, is composed of a loose type of connective tissue, housing some **adipose cells** (AC), **nerves** (N), and **blood vessels** (BV). Collagen fiber bundles of the adventitia secure the trachea to the surrounding structures.

Because each lung contains about 300 million alveoli with a total surface area of approximately 70 m², these small spaces that crowd against each other are separated from one another by walls of various thicknesses known as **interalveolar septa** (Fig. 13-18).

- The thinnest of these portions are comprised of type I pneumocyte of one alveolus and that of the neighboring alveolus, and the extremely thin intervening connective tissue which houses a rich capillary network.

- The thinnest portions often present communicating **alveolar pores (of Kohn)**, whereby air may pass between alveoli.

basal lamina, providing for a minimal blood–air barrier, thus facilitating the exchange of gases. Therefore, the **blood–air barrier** is composed of the attenuated endothelial cell of the capillary, the two combined basal laminae, the attenuated type I pneumocyte, and the surfactant and fluid coating of the alveolus (Fig. 13-17 and Table 13-2).

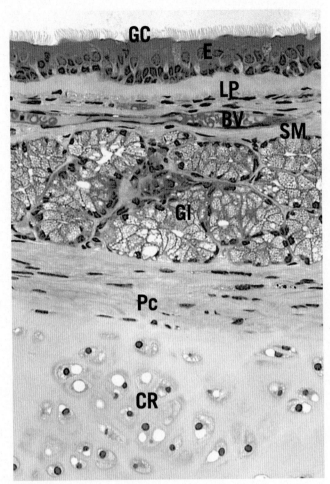

FIGURE 13-9. Trachea. l.s. Monkey. Plastic section. ×270.

The trachea is lined by a pseudostratified ciliated columnar **epithelium** (E), which houses numerous **goblet cells** (GC) that actively secrete a mucous substance. The **lamina propria** (LP) is relatively thin, whereas the **submucosa** (SM) is thick and contains mucous and seromucous **glands** (GI), whose secretory product is delivered to the epithelial surface via ducts that pierce the lamina propria. The **perichondrium** (Pc) of the hyaline cartilage **C-rings** (CR) merges with the submucosal connective tissue. Note a longitudinal section of a **blood vessel** (BV), indicative of the presence of a rich vascular supply.

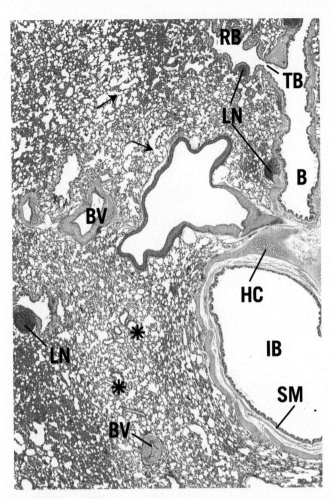

FIGURE 13-10. Lung. Paraffin section. ×14.

This survey photomicrograph presents a section of a lung that permits the observation of the various conduits that conduct air and blood to and from the lung. The **intrapulmonary bronchus** (IB) is recognizable by its thick wall, containing plates of **hyaline cartilage** (HC) and **smooth muscle** (SM). Longitudinal sections of a **bronchiole** (B), **terminal bronchiole** (TB), and **respiratory bronchiole** (RB) are also evident. Smaller bronchioles (*asterisks*) may also be recognized, but their identification cannot be ascertained. *Arrows* point to structures that are probably alveolar ducts leading into alveolar sacs. Several **blood vessels** (BV), branches of the pulmonary circulatory system, may be noted. Observe that **lymphoid nodules** (LN) are also present along the bronchial tree.

- A somewhat thicker septum may possess collagen and elastic fibers as well as smooth muscle fibers and connective tissue cells including the resident macrophages of the lungs, known as **dust cells** (Fig. 13-19).

- These dust cells are derived from monocytes and enter the lungs via the bloodstream.

- Here they mature and become extremely efficient scavengers. It is believed that dust cells are the most numerous of all cell types present in the lungs, even

though they are eliminated from the lungs at a rate of 50 million per day.

- Although it is not known whether they actively migrate to the bronchioles or reach it via fluid flow, it is known that they are transported from there within the mucus layer, via ciliary action of the respiratory epithelium, into the pharynx.

- Once they reach the pharynx, they are either expectorated or swallowed.

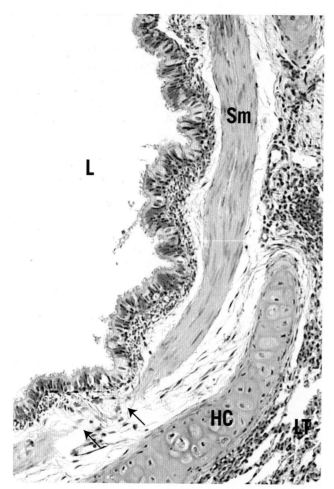

FIGURE 13-11. Intrapulmonary bronchus. x.s. Paraffin section. ×132.

Intrapulmonary bronchi are relatively large conduits for air, whose **lumina** (L) are lined by a typical respiratory epithelium. The **smooth muscle** (Sm) is located beneath the mucous membrane and encircles the entire lumen. Note that gaps (*arrows*) appear in the muscle layer, indicating that two ribbons of smooth muscle wind around the lumen in a helical arrangement. Plates of **hyaline cartilage** (HC) act as skeletal support, maintaining the patency of the bronchus. The entire structure is surrounded by **lung tissue** (LT).

Mechanism of Gaseous Exchange

The partial pressures of O_2 and CO_2 are responsible for the uptake or release of these gases by RBCs. Because cells convert O_2 to CO_2 during their metabolism, the partial pressure of CO_2 is high in tissues, and this gas is preferentially taken up by RBCs. Simultaneously, they release oxygen. The converse is true in the lungs, where O_2 is taken up by RBCs and CO_2 is released. The movement of these gases occurs by **passive diffusion** owing to the partial pressures of oxygen and carbon dioxide in the alveolar spaces of the lung and in the blood.

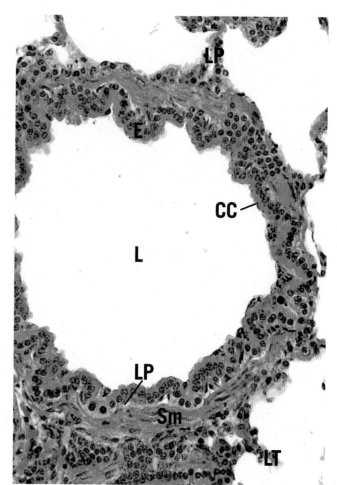

FIGURE 13-12. Bronchiole. x.s. Paraffin section. ×270.

Bronchioles maintain their patent **lumen** (L) without the requirement of cartilaginous support because they are attached to surrounding lung tissue by elastic fibers radiating from their circumference. The lumina of bronchioles are lined by simple columnar to simple cuboidal **epithelium** (E), interspersed with **club cells** (CC), depending on the diameter of the bronchiole. The **lamina propria** (LP) is thin and is surrounded by **smooth muscle** (Sm), which encircles the lumen. Bronchioles have no glands in their walls and are surrounded by **lung tissue** (LT).

The process in the body is similar to the process in the alveoli of the lungs. CO_2 released by cells of the body crosses the capillary endothelium and is dissolved in the blood. About 10% of the dissolved carbon dioxide then remains in the blood and 80% diffuses into the cytosol of the RBCs. Approximately 20% of the *original* volume of CO_2 binds to the heme portion of the hemoglobin molecule, and the remaining 70% forms **carbonic acid**, H_2CO_3, catalyzed by the activity of the **carbonic anhydrase** within the erythrocyte cytosol. The carbonic acid dissociates into H^+ and HCO_3-; the H^+ ion binds to the hemoglobin molecule and the HCO_3- diffuses back into the blood to be replaced by Cl^- to reestablish electrical neutrality—a process known as the **chloride shift**.

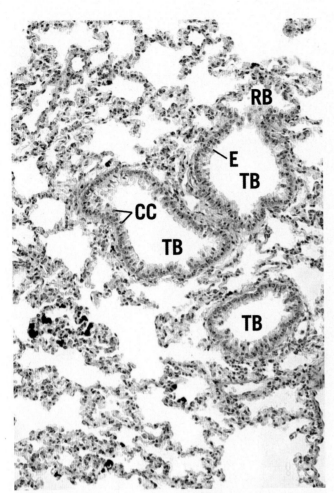

FIGURE 13-13. Terminal bronchioles. x.s. Paraffin section. ×132.

The smallest conducting bronchioles are referred to as **terminal bronchioles** (TB). These have very small diameters, and their lumina are lined with a simple cuboidal **epithelium** (E) interspersed with **club cells** (CC). The connective tissue is much reduced, and the smooth muscle layers are incomplete and difficult to recognize at this magnification. Terminal bronchioles give rise to **respiratory bronchioles** (RB), whose walls resemble those of the terminal bronchioles except that the presence of alveoli permits the exchange of gases to occur. Observe the alveolar duct (not labeled) in the lower right-hand corner.

Once in the lungs, the CO_2-rich blood loses its carbon dioxide, which enters the lumina of the alveoli. This process is the mirror image of the mechanism that occurred in the body. HCO_3^- diffuses from the blood into the RBCs, making the cytosol more negative and prompting Cl^- ions to leave the RBCs (a process known as **chloride shift**) in order to reestablish electrical neutrality. The H^+ and HCO_3^- ions form **carbonic acid**, which, catalyzed by **carbonic anhydrase**, breaks down into CO_2 and H_2O. The carbon dioxide leaves the erythrocytes and enters the blood, and because the concentration of CO_2 in the alveolar spaces of the lung is much less than in the blood, carbon dioxide passively diffuses into the alveolar lumina to be exhaled.

CLINICAL CONSIDERATIONS 13-1

Bronchial Asthma

Bronchial asthma is a condition in which the bronchi become partially and reversibly obstructed by airway spasm (**bronchoconstriction**), mast cell–induced inflammatory response to allergens and/or other stimuli that would not affect a normal lung, and the formation of excess mucus. Some of the most characteristic alterations are the hypertrophy of the bronchial smooth muscle coat as well as the increase in the submucosal mucous glands. Moreover, the epithelium loses its pseudostratified ciliated characteristic and assumes a squamous metaplastic appearance with an increase in basal cell and goblet cell numbers. The basal lamina is also increased in thickness and the submucosa is edematous and infiltrated by eosinophils and other leukocytes. Asthma attacks vary with the individual; in some, it is hardly noticed, whereas in others shortness of breath is very evident, and wheezing accompanies breathing out. Most individuals who suffer from asthmatic conditions use nebulizers containing bronchodilators, such as albuterol, to relieve the attack.

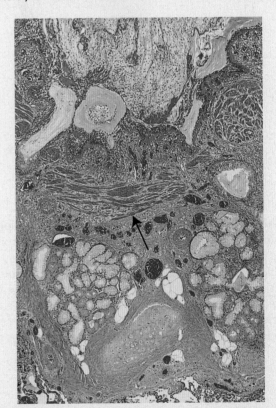

This figure is from the lung of a patient who died of asthma. Note that the lumen of the bronchus is obstructed by a mucous plug. The *arrow* indicates smooth muscle hyperplasia characteristic in advanced cases of asthma. (Reprinted with permission from Strayer DS, et al., eds. *Rubin's Pathology: Mechanisms of Human Disease*, 8th ed. Philadelphia: Wolters Kluwer, 2020. Figure 18-49.)

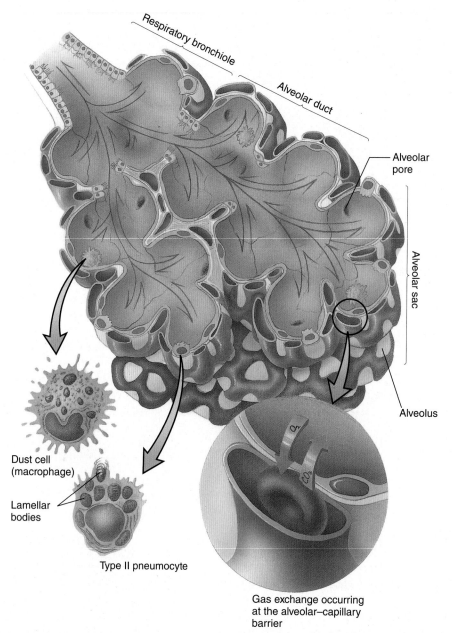

Respiratory bronchiole

Alveolar duct

Alveolar pore

Alveolar sac

Alveolus

Dust cell
(macrophage)

Lamellar
bodies

Type II pneumocyte

Gas exchange occurring
at the alveolar–capillary
barrier

FIGURE 13-14. Respiratory portion. This illustration outlines the structural organization of the respiratory portion of the respiratory system. The inspired air travels from the respiratory bronchioles to alveolar ducts, atrium, alveolar sacs to the alveoli, coming in contact along the way with the thin lining epithelium of the alveoli composed mostly of type I pneumocytes. Note the impressive amount of continuous capillary network in the thin connective tissue outside the thin lining of the alveoli. Gas exchange between the air and blood occurs through the thin membrane called the blood–air barrier composed of the pneumocyte type I, the endothelial cell, and the fused basement membrane between the two cell types. Additional cells of the lung parenchyma include type II pneumocytes, which produce surfactants and the resident macrophages of the lung tissue called dust cells.

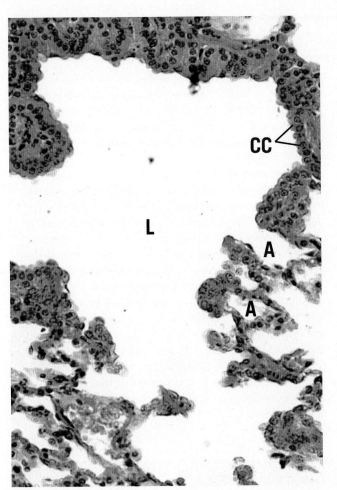

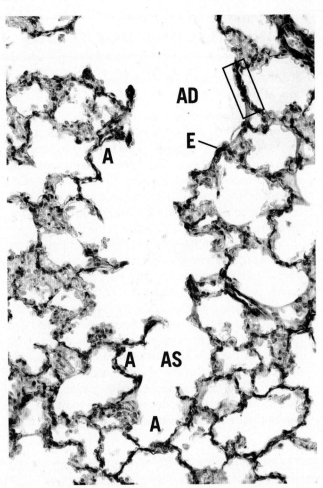

FIGURE 13-15. Respiratory bronchiole. Paraffin section. ×270.

The respiratory bronchiole whose **lumen** (L) occupies the lower half of this photomicrograph presents an apparently thick wall with small outpocketings of **alveoli** (A). It is in these alveoli that gaseous exchanges first occur. The wall of the respiratory bronchiole is composed of a simple cuboidal epithelium consisting of some ciliated cells and **club cells** (CC). The remainder of the wall presents an incomplete layer of smooth muscle cells surrounded by fibroelastic connective tissue. Careful examination of this photomicrograph reveals that the wall of the respiratory bronchiole is folded upon itself, thus giving a misleading appearance of thick walls.

FIGURE 13-16. Alveolar duct. l.s. Human. Paraffin section. ×132.

Alveolar ducts (AD), unlike respiratory bronchioles, do not possess a wall of their own. These structures are lined by a simple squamous **epithelium** (E), composed of highly attenuated cells. AD present numerous outpocketings of **alveoli** (A), and they end in **alveolar sacs** (AS), consisting of groups of alveoli clustered around a common airspace. Individual alveoli possess small smooth muscle cells that, acting like a purse string, control the opening into the alveolus. These appear as small knobs (*arrow*). A region similar to the *boxed area* is presented at a higher magnification in Figure 13-18.

CLINICAL CONSIDERATIONS 13-2

Hyaline Membrane Disease and Cystic Fibrosis

Hyaline membrane disease is frequently observed in premature infants who lack adequate amounts of pulmonary surfactant. This disease is characterized by **labored breathing**, because a high alveolar surface tension, caused by inadequate levels of surfactant, makes it difficult to expand the alveoli. The administration of glucocorticoids prior to birth can induce the synthesis of surfactant, thus circumventing the appearance of the disease.

Although **cystic fibrosis** is viewed as a disease of the lungs, it is really a hereditary condition that alters the secretions of several glands, such as the liver, pancreas, salivary glands, sweat glands, and glands of the reproductive system. In the case of the lungs, liver, pancreas, and intestines, the mucous secretions become abnormally thickened and block the lumina of these organs. In the respiratory system, the walls of the bronchioles thicken with the progression of the disease, areas of the lung become constricted, the thick secretions in the airways become infected, the lungs cease to function, and death ensues. In the most common type of cystic fibrosis, individuals possess two copies of the defective gene that code for altered ion channels, known as **cystic fibrosis transmembrane conductance regulator** (**CFTR**). In normal cells, the CFTR is embedded in the cell membrane and allows Cl^- ions to leave the cell, which decreases the salt concentration inside the cell, causing water molecules to also leave the cell. The water molecules then dilute the mucus that builds up outside the cell. The mucus can then be cleared from the extracellular space. In mutated cells, the defective CFTR is either destroyed by the cells proteasome system or embedded in the cell membrane but remains shut so that Cl^- ions cannot leave the cell. Consequently, water does not leave the cell and the mucus becomes abnormally thick and viscous and cannot be cleared from the extracellular space. In the case of the small respiratory and terminal bronchioles as well as the larger elements of the conducting system of the respiratory system become clogged with mucus and the individual is unable to respire, succumbs to infections, and dies. Prior to the availability of antibiotics, most children with cystic fibrosis died in the first few years of life. However, with current treatment, the median survival rate is age 37 years.

Table 13-2	Components of the Blood–Air Barrier	
Endothelial Component	**Endothelial and Pneumocyte Component**	**Pneumocyte Component**
Attenuated endothelial cell	Combined basal laminae	Attenuated pneumocyte I
		Surfactant and fluid coating of the alveolus

CLINICAL CONSIDERATIONS 13-3

Emphysema

Emphysema is a disease that results from the **destruction of alveolar walls** with the consequent formation of large cyst-like sacs, reducing the surface available for gas exchange. Emphysema is marked by **decreased elasticity** of the lungs, which are unable to recoil adequately during expiration. It is associated with exposure to **cigarette smoke** and other substances that inhibit α1-antitrypsin, a protein that normally protects the lungs from the action of elastase produced by alveolar macrophages. **Panacinar emphysema** is a form of emphysema characterized by uniform damage to the respiratory bronchiole, alveolar ducts, alveolar sacs, and alveoli. The alveolar septa are almost completely destroyed, and the lung tissue takes on a lacy appearance frequently referred to as "cotton candy lung."

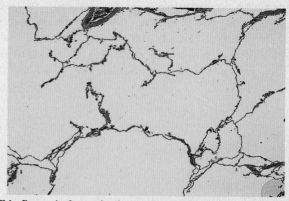

This figure is from the lung of a patient who had panacinar emphysema. Note the large airspaces and the absence of alveolar septa and the limited number of alveolar walls. (Reprinted with permission from Strayer DS, et al., eds. *Rubin's Pathology: Mechanisms of Human Disease*, 8th ed. Philadelphia: Wolters Kluwer, 2020. Figure 18-46.)

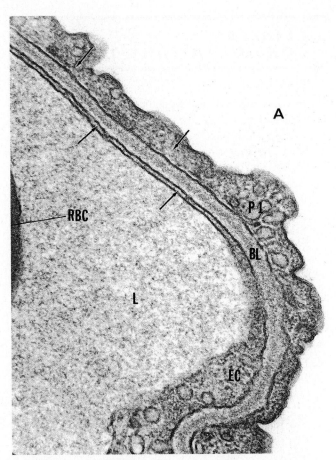

FIGURE 13-17. Blood–air barrier. Dog. Electron microscopy. ×85,500.

The blood–air barrier is composed of highly attenuated **endothelial cells** (EC), **type I pneumocytes** (P1), and an intervening **basal lamina** (BL). Note that the cytoplasm (*arrows*) of both cell types is greatly reduced, as evidenced by the proximity of the plasmalemma on either side of the cytoplasm. The airspace of the **alveolus** (A) is empty, whereas the capillary **lumen** (L) presents a part of a **red blood cell** (RBC). (From DeFouw DO. Vesicle numerical densities and cellular attenuation: comparisons between endothelium and epithelium of the alveolar septa in normal dog lungs. *Anat Rec* 1984;209(1):77–84. Copyright © 1984 Wiley-Liss, Inc. Reprinted by permission of John Wiley & Sons, Inc.)

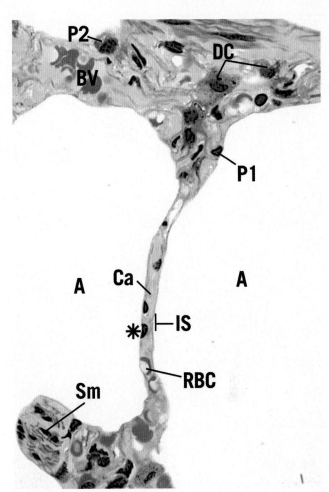

FIGURE 13-18. Interalveolar septum. Monkey. Plastic section. ×540.

This photomicrograph is a higher magnification of a region similar to the *boxed area* of Figure 13-16. Two **alveoli** (A) are presented, recognizable as empty spaces separated from each other by an **interalveolar septum** (IS). The septum contains a **capillary** (Ca), the nucleus (*asterisk*) of whose endothelial lining bulges into the lumen containing **red blood cells** (RBC). The interalveolar septum as well as the entire alveolus is lined by **type I pneumocytes** (P1), which are highly attenuated squamous epithelial cells, interspersed with **type II pneumocytes** (P2). Thicker interalveolar septa house more **blood vessels** (BV) and connective tissue elements including macrophages known as **dust cells** (DC). Note the presence of **smooth muscle cells** (Sm) and connective tissue elements that appear as knobs at the entrance into the alveolus.

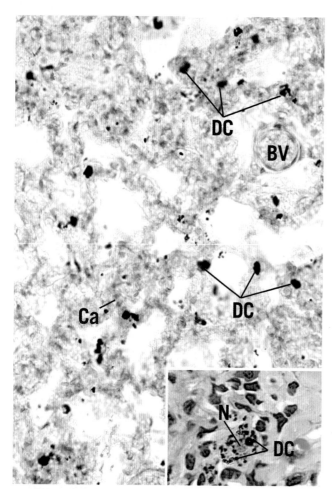

FIGURE 13-19. Lung. Dust cells. Paraffin section. ×270.

The highly vascular nature of the lung is evident in this photomicrograph because the **blood vessels** (BV) and the **capillaries** (Ca) of the interalveolar septa are filled with RBCs. The dark blotches that appear to be scattered throughout the lung tissue represent **dust cells** (DC), macrophages that have phagocytosed particulate matter. *Inset.* **Lung. Dust cell. Monkey. Plastic section.** ×540. The **nucleus** (N) of a **dust cell** (DC) is surrounded by phagosomes containing particulate matter that was probably phagocytosed from an alveolus of the lung.

Pneumonia

Pneumonia is a possibly lethal infection of the alveoli and the connective tissue elements of the lungs. In the United States, of the 2 million people who contract pneumonia annually, approximately 40,000 to 70,000 succumb to this disease. The infection is more dangerous to patients who are immune compromised and/or suffering from chronic diseases. In developing countries, pneumonia and diarrhea-induced dehydration are the two most significant causes of death. There are numerous types of pneumonia depending on the causative agents, namely, bacterial, viral, or fungal, and the organism either is inhaled into the lungs or enters the lungs via the circulatory system. The principal diagnostic features of pneumonia are productive coughs, fever, chills, shallow breathing, hearing rasping sounds amplified by stethoscopes, and the presence of white foci in the lung as observed on chest x-rays.

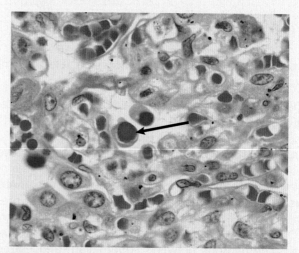

This figure is from the lung of a patient with adenovirus pneumonia. Note that the lumen of the alveolus houses cells with basophilic nuclear inclusions. These cells are referred to as "smudge cells" (*arrow*) and are characterized by a thin rim of cytoplasm surrounding the nucleus housing the basophilic inclusion. (Reprinted with permission from Strayer DS, et al., eds. *Rubin's Pathology: Mechanisms of Human Disease*, 8th ed. Philadelphia: Wolters Kluwer, 2020. Figure 18-30.)

Selected Review of Histologic Images

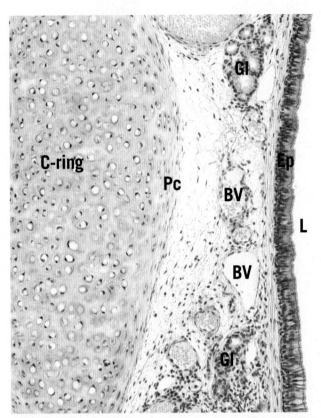

REVIEW FIGURE 13-1-1. Trachea. Monkey l.s. Paraffin section. ×132.

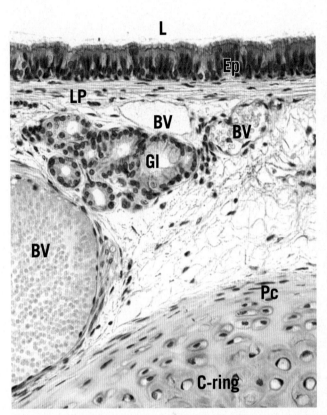

REVIEW FIGURE 13-1-2. Trachea. Monkey l.s. Paraffin section. ×270.

The trachea is lined by a pseudostratified ciliated columnar **epithelium** (Ep) with goblet cells that secrete mucinogen. When mucinogen becomes hydrated, it is known as mucin, and when it is mixed with material in the tracheal **lumen** (L), it becomes known as mucus. The lamina propria is relatively thin, whereas the submucosa is thick and contains mucous and seromucous **glands** (Gl), whose secretory product is delivered to the epithelial surface via ducts that pierce the lamina propria. The **perichondrium** (Pc) of the hyaline cartilage **C-rings** (C-ring) merges with the submucosal connective tissue. Note the rich **vascular supply** (BV).

This photomicrograph is a higher magnification of a region of Review Figure 13-1-1. The pseudostratified, ciliated columnar **epithelium** (Ep) lining the **lumen** (L) is separated from the underlying **glandular** (Gl) **lamina propria** (LP) by the basement membrane. The submucosa and the lamina propria both have a rich **vascular supply** (BV). The **C-ring** (C-ring), with its attendant **perichondrium** (Pc), constitutes the most substantive layer of the tracheal wall. Note that there is no smooth muscle between the C-ring and the epithelium.

KEY					
BV	vascular supply (blood vessel)	**Ep**	epithelium	**LP**	lamina propria
		Gl	gland	**Pc**	perichondrium
C-ring	cartilage C-ring	**L**	lumen		

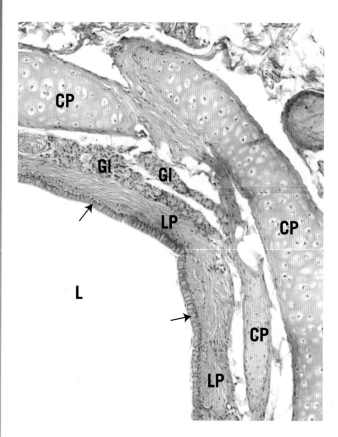

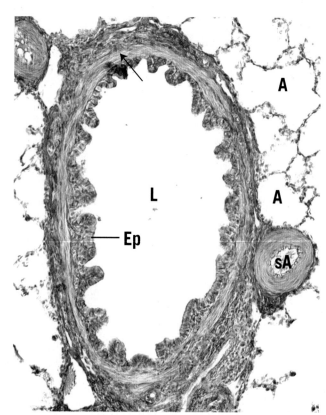

REVIEW FIGURE 13-1-3. Intrapulmonary bronchus. Monkey x.s. Paraffin section. ×132.

Intrapulmonary bronchi are relatively large conduits for air, whose **lumina** (L) are lined by a typical respiratory epithelium (*arrows*). Smooth muscle is located at the junction of the **lamina propria** (LP) and the submucosa. Seromucous **glands** (Gl) are present in the submucosa. Plates of **hyaline cartilage** (CP) act as the skeletal support, maintaining the patency of the bronchus. The entire structure is surrounded by lung tissue.

REVIEW FIGURE 13-1-4. Bronchiole. Opossum x.s. Paraffin section. ×132.

Bronchioles maintain their patent **lumen** (L) by the elastic fibers radiating from their circumference. The lumina of bronchioles are lined by simple columnar to simple cuboidal **epithelium** (Ep), interspersed with club cells, depending on the diameter of the bronchiole. The lamina propria is thin and is surrounded by smooth muscle (*arrow*), which encircles the lumen. Bronchioles have no glands in their walls, are surrounded by **lung tissue** (A), and are accompanied by a well-developed blood supply, as evidenced by the **small arterioles** (sA).

KEY					
A	lung tissue (alveoli)	**Gl**	gland	**LP**	lamina propria
CP	hyaline cartilage	**L**	lumen	**sA**	small arteriole
Ep	epithelium				

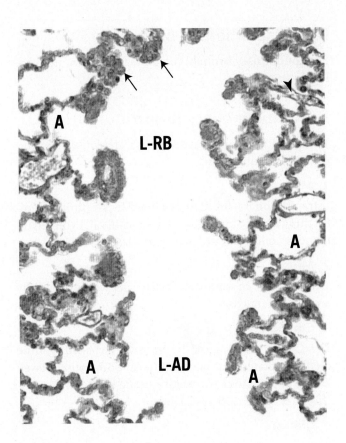

REVIEW FIGURE 13-1-5. Respiratory bronchiole. Monkey l.s. Paraffin section. ×270.

The first regions of the bronchial tree where exchange of gases may occur are the **respiratory bronchioles** (L-RB). These have very small diameters, and their lumina are lined with a simple cuboidal epithelium interspersed with club cells (*arrows*) and occasional **alveoli** (A) open from their walls. Respiratory bronchioles end in an atrium from which **alveolar ducts** (L-AD) emanate. Note the lumen of a capillary (*arrowhead*) housing erythrocytes.

KEY		
A alveoli	**L-AD** alveolar duct	**L-RB** respiratory bronchiole

Summary of Histologic Organization

I. Conducting Portion

A. Nasal Cavity

1. Respiratory Region

The **respiratory region** is lined by **respiratory (pseudostratified ciliated columnar) epithelium**. The subepithelial connective tissue is richly vascularized and possesses seromucous glands.

2. Olfactory Region

The epithelium of the **olfactory region** is thick, **pseudostratified ciliated columnar epithelium** composed of three cell types: **basal cell**, **supporting cells**, and **olfactory cells**. The lamina propria is richly vascularized and possesses **Bowman's glands**, which produce a watery secretion.

B. Larynx

The **larynx** is lined by a **respiratory epithelium** except for certain regions of the **epiglottis** and the **vocal folds** that are lined by **stratified squamous nonkeratinized epithelium**. From superior to inferior, the **lumen** of the larynx presents three regions: the **vestibule**, **the ventricle**, and the **infraglottic cavity**. The **ventricular** and **vocal folds** are the superior and inferior boundaries of the ventricle, respectively. Hyaline and elastic cartilages, extrinsic and intrinsic muscles, as well as mucous and seromucous glands are present in the larynx.

C. Trachea

1. Mucosa

The **mucosa** of the trachea is composed of a **respiratory epithelium** with numerous **goblet cells**, a **lamina propria**, and a well-defined **elastic lamina**.

2. Submucosa

The **submucosa** houses **mucous** and **seromucous glands**.

3. Adventitia

The **adventitia** is the thickest portion of the tracheal wall. It houses the **C-rings** of **hyaline cartilage** (or thick connective tissue between the rings). Posteriorly, the **trachealis muscle** (smooth muscle) fills in the gap between the free ends of the cartilage.

D. Extrapulmonary Bronchi

Extrapulmonary bronchi resemble the trachea in histologic structure.

E. Intrapulmonary Bronchi

These and subsequent passageways are completely surrounded by lung tissue.

1. Mucosa

Intrapulmonary bronchi are lined by **respiratory epithelium** with **goblet cells**. The subepithelial connective tissue is no longer bordered by an elastic lamina.

2. Muscle

Two ribbons of **smooth muscle** are wound helically around the mucosa.

3. Cartilage

The C-rings are replaced by irregularly shaped **hyaline cartilage plates** that encircle the smooth muscle layer. **Dense collagenous connective tissue** connects the perichondria of the cartilage plates.

4. Glands

Seromucous glands occupy the connective tissue between the cartilage plates and smooth muscle. **Lymphatic nodules** (BALTs) and branches of the pulmonary arteries are also present.

F. Bronchioles

Bronchioles are lined by **ciliated simple columnar** to **simple cuboidal epithelium** interspersed with nonciliated **club cells (Clara cells)**. **Goblet cells** are found only in larger bronchioles. The **lamina propria** possesses no glands and is surrounded by **smooth muscle**. The walls of bronchioles are not supported by cartilage. The largest bronchioles are about 1 mm in diameter.

G. Terminal Bronchioles

Terminal bronchioles are usually less than 0.5 mm in diameter. The lumen is lined by **simple cuboidal epithelium** (some ciliated) interspersed with **club cells (Clara cells)**. The connective tissue and smooth muscle of the wall of the terminal bronchioles are greatly reduced.

II. Respiratory Portion

A. Respiratory Bronchiole

Respiratory bronchioles resemble terminal bronchioles, but they possess outpocketings of **alveoli** in their walls. This is the first region where the exchange of gases occurs.

B. Alveolar Ducts

Alveolar ducts possess no walls of their own. They are long, straight tubes lined by **simple squamous epithelium** and display numerous outpocketings of **alveoli**. Alveolar ducts end in alveolar sacs.

C. Alveolar Sacs

Alveolar sacs are composed of groups of **alveoli** clustered around a common airspace.

D. Alveolus

An **alveolus** is a small airspace partially surrounded by a highly attenuated epithelium. Two types of cells are present in the lining: **type I pneumocytes** (lining cells) and **type II pneumocytes** (produce surfactant). The opening of the alveolus is controlled by **elastic fibers**. Alveoli are separated from each other by richly vascularized walls known as **interalveolar septa**, some of which present **alveolar pores** (communicating spaces between alveoli). **Dust cells** (macrophages), **fibroblasts**, and other **connective tissue elements** may be noted in interalveolar septa. The **blood–air barrier** is a part of the interalveolar septum, the thinnest of which is composed of surfactant, **continuous endothelial cells**, **type I pneumocyte**, and their intervening **fused basal laminae**.

Chapter Review Questions

Clinical vignette for questions 13-1 to 13-3: A 38-year-old male patient presents to an emergency room with severe pneumonia and hypoxia. The patient's medical history is significant for infertility diagnosed 10 years ago, dextrocardia, and chronic upper respiratory tract infection since a young age.

13-1. Based on the medical history, dysfunction in which cells is the most likely cause of the patient's severe pneumonia?

A. Brush cells

B. Ciliated cells

C. Dust cells

D. Serous cells

E. Type II pneumocytes

13-2. Which subcellular structure is dysfunctional in this patient's cells?

A. Actin filaments

B. Chloride channels

C. Dynein arms

D. Golgi apparatus

E. Proteasomes

13-3. The patient's hypoxia indicates compromise of which histologic structure in the respiratory system?

A. Cartilage plates

B. Elastic fibers

C. Interalveolar septum

D. Olfactory epithelium

E. Smooth muscles

13-4. Presence of nonkeratinized stratified squamous epithelium is metaplastic in which structure of the respiratory system?

A. Nasal vestibule

B. Tip of epiglottis

C. True vocal folds

D. Primary bronchi

13-5. Which of the following structure is a part of the respiratory portion of the respiratory system?

A. Diaphragm

B. Epiglottis

C. Interalveolar septum

D. Terminal bronchiole

E. Ventricular folds

DIGESTIVE SYSTEM I

The digestive system is modified along its considerable length to ingest, digest, and absorb food as well as to eliminate its undigestible portions and the gases that were either swallowed or produced by the microbial flora resident in the alimentary canal. The digestive system is organized into three major components so that the above functions can be performed. These components are as follows:

1. The **oral cavity**, where the introduced food is reduced in size, is moistened, begins to be digested, and is formed into small spherical portions, each known as a **bolus,** that enters the alimentary canal;

2. A **muscular alimentary (gastrointestinal [GI]) canal,** along whose lumen the ingested foods are converted, both physically and chemically, into absorbable substances; and

3. A **glandular portion**, which provides fluids, enzymes, and emulsifying agents necessary, so that the alimentary canal can perform its manifold functions.

Oral Region: Oral Cavity

The **oral cavity** is subdivided into two smaller cavities: the externally positioned vestibule and the internally placed oral cavity proper.

- The **vestibule** is the space bounded by the **lips** and **cheeks** anteriorly and laterally, whereas its internal boundary is formed by the **dental arches**. The ducts of the parotid glands deliver their secretory products into the vestibule.

- The **oral cavity proper** is bounded by the teeth externally, the floor of the mouth inferiorly, and the hard and soft palates superiorly. At its posterior extent, the oral cavity proper is separated from the oral pharynx at a plane of the palatoglossal folds just anterior to the palatine tonsils. Ducts of the submandibular and sublingual glands deliver their secretions into the oral cavity proper.

- Both the oral cavity proper and the vestibule are lined by **stratified squamous epithelium,** which, in regions that are subject to abrasive forces, is modified into **stratified squamous keratinized (or parakeratinized) epithelium** (Table 14-1).

Oral Mucosa

The wet epithelium and the subepithelial connective tissue of the oral cavity constitute the **oral mucosa**. If the epithelium is keratinized (or parakeratinized), the mucosa is said to be **masticatory mucosa**, and if the epithelium is not keratinized, the mucosa is referred to as **lining mucosa**. Most of the oral cavity is covered by lining mucosa, except the gingiva, and the hard palate, all of which are covered by masticatory mucosa. Additionally, the dorsal surface of the tongue is covered by a **specialized mucosa**, which is characterized by numerous projections called **lingual papillae**. Some of these lingual papillae possess, embedded within their epithelia, special sensory structures, known as **taste buds**. Although most taste buds are located on the dorsal surface of the tongue, the palate and pharynx also possess a few of these structures. Each taste bud recognizes one or more of the five taste sensations: sour, sweet, salt, umami (savory), or bitter. In some individuals, there is an additional type of taste buds that can recognize fat as a specific taste.

Lips

The upper and lower **lips**, forming the anterior boundary of the oral cavity, have three surfaces, the **external (skin)**

Table 14-1	Summary of the Oral Mucosa		
Mucosal Region	**Type of Epithelium**	**Height of Connective Tissue Papillae**	**Special Comments**
Lip			
Skin aspect	Stratified squamous keratinized	Medium	Hair, sebaceous glands, and sweat glands
Vermilion zone	Stratified squamous keratinized	High	Few sebaceous glands? The vermilion zone must be moistened by tongue
Mucosal region*	Lining mucosa	Medium	Mucous (mixed?) salivary glands
Cheek			
Skin aspect	Stratified squamous keratinized	Medium	Hair, sebaceous glands, and sweat glands
Vestibular aspect	Lining mucosa	Medium	Mucous (mixed?) salivary glands; Fordyce's granules
Gingiva			
Free and attached	Masticatory mucosa	High	Tightly bound to periosteum
Sulcular	Lining mucosa	Low	
Junctional epithelium	Lining mucosa	None	Attached to the tooth surface by hemidesmosomes
Col	Lining mucosa (junctional epithelium?)	Low to none	
Alveolar Mucosa			
	Lining mucosa	Low	Some minor salivary glands
Hard Palate			
Anterior lateral	Masticatory mucosa	High	Fat globules
Posterior lateral	Masticatory mucosa	High	Mucous salivary glands
Raphe	Masticatory mucosa	High	Tightly bound to periosteum
Soft Palate			
	Lining mucosa	Low	Elastic lamina; mucous salivary glands
Uvula	Lining mucosa	Low	Mucous salivary glands
Floor of Mouth			
	Lining mucosa	Low	Mucous salivary glands
Tongue			
Dorsal surface	Specialized mucosa		Taste buds; lingual papillae, serous, mucous, and mixed salivary glands; lingual tonsils
Ventral surface	Lining mucosa	Low	Plica fimbriata

Reprinted with permission from Gartner LP. *Essentials of Oral Histology and Embryology*, 3rd ed. Baltimore: Jen House Publishing Company, 1999. p. 118.

*Also referred to as the internal region and the vestibular aspect.

aspect, **vermilion zone**, and the wet, **mucosal (internal) region**, with a skeletal muscle **core** that permits movement of the lips (Fig. 14-1).

- The **external aspect** of the lips is covered by **thin skin**, composed of **epidermis** and **dermis** as well as the normal skin appendages, namely hair follicles, sebaceous glands, and sweat glands. The epidermal–dermal interface displays a shallow rete apparatus.
- The **vermilion zone** is also thin skin but modified in that it has no hair follicles or sweat glands, but it does have

a limited number of nonfunctional sebaceous glands (**Fordyce's granules**). The epidermal–dermal interface is highly developed so that there is a relatively high rete apparatus, where the dermal papillae reach close to the surface of the epidermis and their rich vascular supply imparts a pink coloration to the vermilion zone.

- The **mucosal region** is composed of a wet stratified squamous nonkeratinized epithelium and a subepithelial connective tissue housing mucous, mixed minor salivary glands along with some Fordyce's granules.

CLINICAL CONSIDERATIONS 14-1

Lip Disorders

The **vermillion zone** in a healthy person has a pinkish appearance; however, individuals with reduced blood oxygen levels present with cyanotic (bluish-colored) lips. Of course, even healthy individuals will exhibit a bluish lip coloration in very cold temperatures.

Angular cheilitis, a painful inflammation of the corners of the mouth, occurs in individuals with certain dietary deficiencies, such as low levels of one of the B vitamins, iron, or zinc (especially prevalent in developing countries); irritation as by dentures that no longer fit well; or due to allergies and overexposure to the sun. Usually, both angles of the mouth are involved, and frequently there are exacerbating circumstances, such as infection by bacteria (e.g., *Staphylococcus aureus*) or by yeast (e.g., *Candida albicans*). This painful condition usually lasts a few days but can occasionally last for several years.

Herpetic stomatitis, a relatively common disease caused by the herpes simplex virus (HSV) type I, is distinguished by painful **fever blisters** appearing on or in the vicinity of the lips. This is a recurring disease because the virus, in its dormant phase, inhabits the trigeminal ganglion. It travels along the axon to cause the formation of blisters. During the active stage, the patient is highly contagious, as the virus is shed via the seeping clear exudate.

Individuals with a burning sensation of unknown origin in their mouths, that involve the inside of their cheeks, lips, palate, and especially their tongue, are said to be suffering from **primary burning mouth syndrome** (**BMS**). Visual examination of the affected regions does not reveal any physical symptoms. This condition usually appears suddenly, but, in some patients, it may develop over several days and even weeks. The burning sensation may vary not only in its intensity but also in its duration. In some individuals, it is present all the time, whereas in others, its intensity increases during the day and is most severe in the late evening and at night. In other patients, the intensity of the burning sensation does not vary with the time of day. This painful, or at best uncomfortable, condition may last for years and then suddenly disappear.

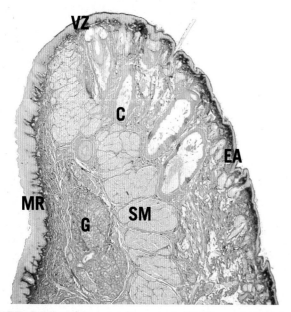

FIGURE 14-1. This very low-magnification photomicrograph of the human lip displays its three regions, the **external aspect** (EA) with its hair follicles, the **vermillion zone** (VZ), and the **mucosal region** (MR) with its minor salivary **glands** (G), as well as the **core** of the lip (C) housing its **skeletal muscle** (SM). ×14.

Salivary Glands

The three (possibly four) pairs of major salivary glands, parotid, sublingual, and submandibular (perhaps also tubarial) deliver their secretions into the oral cavity proper and are discussed in Chapter 16 (Digestive System III).

The connective tissue underlying the epithelium of the oral cavity is richly endowed with **minor salivary glands**. These minor glands secrete **saliva** continuously, producing approximately 5% of the daily total salivary output, and contribute to the maintenance of a moist environment (see Table 14-1). Saliva functions also in assisting in the process of deglutition by acting as a lubricant for dry foods and for holding the bolus together in a semi-solid mass. Moreover, enzymes present in saliva initiate digestion of carbohydrates, whereas **secretory antibodies (IgA)** protect the body against antigenic substances. Additionally, antibacterial agents, **lysozymes** and **lactoferrin**, are secreted by the minor salivary glands.

Palate

The **palate** forms the roof of the mouth and the floor of the nasal cavity because it separates the two cavities from each other. It has three regions, the anterior hard palate, named because of the bony shelf that forms its core, the soft palate, named because of the skeletal muscles in its core, and the uvula, the posterior extension of the soft palate.

- The oral surface of the **hard palate** is covered by a keratinized (or parakeratinized) stratified squamous epithelium that forms extensive rete apparatus with its subjacent dense irregular collagenous connective tissue. Anteriorly, this connective tissue houses **adipose tissue** whereas posteriorly it houses **mucous minor salivary glands**. The core of the hard palate is composed of a bony shelf. The nasal aspect is covered by a respiratory epithelium (ciliated pseudostratified epithelium) with numerous goblet cells. The subepithelial connective tissue is richly endowed by mucous glands.

- The oral surface of the **soft palate** is covered by a stratified squamous nonkeratinized epithelium with shallow rete apparatus. The subepithelial connective tissue is separated into two layers by an intervening, thin **elastic lamina**: a superficial **lamina propria** and a deeper, mucous minor salivary gland-containing **submucosa**. The core of the soft palate is composed of skeletal muscles that elevate the soft palate during swallowing. The nasal aspect of the soft palate is continuous with and identical to that of the hard palate.

- The **uvula** is a conical continuation of the soft palate. The entire surface of the uvula is covered by a stratified squamous nonkeratinized epithelium. Its subepithelial connective tissue resembles that of the soft palate and houses some mucous minor salivary glands. The uvula's core is composed of skeletal muscle fibers that elevate the uvula and presses it against the back of the pharynx during swallowing.

The entrance to the pharynx is guarded against bacterial invasion by the **tonsillar ring,** composed of the lingual, pharyngeal, and palatine tonsils (see Chapter 10, Lymphoid [Immune] System).

Teeth

The contents of the oral cavity are the **teeth** and their supporting apparatus that function in chewing food into small pieces as well as the **tongue** that functions in the preparation of the bolus, tasting of the food, and initiating deglutition (swallowing).

Humans have two sets of dentition: Children have 20 deciduous teeth, and, as they are exfoliated, they are replaced by the permanent dentition, composed of 20 succedaneous teeth and an additional 12 accessional teeth for a total of 32 permanent teeth. At approximately age 6 to 13 years, the dentition is mixed in that both deciduous and permanent teeth are present in the mouth simultaneously. The larger number of permanent dentition is probably a function of the greater space availability in the adult mouth.

Structure of Teeth

Each tooth is composed of a **crown, root**, and the **cervix (neck)**, where the crown and root contact each other (see Figs. 14-2 and 14-3). Three calcified substances, **enamel, dentin,** and **cementum**, form the substance of each tooth. Dentin forms the bulk of each tooth and is located both in the crown (**coronal dentin**) and in the

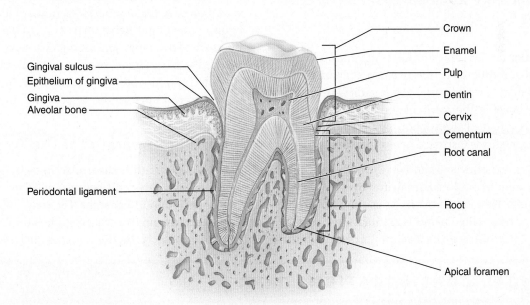

FIGURE 14-2. Schematic diagram of a tooth and its supporting apparatus. The tooth, composed of a crown and root, is suspended in its bony socket, the alveolus, by a dense, collagenous connective tissue, the **periodontal ligament**. The crown of the tooth consists of two calcified tissues, **dentin** and **enamel**, whereas the root is composed of dentin and **cementum**. The pulp chamber of the crown and the root canal of the root are continuous with one another. They are occupied by a gelatinous connective tissue, the **pulp**, which houses blood and lymph vessels, nerve fibers, connective tissue elements, as well as **odontoblasts**, the cells responsible for the maintenance and repair of dentin. Vessels and nerves serving the pulp enter the root canal via the **apical foramen**, a small opening at the apex of the root.

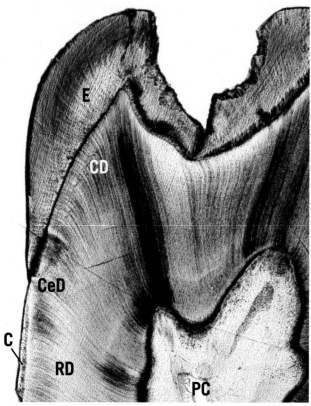

FIGURE 14-3. This very low-magnification photomicrograph of a ground section of a human molar tooth displays the **enamel** (E) overlying the **coronal dentin** (CD). Observe that the **cervical dentin** (CeD) and **radicular dentin** (RD) are both covered by **cementum** (C). The large space surrounded by the dentin is the **pulp cavity** (PC). ×14.

root (**radicular dentin**) and surrounds the **pulp**, a highly vascularized and ordered connective tissue. Enamel covers coronal dentin, **cementum** covers radicular dentin, and the two meet at the cervix. It should be noted that cementum is a part of the supporting apparatus of the tooth even though it is discussed here as part of the tooth.

- **Enamel** is the hardest substance in the body; it is 96% inorganic matrix composed of **calcium hydroxyapatite crystals** and 4% organic matrix consisting mostly of the protein **enamelin**. Enamel is manufactured by cells known as **ameloblasts** which are not present after the

tooth erupts into the oral cavity; therefore, the enamel is acellular posteruption and cannot repair itself.

- **Dentin** is the second hardest tissue in the body, it is 65% to 70% inorganic matrix composed of **calcium hydroxyapatite crystals** and 30% to 35% **type I collagen fibers**. Dentin is elaborated by cells known as **odontoblasts** whose cell bodies reside in the pulp, but their long cytoplasmic extensions occupy narrow tubules in the dentin, called **dentinal tubules**. Odontoblasts, therefore, continue to form and maintain dentin throughout the tooth's life.

- **Cementum** approximates bone in hardness, it is 45% to 50% inorganic matrix composed of **calcium hydroxyapatite crystals** and 50% to 55% type I collagen fibers, glycosaminoglycans, and proteoglycans. It is formed by cementoblasts that continue to manufacture cementum throughout the life of the tooth. Because the addition of cementum compensates for the erosion of enamel, it maintains the length of the tooth for proper occlusion.

- **Pulp** is a gelatinous, highly vascularized connective tissue that fills the **pulp cavity**, composed of the **pulp chamber** in the crown of the tooth and the **root canal** in the root of the tooth. The peripheral layer of the pulp is composed of **odontoblasts**. Deep to the odontoblasts is an acellular layer known as the **cell-free zone** and deep to that is a layer of fibroblasts and mesenchymal cells called the **cell-rich zone**. The **core of the pulp** is a connective tissue proper and houses blood vessels, lymph vessels, and nerve fibers (Fig. 14-4). The nerve fibers are of two types: **autonomic** that serve blood vessels and **sensory fibers** that conduct pain information from the pulp. The odontoblasts of the pulp can manufacture more dentin for the remainder of their lives.

Supporting Apparatus of the Tooth

The root of each tooth is suspended in its bony housing, the **alveolus**, by a dense collagenous connective tissue ligament, the **periodontal ligament**. The cervix of each tooth is surrounded by **gingiva** whose epithelium forms a collar, the **junctional epithelium**, whose attachment to the

CLINICAL CONSIDERATIONS 14-2

Caries

Caries, or cavities, are formed by the action of acid-secreting bacteria that adhere to very small defects or irregularities of the enamel surface. The acids formed by the bacteria decalcify the enamel, providing larger defects that can house a much larger number of the proliferating bacteria with the formation of more acid and

decalcification of more of the enamel. The carious lesion is pain-free until it reaches the underlying dentin. Because the most sensitive region of dentin is at the dentinoenamel junction, the tooth is sensitive to heat, cold, mechanical contact, and sweets. Continued bacterial activity, without the intervention of a dental health professional, could cause eventual loss of the tooth and perhaps even more serious sequelae.

CLINICAL CONSIDERATIONS 14-3

Pulp Disorders

Darkening of a tooth may be caused by **hemorrhage of the pulp**. Although, frequently, the pulp is damaged severely enough that it can no longer be saved, a dental professional should be consulted because tooth discoloration does not necessarily require root canal therapy.

As the individual ages, the pulp becomes more fibrotic with a concomitant reduction in the amounts of fine fibrils, extracellular matrix, and cellular elements. Other **age-related changes in the pulp** arise because the odontoblasts of the pulp continue to manufacture dentin, thereby decreasing the size of the pulp cavity. This decrease is especially noted in the roof of the pulp chamber as well as in the width of the root canal.

There are two types of **calcifications of the pulp**: dystrophic calcification and denticles. The former is located mostly in the pulp chamber and occurs along the collagenous sheaths that surround nerve fiber bundles and blood vessels. Denticles are present mostly in the root canals, and, as they grow, they may occlude most of the canal. The obstruction occasionally causes problems for endodontists as they are performing root canal treatments.

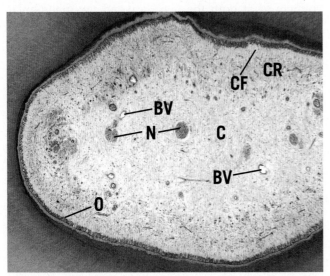

FIGURE 14-4. This very low-magnification photomicrograph displays the four layers of the pulp; the peripheral-most **odontoblastic layer** (O), surrounding the **cell-free zone** (CF), which surrounds the **cell-rich zone** (CR) and the bulk of the pulp, known as the **core** (C). Observe the numerous **blood vessels** (BV) and the **nerve fiber bundles** (N) throughout the core of the pulp. ×56.

cervical enamel creates occluding junctions, thus isolating the connective tissue of the gingiva from the oral cavity.

- The **alveolar process** is a bony extension of the mandible and the maxillae, in which the teeth are located. This bony process is partitioned into individual spaces, each known as an **alveolus**. The root of each tooth has its own alveolus, and the alveoli of adjacent teeth are separated from one another by an **interalveolar (interdental) septum**. The alveoli of teeth with two or more roots are modified so that bony septa, known as **interradicular septa**, are interposed between individual roots of the same tooth.

- Each alveolus has three component parts:

- cortical plate, the compact bone that is the lingual and labial continuation of the alveolar process,
- spongiosa, the cancellous bone that intervenes between the cortical plate and the alveolar bone proper, and
- alveolar bone proper, the conical-shaped plate of compact bone that immediately surrounds the root.

The **periodontal ligament (PDL)**, a dense irregular collagenous connective tissue whose type I collagen fibers are arranged in five named patterns (alveolar crest, horizontal, oblique, apical, and interradicular fiber groups), suspends the tooth in its alveolus. It is assisted in this function by the **gingiva** and its gingival fiber groups. The PDL is located in the **periodontal ligament space**, a very narrow space between the alveolar bone proper and the cementum of the root although the PDL space is somewhat wider apically and cervically than in the mid-length of the root (where, in a healthy mouth, it is ~1 mm wide). The terminus of each fiber group is embedded in cementum on the tooth side and the alveolar bone proper on the alveolar side, thereby suspending the tooth in its socket and preventing contact, and fusion, of the cementum of the tooth with the alveolar bone proper (Fig. 14-5).

The **gingiva (gum)** is covered by a stratified squamous (para-)keratinized epithelium. Its dense irregular collagenous connective tissue possesses type I collagen fibers that are arranged in five principal gingival fiber groups (alveologingival, dentogingival, circular, dentoperiosteal, and transseptal fiber groups). The gingiva has two regions, the coronally positioned **free gingiva** and the apically positioned **attached gingiva**.

- The free gingiva covers the **gingival sulcus** (less than 3 mm deep in a healthy mouth), a shallow groove between the soft tissue and enamel.

- The attached gingiva extends apically to the alveolar mucosa, the lining of the mouth that is covered by

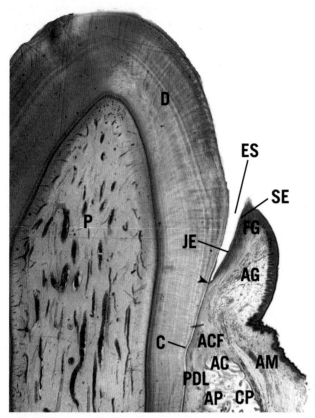

FIGURE 14-5. This very low-magnification photomicrograph of a decalcified tooth in its alveolus displays its **dentin** (D) and **pulp** (P). Because enamel is composed of 96% calcified material, decalcification removes almost all the enamel, leaving an empty **enamel space** (ES) that is most evident between the gingiva and the dentin, making it appear as if the gingival sulcus extended to the cementoenamel junction (*arrowhead*). The **sulcular epithelium** (SE) lines the sulcus and its apical continuation, the **junctional epithelium** (JE) adheres very tightly to the enamel surface. Observe the locations of the **free gingiva** (FG), **attached gingiva** (AG), and the **alveolar mucosa** (AM). Note that the **periodontal ligament** (PDL) is located between the **cementum** (C) and the **alveolar bone proper** (AP). The coronal-most region of the alveolus is the **alveolar crest** (AC), where the alveolar bone proper meets the **cortical plate** (CP). Observe the **alveolar crest fibers** (ACF) that extend from the cementum to insert into the alveolar crest. ×14.

a nonkeratinized stratified squamous epithelium. The attached gingiva adheres to the enamel surface by the formation of the **junctional epithelium** that adheres to a **basal lamina** that is located between the enamel surface and the junctional epithelium. This powerful attachment, mediated by hemidesmosomes, ensures that material in the oral cavity of a healthy mouth has no access to the PDL, maintaining the sterility of the connective tissue surrounding the teeth.

Odontogenesis

Morphology of Odontogenesis

Odontogenesis, tooth formation, begins at 6 1/2 weeks of development as a horseshoe-shaped epithelial band, known as the **dental lamina**, that arises from the oral epithelium of both the maxillary and the mandibular processes.

- Ten epithelial swellings, known as **tooth buds**, form on the lingual aspect of each dental lamina and press into the surrounding neural crest-derived ectomesenchyme (Fig. 14-6).

- Each tooth bud develops at a different rate, but all tooth buds initially form a three-dimensional hemispherical dome during the **cap stage** of tooth development as the concavity forms in the distal end of the bud. The epithelial hemispherical dome is called the **enamel organ** and it surrounds the neural crest-derived ectomesenchyme known as the **dental papilla**. The enamel organ and dental papilla together form the **tooth germ**.

- The enamel organ during the cap stage is composed of three epithelial layers: the **outer enamel epithelium**, the **inner enamel epithelium** separated by the third layer, the **stellate reticulum**, an ectoderm-derived mesenchyme. The region where the outer and inner enamel epithelia are continuous forms a rim called the **cervical loop**.

- The concavity of the inner enamel epithelial layer is filled with neural crest-derived ectomesenchymal cells, the **dental papilla**, which is responsible for the formation of **dentin** and the **pulp**.

CLINICAL CONSIDERATIONS 14-4

Necrotizing Ulcerative Gingivitis

Necrotizing ulcerative gingivitis is an acute ulcerative condition of the gingiva with accompanying necrosis, halitosis, erythematous appearance, and moderate to severe pain. Fever and regional lymphadenopathy may also be evident. This is usually a disease of the young adult who is experiencing stress and is not particularly attentive to dental hygiene. Frequently, *Treponema vincentii* and fusiform bacillus are present in large numbers, and they are also believed to be causative agents of the condition.

CLINICAL CONSIDERATIONS 14-5

Spindle Cell Carcinoma

Spindle cell carcinoma is a modified type of squamous cell carcinoma in which the histologic appearance of the malignant epithelial cells is spindle-shaped, resembling fibroblasts. It is highly aggressive, resulting in a survival rate of only 40% after 2 years. Spindle cell carcinoma is more common in males aged 60 years or older, and, in the oral region, this tumor is usually restricted to the gingiva, tongue, and lower lip. The most common causative agents of spindle cell carcinoma are alcoholism, tobacco use, and poor oral hygiene. Diagnostic features include painful inflammation, ulcers that do not heal readily, and growths that may be as large as 10 cm in diameter.

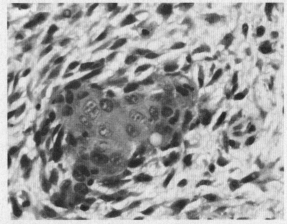

This light microscopic image from a patient with spindle cell carcinoma displays both epithelioid and spindle-shaped malignant cells. (Reprinted with permission from Mills SE, et al., eds. *Sternberg's Diagnostic Surgical Pathology*, 6th ed. Philadelphia: Wolters Kluwer, 2015. p. 872, Figure 19-42.)

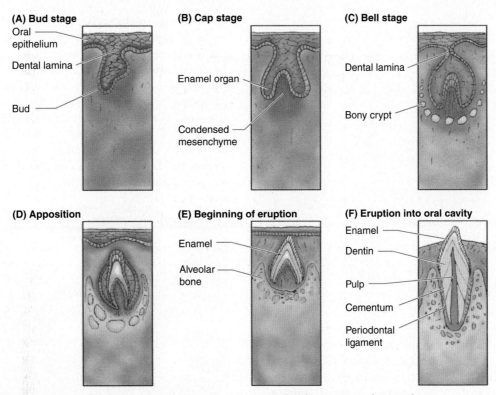

FIGURE 14-6. This schematic diagram presents the stages in the formation of a tooth.

• Ectomesenchymal cells surrounding the tooth germ condense to form a connective tissue capsule, the **dental sac**, around the developing tooth germ. The dental sac is responsible for the formation of cementum, the PDL, and the bony alveolus.

• A new epithelial growth develops from the dental lamina just lingually directed from the cap, known as the **succedaneous lamina**. This lamina grows deep into the ectomesenchyme, its distal terminus will form a tooth bud that will give rise to the permanent replacement of the forming deciduous tooth.

- A group of cells, most probably derived from the stellate reticulum, form a cluster against the inner enamel epithelium known as the **primary enamel knot**. These cells will either undergo apoptosis during the cap stage or survive into the next stage of tooth development.

- The inner enamel epithelial cells will differentiate into ameloblasts and will form the **enamel** of the tooth.

- As the cap enlarges and forms the fourth layer of cells, the stratum intermedium, located between the stellate reticulum and the inner enamel epithelium, the tooth germ enters the **bell stage** of odontogenesis (Fig. 14-7). If the enamel knot survives into the bell stage, the enamel organ rearranges itself to form a **premolar** or a **molar tooth**. If the enamel knot undergoes apoptosis during the cap stage, the developing tooth will be an **incisor or a canine tooth**.

- During the late bell stage, the peripheral-most cells of the dental papilla begin to differentiate into **odontoblasts** to start forming **dentin**. In response to the formation of the odontoblasts, the cells of the inner enamel epithelium differentiate into **ameloblasts** to start forming **enamel**.

- Once the tooth germ forms dentin as well as enamel, odontogenesis has progressed into a new stage known as **apposition**. The **appositional stage** of tooth development is responsible for the formation of the crown of the tooth.

- After the enamel of the crown is completely formed, odontogenesis enters its new phase, namely **root formation**. This process occurs simultaneously with **eruption**, in that as the root of the tooth increases in length the tooth moves toward the oral cavity and will erupt through the connective tissue and eventually the

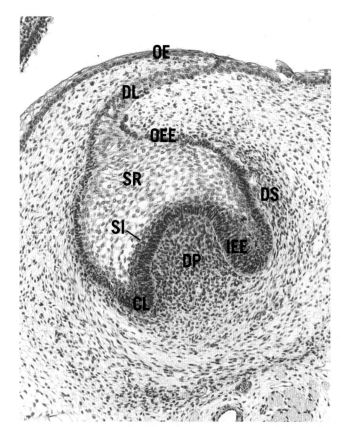

FIGURE 14-7. This low-magnification photomicrograph of a developing mandibular tooth displays the early to mid-bell stage of odontogenesis. Observe the **dental lamina** (DL) connecting the tooth germ to the **oral epithelium** (OE). The **outer enamel epithelium** (OEE) contacts the **inner enamel epithelium** (IEE) at the **cervical loop** (CL), and most of the space between these two layers is occupied by cells of the **stellate reticulum** (SR). Between the stellate reticulum and the IEE are cells of the **stratum intermedium** (SI). The concavity of the enamel organ is filled with cells of the **dental papilla** (DP), and the entire tooth germ is invested by cells of the **dental sac** (DS). ×132.

CLINICAL CONSIDERATIONS 14-6

Odontomas

Odontomas are hamartomatous anomalies (developmental malformations) that appear to be malignant but, fortunately, they are benign. These are the most frequent tumor-like structures of the maxillary and mandibular arches, and they arise from remnants of embryonic odontogenic tissues, forming tooth-like structures that are frequently calcified and display a haphazard arrangement. They are usually asymptomatic and are discovered on radiographs taken during routine dental examinations. Complex odontomas do not pose a significant health risk.

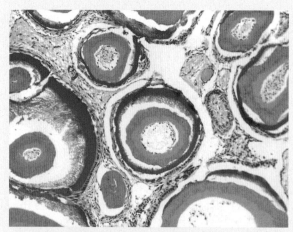

This light microscopic image from a patient with complex odontoma displays the presence of dentin, enamel, and pulp-like tissues scattered in a haphazard manner. (Reprinted with permission from Mills SE, et al., eds. *Sternberg's Diagnostic Surgical Pathology*, 6th ed. Philadelphia: Wolters Kluwer, 2015. p. 886, Figure 19-73.)

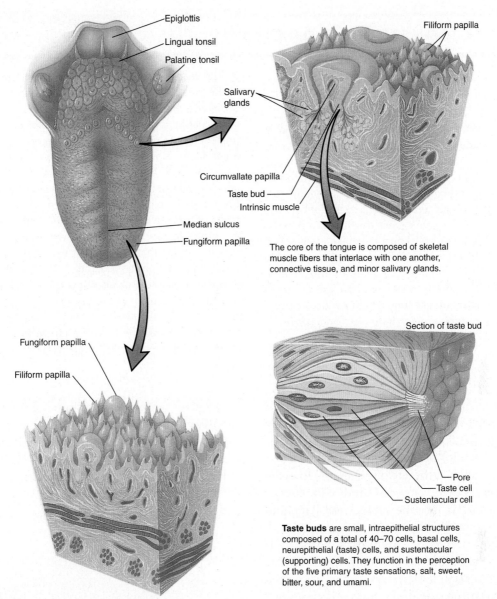

The core of the tongue is composed of skeletal muscle fibers that interlace with one another, connective tissue, and minor salivary glands.

Taste buds are small, intraepithelial structures composed of a total of 40–70 cells, basal cells, neurepithelial (taste) cells, and sustentacular (supporting) cells. They function in the perception of the five primary taste sensations, salt, sweet, bitter, sour, and umami.

FIGURE 14-8. Schematic representation of the tongue, its lingual papillae, and a taste bud. The dorsal surface of the tongue is subdivided into an anterior two-thirds, populated by the four types of lingual papillae, and a posterior third housing the lingual tonsils. The two regions are separated from one another by a V-shaped depression, the sulcus terminalis. **Filiform papillae** are short, conical, and highly keratinized. **Fungiform papillae** are mushroom-shaped, and the dorsal aspect of their epithelia houses 3 to 5 taste buds. **Circumvallate papillae**, the largest of the lingual papillae, are 6 to 12 in number. Each circumvallate papilla is depressed into the surface of the tongue and is surrounded by a moat-like trough. The lateral aspect of the papillae as well as the lining of the trough houses numerous taste buds. **Foliate papillae** are located on the lateral aspect of the tongue.

oral epithelium. Once the tooth reaches the oral cavity, it will continue to erupt at a rapid pace until it contacts its opposite in the other arch.

- It is important to understand that the root does not push the tooth into its position in the oral cavity; instead, osteoblasts on the floor of the alveolus form more bone, and this osteogenesis places forces on the developing root that cause its eruption.

- Additionally, the roof of the bony crypt surrounding the developing bone becomes resorbed by osteoclastic activity providing space for the erupting tooth.

Tongue

The tongue is a mucosal-invested movable, muscular structure that has two regions, the root (base) and the body (Fig. 14-8).

The **root** anchors the tongue into the hyoid bone, the posterior aspect of the oral cavity and the pharynx. The **body** is freely moving in the oral cavity, and its dorsal surface (facing the palate) is divided into anterior two-thirds and a posterior one-third by a shallow, posteriorly directed V-shaped groove, the **sulcus terminalis**, whose apex is a shallow depression, the **foramen cecum**.

CLINICAL CONSIDERATIONS 14-7

Tongue Disorders

During early embryogenesis of the head and neck, the thyroid gland begins its formation at the junction of the anterior two-thirds and posterior one-third of the tongue, at the apex of the future sulcus terminalis, the location of the foramen cecum. The thyroid gland, as any other endocrine gland, begins its development with the formation of a duct, the **thyroglossal duct**, that penetrates the substance of the tongue and descends to its normal location, just inferior to the larynx. Once the thyroid reaches its final location, the thyroglossal duct degenerates, although occasionally its remnant is evident in the anterior neck. In certain cases, the thyroid does not descend; instead, it remains on the surface of the tongue or within the substance of the tongue as a normally functioning endocrine gland manufacturing normal thyroid hormones and known as **lingual thyroid**.

The inferior aspect of the tongue is attached to the floor of the mouth by a slender, epithelially covered, connective tissue element known as the **lingual frenulum**. In some individuals, this frenulum is shorter and thicker than normal, preventing the normal range of movement of the tongue, a condition known as **ankyloglossia (tongue-tie)**. Infants born with this disorder may have difficulties nursing, and, as they get older, they may be unable to stick the tongue even to the occlusal surfaces of the mandibular teeth or even to reach the maxillary teeth. Children may be unable to pronounce certain words, especially if they contain sounds that require that the tongue interact with the teeth or the palate (e.g., "th," "d," and the letter "l"). In many cases, the problem corrects itself as children grow because the frenulum becomes looser, permitting a greater range of motion. However, in some cases, it may become necessary to incise the frenulum **(frenotomy)** or maybe even surgically remove the frenulum **(frenuloplasty)**.

During embryogenesis, the **thyroglossal duct** forms from the epithelial downgrowth at the foramen cecum and gives rise to the thyroid gland. Once thyroid is established, the thyroglossal duct degenerates but leaves behind an indentation at the site of origin, the foramen cecum. The dorsum of the posterior third of the tongue has crypts that burrow into the submucosal lymphoid tissue, the **lingual tonsil**.

The dorsum of the anterior two-thirds of the tongue is covered by **specialized mucosa** sporting **lingual papillae** some with taste buds, and the ventral surface is covered by **lining mucosa**. The core of the tongue is composed of two groups of skeletal muscle, the **intrinsic group** and the **extrinsic group**, interspersed with connective tissue and three pairs of minor salivary glands, **posterior mucous glands, glands of von Ebner** (purely **serous glands**), and **Blandin–Nuhn glands (mixed glands)**.

Lingual Papillae

The four types of **lingual papillae** are outgrowths of the mucosa of the dorsal surface.

Filiform papillae are the most numerous and are conical in shape, have no taste buds, and their stratified squamous epithelium is **highly keratinized. Fungiform papillae** are mushroom-shaped and possess a few **taste buds** on their free surface located within the nonkeratinized stratified squamous epithelium. **Foliate papillae** are located on the posterolateral aspects of the anterior two-thirds of the tongue. They present as shallow furrows that possess taste buds for the first 2 years of life, after which, the taste buds degenerate. Glands of von Ebner

release their serous secretion into the furrows. The 12 or so **circumvallate papillae**, located just anterior to the sulcus, possess numerous **taste buds** and are surrounded by a deep, moat-like furrow (Fig. 14-9). Glands of von Ebner release their serous secretion into the bottom of the moat-like depression.

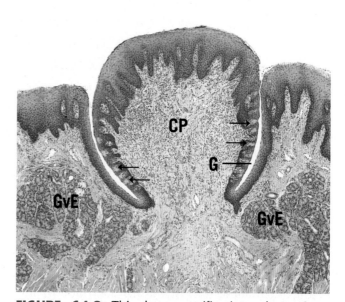

FIGURE 14-9. This low-magnification photomicrograph of a **circumvallate papilla** (CP) displays its associated **glands of von Ebner** (GvE), minor serous salivary glands that discharge their watery saliva into the bottom of the epithelially lined **groove** (G) that surrounds the papilla. Note that all the taste buds (*arrows*) are located in the epithelium along the lateral aspect of the circumvallate papilla. ×56.

Taste Buds and Taste Perception

Taste perception is performed by cells of the intraepithelial structures known as **taste buds**, located mostly on the dorsal surface of the tongue, although present also on the soft palate and pharynx (Fig. 14-10). They are composed of 60 to 80 spindle-shaped **neuroepithelial cells** that are of four types, **basal cells** (type IV) that act as regenerative cells, **dark cells** (type I cells, neuroepithelial cells) that probably arise directly from basal cells and mature into **light cells** (type II, sustentacular cells), and **intermediate cells** (type III cells) that will undergo apoptosis. The complete life cycle of these cells is about 10 days to 2 weeks, and they are continuously replaced by basal cell derivatives.

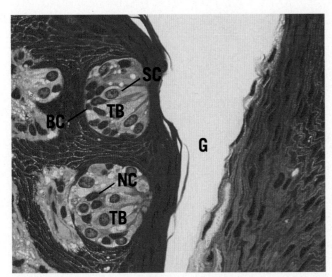

FIGURE 14-10. This high-magnification photomicrograph displays **taste buds** (TB) opening, via their taste pore, into the **groove** (G) surrounding the circumvallate papilla. With light microscopy three types of cells can be recognized, regenerative **basal cells** (BC), large **sustentacular cells** (SC), also known as light cells, and narrow **neuroepithelial cells** (NC), also known as dark cells. ×540.

The cells of the taste bud are compacted together and form an opening known as a **taste pore** at the epithelial surface. Basally, cell types I, II, and III form **synaptic contacts** with nerve fibers, and apically they possess long microvilli, known as **taste hairs,** that pass through the taste pore and are exposed to the moist environment of the oral cavity. The taste hairs have **taste receptors** that bind dissolved chemicals from the food, known as **tastants,** and the binding results in the opening of ion channels, thereby activating neuroepithelial cells which release neurotransmitter substances at their synaptic junctions with the nerve fibers. The central nervous system then registers the signal and interprets the taste that was sensed by the taste bud.

There are several types of taste receptors, some of which (**sweet**, **bitter**, and **umami**) require **G protein–linked receptors** embedded in the plasmalemmae of the taste hairs. Two of the following genes are responsible for the synthesis of receptors that recognize the tastes sweet and umami, namely **T1R1, T1R2**, and **T1R3**, whereas bitter taste is recognized by a large number of **T2R** receptors, the most common of which is **T2R38**. Sour and salt tastes are recognized by taste hair that possesses **hydrogen ion channels** and **sodium ion channels**, respectively. Individuals who can taste fat possess a **cluster of differentiation molecules 36 (CD36)** in the plasmalemmae of their taste hairs.

PLATE 14-1A Lip

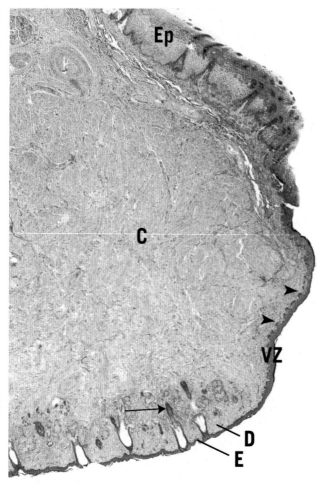

FIGURE 14-1-1. Lip. Human. Paraffin section. ×14.

The human lip presents three surfaces and a **core** (C). The external surface is covered by skin, composed of **epidermis** (E) and **dermis** (D). Associated hair follicles (*arrow*) and glands are evident. The **vermilion (red) zone** (VZ) is only found in humans. The high dermal papillae (*arrowheads*) carry blood vessels close to the surface, accounting for the pinkish coloration of this region. The internal aspect is lined by a wet, stratified, squamous, nonkeratinized **epithelium** (Ep), and the underlying connective tissue houses minor salivary glands. The core of the lip is composed of skeletal muscle interspersed with fibroelastic connective tissue.

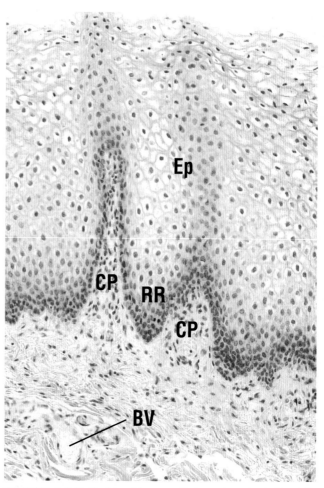

FIGURE 14-1-2. Lip. Human. Internal aspect. Paraffin section. ×270.

The internal aspect of the lip is lined by a mucous membrane that is continuously kept moist by saliva secreted by the three major and numerous minor salivary glands. The thick **epithelium** (Ep) is a stratified squamous nonkeratinized type, which presents deep **rete ridges** (RR) that interdigitate with the **connective tissue papillae** (CP). The connective tissue is fibroelastic in nature, displaying a rich **vascular supply** (BV).

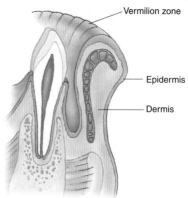

Lip

KEY					
BV	vascular supply	**D**	dermis	**RR**	rete ridges
C	core	**E**	epidermis	**VZ**	vermilion (red) zone
CP	connective tissue papillae	**Ep**	epithelium		

PLATE 14-1B Lip

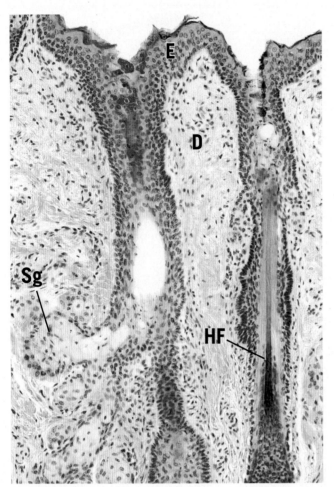

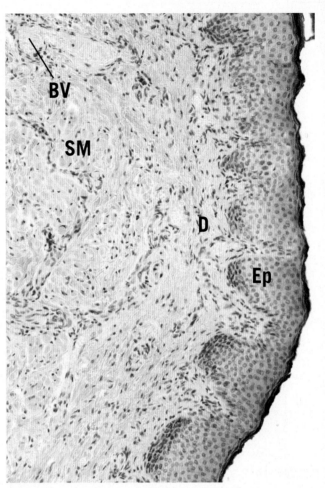

FIGURE 14-1-3. Lip. Human. External aspect. Paraffin section. ×132.

The external aspect of the lip is covered by thin skin. Neither the **epidermis** (E) nor the **dermis** (D) presents any unusual features. Numerous **hair follicles** (HF) populate this aspect of the lip, and **sebaceous glands** (Sg) and sweat glands are noted in abundance.

FIGURE 14-1-4. Lip. Human. Vermilion zone. Paraffin section. ×132.

The vermilion zone of the lip is covered by a modified skin composed of stratified squamous keratinized **epithelium** (Ep) that forms extensive interdigitations with the underlying **dermis** (D). Neither hair follicles nor sweat glands populate this area (though occasional sebaceous glands may be present). Note the cross-sectional profiles of **skeletal muscle fibers** (SM) and the rich **vascular supply** (BV) of the lip.

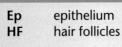

KEY					
BV	vascular supply	Ep	epithelium	Sg	sebaceous glands
D	dermis	HF	hair follicles	SM	skeletal muscle fibers
E	epidermis				

PLATE 14-2A Tooth

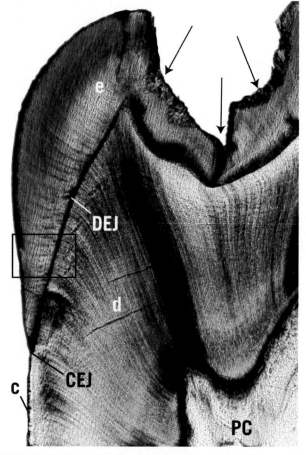

FIGURE 14-2-1. Tooth. Human. Ground section. ×14.

The tooth consists of a crown, neck, and root, composed of calcified tissue surrounding a chamber housing a soft, gelatinous pulp. In ground section, only the hard tissues remain. The crown is composed of **enamel** (e) and **dentin** (d), whose interface is known as the **dentinoenamel junction** (DEJ). At the neck of the tooth, enamel meets **cementum** (c), forming the **cementoenamel junction** (CEJ). The **pulp chamber** (PC) is reduced in size as the individual ages. The gap in the enamel (*arrows*) is caused by the presence of a carious lesion (cavity). A region similar to the *boxed area* is presented at a higher magnification in Figure 14-2-2.

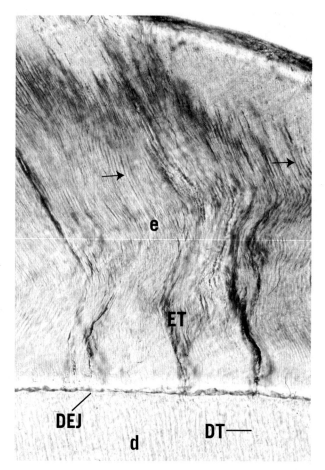

FIGURE 14-2-2. Tooth. Human. Ground section. ×132.

This photomicrograph is a higher magnification of a region similar to the *boxed area* of Figure 14-2-1. The **enamel** (e) is composed of enamel rods (*arrows*), each surrounded by a rod sheath. Hypomineralized regions of enamel present the appearance of tufts of grass, **enamel tufts** (ET), which extend from the **dentinoenamel junction** (DEJ) partway into the enamel. **Dentin** (d), not as highly calcified as enamel, presents long, narrow canals, **dentinal tubules** (DT), which, in the living tooth, house processes of odontoblasts, cells responsible for the formation of dentin.

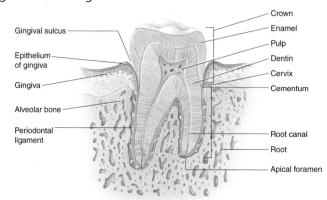

KEY					
c	cementum	**DEJ**	dentinoenamel junction	**ET**	enamel tufts
CEJ	cementoenamel junction	**DT**	dentinal tubules	**PC**	pulp chamber
d	dentin	**e**	enamel		

PLATE 14-2B   Pulp

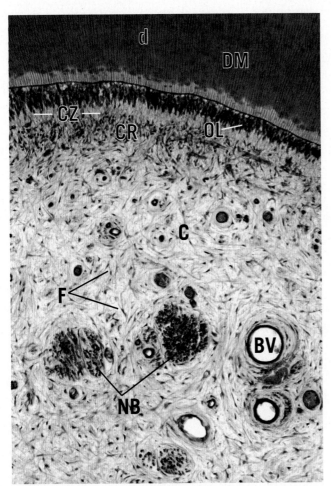

FIGURE 14-2-3. Pulp. Human. Paraffin section. ×132.

The pulp is surrounded by **dentin** (d) from which it is separated by a noncalcified **dentin matrix** (DM). The pulp is said to possess four regions: the **odontoblastic layer** (OL), the **cell-free zone** (CZ), the **cell-rich zone** (CR), and the **core** (C). The core of the pulp is composed of **fibroblasts** (F), delicate collagen fibers, numerous **nerve bundles** (NB), and **blood vessels** (BV). Branches of these neurovascular structures reach the periphery of the pulp, where they supply the cell-rich zone and the odontoblasts with capillaries and fine nerve fibers.

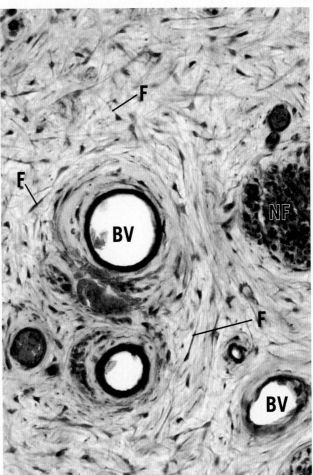

FIGURE 14-2-4. Pulp. Human. Paraffin section. ×270.

This is a higher magnification of the lower right corner of Figure 14-2-3. Note the presence of **blood vessels** (BV) and **nerve fibers** (NF), as well as the numerous **fibroblasts** (F) of this gelatinous connective tissue.

KEY						
BV	blood vessel	**d**	dentin	**NB**	nerve bundles
C	core	**DM**	dentin matrix	**NF**	Nerve fibers
CR	cell-rich zone	**F**	fibroblasts	**OL**	odontoblastic layer
CZ	cell-free zone				

PLATE 14-3A   Periodontal Ligament

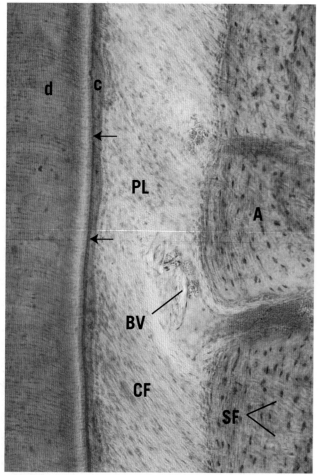

FIGURE 14-3-1. Periodontal ligament. Human. Paraffin section. ×132.

The root of the tooth, composed of **dentin** (d) and **cementum** (c), is suspended in its **alveolus** (A) by a collagenous tissue, the **periodontal ligament** (PL). The strong bands of **collagen fibers** (CF) are embedded in the bone via **Sharpey's fibers** (SF). **Blood vessels** (BV) from the bone enter and supply the PL. The dentinocemental junction (*arrows*) is clearly evident. Near the apex of the root, the cementum becomes thicker and houses cementocytes.

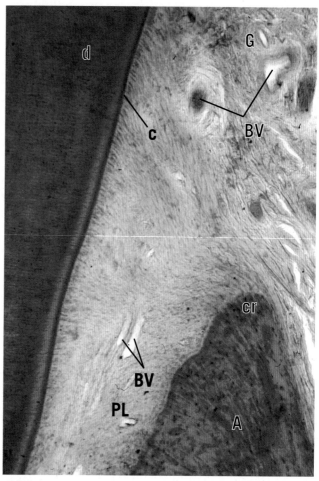

FIGURE 14-3-2. Periodontal ligament. Human. Paraffin section. ×270.

The root of the tooth, composed of **dentin** (d) and **cementum** (c), is suspended in its bony **alveolus** (A) by fibers of the **periodontal ligament** (PL). Note that this photomicrograph is taken in the region of the **crest** (cr) of the alveolus, above which the PL is continuous with the connective tissue of the **gingiva** (G). Note that both the gingiva and the periodontal ligament are highly vascular, as evident from the abundance of **blood vessels** (BV).

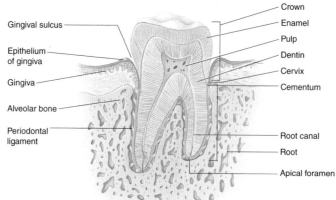

Gingival sulcus	Crown
	Enamel
Epithelium of gingiva	Pulp
	Dentin
Gingiva	Cervix
	Cementum
Alveolar bone	
Periodontal ligament	Root canal
	Root
	Apical foramen

KEY					
A	alveolus	**CF**	collagen fibers	**PL**	periodontal ligament
BV	blood vessels	**cr**	crest	**SF**	Sharpey's fibers
c	cementum	**G**	gingiva		

PLATE 14-3B Gingiva

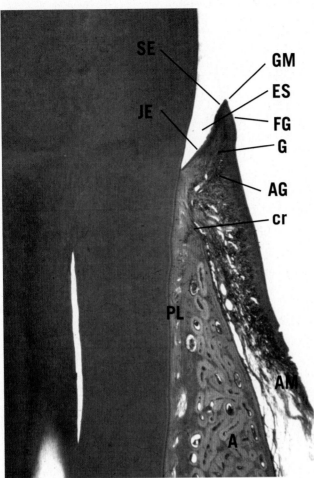

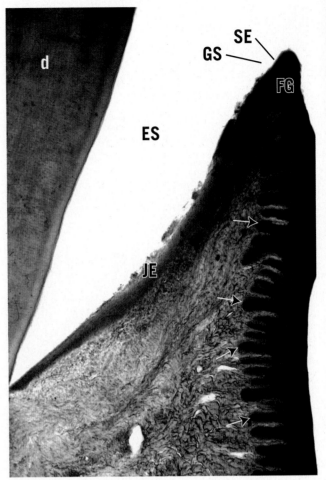

FIGURE 14-3-3. Gingiva. Human. Paraffin section. ×14.

This is a decalcified longitudinal section of an incisor tooth; thus, all the calcium hydroxyapatite crystals have been extracted from the tooth and from its bony **alveolus** (A). Because enamel is composed almost completely of calcium hydroxyapatite crystals, only the space where enamel used to be, the **enamel space** (ES), is represented in this photomicrograph. The **crest** (cr) of the alveolus is evident, as are the **periodontal ligament** (PL) and the **gingiva** (G). The **gingival margin** (GM), **free gingiva** (FG), **attached gingiva** (AG), **sulcular epithelium** (SE), **junctional epithelium** (JE), and **alveolar mucosa** (AM) are also identified.

FIGURE 14-3-4. Gingiva. Human. Paraffin section. ×132.

This photomicrograph is a higher magnification of the gingival margin region of Figure 14-3-3. Note that the **enamel space** (ES) is located between the **dentin** (d) of the incisor tooth's crown and the **junctional epithelium** (JE). The **sulcular epithelium** (SE) of the **free gingiva** (FG) borders a space known as the **gingival sulcus** (GS), which would be clearly evident if the enamel were still present in this photomicrograph. Observe the well-developed interdigitations of the epithelium and connective tissue, known as the rete apparatus (*arrows*) of the **free gingiva** (FG) and **attached gingiva**, indicative of the presence of abrasive forces that act on these regions of the oral cavity.

KEY							
A	alveolus	**ES**	enamel space	**GS**	gingival sulcus		
AG	attached gingiva	**FG**	free gingiva	**JE**	junctional epithelium		
AM	alveolar mucosa	**G**	gingiva	**PL**	periodontal ligament		
cr	crest	**GM**	gingival margin	**SE**	sulcular epithelium		
d	dentin						

PLATE 14-4A Tooth Development

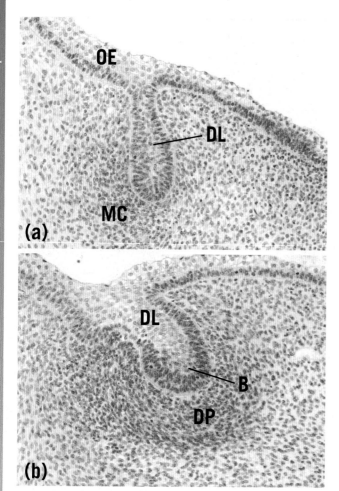

(a)

(b)

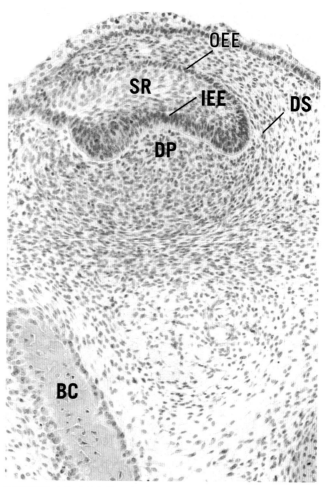

FIGURE 14-4-1A. Tooth development. Dental lamina. Frontal section. Pig. Paraffin section. ×132.

The **dental lamina** (DL) is a horseshoe-shaped band of epithelial tissue that arises from the **oral epithelium** (OE) and is surrounded by **mesenchymal cells** (MC). A frontal section of the dental lamina is characterized by the club-shaped appearance in this photomicrograph. The MC in discrete regions at the distal aspect of the dental lamina become rounded and congregate to form the precursor of the dental papilla responsible for the formation of the pulp and dentin of the tooth.

FIGURE 14-4-1B. Tooth development. Bud stage. Frontal section. Pig. Paraffin section. ×132.

At various discrete locations along the **dental lamina** (DL), an epithelial thickening, the **bud** (B), makes its appearance. Each bud will provide the cells necessary for enamel formation for a single tooth. The **dental papilla** (DP) forms a crescent-shaped area at the distal aspect of the bud.

FIGURE 14-4-2. Tooth development. Cap stage. Frontal section. Pig. Paraffin section. ×132.

Increased mitotic activity transforms the bud into a cap-shaped structure. Observe that three epithelial layers of the enamel organ may be recognized: the **outer enamel epithelium** (OEE), the **inner enamel epithelium** (IEE), and the intervening **stellate reticulum** (SR). The inner enamel epithelium has begun to enclose the **dental papilla** (DP). Note that mesenchymal cells become elongated, forming the **dental sac** (DS), which will envelop the enamel organ and dental papilla. Moreover, a **bony crypt** (BC) will enclose the dental sac.

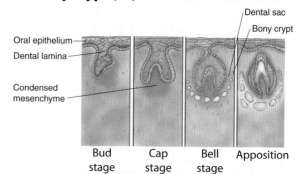

Bud stage	Cap stage	Bell stage	Apposition

KEY					
B	bud	**DS**	dental sac	**OE**	oral epithelium
BC	bony crypt	**IEE**	inner enamel epithelium	**OEE**	outer enamel epithelium
DL	dental lamina	**MC**	mesenchymal cells	**SR**	stellate reticulum
DP	dental papilla				

PLATE 14-4B Tooth Development

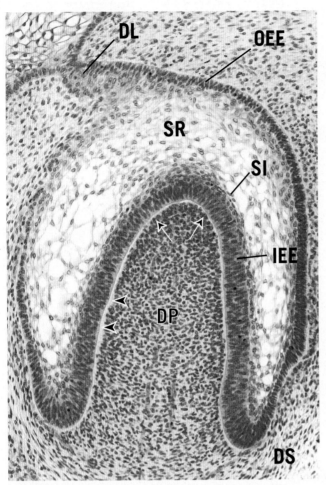

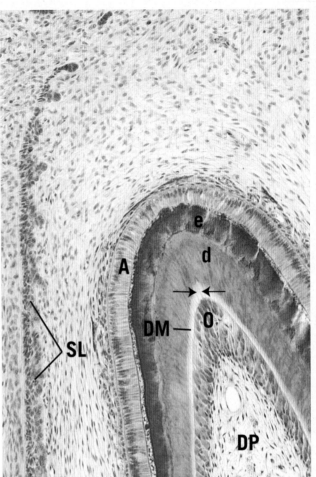

FIGURE 14-4-3. Tooth development. Bell stage. Frontal section. Pig. Paraffin section. ×132.

As the enamel organ expands in size, it resembles a bell, hence the bell stage of tooth development. This stage is characterized by four cellular layers: **outer enamel epithelium** (OEE), **stellate reticulum** (SR), **inner enamel epithelium** (IEE), and **stratum intermedium** (SI). Observe that the enamel organ is still connected to the **dental lamina** (DL). The **dental papilla** (DP) is composed of rounded mesenchymal cells, whose peripheral-most layer (*arrows*) will differentiate to form odontoblasts. Note the wide basement membrane (*arrowheads*) between the future odontoblasts and inner enamel epithelium (the future ameloblasts). Observe also the spindle-shaped cells of the **dental sac** (DS).

FIGURE 14-4-4. Tooth development. Apposition. Frontal section. Pig. Paraffin section. ×132.

The elaboration of **dentin** (d) and **enamel** (e) is indicative of apposition. Dentin is manufactured by **odontoblasts** (O), the peripheral-most cell layer of the **dental papilla** (DP). The odontoblastic processes (*arrows*) are visible in this photomicrograph as they traverse the **dentin matrix** (DM). **Ameloblasts** (A) are highly elongated, columnar cells that manufacture enamel. The long, epithelial structure located to the left is the **succedaneous lamina** (SL), which is responsible for the development of the permanent tooth.

KEY					
A	ameloblast	DS	dental sac	OEE	outer enamel epithelium
d	dentin	e	enamel	SI	stratum intermedium
DL	dental lamina	IEE	inner enamel epithelium	SL	succedaneous lamina
DM	dentin matrix	O	odontoblasts	SR	stellate reticulum
DP	dental papilla				

PLATE 14-5A Tongue

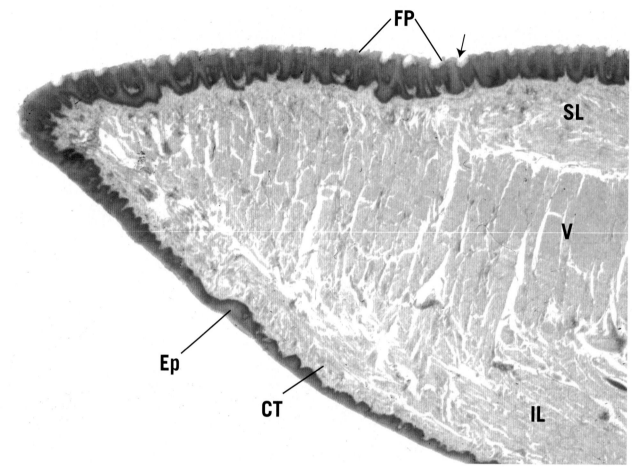

FIGURE 14-5-1. Tongue. Human. l.s. Paraffin section. ×20.

Part of the anterior two-thirds of the tongue is presented in this photomicrograph. This muscular organ bears numerous **filiform papillae** (FP) on its dorsal surface, whose stratified squamous epithelium is keratinized (*arrow*). The ventral surface of the tongue is lined by stratified squamous nonkeratinized **epithelium** (Ep). The intrinsic muscles of the tongue are arranged in four layers: **superior longitudinal** (SL), **vertical** (V), **inferior longitudinal** (IL), and horizontal (not shown here). The mucosa of the tongue tightly adheres to the perimysium of the intrinsic tongue muscles by the subepithelial **connective tissue** (CT).

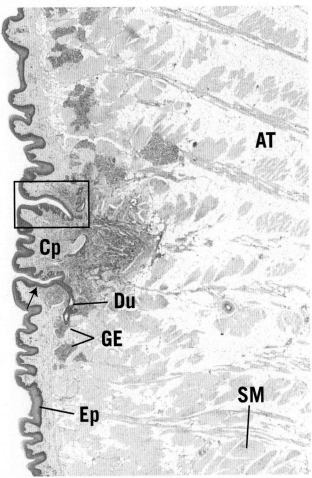

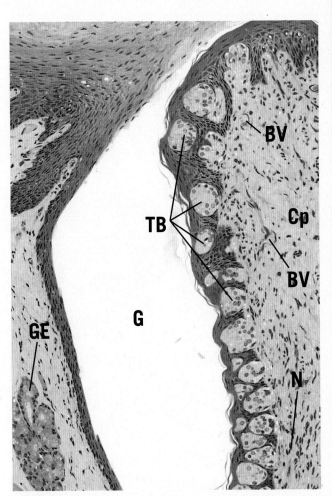

FIGURE 14-5-2. Tongue. Human. l.s. Paraffin section. ×14.

The posterior aspect of the anterior two-thirds of the tongue presents **circumvallate papillae** (Cp). These papillae are surrounded by a deep groove (*arrow*), the base of which accepts a serous secretion via the **ducts** (Du) of the **glands of von Ebner** (GE). The **epithelium** (Ep) of the papilla houses taste buds along its lateral aspects but not on its superior surface. The core of the tongue contains **skeletal muscle** (SM) fibers as well as glands and **adipose tissue** (AT). A region similar to the *boxed area* is presented at a higher magnification in Figure 14-5-3.

FIGURE 14-5-3. Circumvallate papilla. Monkey. x.s. Plastic section. ×132.

This photomicrograph is a higher magnification of a region similar to the *boxed area* of Figure 14-5-2, rotated 90°. Note the presence of the **groove** (G) separating the **circumvallate papilla** (Cp) from the wall of the groove. **Glands of von Ebner** (GE) deliver a serous secretion into this groove, whose contents are monitored by numerous intraepithelial **taste buds** (TB). Observe that taste buds are not present on the superior surface of the circumvallate papilla, only on its lateral aspect. The connective tissue core of the papilla is richly endowed by **blood vessels** (BV) and **nerves** (N).

KEY					
AT	adipose tissue	**Ep**	epithelium	**SL**	superior longitudinal muscle
Cp	circumvallate papillae	**FP**	filiform papillae		
CT	connective tissue	**GE**	glands of von Ebner	**SM**	skeletal muscle
Du	ducts	**IL**	inferior longitudinal muscle	**V**	vertical muscle

KEY					
BV	blood vessels	**G**	groove	**N**	nerves
Cp	circumvallate papilla	**GE**	glands of von Ebner	**TB**	taste buds

PLATE 14-6A Tongue

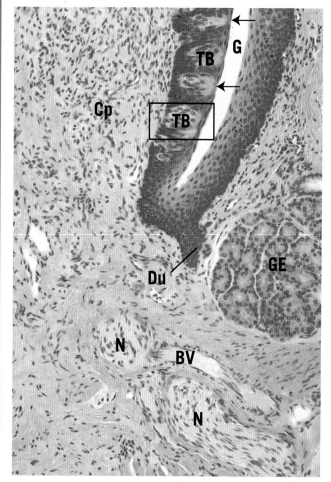

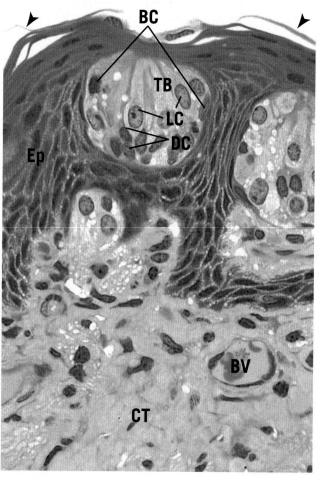

FIGURE 14-6-1. Circumvallate papilla. Monkey. Paraffin section. ×132.

The base of the **circumvallate papilla** (Cp), the surrounding **groove** (G), and the wall of the groove are evident in this photomicrograph. The **glands of von Ebner** (GE) deliver their serous secretions via short **ducts** (Du) into the base of the groove. Observe the rich **vascular** (BV) and **nerve** (N) supply to this region. Numerous **taste buds** (TB) populate the epithelium of the lateral aspect of the circumvallate papilla. Each taste bud possesses a taste pore (*arrows*) through which taste hairs (microvilli) protrude into the groove. A region similar to the *boxed area* is presented at a higher magnification in Figure 14-6-2.

FIGURE 14-6-2. Taste bud. Monkey. Paraffin section. ×540.

This is a higher magnification of a region similar to the *boxed area* of Figure 14-6-1. Note that the stratified squamous parakeratinized **epithelium** (Ep) displays squames in the process of desquamation (*arrowheads*). The **taste buds** (TB) are composed of four cell types. **Basal** (lateral) **cells** (BC) are believed to be regenerative in nature, whereas **light cells** (LC), intermediate cells, and **dark cells** (DC) are gustatory. Observe the presence of **blood vessels** (BV) in the subepithelial **connective tissue** (CT).

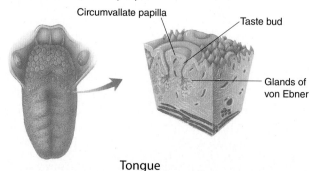

Circumvallate papilla

Taste bud

Glands of von Ebner

Tongue

KEY					
BC	basal cells	**DC**	dark cells	**GE**	glands of von Ebner
BV	blood vessels	**Du**	ducts	**LC**	light cells
Cp	circumvallate papilla	**Ep**	epithelium	**N**	Nerves
CT	connective tissue	**G**	groove	**TB**	taste buds

PLATE 14-6B   Palate

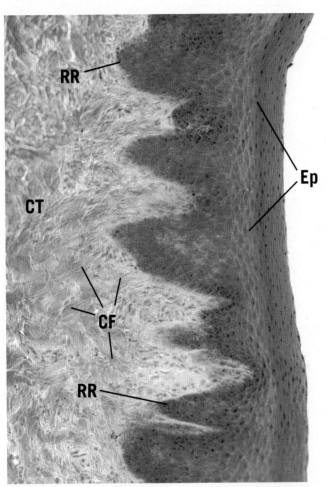

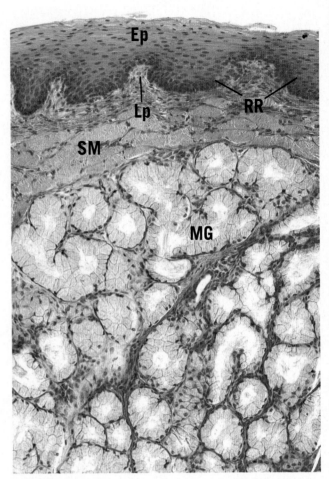

FIGURE 14-6-3. Hard palate. Human. Paraffin section. ×132.

The hard palate possesses a nasal and an oral surface. The stratified squamous parakeratinized **epithelium** (Ep) of the oral surface forms deep invaginations, **rete ridges** (RR), which interdigitate with the subepithelial **connective tissue** (CT). The thick **collagen fiber bundles** (CF) firmly bind the palatal mucosa to the periosteum of the underlying bone. The hard palate also houses large deposits of adipose tissue and mucous glands.

FIGURE 14-6-4. Soft palate. Human. Paraffin section. ×132.

The oral surface of the soft palate is lined by a stratified squamous nonkeratinized **epithelium** (Ep), which interdigitates with the **lamina propria** (LP) by the formation of shallow **rete ridges** (RR). The soft palate is a movable structure, as attested by the presence of **skeletal muscle fibers** (SM). The core of the soft palate also houses numerous **mucous glands** (MG) that deliver their secretory products into the oral cavity via short, straight ducts.

KEY

CF	collagen fiber bundles	LP	lamina propria	RR	rete ridges
CT	connective tissue	MG	mucous glands	SM	skeletal muscle
Ep	epithelium				

PLATE 14-7A   Teeth

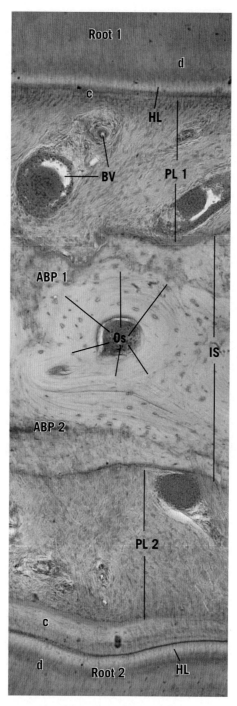

FIGURE 14-7-1. Human central incisor roots. Paraffin section. ×132.

The roots of two human central incisors and their supporting tissues are noted in this composite photomicrograph. Note that the root of one incisor, root 1, is at the top of the figure, and progressing down the page, the **hyaline layer of Hopewell–Smith** (HL) separates the **dentin** (d) of the root from the **cementum** (c). The **periodontal ligament** (PL 1), with its attendant **blood vessels** (BV), of this tooth suspends tooth 1 in its alveolus. The **interdental septum** (IS), positioned between the two incisors and composed of woven bone, is formed by the fusion of the **alveolar bones proper** (ABP 1 and 2) of each root. Note the presence of **osteons** (Os) in the woven bone; the center of these osteons approximates the line of fusion between the two ABP. The **periodontal ligament** of the other incisor (PL 2) is located between the **alveolar bone proper** (ABP 2) and the **cementum** of this tooth. Its **dentin** (d) and **hyaline layer of Hopewell–Smith** (HL) of root 2 are evident.

KEY					
ABP	alveolar bone proper	**d**	dentin	**IS**	interdental septum
BV	blood vessels	**HL**	hyaline layer of	**Os**	osteons
c	cementum		Hopewell–Smith	**PL**	periodontal ligament

PLATE 14-7B   Nasal Aspect of the Hard Palate

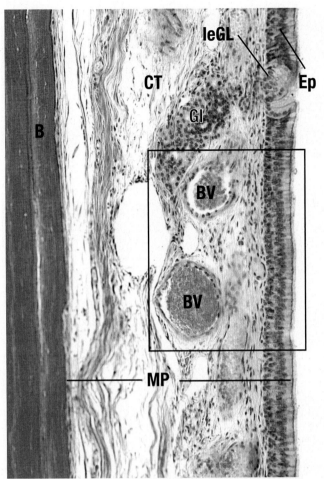

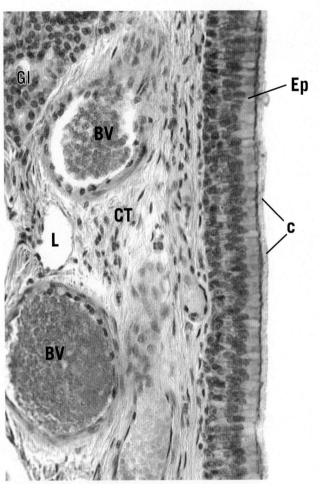

FIGURE 14-7-2. Hard palate. Human. Paraffin section. ×132.

The hard palate possesses a nasal and an oral surface. Note that the pseudostratified ciliated columnar **epithelium** (Ep) displays cilia and an **intraepithelial gland** (IeGL). Observe the presence of **glands** (Gl) and **blood vessels** (BV) in the subepithelial **connective tissue** (CT). The epithelium and the subepithelial connective tissue are collectively referred to as the **mucoperiosteum** (MP), which is firmly attached to the **bony shelf** (B) of the palate. A higher magnification of the *boxed area* is presented in Figure 14-7-3.

FIGURE 14-7-3. Hard palate. Human. Paraffin section. ×132.

This is a higher magnification of a region similar to the *boxed area* of Figure 14-7-2. Note the presence of **glands** (Gl), **blood vessels** (BV), and **lymph vessels** (LV) within the subepithelial **connective tissue** (CT). Observe the clearly visible **cilia** (c) of the pseudostratified ciliated columnar **epithelium** (Ep) covering the nasal surface of the hard palate.

KEY					
B	bony shelf	**CT**	connective tissue	**LV**	lymph vessel
BV	blood vessels	**Ep**	epithelium	**MP**	mucoperiosteum
c	cilia	**Gl**	glands		
CF	collagen fiber bundles	**IeGL**	intraepithelial gland		

PLATE 14-8 Scanning Electron Micrograph of Tooth Enamel

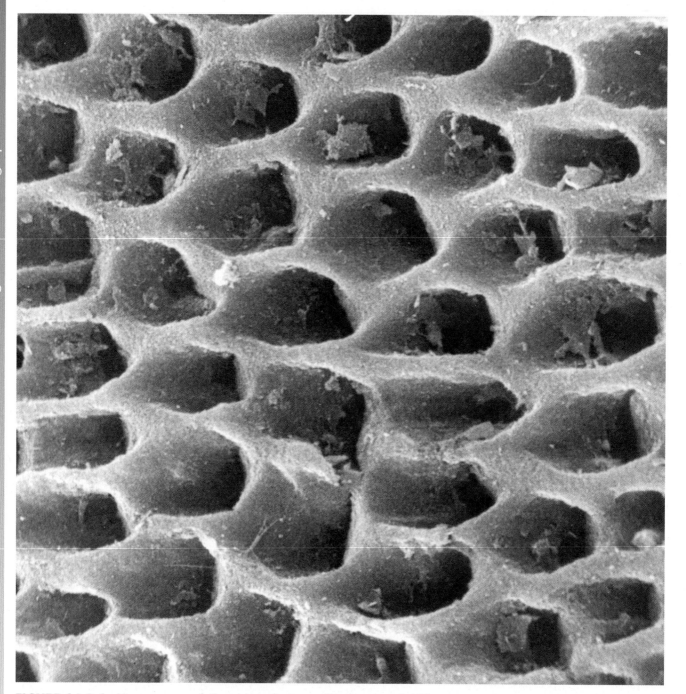

FIGURE 14-8-1. Human enamel. Scanning electron microscopy. ×3,150.

This three-dimensional view of the forming mineralized human enamel displays rod spaces (the recesses) surrounded by the inter-rod enamel. The rod spaces were occupied by Tomes' processes of the ameloblasts, and, as the ameloblasts recede, rod spaces are filled in by the secretory mechanism and the spaces are filled by enamel known as rod segments. The arched aspects of the rod spaces are directed occlusally. As rod segments are positioned on top of each other, they form an enamel rod whose shape resembles a keyhole. (From Fejerskov O. Human dentition and experimental animals. *J Dent* Res 1979;58(Special Issue B):725–734. Copyright © 1979 SAGE Publications. Reprinted by permission of SAGE Publications, Inc.)

PLATE 14-9 Scanning Electron Micrograph of Tooth Dentin

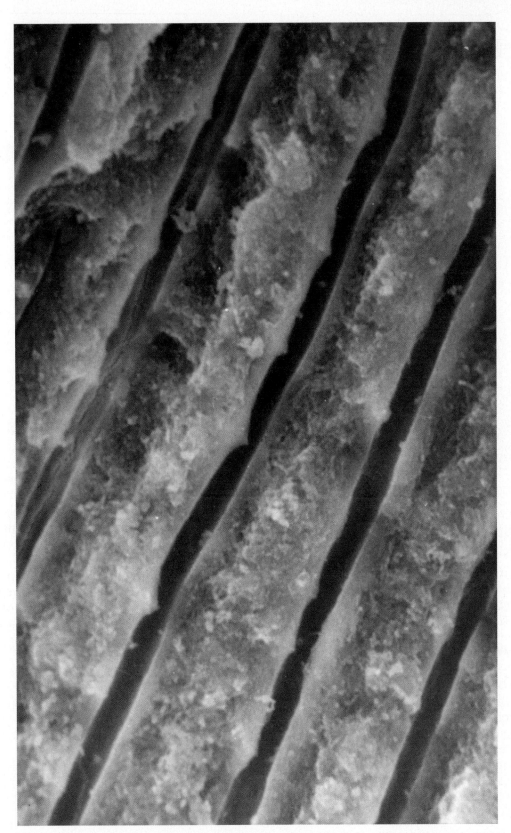

FIGURE 14-9-1. Human dentin. Scanning electron microscopy. ×3,800.

This three-dimensional view of mineralized human dentin displays a longitudinal section of dentinal tubules. In healthy, living dentin, the tubules house the processes of odontoblasts that extend at least 1 mm into the dentinal tubule. Additionally, some of the tubules also house nerve fibers, and all the tubules are filled completely with an extracellular fluid that originates in the pulp of the tooth. (From Thomas HF. The dentin-predentin complex and its permeability: anatomical overview. *J Dent* Res 1985;64(4):607–612. Copyright © 1985 SAGE Publications. Reprinted by permission of SAGE Publications, Inc.)

Selected Review of Histologic Images

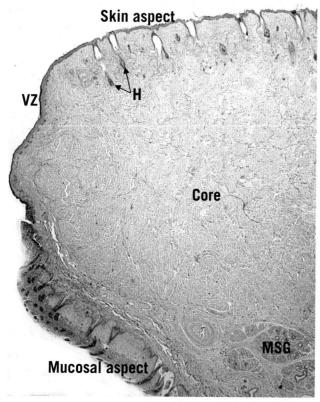

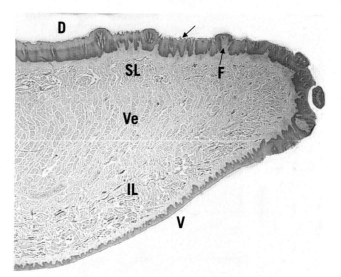

REVIEW FIGURE 14-1-1. Lip. Human l.s. Paraffin section. ×14.

This is a low-magnification photomicrograph of the human lip showing that its **core** of skeletal muscle and some connective tissue is covered by a stratified squamous epithelium whose structure determines the three aspects of the lip. The internal, or **mucosal aspect**, is a wet epithelium that is not cornified. The subepithelial connective tissue houses minor **mucous salivary glands** (MSG). The middle aspect of the lip—where the lipstick is placed—is the **vermilion zone** (VZ), devoid of hair follicles but is keratinized. Its rete apparatus is highly convoluted, permitting capillary loops to reach near the surface, imparting a pink coloration to this region. The external, or **skin aspect**, is a thin skin displaying **hair follicles** (H). (Reprinted with permission from Gartner LP. *Oral Histology and Embryology*, 3rd ed. Baltimore: Jen House Publishing Company, 2014.)

REVIEW FIGURE 14-1-2. Tongue tip. Human l.s. Paraffin section. ×14.

This is a low magnification of the tip of a human tongue showing that its core is composed of skeletal muscle fibers, arranged in four different orientations, **superior longitudinal** (SL), **vertical** (Ve), **inferior longitudinal** (IL), and horizontal (not shown). The epithelial covering of the tongue is stratified squamous. It is keratinized on its **dorsal surface** (D) and nonkeratinized on its **ventral surface** (V). The dorsal surface of the tongue presents with lingual papillae, two types of which are visible in this photomicrograph, the highly keratinized and most numerous filiform papillae (*arrow*), and the mushroom-shaped **fungiform papillae** (F). (Reprinted with permission from Gartner LP. *Oral Histology and Embryology*, 3rd ed. Baltimore: Jen House Publishing Company, 2014.)

KEY					
D	dorsal surface	**MSG**	mucous salivary glands	**Ve**	vertical muscle
F	fungiform papilla	**SL**	superior longitudinal muscle	**VZ**	vermilion zone
H	hair follicles				
IL	inferior longitudinal muscle	**V**	ventral surface		

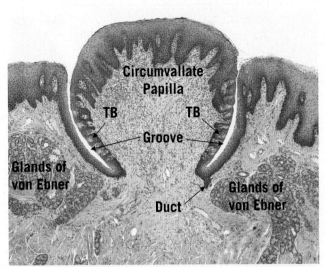

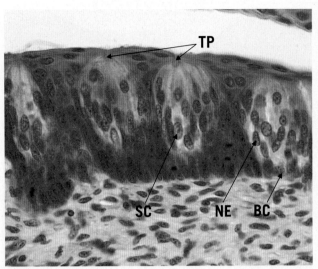

REVIEW FIGURE 14-1-3. Tongue tip. Human l.s. Paraffin section. ×14.

This is a low-magnification photomicrograph of a **circumvallate papilla** from a human tongue. Note that the subepithelial connective tissue of this region of the dorsal tongue surface has **glands of von Ebner** whose **ducts** deliver their serous secretion into the **groove** that surrounds the circumvallate papilla. Observe that the wall of the circumvallate papilla is rich in **taste buds** (TB). (Reprinted with permission from Gartner LP. *Oral Histology and Embryology*, 3rd ed. Baltimore: Jen House Publishing Company, 2014.)

REVIEW FIGURE 14-1-4. Tongue tip. Human l.s. Paraffin section. ×540.

This photomicrograph presents four taste buds located on the wall of the circumvallate papilla in the previous figure. Note that the orientation of this photomicrograph is perpendicular to that of Review Figure 14-1-3. The classical description, as viewed with the light microscope, describes three types of cells, short **basal cells** (BC), lightly staining **sustentacular cells** (SC), and dark **neuroepithelial cells** (NE). Observe the **taste pores** (TP) that open into the groove surrounding the circumvallate papilla. (Reprinted with permission from Gartner LP. *Oral Histology and Embryology*, 3rd ed. Baltimore: Jen House Publishing Company, 2014.)

KEY					
BC	basal cells	**SC**	sustentacular cells	**TP**	taste pores
NE	neuroepithelial cells	**TB**	taste buds		

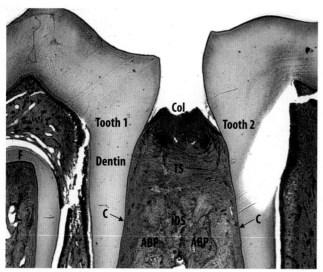

REVIEW FIGURE 14-2-1. Adjoining first and second molar teeth. Human l.s. Paraffin section. ×14.

The two molars (tooth 1 and tooth 2) are separated from each other by a bony **interdental septum** (IDS) whose region that surrounds the root of each tooth is known as the **alveolar bone proper** (ABP). The gingival tissue between the two teeth has a depression in its apex, known as the **col**. The two molars are secured to each other via a gingival ligament, known as the **transseptal fiber group** (TS). The **dentin** and **cementum** (C) of the teeth are readily visible, but the enamel has been removed during the decalcification process. Observe the **furcation** (F) of tooth 1. (Reprinted with permission from Gartner LP. *Oral Histology and Embryology*, 3rd ed. Baltimore: Jen House Publishing Company, 2014.)

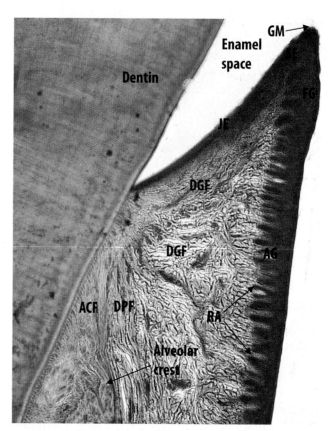

REVIEW FIGURE 14-2-2. Incisor tooth. Human l.s. Paraffin section. ×14.

This low-magnification photomicrograph of a human incisor tooth and its adjacent gingiva displays the **dentin** of the tooth and the empty space (**enamel space**) occupied by the enamel prior to its removal during the decalcification of the specimen. The gingiva, whose **margin** (GM) dips into the depression, is known as the sulcus between the enamel and the soft tissue. The **sulcular epithelium** (SE) is continuous with the **junctional epithelium** (JE). On the oral aspect, the gingiva is separated into the **free gingiva** (FG) and the **attached gingiva** (AG). The attached gingiva has a great deal of frictional forces acting on it; therefore, its **rete apparatus** (RA) is highly developed. The **crest of the alveolus** is clearly evident. The **alveolar crest fibers** (ACF) of the periodontal ligament attach to the cementum of the root and to the crest of the alveolus. The **dentogingival** (DGF) and **dentoperiosteal fibers** (DPF) of the gingiva are also evident. (Reprinted with permission from Gartner LP. *Oral Histology and Embryology*, 3rd ed. Baltimore: Jen House Publishing Company, 2014.)

KEY					
ABP	alveolar bone proper	**DPF**	dentoperiosteal fibers	**JE**	junctional epithelium
ACF	alveolar crest fibers	**F**	furcation	**RA**	rete apparatus
AG	attached gingiva	**FG**	free gingiva	**SE**	sulcular epithelium
C	cementum	**GM**	gingival margin	**TS**	transseptal fiber group
DGF	dentogingival fibers	**IDS**	interdental septum		

Summary of Histologic Organization

I. Lips

The **lips** control access to the **oral cavity** from the outside environment.

A. External Surface

The external surface is covered with thin **skin** and therefore possesses **hair follicles, sebaceous glands,** and **sweat glands**.

B. Transitional Zone

The **transitional zone (vermilion zone)** is the pink area of the lip. Here the connective tissue papillae extend deep into the epidermis. Hair follicles and sweat glands are absent, whereas sebaceous glands are occasionally present.

C. Mucous Membrane

The vestibular aspect of the lip is lined by a **wet epithelium** (stratified squamous nonkeratinized) with numerous **minor mixed salivary glands** in the subepithelial connective tissue.

D. Core of the Lip

The core of the lip contains **skeletal muscle** surrounded by connective tissue.

II. Teeth

Teeth are composed of three calcified tissues and a loose connective tissue core, the pulp.

A. Enamel

Enamel is the hardest substance in the body. It is made by **ameloblasts,** cells no longer present in the erupted tooth. Enamel is present only in the crown.

B. Dentin

Dentin is a calcified, collagen-based material that constitutes the bulk of the **crown** and **root**; it surrounds the pulp. Dentin is made by **odontoblasts,** whose long processes remain in channels, the **dentinal tubules,** traversing dentin. The odontoblast cell body forms the peripheralmost extent of the pulp.

C. Cementum

Cementum is located on the **root** of the tooth, surrounding **dentin**. Cementum is a collagen-based, calcified material manufactured by **cementoblasts,** which may become entrapped in the cementum and then are referred to as **cementocytes**. Fibers of the **periodontal ligament** are embedded in cementum and bone, thus suspending the tooth in its **bony socket,** the **alveolus**.

D. Pulp

The **pulp** is a gelatinous type of mesenchymal-appearing connective tissue that occupies the **pulp cavity**. It is richly supplied by **nerves** and **blood vessels**.

III. Gingiva

The **gingiva** (gum) is that region of the oral mucosa that is closely applied to the **neck of the tooth** and is attached to the **alveolar bone**. It is covered by a **stratified squamous partially keratinized (parakeratotic) epithelium**. The underlying connective tissue is densely populated with thick bundles of collagen fibers.

IV. Tongue

The **tongue** is a **muscular organ** whose oral region is freely moving; its root is attached to the floor of the pharynx. **Skeletal muscle** forms the core of the tongue, among which groups of serous and seromucous glands are interspersed.

A. Oral Region (Anterior Two-Thirds)

The mucosa of the dorsal surface of the anterior two-thirds of the tongue is modified to form four types of lingual papillae.

1. Filiform Papillae

Filiform papillae are long, slender, and the most numerous projections. They form a roughened surface (especially in animals such as cats) and are distributed in parallel rows along the entire surface. They are covered by a **parakeratinized stratified squamous epithelium** (but bear no taste buds) over a **connective tissue core**.

2. Fungiform Papillae

Fungiform papillae are mushroom-shaped, are scattered among the filiform papillae, and may be recognized grossly by their appearance as red dots owing to the vascular core. The epithelium contains **taste buds** on the dorsal aspect of the fungiform papilla.

3. Foliate Papillae

Foliate papillae appear as longitudinal furrows along the side of the tongue near the posterior aspect of the anterior two-thirds. Their **taste buds** degenerate at an early age in humans. Serous **glands of von Ebner** are associated with these papillae.

4. Circumvallate Papillae

Circumvallate papillae are very large and form a V-shaped row at the border of the oral and pharyngeal portions of the tongue. Circumvallate papillae are each surrounded by a moat or groove, the walls of which contain **taste buds** in their **stratified squamous nonkeratinized epithelium**. Serous **glands of von Ebner** open into the base of the groove. The connective tissue core of the circumvallate papilla possesses a rich nerve and vascular supply.

5. Taste Buds

The classical description, as viewed with the light microscope describes three types of cells, short basal cells (type IV), lightly staining sustentacular cells (types II and III), and dark neuroepithelial cells (type I).

B. Pharyngeal Region (Posterior One-Third)

The **mucosa** of the posterior one-third of the tongue presents numerous **lymphatic nodules** that constitute the **lingual tonsils**.

V. Palate

The **palate**, composed of hard and soft regions, separates the **oral** and **nasal cavities** from each other. Therefore, the palate possesses a **nasal** and an **oral aspect**. The **oral** aspect is covered by **stratified squamous epithelium** (**partially keratinized** on the hard palate), whereas the **nasal** aspect is covered by **respiratory epithelium**. The **subepithelial connective tissue** presents dense collagen fibers interspersed with **adipose tissue** and **mucous glands**. The **core** of the hard palate houses a **bony shelf**, whereas that of the soft palate is composed of **skeletal muscle** as well as **minor mucous salivary glands**.

VI. Tooth Development

Tooth development (**odontogenesis**) may be divided into several stages (see Fig. 14-6). These are named according to the morphology and/or the functional state of the developing tooth. **Dental lamina**, the first sign of odontogenesis, is followed by **bud**, **cap**, and **bell stages**. Dentin formation initiates the **apposition stage**, followed by **root formation** and **eruption**. These stages occur in both **primary** (deciduous teeth) and **secondary** (permanent teeth) **dentition**.

Chapter Review Questions

14-1. The microorganism, *Staphylococcus aureus*, is the cause of which of the following conditions?

A. Primary burning mouth syndrome

B. Fever blisters

C. Angular cheilitis

D. Carious lesions

E. Hemorrhage of the pulp

14-2. Which of the following is the location of the periodontal ligament?

A. Labial to the cortical plate

B. Between the cortical plate and alveolar bone proper

C. Coronal to the crest of the alveolus

D. Between the cementum and the alveolar bone proper

E. Between the sulcular epithelium and the junctional epithelium

14-3. Which of the following structures has an epithelial rather than a neural crest origin?

A. Enamel

B. Dentin

C. Cementum

D. Periodontal ligament

E. Pulp

14-4. Which congenital condition is associated with an inability to stick out one's tongue and difficulties in pronouncing certain letters, such as "th"?

A. Lingual thyroid

B. Macroglossia

C. Microglossia

D. Ankyloglossia

14-5. Individuals who can discern the taste of lipids possess which of the following receptors on the plasmalemmae of their taste hairs?

A. CD36

B. T1R1

C. T1R2

D. T1R3

E. T2R38

CHAPTER
15

DIGESTIVE SYSTEM II

CHAPTER OUTLINE

The approximately 9-meter-long **alimentary canal** (**digestive** or **gastrointestinal [GI] tract**) is a hollow, tubular structure that extends from the oral cavity to the anus, and its wall is modified along its length to perform the various facets of digestion.

- The oral cavity receives food, reduces it in size via mastication, and delivers the small, ball-shaped, slippery structure known as a **bolus** into the oral pharynx from where, via deglutition (swallowing), the bolus enters the esophagus and eventually the stomach.

- The gastric contents are reduced to an **acidic chyme**, which is transferred in small aliquots into the small intestine (duodenum, jejunum, and ileum), where most digestion and absorption occur.

- The liquefied food residue passes into the large intestine (cecum; ascending, transverse, descending, and sigmoid colon; rectum and anal canal; and the appendix) where the digestion is completed and water is resorbed.

- The solidified **feces** are then passed to the rectum for elimination through the anus.

A common architectural plan is evident for the alimentary tract from the esophagus to the anus, in that four distinct concentric layers constitute the wall of this long tubular structure. These layers are described from the lumen outward, and they form the general plan of the **digestive tract**. The cellular composition and the general plan are modified along the digestive tract, proceeding from the esophagus to the anus (see Table 15-1 which depicts these alterations).

Layers of the Wall of the Alimentary Canal

The layers of a generalized plan of the alimentary canal, as illustrated by a cross section of the esophagus (Fig. 15-1), consist of the mucosa, submucosa, muscularis externa, and the serosa (or adventitia).

Mucosa

The innermost layer directly surrounding the lumen is known as the **mucosa**, which is composed of three concentric layers: a **wet epithelial lining** with secretory and absorptive functions; a loose connective tissue **lamina propria** housing glands and components of the blood and lymph circulatory systems; and **muscularis mucosae**, usually consisting of two thin smooth muscle layers, responsible for the mobility of the mucosa.

Submucosa

The **submucosa** is a coarser fibroelastic connective tissue component that physically supports and provides neural, vascular, and lymphatic supply to the mucosa. Moreover, in some regions of the alimentary canal (esophagus and duodenum), the submucosa houses glands. Neural plexuses (**Meissner's submucosal plexus**) and vascular plexuses are located at the interface between the submucosa and muscularis externa.

Table 15-1   Principal Histologic Features of the Digestive Tract

Region	Epithelium	Epithelial Cell Types	Lamina Propria	Muscularis Mucosae	Submucosa	Muscularis Externa	Serosa/ Adventitia
Esophagus	Stratified squamous nonkeratinized		Esophageal cardiac glands	Longitudinal only	Esophageal glands proper	Inner circular; outer longitudinal; skeletal muscle in upper 1/3; mixed skeletal and smooth muscles in middle 1/3; smooth muscle in lower 1/3 of the esophagus	Adventitia except within the abdominal cavity where it is the serosa
Cardiac stomach			Gastric glands; shallow gastric pits	Inner circular; outer longitudinal; some outermost circular		Inner oblique, middle circular, (well developed in pyloric region where it forms the pyloric sphincter) outermost longitudinal	
Fundic stomach	Simple columnar	Surface lining cells			No glands		Serosa
Pyloric stomach			Deep gastric pits				
Duodenum		Surface absorptive cells, goblet cells, DNES cells, Paneth cells	Villi and Crypts of Lieberkühn in small intestine		Brunner glands		Both serosa and adventitia
				Inner circular; outer longitudinal		Inner circular; outer longitudinal	
Jejunum							Serosa
Ileum	Simple columnar		Peyer's patches, lymphoid nodules				Serosa
Colon		Same as small intestine but no Paneth cells in the large intestine	Crypts of Lieberkühn in colon but no villi	Inner circular and outer longitudinal	No glands	Inner circular; outer longitudinal (modified to taeniae coli)	Both serosa and adventitia
Rectum			Shallow crypts of Lieberkühn			Inner circular; outer longitudinal	Adventitia
Anal canal	Simple cuboidal proximal to anal valves; Stratified squamous nonkeratinized distal to anal valves; stratified squamous keratinized at anus		Rectal columns; circumanal glands; hair follicles at anus with sebaceous glands	Inner circular; outer longitudinal	No glands; Internal and external hemorrhoidal plexuses, fibroelastic CT	Inner circular forms internal anal sphincter; outer longitudinal loses its muscular characteristic to form a fibroelastic sheet	

Table 15-1	Principal Histologic Features of the Digestive Tract (*continued*)						
Region	**Epithelium**	**Epithelial Cell Types**	**Lamina Propria**	**Muscularis Mucosae**	**Submucosa**	**Muscularis Externa**	**Serosa/ Adventitia**
Appendix	Simple columnar with goblet cells	Surface absorptive cells, goblet cells, DNES cells	Shallow crypts of Lieberkühn; lymphoid nodules extend into submucosa	Inner circular and outer longitudinal	No glands; lymphoid nodules; fibroelastic CT	Inner circular; outer longitudinal	Serosa

Muscularis externa are all smooth muscles except in the esophagus where the superior third is skeletal, middle third mixed, and inferior third is smooth.
CT, connective tissue; DNES, diffuse neuroendocrine system.

Muscularis Externa

The **muscularis externa** usually consists of an **inner circular** and an **outer longitudinal smooth muscle layer**, which is modified in certain regions of the alimentary canal. Although these layers are described as circularly or longitudinally arranged, they are actually wrapped around the alimentary canal in tight and loose helices, respectively, giving, in cross or longitudinal sections, the appearance of a circular and a longitudinal orientation of the muscle fibers. Vascular and neural (**Auerbach's myenteric plexus**) plexuses reside between the muscle layers. The muscularis externa functions in churning and propelling the luminal contents along the digestive tract via peristaltic action. Thus, as the circular muscles reduce the diameter of the lumen, preventing the movement of the luminal contents in a proximal direction (toward the mouth), the longitudinal muscles contract in such a fashion as to push the luminal contents in a distal direction (toward the anus).

Serosa or Adventitia

The outermost layer of the alimentary canal is either a serosa or an adventitia. The intraperitoneal regions of the alimentary canal, for example, those that are suspended by peritoneum, possess a **serosa**. This structure consists of connective tissue covered by a **mesothelium** (simple squamous epithelium), which reduces frictional forces with other intraperitoneal organs during digestive movements. The retroperitoneal regions (i.e., those that are behind the peritoneal cavity and firmly attached to surrounding structures by connective tissue) possess a serosa on the anterior surface, but the posterior surface without a mesothelium is called **adventitia**.

Regions of the Alimentary Canal

Esophagus

The **esophagus** (Fig. 15-2; also see Fig. 15-1) is a muscular tube whose lumen is usually collapsed unless a bolus

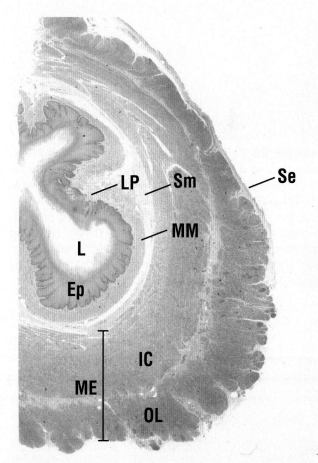

FIGURE 15-1. This photomicrograph of a cross section near the distal end of the lower one-third of the esophagus, after it passed through the abdominal surface of the diaphragm, displays the general structure of the digestive tract. The **lumen** (L) is lined by a wet **epithelium** (Ep), stratified squamous nonkeratinized in this case, lying on a thin **lamina propria** (LP) that is surrounded by the **muscularis mucosae** (MM). The **submucosa** (Sm) is surrounded by the **muscularis externa** (ME), composed of an **inner circular** (IC) and an **outer longitudinal** (OL) layer. The outermost tunic of the alimentary canal is either serosa or adventitia; in this section of the esophagus is **serosa** (Se). ×14.

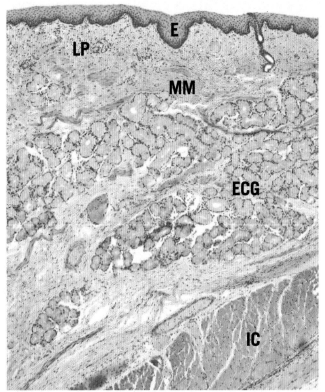

FIGURE 15-2. This very low-magnification photomicrograph of a longitudinal section of the esophagus displays its stratified squamous nonkeratinized **epithelium** (E) with its underlying **lamina propria** (LP) and the single layer of longitudinally disposed smooth muscle of the **muscularis mucosae** (MM). Note the **esophageal cardiac glands** (ECG) of the submucosa and the **inner circular layer** (IC) of the muscularis externa. ×56.

of food is traversing its length for delivery from the pharynx into the stomach.

- The **mucosa** is composed of a **stratified squamous nonkeratinized epithelium**; a loose connective tissue, the **lamina propria**, housing small blood and lymph vessels, mucus-producing **esophageal cardiac glands**, infrequent lymphoid nodules; and a **muscularis mucosae**, composed solely of longitudinally oriented smooth muscle fibers.

- The **submucosa** of the esophagus is composed of a fibroelastic connective tissue interspersed with elastic fibers. This is one of the two regions of the alimentary canal (the other is the duodenum) that houses glands in its submucosa. These glands produce a mucous secretion and are known as the **esophageal glands proper**.

- The **muscularis externa** of the esophagus is composed of **inner circular** and **outer longitudinal** layers. Those in the proximal (upper) third of the esophagus are composed of **skeletal muscle fibers**, those in the middle third of the esophagus consist of a combination of **skeletal** and **smooth muscle fibers**, whereas those in the distal (lower, near the stomach) third of the esophagus consist of **smooth muscle fibers**. The muscularis externa functions in conveying boluses of food from the pharynx into the stomach.

- Two **physiologic sphincters**, one near the pharynx and the other near the stomach, ensure that the bolus moves in one direction only, toward the stomach.

- The entire esophagus is covered by an **adventitia**, except after it pierces the diaphragm and joins the stomach where it is covered by a **serosa**.

CLINICAL CONSIDERATIONS 15-1

Stomach Disorders

Normally when the bolus is pushed into the pharynx by the back of the tongue, the pharyngeal musculature begins its peristaltic movement forcing the bolus into the esophagus, and, within 5 seconds, the bolus enters the stomach. The two physiologic sphincters, pharyngoesophageal and gastroesophageal, prevent the bolus from reversing its direction. However, after the bolus enters the stomach and contains noxious materials, or if the person swallowing the food discerns something disgusting, the emetic center of the brain is activated, triggering violent contractions of the stomach, relaxation of the physiologic sphincters, and the gastric content is forced out of the stomach, back up the esophagus into the oral cavity to be eliminated as vomitus. This process of vomiting is referred to as **reverse peristalsis**.

Approximately 4% to 6% of upper GI bleeding is attributable to **Mallory–Weiss syndrome**. This is a laceration of the lower esophagus or the cardiac/fundic region of the stomach from powerful vomiting or sometimes strenuous hiccupping. Usually, the bleeding is self-limiting, but occasionally it requires surgical intervention.

Hiatal hernia is a condition in which a region of the stomach herniates through the **esophageal hiatus** of the diaphragm. It may be of two types. In sliding hiatal hernia, the cardioesophageal junction and the cardiac region of the stomach slide in and out of the thorax, whereas in paraesophageal hiatal hernia, the cardioesophageal junction remains in its normal place, below the diaphragm, but a part (or occasionally all) of the stomach pushes into the thorax and is positioned next to the esophagus. Usually, hiatal hernia is asymptomatic, although acid reflux disease is common in patients afflicted with this condition.

Stomach

The **stomach** not only secretes low pH gastric juices (water, HCl, mucus) that acidify and alter the semisolid **bolus** into a viscous, acidic fluid that resembles, visually, split pea soup and is called **chyme**, but it also produces enzymes (pepsinogen, gastric lipase, and rennin) and releases hormones (gastrin, histamine, somatostatin, and gastric intrinsic factor). Once chyme reaches the proper consistency, it is delivered in 1 to 2 mL aliquots into the duodenum for thorough digestion.

Gastric Mucosa

The **gastric mucosa** is lined by a **simple columnar epithelium** whose **surface lining cells** (they are *not* goblet cells) produce a mucous secretion, known as **visible mucus**, that coats and protects the gastric lining from the highly acidic environment (pH 2.0) and from autodigestion (Fig. 15-3).

The mucosa of the empty stomach exhibits longitudinal folds known as **rugae**. The luminal surface displays **foveolae (gastric pits)** whose base is perforated by several gastric glands of the lamina propria. The **lamina propria** houses simple, branched, tubular glands known as **gastric glands**; depending on the region of the stomach that these glands occupy, they are known as **cardiac**, **fundic**, or **pyloric glands** (Figs. 15-4 and 15-5; also see Fig. 15-3). All **gastric glands** are composed of **parietal (oxyntic) cells, mucous neck cells, surface lining cells, diffuse neuroendocrine system cells (DNES cells,** formerly

CLINICAL CONSIDERATIONS 15-2

Peptic Ulcers and Zollinger–Ellison Syndrome

Peptic ulcers are areas of the stomach, but mostly of the duodenum, that are denuded of the epithelial lining due to the action of the acidic chyme. Most commonly, the underlying reasons are *Helicobacter pylori* infections and the use of aspirin, corticosteroids, and nonsteroidal anti-inflammatory drugs (NSAIDs). *H. pylori* are able to live in the visible mucous lining the gastric epithelium probably by forming a protective envelope of bicarbonate buffer around themselves that neutralizes the acidic milieu. It is now believed that strains of this bacterium that possess *cagA* gene are the causative agents of peptic ulcers. Interestingly, people who smoke and/or drink alcoholic beverages develop peptic ulcers more frequently than do nonsmokers and nondrinkers. The symptoms involve mild to sharp pain in the midline of the lower thoracic and upper abdominal regions.

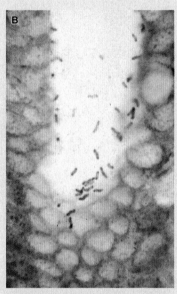

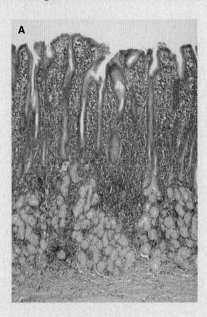

A. This figure is from a patient with an active *H. pylori* infection that resulted in chronic gastritis, a condition that may progress to peptic ulcer disease. Observe that the lamina propria has a heavy infiltrate of lymphocytes and plasma cells. **B.** A high magnification of the surface lining cells stained with silver displays the presence of *H. pylori* as small, curved rods. (Reprinted with permission from Strayer DS, et al., eds. *Rubin's Pathology: Mechanisms of Human Disease*, 8th ed. Philadelphia: Wolters Kluwer, 2020. Figure 19-16A and Reprinted with permission from Rubin R, et al., eds. *Rubin's Pathology: Clinicopathologic Foundations of Medicine*, 5th ed. Philadelphia: Wolters Kluwer Health/Lippincott Williams & Wilkins, 2008. Figure 13-12B.)

Zollinger-Ellison syndrome is a cancerous lesion of gastrin–producing cells in the stomach, duodenum, or the pancreas, resulting in the overproduction of HCl by parietal cells of the stomach and the formation of numerous recurrent peptic ulcers. A high blood level of gastrin, especially after intravenous administration of secretin, usually is a strong indicator of this syndrome.

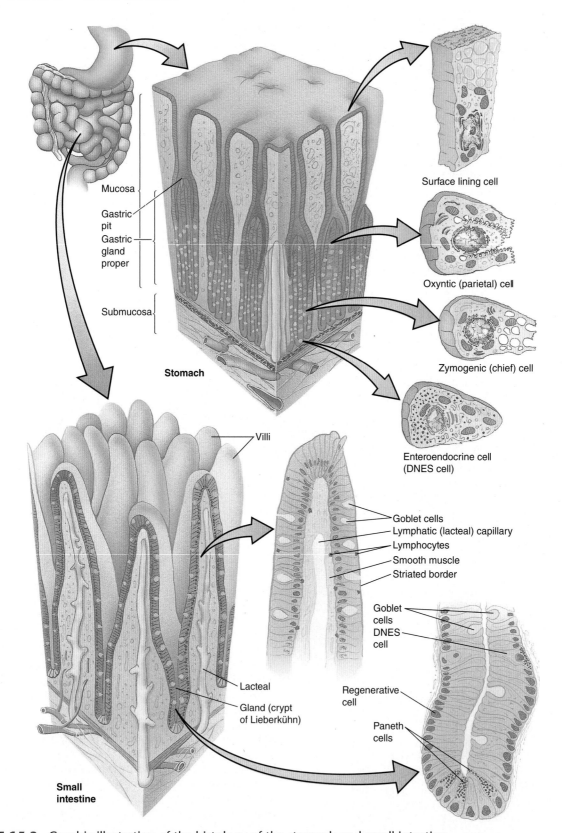

FIGURE 15-3. Graphic illustration of the histology of the stomach and small intestine.

known as **enteroendocrine or APUD [amine precursor uptake and decarboxylation] cells)**, and **regenerative cells. Fundic glands**, in addition, also possess **chief (zymogenic) cells** (see Table 15-2). Despite the common cellular components, the proportion of these cells that comprise the glands varies in the different regions of the stomach, thereby conferring variations in the glandular histology, density, and function. The cardiac and pyloric glands are composed of more mucus-secreting cells and interspersed DNES cells, and are not as densely packed

Table 15-2	Life Spans and Principal Secretions of the Epithelial Cells of the Stomach	
Gastric Glands of the Stomach	**Approximate Life Span of the Cells**	**Secretions**
Surface lining cells	3–5 days	Visible mucus
Mucous neck cells	6 days	Soluble mucus
Parietal cells	200 days	Hydrochloric acid, gastric intrinsic factor
Chief cells	60–90 days	Pepsin, rennin, lipase precursors
DNES cells	60–90 days	Gastrin, somatostatin, secretin, cholecystokinin
Regenerative cells	Function to replace the epithelial lining of stomach and cells of glands	

DNES, diffuse neuroendocrine system.

as the fundic glands. The densely packed fundic glands are composed mostly of parietal cells concentrated in the mid-region of the glands and chief cells at the base of

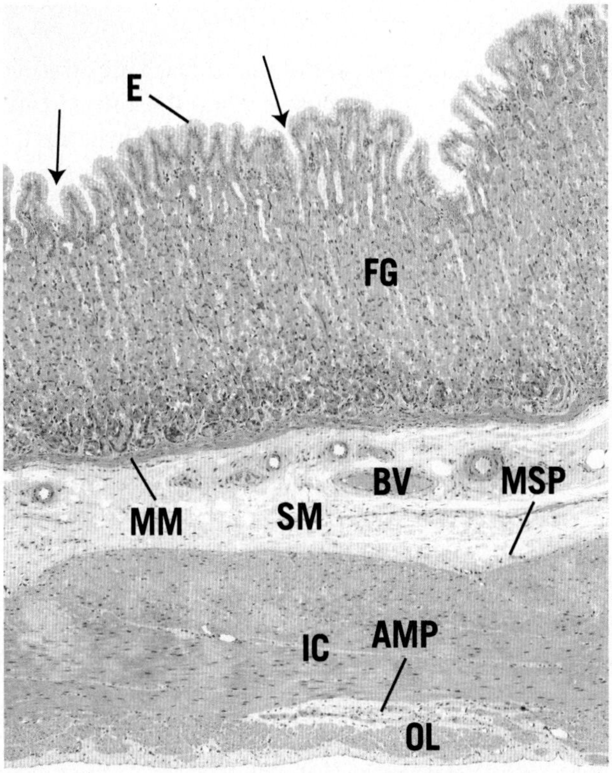

FIGURE 15-4. Low magnification of the fundic stomach. Note that the lumen is lined by a simple columnar **epithelium** (E) composed of surface lining cells and that these cells continue into the gastric pits (*arrows*). The lamina propria is packed with **fundic glands** (FG) that extend from the bases of the gastric pits to the **muscularis mucosae** (MM). The **submucosa** (SM) consists of a highly **vascular** (BV) dense fibroelastic connective tissue. **Meissner's submucosal plexus** (MSP) is barely visible as it is couched by the **inner circular** (IC) layer of the muscularis externa. Observe the well-defined **Auerbach's myenteric plexus** (AMP) situated between the inner circular and **outer longitudinal** (OL) layers of the muscularis externa. The stomach is covered by a serosa. ×56.

the glands. Moreover, cardiac glands are the shortest and pyloric glands are the longest of the gastric glands.

- **Parietal cells** live for ~200 days before they are replaced by regenerative cells.
  - These pyramidal, eosinophilic cells have deep apical plasmalemma invaginations, known as

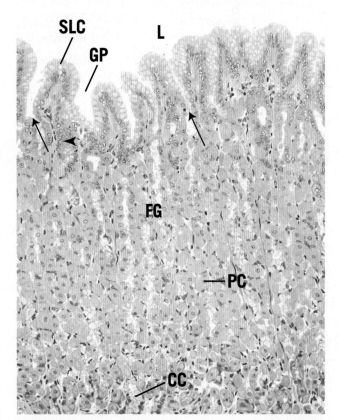

FIGURE 15-5. This low-magnification photomicrograph of the fundic stomach displays part of the mucosa of the fundic stomach. Note that the **lumen** (L) is lined by **surface lining cells** (SLC), which also line the **gastric pits** (GP). The simple tubular **fundic glands** (FG) open into the bases of the gastric pits (*arrows*) and are composed of several types of cells, three of which are clearly evident, namely mucous neck cells (*arrowhead*), *parietal cells* (PC), and **chief cells** (CC). The scant interglandular connective tissue is occupied by capillaries and connective tissue cells. ×132.

intracellular canaliculi, that traverse the cell body and into which **hydrochloric acid (HCl)** is secreted. Microvilli extend into these intracellular canalicular spaces to increase surface area for HCl secretion. It is believed that these microvilli are stored intracellularly as tubules and vesicles, known as the **tubulovesicular system**, that reside alongside the intracellular canaliculi when the cell is not secreting HCl. The production of HCl is dependent on gastrin, histamine, and acetylcholine binding to their respective receptors on the parietal cell basal plasmalemma.

- Parietal cells also secrete **gastric intrinsic factor**, a glycoprotein that binds to and forms a complex with vitamin B_{12} in the gastric lumen. When this complex reaches the ileum, it binds to specific receptors on the surface absorptive cells and the vitamin becomes absorbed.

- **Mucous neck cells**, situated in the neck of the glands, secrete **soluble mucus** (different from the visible mucus produced by the surface lining cells), which becomes part of chyme, lubricating it and easing its movement within the lumen of the stomach.

- The various types of **DNES cells** located in the stomach produce hormones such as **gastrin**, **somatostatin**, **secretin**, and **cholecystokinin** (Table 15-3). It is believed that each DNES cell type manufactures only a single hormone, but some may manufacture two different hormones. Although some of these hormones enter blood or lymph vessels to be delivered to their target cells, most of them act locally and are, therefore, known as **paracrine hormones**.

- **Regenerative cells**, located mainly in the neck and isthmus, replace the epithelial lining of the stomach and the cells of the glands. They have a very high mitotic rate because they replace mucous neck cells, DNES cells, and surface lining cells every 5 to 7 days. They also replace parietal cells and chief cells every 200 days and 60 to 90 days, respectively.

- **Chief cells**, located in the base of the fundic glands, have a 60- to 90-day life span and produce precursors of enzymes (**pepsin**, **rennin**, **lipase**). Chief cells also manufacture **leptin**, the hormone that inhibits hunger sensations.

The **muscularis mucosae** of the stomach are arranged in three layers of smooth muscle, where the inner circular and outer longitudinal layers are well defined, whereas the outermost circular layer is either poorly defined or absent.

Gastric Submucosa

The **submucosa** of the stomach is composed of a fibroelastic connective tissue richly supplied by blood and

Table 15-3	Hormones Produced by Cells of the Digestive Tract	
Hormone	**Location**	**Action**
Cholecystokinin (CKK)	Small intestine	Contraction of the gallbladder; release of pancreatic enzymes
Gastric inhibitory peptide	Small intestine	Inhibits HCl secretion
Gastrin	Stomach	Stimulates secretion of HCl and gastric enzymes
Ghrelin	Stomach	Maintains constant intraluminal pressure in the stomach; induces hunger; modulates smooth muscle tension in muscularis externa
Glicentin	Stomach; large intestine	Stimulates hepatocytic glycogenolysis
Glucagon	Stomach; duodenum	Stimulates hepatocytic glycogenolysis
Motilin	Small intestine	Increases intestinal peristalsis
Neurotensin	Small intestine	Decreases intestinal peristalsis; stimulates blood flow to the ileum
Secretin	Small intestine	Stimulates bicarbonate secretion by the pancreas
Serotonin	Stomach; small intestine; large intestine	Increases intestinal peristalsis
Somatostatin	Stomach; duodenum	Inhibits DNES cells in the vicinity of the release
Substance P	Stomach; small intestine; large intestine	Increases intestinal peristalsis
Human epidermal growth factor (urogastrone)	Duodenal (Brunner's) glands	Inhibits HCl secretion; increases epithelial cell mitosis
Vasoactive intestinal peptide	Stomach; small intestine; large intestine	Increases intestinal peristalsis; stimulates the secretion of ions and water by the digestive tract

DNES, diffuse neuroendocrine system; HCl, hydrochloric acid.

lymphatic vessels. **Meissner's submucosal plexus** is present near the inner circular layer of the muscularis externa.

Gastric Muscularis Externa

The muscularis externa of the stomach is composed of three layers of smooth muscle, an innermost oblique, middle circular (which becomes modified in the pyloric region to form the pyloric sphincter), and an outer longitudinal layer. **Auerbach's myenteric plexus** is present between the inner circular and outer longitudinal muscle layers.

Gastric Serosa

The entire stomach is covered by a **serosa**.

Small Intestine

The luminal aspect of the **small intestine** is modified to increase its surface area. These modifications range from the macroscopic, **plicae circulares** (increase 2 to 3×), through the microscopic, **villi** (increase 10×), to the electron microscopic, **microvilli** (increase 20×) for a total increase of the surface area by approximately 400 to 600×. The small intestine has three regions: the duodenum, jejunum, and ileum.

Mucosa of the Small Intestine

The mucosa of all three regions displays villi, extensions of the lamina propria, covered by a simple columnar epithelium composed of enterocytes (surface absorptive), goblet, DNES cells, M cells, and tuft cells (see Fig. 15-3).

- Each tall columnar **enterocyte (surface absorptive cell)** possesses as many as 3,000 microvilli covered by a thick **glycocalyx** coat rich in **disaccharidases** and **dipeptidases**.
  - These cells function in the absorption of sugars, amino acids, fatty acids, monoglycerides, electrolytes, and water as well as several additional substances (see below in the section on Digestion and Absorption).
  - Enterocytes also participate in the immune defense of the body. They do so by manufacturing **secretory protein**, which binds to the J protein component of the antibody dimer and protects what is known as **secretory immunoglobulin A (sIgA)** as it traverses the enterocyte and enters the intestinal lumen. A small fraction of the sIgA acts within the lumen of the small intestine to eliminate antigenic invaders, but the bulk of the sIgA is reabsorbed by the enterocytes, which release them into the blood vessels of the lamina propria. The blood vessels deliver the sIgA into the liver where hepatocytes transfer it into the forming bile and eventually into the lumen of the duodenum to combat antigens. This path of the sIgA is referred to as the enterohepatic circulation of the secretory IgA.

- **Goblet cells** produce **mucinogen** that becomes hydrated to form **mucin**, which, when mixed with the luminal contents of the duodenum, becomes known as **mucus**.

- **DNES cells** release various hormones (e.g., secretin, motilin, neurotensin, cholecystokinin, gastric inhibitory peptide, and gastrin; see Table 15-3). A small population of **DNES cells** of the lining of the small intestine appears to function as taste cells because they possess receptor proteins on their cell processes that contact the intestinal lumen. These receptors can distinguish umami, sweet, and bitter tastes and prompt β cells of the islets of Langerhans to release insulin.

- **M cells (microfold cells)** replace those simple columnar cells of the epithelia of the small intestine that abut **lymphoid nodules**. These cells phagocytose antigens present in the intestinal lumen and transfer them, without processing them first, into the lamina propria to be phagocytosed by **dendritic** and **antigen-presenting cells** residing in their vicinity. The phagocytosed antigens are processed by these cells, and the resultant epitopes are presented to lymphocytes to generate an immune response.

- **Tuft cells**, whose clusters of microvilli project into the intestinal lumen, recognize the presence of parasitic worms and initiate an immune response against them.

The **lamina propria** of the small intestine, a loose connective tissue, extends from the epithelial lining to the muscularis mucosae and forms the core of the villi as well as the connective tissue elements interspersed among the **crypts of Lieberkühn (intestinal crypts or glands)**, the simple tubular glands that open, at the base of the villi, into the intervillar spaces.

- The **cores of the villi** are richly endowed by blood vessels, fibroblasts, and lymphoid elements, including **lymphocytes**, **plasma cells**, and **mast cells**, as well as blindly ending lymphatic vessels, known as **lacteals**, that collect most of the lipids absorbed during the digestive process (see the section on Digestion and Absorption). Smooth muscle cells, derived from the muscularis mucosae, are located in the core of each villus and, by contracting occasionally, "inject" the contents of the lacteals into a plexus of lymph vessels located in the submucosa.

- The **crypts of Lieberkühn (intestinal crypts or glands)** are composed of simple columnar cells (like surface absorptive cells), goblet (and oligomucous) cells, DNES, and regenerative cells, as well as **Paneth cells**. The last are located in the base of the glands and house in their apical compartment, large secretory granules containing the antibacterial enzyme **lysozyme** as well as other agents, such as **defensin** and **tumor necrosis factor-α**.

The **muscularis mucosae** are composed of an inner circular and an outer longitudinal smooth muscle layer.

Submucosa of the Small Intestine

The **submucosa** of the small intestine is a fibroelastic connective tissue that has a rich vascular, lymphatic, and neural supply. Meissner's submucosal plexus occupies its normal location in the submucosa.

Muscularis Externa of the Small Intestine

The muscularis externa is composed of an **inner circular** and an **outer longitudinal smooth muscle layer** with **Auerbach's myenteric plexus** located between them.

Serosa and Adventitia of the Small Intestine

Except for a retroperitoneal segment of the duodenum that is covered on the posterior aspect by an **adventitia**, the entire small intestine is covered by a **serosa**.

Regional Differences in the Histology of the Small Intestine

The three regions of the small intestine, duodenum (Fig. 15-6), jejunum, and ileum (Fig. 15-7), present histologic differences that permit them to be differentiated from each other. Villi are tallest and proportionally most numerous in the duodenum, are shorter and fewer in the jejunum, and the shortest and least numerous in the ileum. The number of goblet cells increases from the duodenum through the ileum.

- The submucosa of the **duodenum** contains numerous glands, **duodenal (Brunner's) glands**, that produce an alkaline, mucin-containing fluid that buffers the acidic chyme entering from the stomach, thereby protecting the intestinal lining (see Fig. 15-6). These glands also manufacture **urogastrone (human epidermal growth factor)**, a polypeptide that inhibits HCl production and enhances cell division of regenerative cells. These glands are *not* present in the jejunum or the ileum.

- The lamina propria of the **ileum** houses large accumulations of lymphatic nodules, **Peyer's patches**. The surface epithelium covering Peyer's patches is composed of **M cells** (see above) instead of simple columnar cells. Peyer's patches are *not* present in the duodenum or the jejunum.

- The jejunum possesses the most prominent plicae circularis, but neither Brunner's glands nor Peyer's patches.

Large Intestine

The **large intestine** is subdivided into the **cecum**, the **ascending**, **transverse**, **descending**, and **sigmoid colons**, the **rectum**, the **anal canal**, and the **appendix** (Figs. 15-8 and 15-9). The large intestine possesses no villi but does house **crypts of Lieberkühn (intestinal glands)** in its lamina propria. The epithelial lining of the lumen and the crypts is composed of **enterocytes (surface absorptive cells)**, **goblet** (and oligomucous) cells, **regenerative cells**, and occasional **DNES cells**. There are no Paneth cells in the large intestine, with the possible exception of the crypts of Lieberkühn of the appendix. The population of enterocytes (surface absorptive cells) is the largest followed by goblet cells. The number of regenerative cells is considerable, and they possess a high rate of mitotic activity because they must replace the epithelial cell population every 6 to 7 days. The muscularis mucosae and the submucosa do not vary from the general pattern of

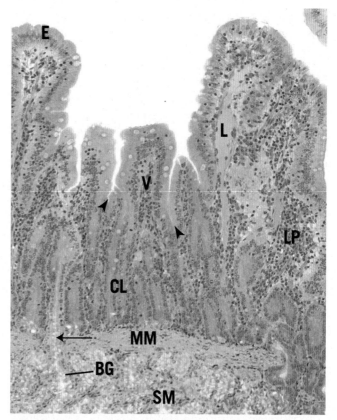

FIGURE 15-6. This low-magnification photomicrograph of the monkey duodenum displays the simple columnar **epithelial** (E) lining of the **villi** (V) and the **crypts of Lieberkühn** (CL) opening into the intervillar spaces (*arrowheads*). Observe the limited number of goblet cells among the epithelial cells. Note the presence of a **lacteal** (L) as well as the numerous lymphoid cells in the core of one of the villi. The **muscularis mucosae** (MM) separates the **lamina propria** (LP) from the **submucosa** (SM). Observe that **Brunner's glands** (BG) open into the base of the crypts of Lieberkühn (*arrow*). ×132.

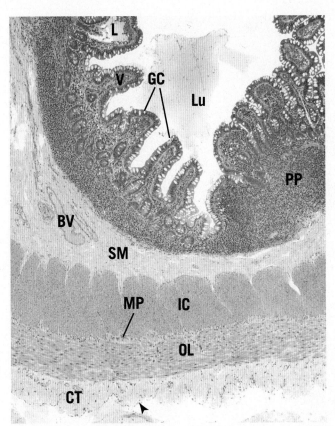

FIGURE 15-7. This is a very low-magnification photomicrograph of the monkey ileum. Note that the **villi** (V) are shorter and sparser than those of the duodenum but that there are more **goblet cells** (GC) among the epithelial cells lining the **lumen** (Lu). There is a **lacteal** (L) in the core of the villus on the upper left-hand side. Observe that the lamina propria is populated by lymphoid elements that constitute **Peyer's patches** (PP) of the ileum, but the richly **vascularized** (BV) **submucosa** (SM) has limited lymphoid infiltration. The **inner circular** (IC) and **outer longitudinal** (OL) layers of the muscularis externa are well differentiated. Note the presence of **Auerbach's myenteric plexus** (MP) between the two layers of the muscularis externa. The serosa (*arrowhead*) and the subserosal **connective tissue** (CT) are well displayed. ×56.

the alimentary canal; however, the muscularis externa is atypical because the outer longitudinal layer is arranged in three slender bands, called **taeniae coli**, that extend along the entire length of the large intestine. These three bands of smooth muscle fibers are in a constant state of partial contraction causing sequential "pouching" of the large intestine, where each small pouch is referred to as **haustra coli**. The serosa is also modified in the large intestine in that slender fat-filled pockets, **appendices epiploicae (epiploic appendages)**, are suspended along much of the length of the large intestine.

The large intestine functions in the absorption of the remaining amino acids, lipids, and carbohydrates as well as fluids, electrolytes, gases, and certain vitamins. It is also responsible for the compaction of **feces**.

Rectum, Anal Canal, and Appendix

The **rectum**, the most distal region of the colon, has fewer but longer crypts of Lieberkühn than most other regions of the colon.

The **anal canal**, ~4 cm in length, is narrower than the rectum, has fewer and shorter crypts of Lieberkühn. Its mucosa forms long folds, known as **anal columns**, that join distally, forming the **anal valves**, that function in buttressing the feces. The inner circular layer of the **muscularis externa** of the anal canal, composed of smooth muscle fibers, forms the **internal anal sphincter**, whereas the outer longitudinal smooth muscle layer loses its smooth muscle to be replaced by a fibroelastic sheath that supports the internal sphincter. Because the internal anal sphincter is composed of smooth muscle cells, there is no voluntary control over them. However, the floor of the pelvis, formed by skeletal muscles, organizes the **external anal sphincter** around the outer longitudinal muscle's fibroelastic sheath, and that is under voluntary control.

The **appendix**, a short, narrow tubular extension of the cecum, resembles the colon. It has a few, shallow crypts of Lieberkühn, lined by a simple columnar epithelium composed of enterocytes, goblet cells, regenerative cells, many DNES cells, and, unlike the colon, it sports occasional Paneth cells. The **lamina propria** displays an abundance of **lymphoid nodules** with their associated M cells where the nodules contact the epithelium. The muscularis mucosae and submucosa present a normal appearance. The outer longitudinal layer of the muscularis externa is not organized into three bands; therefore, there are no taeniae coli in the appendix. The entire appendix is covered by a **serosa**. The appendix, once considered a vestigial organ, has been shown to house bacterial biofilms that are believed to be a reservoir of microbiota, to reestablish the normal bacterial flora of the colon in case it is partially or completely eradicated as a result of certain disease processes.

Progress of Food Through the Alimentary Canal

The amount of time that the ingested food spends in various regions of the alimentary canal depends on a multitude of factors, including the chemical components of the food. For instance, the more fat the food contains, the longer time it spends being digested. The average meal ingested spends 3 to 5 hours in the stomach, 6 to 12 hours in the small intestine, and 30 to 40 hours in the large intestine. For the sake of completeness, it should be noted that once a bolus enters the esophagus it takes it ~5 seconds to reach the stomach.

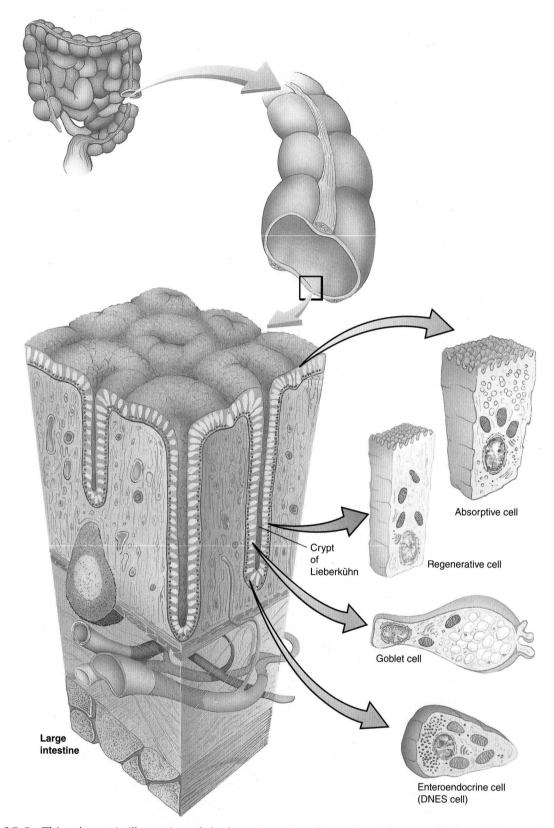

Absorptive cell

Regenerative cell

Crypt
of
Lieberkühn

Goblet cell

Enteroendocrine cell
(DNES cell)

**Large
intestine**

FIGURE 15-8. This schematic illustration of the large intestine shows that it has no villi, but it does possess crypts of Lieberkühn. The outer longitudinal layer of the muscularis externa is gathered into the taeniae coli. Lymphoid nodules and lymphoid infiltration are frequently noted in the large and small intestines. The crypts of Lieberkühn are glands composed of a simple columnar type of epithelium. Four types of cells constitute this epithelium: mucus-producing goblet cells; absorptive cells that function in absorbing nutrients, electrolytes, and fluid; regenerative cells that proliferate and replace the other cells of the epithelium; and enteroendocrine cells that release paracrine hormones.

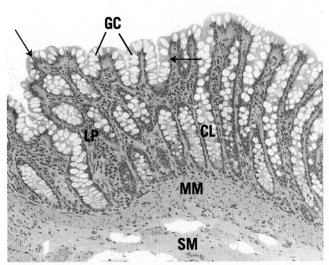

FIGURE 15-9. This photomicrograph of a monkey colon displays the **crypts of Lieberkühn** (CL) with its numerous **goblet cells** (GC). Although the enterocytes (*arrows*) outnumber the goblet cells, they are not easily seen because the goblet cell theca compresses them. Note that the **lamina propria** (LP) is infiltrated with lymphocytes, plasma cells, and mast cells. The **muscularis mucosae** (MM) and the **submucosa** (SM) are clearly evident. ×132.

Microbiota of the Large Intestine

The colon is inhabited by trillions of mostly **commensal microorganisms**, which form a significant portion of the microorganism population, collectively known as the **microbiota**. According to recent investigations, the microbiota has a direct effect on the individual's well-being. Although numerous reports have been published concerning the human microbiota, including its combined genome, known as the **microbiome**, the roles of these microorganisms are just becoming understood. It appears that the principal inhabitants of the human colon belong to two phyla, *Bacteroides* and *Prevotella*, and, depending on the individual, one or the other is more common. It has been reported that as individuals alter their diet, become more infirm, or age, the predominant flora may be displaced by members of other phyla. These changes in the microbiota may be responsible for obesity and type 2 diabetes in some individuals.

Digestion and Absorption

Carbohydrates

Amylases in the saliva and the pancreatic secretion hydrolyze carbohydrates to disaccharides. **Oligo- and disaccharidases**, present in the glycocalyx of enterocytes, break down oligo- and disaccharides into monosaccharides (mainly glucose, fructose, and galactose) that enter the enterocytes requiring active transport using a specific transporter enzyme. The cells then release the sugars into the lamina propria where these sugars enter the circulatory system for transport to the liver.

Proteins

Proteins, denatured by HCl in the lumen of the stomach, are hydrolyzed (by the enzyme **pepsin**) into **polypeptides**. These are further broken down into **tri- and dipeptides** by proteases of the pancreatic secretions. **Tri- and dipeptidases** of the glycocalyx hydrolyze dipeptides into individual amino acids, which enter the enterocytes involving active transport and are transferred into the lamina propria where they enter the capillary network to be transported to the liver.

Lipids

Pancreatic lipase breaks lipids down into **fatty acids**, **monoglycerides**, and **glycerol** within the lumen of the duodenum and proximal jejunum. Bile salts, delivered from the liver and the gallbladder, emulsify the fatty acids and monoglycerides, forming **micelles**, which, along with glycerol, diffuse into the enterocytes. Within these cells, they enter the **smooth endoplasmic reticulum**, are re-esterified to **triglycerides**, and are covered by a coat of protein within the Golgi apparatus, forming lipoprotein droplets known as **chylomicrons**. Chylomicrons exit these cells at their basolateral membranes and enter the **lacteals** of the villi, contributing to the formation of **chyle**. Chyle enters the lymph vascular system, makes its way to the thoracic duct, and then into the venous system at the junction of the left internal jugular vein and left brachiocephalic vein.

Fatty acids that are shorter than 12 carbon chains in length pass through the enterocytes without being re-esterified and gain entrance to the blood capillaries of the villi.

Water and Ions

Water and ions are absorbed through the surface absorptive cells of the small and the large intestine.

Composition of Feces

Feces is compacted in the large intestine where terminal digestion occurs, and water, along with various ions, is removed during the compaction process but mucus is added to permit the components of feces to adhere to each other. Even though water and electrolytes are absorbed through the enterocytes of the small and the large intestines, feces is still composed mostly of water. In fact, of the ~100 mL of feces eliminated daily, 75% is water. The remainder is roughage (7%), dead bacteria (7%), lipids (5%), inorganic material (5%), and the three residual components, bile pigment, proteins, and dead cells, that constitute the final 1%.

CLINICAL CONSIDERATIONS 15-3

Crohn's Disease and Antibiotic-Associated Colitis

Crohn's disease is a subcategory of **inflammatory bowel disease**, a condition of unknown etiology. It usually involves the small intestine or the colon but may affect any region of the digestive tract, from the esophagus to the anus, as well as extra-alimentary canal structures such as the skin, the kidney, and the larynx. It is characterized by patchy ulcers and deep fistulas in the intestinal wall. Clinical manifestations include abdominal pain, diarrhea, and fever, and these recur after various periods of ever-shortening remission.

In **antibiotic-associated colitis**, antibiotics such as ampicillin, cephalosporin, and clindamycin often cause an imbalance in the intestinal bacterial flora, permitting the vigorous proliferation of *Clostridioides difficile*, resulting in infection by this organism. The two major toxins (Toxin A and Toxin B) produced by *C. difficile* frequently cause inflammation of the sigmoid colon. Depending on the severity of the infection, the patient will suffer from abdominal cramps, loose stool, bloody diarrhea, fever, and, in extreme cases, dehydration and perforation of the bowel.

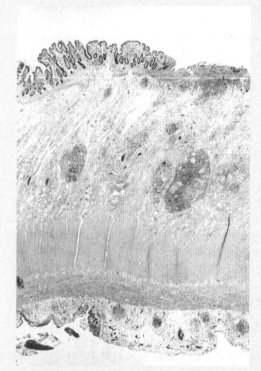

This figure is from the colon of a patient with Crohn's disease displaying ulceration of the mucosa, a hypertrophied submucosa with clusters of lymphoid elements, as well as smaller aggregates of lymphoid elements in the subserosal connective tissue adjacent to the muscularis externa. (Reprinted with permission from Rubin R, et al., eds. *Rubin's Pathology: Clinicopathologic Foundations of Medicine*, 5th ed. Philadelphia: Wolters Kluwer Health/Lippincott Williams & Wilkins, 2008. Figure 13-43A.)

PLATE 15-1A Esophagus

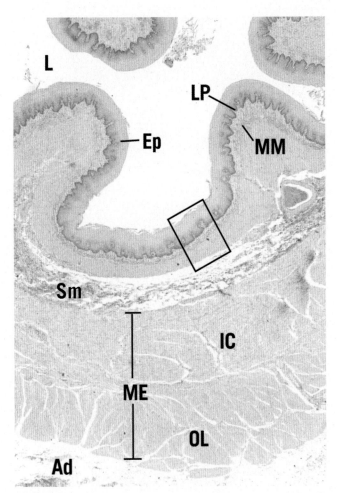

FIGURE 15-1-1. Esophagus. x.s. Paraffin section. ×14.

This photomicrograph of a cross section of the lower third of the esophagus displays the general structure of the digestive tract. The **lumen** (L) is lined by a stratified squamous nonkeratinized **epithelium** (Ep) lying on a thin **lamina propria** (LP) that is surrounded by the **muscularis mucosae** (MM). The **submucosa** (Sm) contains glands and is surrounded by the **muscularis externa** (ME) composed of an **inner circular** (IC) and an **outer longitudinal** (OL) layer. The outermost tunic of the esophagus is the fibroelastic **adventitia** (Ad). A region similar to the *boxed area* is presented at a higher magnification in Figure 15-12.

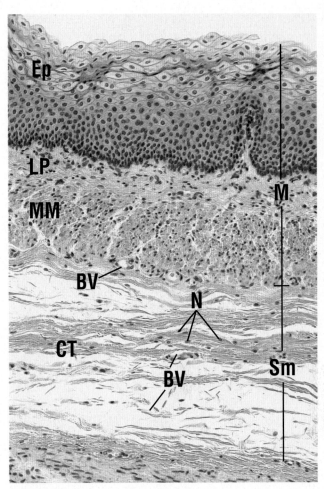

FIGURE 15-1-2. Esophagus. Human. x.s. Paraffin section. ×132.

This photomicrograph is a higher magnification of a region similar to the *boxed area* of Figure 15-1-1. The **mucosa** (M) of the esophagus consists of a stratified squamous nonkeratinized **epithelium** (Ep), a loose collagenous connective tissue layer, the **lamina propria** (LP), and a longitudinally oriented smooth muscle layer, the **muscularis mucosae** (MM). The **submucosa** (Sm) is composed of a coarser collagenous **connective tissue** (CT), housing **blood vessels** (BV) and various connective tissue cells whose **nuclei** (N) are evident.

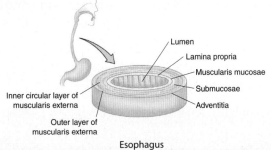

Lumen
Lamina propria
Muscularis mucosae
Submucosae
Adventitia
Inner circular layer of muscularis externa
Outer layer of muscularis externa

Esophagus

KEY					
Ad	adventitia	**L**	lumen	**MM**	muscularis mucosae
BV	blood vessels	**LP**	lamina propria	**N**	nuclei
CT	connective tissue	**M**	mucosa	**OL**	outer longitudinal layer
Ep	epithelium	**ME**	muscularis externa	**Sm**	submucosa
IC	inner circular layer				

PLATE 15-1B   Esophagus and Esophagogastric Junction

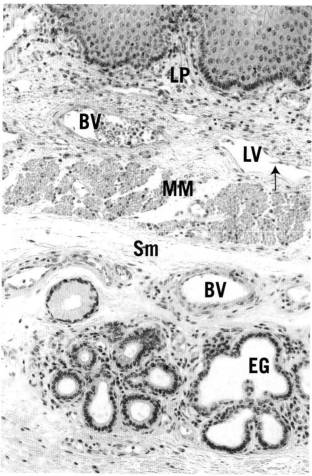

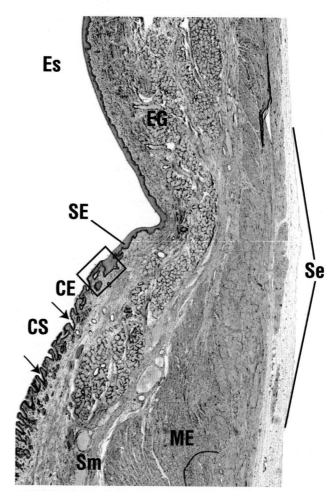

FIGURE 15-1-3. Esophagus. Human. x.s. Paraffin section. ×132.

The **lamina propria** (LP) and **submucosa** (Sm) of the esophagus are separated from each other by the longitudinally oriented smooth muscle bundles, the **muscularis mucosae** (MM). Observe that the lamina propria is a very vascular connective tissue, housing numerous **blood vessels** (BV) and **lymph vessels** (LV), whose valves (*arrow*) indicate the direction of lymph flow. The submucosa also displays numerous **blood vessels** (BV) as well as the presence of the **esophageal glands proper** (EG), which produce a mucous secretion to lubricate the lining of the esophagus.

FIGURE 15-1-4. Esophagogastric junction. l.s. Dog. Paraffin section. ×14.

The junction of the **esophagus** (Es) and **cardiac stomach** (CS) is very abrupt, as evidenced by the sudden change of the **stratified squamous epithelium** (SE) to the **simple columnar epithelium** (CE) of the stomach. Note that the **esophageal glands proper** (EG) continue for a short distance into the **submucosa** (Sm) of the stomach. Also observe the presence of gastric pits (*arrows*) and the increased thickness of the **muscularis externa** (ME) of the stomach compared with that of the esophagus. The outermost tunic of the esophagus inferior to the diaphragm is a **serosa** (Se) rather than an adventitia. The *boxed area* is presented at a higher magnification in Figure 15-2-1.

KEY					
BV	blood vessels	Es	esophagus	Se	serosa
CE	simple columnar epithelium	LP	lamina propria	SE	stratifies squamous epithelium
CS	cardiac stomach	LV	lymph vessels	Sm	submucosa
EG	esophageal glands proper	ME	muscularis externa		
		MM	muscularis mucosae		

PLATE 15-2A Stomach

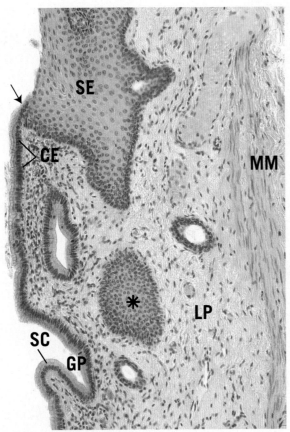

FIGURE 15-2-1. Esophagogastric junction. l.s. Dog. Paraffin section. ×132.

FIGURE 15-2-2. Fundic stomach. l.s. Paraffin section. ×14.

This photomicrograph is a higher magnification of the *boxed region* of Figure 15-1-4. The **stratified squamous epithelium** (SE) of the esophagus is replaced by the **simple columnar epithelium** (CE) of the stomach in a very abrupt fashion (*arrow*). The **lamina propria** (LP) displays **gastric pits** (GP), lined by the visible mucus-secreting **surface lining cells** (SC), characteristic of the stomach. The structure labeled with an *asterisk* is not a lymphoid nodule but is a more or less tangential section through the esophageal epithelium. Note the presence of the **muscularis mucosae** (MM).

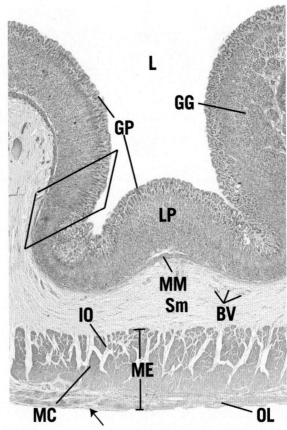

The fundic region presents all the characteristics of the stomach, as demonstrated by this low-power photomicrograph. The **lumen** (L) is lined by a simple columnar epithelium, deep to which is the **lamina propria** (LP), housing numerous **gastric glands** (GG). Each gland opens into the base of a **gastric pit** (GP). The **muscularis mucosae** (MM) separate the lamina propria from the **submucosa** (Sm), a richly **vascularized** (BV) connective tissue, thrown into folds (rugae) in the empty stomach. The **muscularis externa** (ME) is composed of three poorly defined layers of smooth muscle: **innermost oblique** (IO), **middle circular** (MC), and **outer longitudinal** (OL). Serosa (*arrow*) forms the outermost tunic of the stomach. A region similar to the *boxed area* is presented at a higher magnification in Figure 15-2-3.

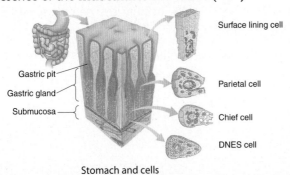

Stomach and cells

KEY					
BV	blood vessels	**L**	lumen	**SC**	surface lining cells
CE	simple columnar epithelium	**LP**	lamina propria	**SE**	stratified squamous epithelium
GC	gastric glands	**MC**	middle circular layer	**Sm**	submucosa
GP	gastric pit	**ME**	muscularis externa		
IO	innermost oblique layer	**MM**	muscularis mucosae		
		OL	outer longitudinal layer		

PLATE 15-2B Stomach

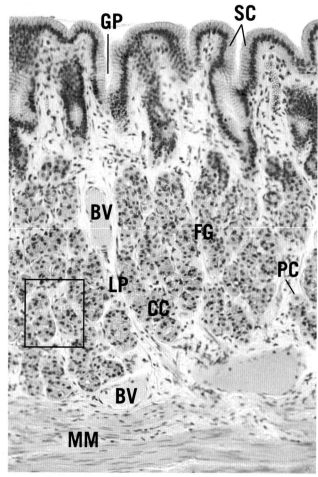

FIGURE 15-2-3. Fundic stomach. x.s. Dog. Paraffin section. ×132.

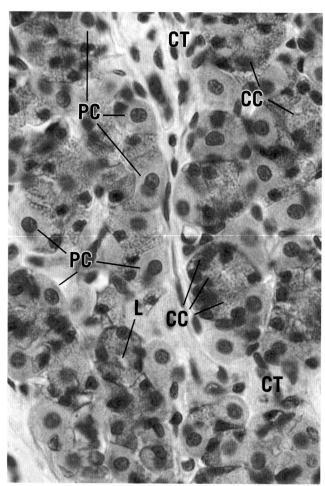

FIGURE 15-2-4. Fundic glands. x.s. Paraffin section. ×540.

This photomicrograph presents a higher magnification of a region similar to the *boxed area* of Figure 15-2-2. The mucosa of the fundic stomach displays numerous **gastric pits** (GP) that are lined by a simple columnar epithelium, consisting mostly of visible mucus-producing **surface lining** (surface mucous) **cells** (SC). The base of each pit accepts the isthmus of two to four **fundic glands** (FG). Although fundic glands are composed of several cell types, only two, **parietal cells** (PC) and **chief cells** (CC), are readily distinguishable in this preparation. The **lamina propria** (LP) is richly **vascularized** (BV). Note the **muscularis mucosae** (MM) beneath the lamina propria. A region similar to the *boxed area* is presented at a higher magnification (positioned at an angle) in Figure 15-2-4.

This photomicrograph presents a higher magnification (positioned at an angle) of a region similar to the *boxed area* of Figure 15-2-3. The **lumina** (L) of several glands can be recognized. Note that **chief cells** (CC) are granular in appearance and are much smaller than the round, plate-like **parietal cells** (PC). Parietal cells, as their name implies, are located at the periphery of the gland. Slender **connective tissue elements** (CT), housing blood vessels, occupy the narrow spaces between the closely packed glands.

KEY					
BV	blood vessels	**FG**	fundic glands	**MM**	muscularis mucosae
CC	chief cells	**GP**	gastric pit	**PC**	parietal cells
CT	connective tissue elements	**L**	lumina	**SC**	surface lining cells
		LP	lamina propria		

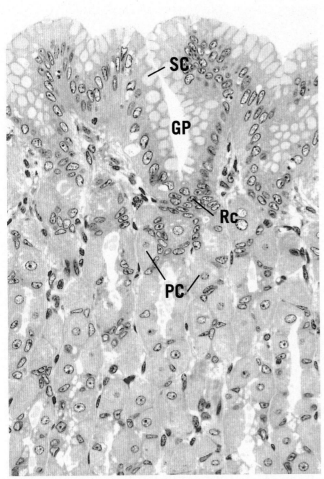

FIGURE 15-3-1. Fundic stomach. x.s. Monkey. Plastic section. ×270.

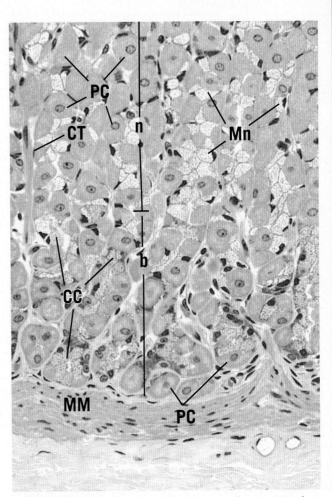

FIGURE 15-3-2. Fundic gland. Stomach. x.s. Monkey. Plastic section. ×270.

The **gastric pits** (GP) of the fundic stomach are lined mostly by visible mucus-producing **surface lining cells** (SC). Each gastric pit receives two to four fundic glands, simple tubular structures that are subdivided into three regions: isthmus, neck, and base. The isthmus opens directly into the gastric pit and is composed of **regenerative cells** (Rc), which are responsible for the renewal of the lining of the gastric mucosa, **surface lining cells** (SC), and **parietal cells** (PC). The neck and base of these glands are presented in Figure 15-3-2.

Both the **neck** (n) and **base** (b) of the fundic gland contain large, plate-shaped **parietal cells** (PC). The neck also possesses a few immature cells as well as **mucous neck cells** (Mn), which manufacture soluble mucus. The base of the fundic glands contains numerous acid-manufacturing **parietal cells** (PC) and **chief cells** (CC), which produce digestive enzymes. Note that the lamina propria is tightly packed with glands and that the intervening **connective tissue** (CT) is flimsy. The bases of these glands extend to the **muscularis mucosae** (MM).

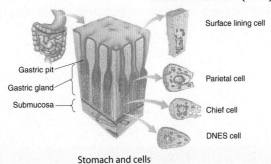

KEY					
b	base	**MM**	muscularis mucosae	**PC**	parietal cells
CC	chief cells	**Mn**	mucous neck cells	**Rc**	regenerative cells
CT	connective tissue	**n**	neck	**SC**	surface lining cells
GP	gastric pit				

PLATE 15-3B Stomach

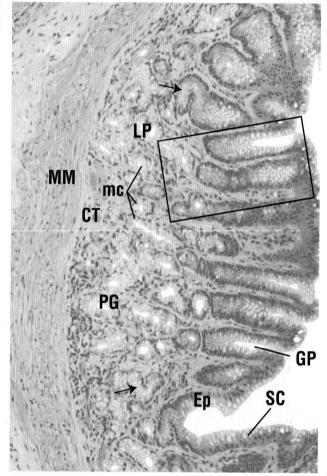

FIGURE 15-3-3. Pyloric gland. Stomach. x.s. Monkey. Plastic section. ×132.

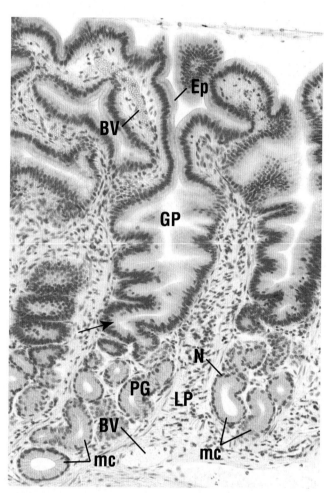

FIGURE 15-3-4. Pyloric gland. Stomach. x.s. Human. Paraffin section. ×270.

The mucosa of the pyloric region of the stomach presents **gastric pits** (GP) that are deeper than those of the cardiac or fundic regions. The deep aspects of these pits are coiled (*arrows*). As in the other regions of the stomach, the **epithelium** (Ep) is simple columnar, consisting mainly of **surface lining cells** (SC). Note that the **lamina propria** (LP) is loosely packed with **pyloric glands** (PG) and that considerable **connective tissue** (CT) is present. The pyloric glands are composed mainly of **mucous cells** (mc). Observe the two muscle layers of the **muscularis mucosae** (MM). A region similar to the *boxed area* is presented in Figure 15-3-4.

This is a photomicrograph of a region similar to the *boxed area* of Figure 15-3-3. The simple columnar **epithelium** (Ep) of the **gastric pit** is composed mostly of surface lining cells. These pits are not only much deeper than those of the fundic or cardiac regions but are also somewhat coiled (*arrow*), as are the **pyloric glands** (PG), which empty into the base of the pits. These glands are populated by **mucus-secreting cells** (mc) similar to mucous neck cells, whose **nuclei** (N) are flattened against the basal cell membrane. Note that the glands are not closely packed and that the **lamina propria** (LP) is very cellular and possesses a rich **vascular supply** (BV).

KEY					
BV	blood vessels	**LP**	lamina propria	**N**	nuclei
CT	connective tissue	**mc**	mucous,	**PG**	pyloric glands
Ep	epithelium		mucus-secreting cells	**SC**	surface lining cells
GP	gastric pit	**MM**	muscularis mucosae		

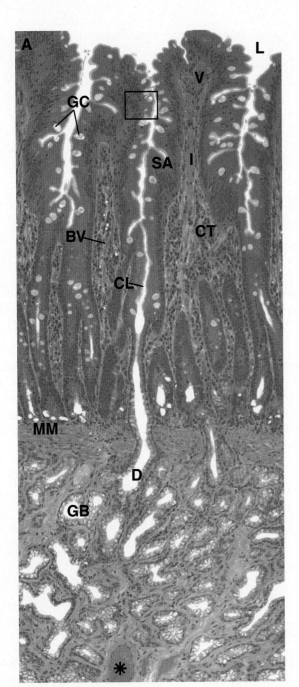

FIGURE 15-4-1A. Duodenum. l.s. Monkey. Plastic section. Montage. ×132.

The lamina propria of the duodenum possesses finger-like evaginations known as **villi** (V), which project into the **lumen** (L). The villi are covered by **surface absorptive cells** (SA): enterocytes forming a simple columnar epithelium with a brush border. Interspersed among these surface absorptive cells are **goblet cells** (GC) as well as occasional DNES cells. The **connective tissue** (CT) core (lamina propria) of the villus is composed of lymphoid and other cellular elements whose nuclei stain very intensely. **Blood vessels** (BV) also abound in the lamina propria, as do large, blindly ending lymphatic channels known as **lacteals** (I), recognizable by their large size and lack of red blood cells. Frequently, these lacteals are collapsed. The deeper aspect of the lamina propria houses glands, the **crypts of Lieberkühn** (CL). These simple tubular glands deliver their secretions into the intervillar spaces. The bases of these crypts reach the **muscularis mucosae** (MM), composed of inner circular and outer longitudinal layers of smooth muscle. Deep to this muscle layer is the submucosa, which, in the duodenum, is occupied by compound tubular **glands of Brunner** (GB). These glands deliver their mucous secretion via **ducts** (D), which pierce the muscularis mucosae, into the crypts of Lieberkühn. A region similar to the *boxed area* is presented at a higher magnification in Figure 15-4-1B. Figure 15-4-2 is the continuation of this montage (compare asterisks).

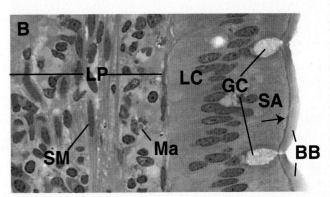

FIGURE 15-4-1B. Epithelium and core of villus. Monkey. Plastic section. ×540.

This higher magnification of a region similar to the *boxed area* in Figure 15-4-1A presents the epithelium and part of the connective tissue core of a villus. Note that the **surface absorptive cells** (SA) display a **brush border** (BB), terminal bars (*arrow*), and **goblet cells** (GC). Although DNES cells are also present, they constitute only a small percentage of the cell population. The **lamina propria** (LP) core of the villus is highly cellular, housing **lymphoid cells** (LC), **smooth muscle cells** (SM), mast cells, **macrophages** (Ma), and fibroblasts, among others.

KEY					
BB	brush border	**GC**	goblet cells	**Ma**	macrophages
CL	crypts of Lieberkühn	**I**	lacteals	**MM**	muscularis mucosae
CT	connective tissue	**L**	lumen	**SA**	surface absorptive cells
D	ducts	**LC**	lymphoid cells	**SM**	smooth muscle cells
GB	glands of Brunner	**LP**	lamina propria	**V**	villi

PLATE 15-4B Duodenum

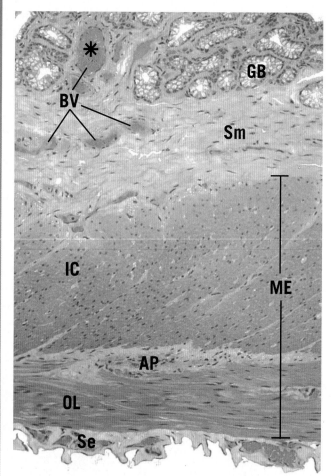

FIGURE 15-4-2. Duodenum. l.s. Monkey. Plastic section. ×132.

This photomicrograph is a continuation of the montage presented in Figure 15-4-1A (compare *asterisks*). Note that the **submucosa (Sm)**, occupied by **glands of Brunner** (GB), is a **vascular** structure (BV) and houses Meissner's submucosal plexus. The submucosa extends to the **muscularis externa (ME)**, composed of an **inner circular** (IC) and **outer longitudinal** (OL) smooth muscle layer. Note the presence of **Auerbach's myenteric plexus** (AP) between these two muscle layers. The duodenum, in part, is covered by a **serosa** (Se), whose mesothelium provides this organ with a smooth, moist surface.

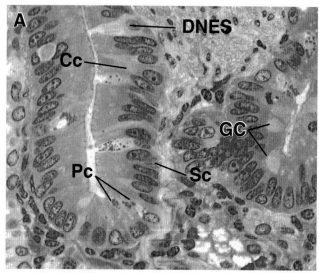

FIGURE 15-4-3A. Duodenum. x.s. Monkey. Plastic section. ×540.

The base of the crypt of Lieberkühn displays the several types of cells that compose this gland. **Paneth cells** (Pc) are readily recognizable due to the large granules in their apical cytoplasm. **DNES cells** (DNES) are clear cells with fine granules usually located basally. **Goblet cells** (GC), **columnar cells** (Cc), and **stem cells** (Sc) constitute the remaining cell population.

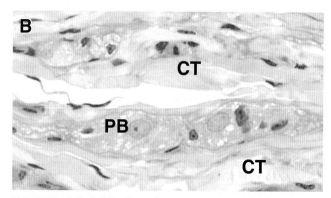

FIGURE 15-4-3B. Duodenum. x.s. Monkey. Plastic section. ×540.

The submucosa of the intestinal tract displays small parasympathetic ganglia, Meissner's submucosal plexus. Note the large **postganglionic cell bodies** (PB) surrounded by elements of **connective tissue** (CT).

KEY					
AP	Auerbach's myenteric plexus	**GB**	glands of Brunner	**PB**	postganglionic cell bodies
		GC	goblet cells	**Pc**	Paneth cells
BV	blood vessels	**IC**	inner circular layer	**Sc**	stem cells
Cc	columnar cells	**ME**	muscularis externa	**Se**	serosa
CT	connective tissue	**OL**	outer longitudinal layer	**Sm**	submucosa
DNES	DNES cells				

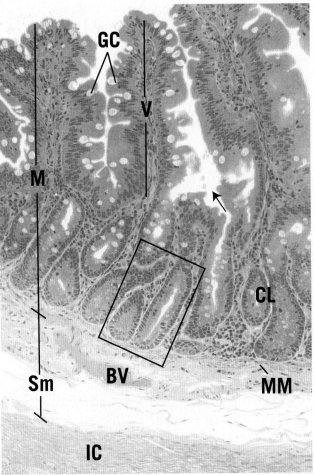

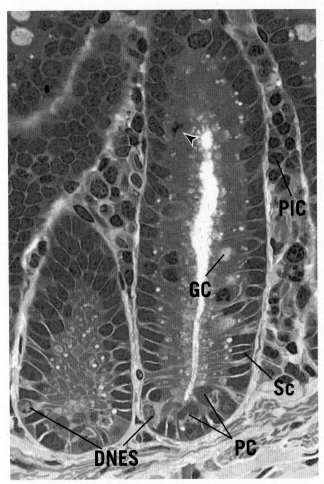

FIGURE 15-5-1. Jejunum. x.s. Monkey. Plastic section. ×132.

FIGURE 15-5-2. Jejunum. x.s. Monkey. Plastic section. ×540.

The **mucosa** (M) and **submucosa** (Sm) of the jejunum are presented in this photomicrograph. The **villi** (V) of this region possess more **goblet cells** (GC) than those of the duodenum. Observe that the **crypts of Lieberkühn** (CL) open into the intervillar spaces (*arrow*) and that the lamina propria displays numerous dense nuclei, evidence of lymphatic infiltration. The flimsy **muscularis mucosae** (MM) separate the lamina propria from the submucosa. Large **blood vessels** (BV) occupy the submucosa, which is composed of a loose type of collagenous connective tissue. The **inner circular** (IC) layer of the muscularis externa is evident at the bottom of the photomicrograph. The *boxed region* is presented at a higher magnification in Figure 15-5-2.

This photomicrograph is a higher magnification of the *boxed area* of Figure 15-5-1. The crypts of Lieberkühn are composed of several cell types, some of which are evident in this figure. **Goblet cells** (GC) that manufacture mucus may be noted in various degrees of mucus production. Narrow **stem cells** (Sc) undergo mitotic activity (*arrowhead*), and newly formed cells reconstitute the cell population of the crypt and villus. **Paneth cells** (PC) are located at the base of crypts and may be recognized by their large granules. **DNES cells** (DNES) appear as clear cells, with fine granules usually basally located. The lamina propria displays numerous **plasma cells** (PlC).

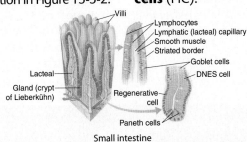

KEY					
BV	blood vessels	**IC**	inner circular layer	**PLC**	plasma cells
CL	crypts of Lieberkühn	**M**	mucosa	**Sc**	stem cells
DNES	DNES cells	**MM**	muscularis mucosae	**Sm**	submucosa
GC	goblet cells	**Pc**	Paneth cells	**V**	villi

PLATE 15-5B   Ileum

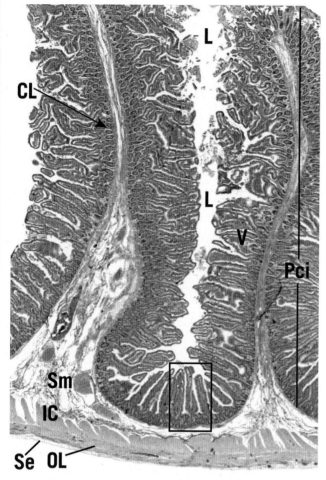

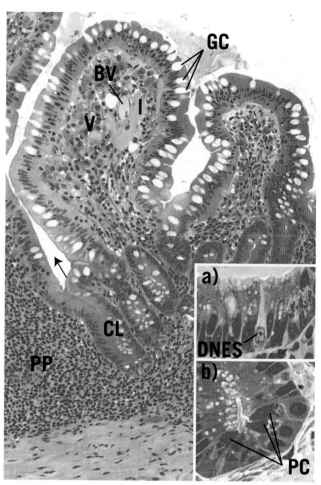

FIGURE 15-5-3. Ileum. l.s. Human. Paraffin section. ×14.

The entire wall of the ileum is presented, displaying spiral folds of the submucosa that partially encircle the lumen. These folds, known as **plicae circulares** (Pci), increase the surface area of the small intestines. Note that the lamina propria is clearly delineated from the **submucosa** (Sm) by the muscularis mucosae. The lamina propria forms numerous **villi** (V) that protrude into the **lumen** (L); glands known as **crypts of Lieberkühn** (CL) deliver their secretions into the intervillar spaces. The submucosa abuts the **inner circular** (IC) layer of smooth muscle that, in turn, is surrounded by the **outer longitudinal** (OL) smooth muscle layer of the muscularis externa. Observe the **serosa** (Se) investing the ileum. A region similar to the *boxed area* is presented at a higher magnification in Figure 15-5-4.

FIGURE 15-5-4. Ileum. x.s. Monkey. Plastic section. ×132.

This is a higher magnification of a region similar to the *boxed area* of Figure 15-5-3. Note that the **villi** (V) are covered by a simple columnar epithelium, whose cellular constituents include numerous **goblet cells** (GC). The core of the villus displays **blood vessels** (BV) as well as a large lymphatic vessel known as a **lacteal** (I). The **crypts of Lieberkühn** (CL) open into the intervillar spaces (*arrow*). The group of lymphoid nodules of the ileum is known as **Peyer's patches** (PP). *Inset a.* **Crypt of Lieberkühn. l.s. Monkey. Plastic section.** ×540. The crypts of Lieberkühn also possess **DNES cells** (DNES), recognizable by their clear appearance and usually basally oriented fine granules. *Inset b.* **Crypt of Lieberkühn. l.s. Monkey. Plastic section.** ×540. The base of the crypt of Lieberkühn displays cells with large granules. These are **Paneth cells** (PC), which produce the bactericidal agent lysozyme.

KEY					
BV	blood vessels	**L**	lumen	**PP**	Peyer's patches
CL	crypts of Lieberkühn	**OL**	outer longitudinal layer	**Se**	serosa
GC	goblet cells	**PC**	Paneth cells	**Sm**	submucosa
IC	inner circular layer	**Pci**	plicae circulares	**V**	villi
I	lacteal				

PLATE 15-6A Colon

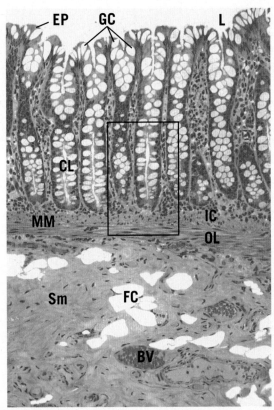

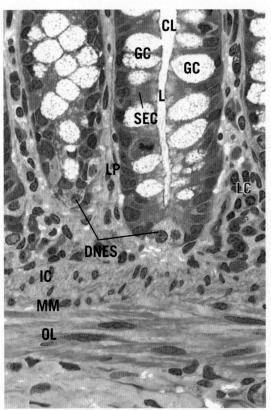

FIGURE 15-6-1. Colon. l.s. Monkey. Plastic section. ×132.

This photomicrograph depicts the mucosa and part of the submucosa of the colon. Note the absence of surface modifications such as pits and villi, which indicate that this section is not of the stomach or small intestines. The **epithelium** (Ep) lining the **lumen** (L) is simple columnar with numerous **goblet cells** (GC). The straight simple tubular glands are **crypts of Lieberkühn** (CL), which extend down to the **muscularis mucosae** (MM). The **inner circular** (IC) and **outer longitudinal** (OL) layers of smooth muscle comprising this region of the mucosa are evident. The **submucosa** (Sm) is very **vascular** (BV) and houses numerous **fat cells** (FC). The *boxed area* is presented at a higher magnification in Figure 15-6-2.

FIGURE 15-6-2. Colon. l.s. Monkey. Plastic section. ×540.

This photomicrograph is a higher magnification of the *boxed area* of Figure 15-6-1. The cell population of the **crypts of Lieberkühn** (CL) is composed of numerous **goblet cells** (GC), which deliver their mucus into the **lumen** (L) of the crypt. **Surface epithelial cells** (SEC) as well as undifferentiated stem cells are also present. The latter undergo mitosis to repopulate the epithelial lining. **DNES cells** (DNES) constitute a small percentage of the cell population. Note that Paneth cells are not present in the colon. The **lamina propria** (LP) is very cellular, housing many **lymphoid cells** (LC). The **inner circular** (IC) and **outer longitudinal** (OL) smooth muscle layers of the **muscularis mucosae** (MM) are evident.

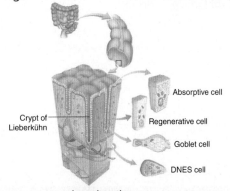

Crypt of Lieberkühn

Absorptive cell

Regenerative cell

Goblet cell

DNES cell

Large intestine

KEY					
BV	blood vessels	**GC**	goblet cells	**MM**	muscularis mucosae
CL	crypts of Lieberkühn	**IC**	inner circular layer	**OL**	outer longitudinal layer
DNES	DNES cells	**L**	lumen	**SEC**	surface epithelial cells
Ep	epithelium	**LC**	lymphoid cells	**Sm**	submucosa
FC	fat cells	**LP**	lamina propria		

PLATE 15-6B   Appendix

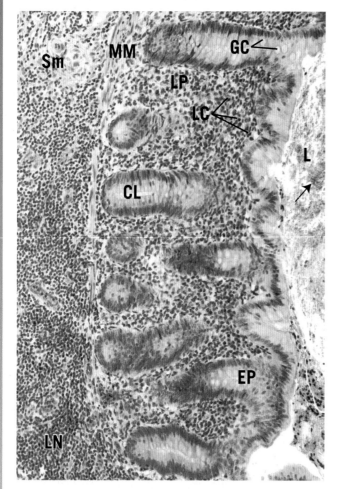

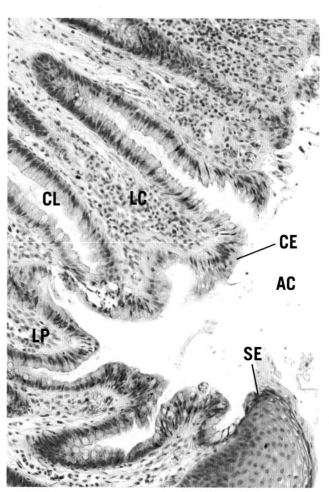

FIGURE 15-6-3. Appendix. x.s. Paraffin section. ×132.

The cross section of the appendix displays a **lumen** (L) that frequently contains debris (*arrow*). The lumen is lined by a simple columnar **epithelium** (Ep), consisting of many **goblet cells** (GC). **Crypts of Lieberkühn** (CL) are relatively shallow in comparison with those of the colon. The **lamina propria** (LP) is highly infiltrated with **lymphoid cells** (LC), derived from **lymphoid nodules** (LN) of the **submucosa** (Sm) and lamina propria. The **muscularis mucosae** (MM) delineate the border between the lamina propria and the submucosa.

FIGURE 15-6-4. Anorectal junction. l.s. Human. Paraffin section. ×132.

The anorectal junction presents a superficial similarity to the esophagogastric junction because of the abrupt epithelial transition. The **simple columnar epithelium** (CE) of the rectum is replaced by the stratified squamous epithelium of the **anal canal** (AC). The **crypts of Lieberkühn** (CL) of the AC are shorter than those of the colon. The **lamina propria** (LP) is infiltrated by **lymphoid cells** (LC).

KEY					
AC	anal canal	**Ep**	epithelium	**LN**	lymphatic nodules
CE	simple columnar	**GC**	goblet cells	**LP**	lamina propria
	epithelium	**L**	lumen	**MM**	muscularis mucosae
CL	crypts of Lieberkühn	**LC**	lymphoid cells	**Sm**	submucosa

PLATE 15-7   Colon, Electron Microscopy

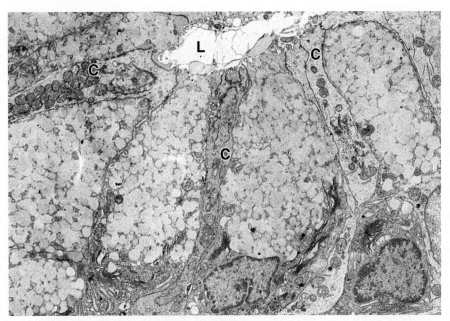

FIGURE 15-7-1. Colon. Rat. Electron microscopy. ×3,780.

The deep aspect of the crypt of Lieberkühn presents **columnar cells** (C) and deep crypt cells that produce a mucous type of secretion that is delivered into the **lumen** (L) of the crypt. (From Altmann GG. Morphological observations on mucus-secreting non-goblet cells in the deep crypts of the rat ascending colon. *Am J Anat* 1983;167(1):95–117. Copyright © 1983 Wiley-Liss, Inc. Reprinted by permission of John Wiley & Sons, Inc.)

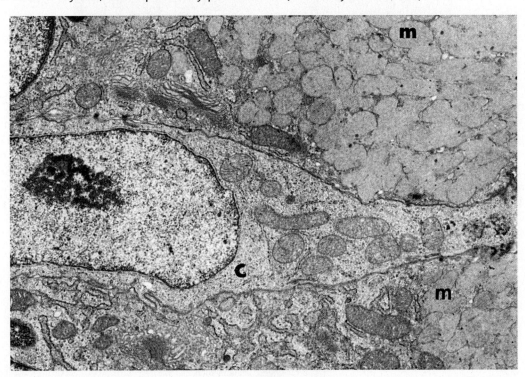

FIGURE 15-7-2. Colon. Rat. Electron microscopy. ×12,600.

At higher magnification of the deep aspect of the crypt of Lieberkühn, the deep crypt cells present somewhat electron-dense **vacuoles** (m). Note that many of these vacuoles coalesce, forming amorphous vacuolar profiles. The slender **columnar cell** (C) displays no vacuoles but does possess numerous mitochondria and occasional profiles of rough endoplasmic reticulum. Observe the large, oval nucleus and clearly evident nucleolus. (From Altmann GG. Morphological observations on mucus-secreting non-goblet cells in the deep crypts of the rat ascending colon. *Am J Anat* 1983;167(1):95–117. Copyright © 1983 Wiley-Liss, Inc. Reprinted by permission of John Wiley & Sons, Inc.)

KEY					
C	columnar cells	L	lumen	m	vacuoles

PLATE 15-8 Colon, Scanning Electron Microscopy

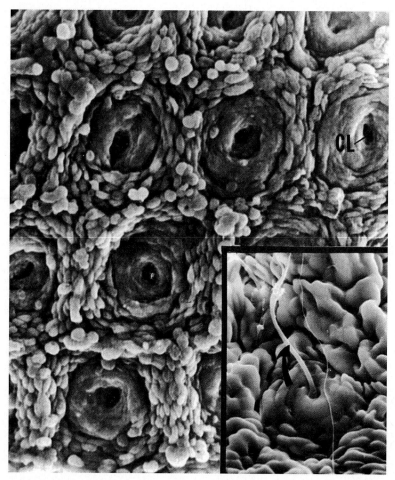

FIGURE 15-8-1. Colon. Monkey. Scanning electron microscopy. ×614.

This scanning electron micrograph displays the openings of the **crypts of Lieberkühn** (CL) as well as the cells lining the mucosal surface. (From Specian RD, et al. The surface topography of the colonic crypt in rabbit and monkey. *Am J Anat* 1981;160(4):461–472. Copyright © 1981 Wiley-Liss, Inc. Reprinted by permission of John Wiley & Sons, Inc.) *Inset.* **Colon. Rabbit. Scanning electron microscopy**. ×778. The openings of the crypts of Lieberkühn are not as regularly arranged in the rabbit as in the monkey. Observe the mucus arising from the crypt opening (*arrow*). (From Specian RD, et al. The surface topography of the colonic crypt in rabbit and monkey. *Am J Anat* 1981;160(4):461–472. Copyright © 1981 Wiley-Liss, Inc. Reprinted by permission of John Wiley & Sons, Inc.)

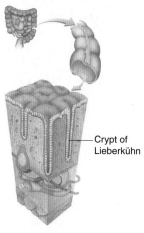

Crypt of
Lieberkühn

Large intestine

KEY	
CL	crypts of Lieberkühn

Selected Review of Histologic Images

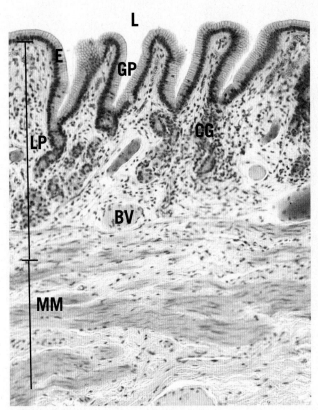

REVIEW FIGURE 15-1-1. Cardiac stomach. x.s. Dog. Paraffin section. ×132.

Note the **simple columnar epithelium** (E) lining both the stomach and the **gastric pits** (GP) and that these gastric pits open into the **lumen** (L) of the cardiac stomach. The **lamina propria** (LP) houses **cardiac glands** (CG) and is richly **vascularized** (BV). The inner circular muscle fibers of the **muscularis mucosae** (MM) are shown to advantage.

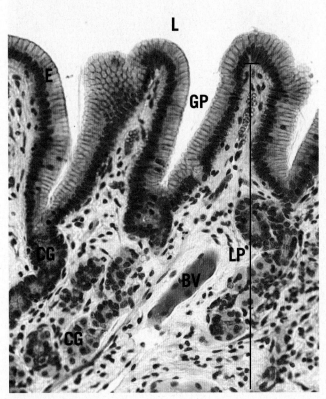

REVIEW FIGURE 15-1-2. Cardiac stomach. x.s. Dog. Paraffin section. ×270.

This is a higher magnification of the left-hand side of Review Figure 15-1-1. Note that the **lumen** (L) is lined by a simple columnar epithelium and that this epithelial lining continues into the **gastric pits** (GP). The **vascular** (BV) **lamina propria** (LP) houses **cardiac glands** (CG) which deliver their secretion into the bottom of the gastric pits.

KEY					
BV	blood vessels	GP	gastric pits	LP	lamina propria
CG	cardiac glands	L	lumen	MM	muscularis mucosae
E	simple columnar epithelium				

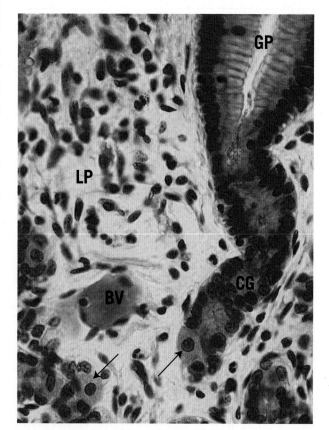

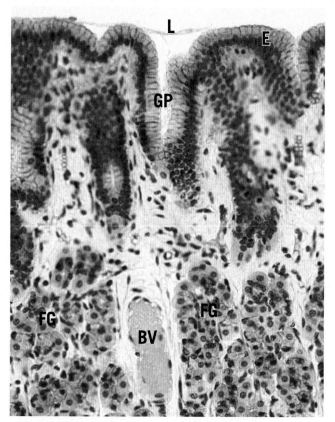

REVIEW FIGURE 15-1-3. Cardiac stomach. x.s. Dog. Paraffin section. ×540.

This is a higher magnification of the left-hand side of Review Figure 15-1-2. Note that the base of the **gastric pit** (GP) receives a **cardiac gland** (CG). The **lamina propria** (LP) of the mucosa is rich in **blood vessels** (BV). The arrows depict **parietal cells** (PC) of the cardiac glands.

REVIEW FIGURE 15-1-4. Fundic stomach. x.s. Dog. Paraffin section. ×270.

The **simple columnar epithelium** (E) that lines the **lumen** (L) of the fundic stomach continues into the **gastric pits** (GP). The **vascular** (BV) lamina propria is crowded with **fundic glands** (FG).

KEY					
BV	blood vessels	**FG**	fundic glands	**LP**	lamina propria
CG	cardiac glands	**GP**	gastric pits	**PC**	parietal cells
E	simple columnar epithelium	**L**	lumen		

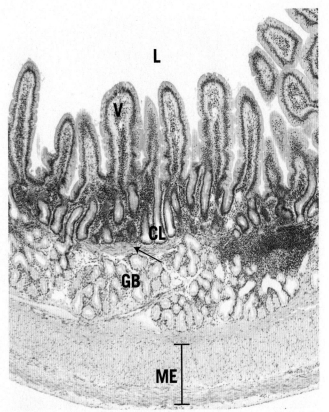

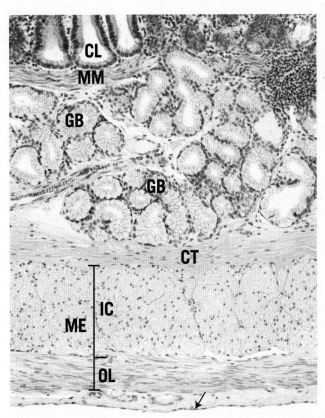

REVIEW FIGURE 15-2-1. Duodenum. x.s. Paraffin section. ×56.

This low-power photomicrograph of the duodenum displays its entire extent from the **lumen** (L) to the outer longitudinal layer of its **muscularis externa** (ME). Note the presence of the finger-like **villi** (V) and that the **crypts of Lieberkühn** (CL) extend to the **muscularis mucosae** (*arrow*). The **glands of Brunner** (GB) occupy most of the submucosa.

REVIEW FIGURE 15-2-2. Duodenum. x.s. Paraffin section. ×132.

This photomicrograph of the duodenum displays the submucosa, housing the **glands of Brunner** (GB), **muscularis externa** (ME), and the **serosa** (*arrow*). The bases of the **crypts of Lieberkühn** (CL) are evident as they nestle against the **muscularis mucosae** (MM) and the **connective tissue** (CT) of the submucosa contacts the **inner circular layer** (IC) of the muscularis externa. The **outer longitudinal** (OL) **layer** abuts the subserosal connective tissue.

KEY					
CL	crypts of Lieberkühn	**IC**	inner circular layer	**MM**	muscularis mucosae
CT	connective tissue	**L**	lumen	**OL**	outer longitudinal layer
GB	glands of Brunner	**ME**	muscularis externa	**V**	villi

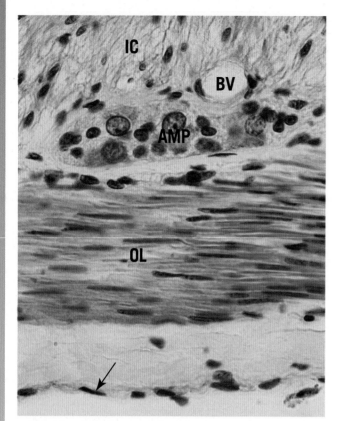

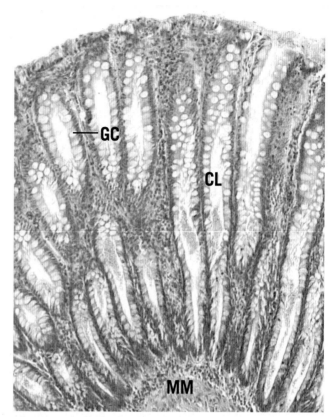

REVIEW FIGURE 15-2-3. Duodenum. Auerbach's myenteric plexus. l.s. Paraffin section. ×540.

This photomicrograph of a longitudinal section of the duodenum displays the smooth muscle cells of the **inner circular layer** (IC) of the muscularis externa cut in cross section and the smooth muscle cells of the **outer longitudinal layer** (OL) cut along their longitudinal axis. The subserosal connective tissue and the **serosa** (*arrow*) are evident. Note that **Auerbach's myenteric plexus** (AMP) is lodged between the inner circular and outer longitudinal muscle layers of the muscularis externa. Observe the **blood vessels** (BV) that serve the muscularis externa as well as the autonomic nerve plexus.

REVIEW FIGURE 15-2-4. Colon. x.s. Paraffin section. ×132.

This photomicrograph of the large intestine displays that there are no villi in the colon. Observe that the **crypts of Lieberkühn** (CL) are richly endowed by **goblet cells** (GC). Note the presence of the **muscularis mucosae** (MM).

KEY					
AMP	Auerbach's myenteric plexus	**CL**	crypts of Lieberkühn	**MM**	muscularis mucosae
BV	blood vessels	**GC**	goblet cells	**OL**	outer longitudinal layer
		IC	inner circular layer		

Summary of Histologic Organization

I. Esophagus

The **esophagus** is a long, muscular tube that delivers the **bolus** of food from the **pharynx** to the **stomach**. The esophagus, as well as the remainder of the digestive tract, is composed of four concentric layers: **mucosa**, **submucosa**, **muscularis externa**, and **adventitia**. The **lumen** of the esophagus is normally collapsed.

A. Mucosa

The **mucosa** has three regions: **epithelium**, **lamina propria**, and **muscularis mucosae**. It is thrown into longitudinal folds.

1. Epithelium

The **epithelium** is **stratified squamous nonkeratinized**.

2. Lamina Propria

The **lamina propria** is a loose connective tissue that contains mucus-producing **esophageal cardiac glands** in some regions of the esophagus.

3. Muscularis Mucosae

The **muscularis mucosae** is composed of a single layer of **longitudinally** oriented **smooth muscle**.

B. Submucosa

The **submucosa**, composed of fibroelastic connective tissue, is thrown into longitudinal folds. The **esophageal glands proper** of this layer produce a mucous secretion. **Meissner's submucosal plexus** houses postganglionic parasympathetic neurons.

C. Muscularis Externa

The **muscularis externa** is composed of **inner circular** (tight helix) and **outer longitudinal** (loose helix) **muscle layers**. In the upper third of the esophagus, these consist of **skeletal muscle**; in the middle third, they consist of **skeletal** and **smooth muscle**; and in the lower third, they consist of **smooth muscle**. **Auerbach's myenteric plexus** is located between the two layers of muscle.

D. Adventitia

The **adventitia** of the esophagus is composed of fibrous connective tissue. Inferior to the diaphragm, the esophagus is covered by a **serosa**.

II. Stomach

The **stomach** is a sac-like structure that receives food from the **esophagus** and delivers its contents, known as chyme, into the **duodenum**. The stomach has three histologically recognizable regions: **cardiac**, **fundic**, and **pyloric**. The **mucosa** and **submucosa** of the empty stomach are thrown into folds, known as **rugae**, that disappear in the distended stomach.

A. Mucosa

The **mucosa** presents **gastric pits**, the bases of which accept the openings of **gastric glands**.

1. Epithelium

The **simple columnar epithelium** has no goblet cells. The cells composing this epithelium are known as **surface lining cells** and extend into the gastric pits.

2. Lamina Propria

The **lamina propria** houses numerous **gastric glands**, slender blood vessels, and various connective tissue and **lymphoid cells**.

a. *Cells of Gastric Glands*

Gastric glands are composed of the following cell types: **parietal (oxyntic) cells**, **chief (zymogenic) cells**, **mucous neck cells**, **DNES (enteroendocrine) cells**, and **stem cells**. Glands of the **cardiac region** have no **chief** and only a few **parietal cells**. Glands of the **pyloric region** are short and possess no chief cells and only a few parietal cells. Most of the cells are mucus-secreting cells resembling **mucous neck cells**. Glands of the **fundic region** possess all five cell types.

3. Muscularis Mucosae

The **muscularis mucosae** is composed of an **inner circular** and an **outer longitudinal smooth muscle** layer. A third layer may be present in certain regions.

B. Submucosa

The **submucosa** contains no glands. It houses a vascular plexus as well as **Meissner's submucosal plexus**.

C. Muscularis Externa

The **muscularis externa** is composed of three smooth muscle layers: the **inner oblique**, the **middle circular**, and the **outer longitudinal**. The middle circular forms the **pyloric sphincter**. **Auerbach's myenteric plexus** is located between the circular and longitudinal layers.

D. Serosa

The stomach is covered by a connective tissue coat enveloped in visceral peritoneum (mesothelium), the **serosa**.

III. Small Intestine

The **small intestine** is composed of three regions: **duodenum**, **jejunum**, and **ileum**. The **mucosa** of the small intestine presents folds, known as **villi**, that change their morphology and decrease in height from the duodenum to the ileum. The submucosa displays spiral folds, **plicae circulares** (valves of Kerckring).

A. Mucosa

The **mucosa** presents **villi**, evaginations of the **lamina propria** covered with epithelium.

1. Epithelium

The **simple columnar epithelium** consists of **goblet**, **surface absorptive (enterocytes)**, and **DNES cells**. The number of goblet cells increases from the duodenum to the ileum.

2. Lamina Propria

The **lamina propria**, composed of **loose connective tissue**, houses glands, known as the **crypts of Lieberkühn**, that extend to the muscularis mucosae. The cells composing these glands are **goblet cells**, **columnar cells**, and, especially at the base, **Paneth cells**, **DNES cells**, and **stem cells**. An occasional **caveolated cell** may also be noted. A central **lacteal**, a blindly ending lymphatic vessel, **smooth muscle cells**, **blood vessels**, solitary **lymphatic nodules**, and **lymphoid cells** are also present. **Lymphatic nodules**, with M cell epithelial caps, are especially abundant as **Peyer's patches** in the ileum.

3. Muscularis Mucosae

The **muscularis mucosae** consists of an **inner circular** and an **outer longitudinal** layer of **smooth muscle**.

B. Submucosa

The **submucosa** is not unusual except in the **duodenum**, where it contains **Brunner's glands**.

C. Muscularis Externa

The **muscularis externa** is composed of the usual **inner circular** and **outer longitudinal** layers of **smooth muscle**, with **Auerbach's myenteric plexus** intervening.

D. Serosa

The duodenum is covered by **serosa** and **adventitia**, whereas the jejunum and ileum are covered by a serosa.

IV. Large Intestine

The **large intestine** is composed of the **appendix**, the **cecum**, the **colon (ascending, transverse, and descending)**, the **rectum**, and the **anal canal**. The appendix and AC are described separately, although the remainder of the large intestine presents identical histologic features.

A. Colon

1. Mucosa

The **mucosa** presents no specialized folds. It is thicker than that of the small intestine.

a. *Epithelium*

The **simple columnar epithelium** has goblet cells and columnar cells.

b. *Lamina Propria*

The **crypts of Lieberkühn** of the **lamina propria** are longer than those of the small intestine. They are composed of numerous **goblet cells**, a few **DNES cells**, and **stem cells**. **Lymphoid nodules** are frequently present.

c. *Muscularis Mucosae*

The **muscularis mucosae** consists of **inner circular** and **outer longitudinal smooth muscle** layers.

2. Submucosa

The **submucosa** resembles that of the jejunum or ileum.

3. Muscularis Externa

The **muscularis externa** is composed of **inner circular** and **outer longitudinal smooth muscle** layers. The outer longitudinal muscle is modified into **taeniae coli**, three flat ribbons of longitudinally arranged smooth muscles. These are responsible for the formation of **haustra coli** (sacculations). **Auerbach's plexus** occupies its position between the two layers.

4. Serosa

The colon possesses both **serosa** and **adventitia**. The serosa presents small, fat-filled pouches, the **appendices epiploicae**.

B. Appendix

The **lumen** of the **appendix** is usually stellate-shaped, and it may be obliterated. The **simple columnar epithelium** covers a **lamina propria** rich in **lymphoid nodules** and some **crypts of Lieberkühn**. The **muscularis mucosae**, **submucosa**, and **muscularis externa** conform to the general plan of the digestive tract but unlike the rest of the colon, the outer longitudinal layer does not form taeniae coli. It is covered by a **serosa**.

C. Anal Canal

The **anal canal** presents longitudinal folds; **anal columns**, which become joined at the orifice of the anus to form **anal valves**; and intervening **anal sinuses**. The epithelium changes from the **simple columnar** of the rectum, to **simple cuboidal** at the **anal valves**, to **stratified squamous** distal to the anal valves, to **epidermis** at the orifice of the anus. **Circumanal glands**, **hair follicles**, and **sebaceous glands** are present here. The **submucosa** is rich in vascular supply. The **muscularis externa** forms the internal anal sphincter muscle. An **adventitia** connects the anus to the surrounding structures.

Chapter Review Questions

15-1. Bleeding caused by Mallory–Weiss syndrome is usually self-limiting, but occasionally surgery is required to stop the bleeding. Which region of the alimentary canal is surgically repaired in patients with this syndrome?

A. Stomach

B. Duodenum

C. Cecum

D. Sigmoid colon

E. Appendix

15-2. *Helicobacter pylori* infection is a common cause of peptic ulcers. These organisms are protected from the acidic milieu by secretions produced by which of the following cells?

A. Paneth cells

B. Parietal cells

C. Surface lining cells

D. DNES cells

E. Goblet cells

15-3. An individual suffering from Zollinger–Ellison syndrome has a high elevation of which of the following?

A. Leptin

B. Gastrin

C. Glicentin

D. Ghrelin

E. Secretin

15-4. A bacterial biofilm that is believed to act as a reservoir to reestablish normal bacterial flora has been discovered in which of the following structures?

A. Cecum

B. Appendix

C. Sigmoid colon

D. Rectum

15-5. Vitamin B_{12} absorption is dependent on a glycoprotein manufactured by which of the following cells?

A. Paneth cells

B. Surface absorptive cells

C. Microfold cells

D. Parietal cells

E. Surface lining cells

DIGESTIVE SYSTEM III

CHAPTER OUTLINE

The **major salivary glands**, **pancreas**, and **liver** (and its accompanying **gallbladder**) are the extramural glands of the digestive system. They are located outside the wall of the alimentary canal, and they deliver their exocrine secretions into the lumen of the digestive tract via ducts. These glands manufacture digestive enzymes, endocrine and paracrine hormones, and blood proteins as well as numerous other products.

Major Salivary Glands

The three (perhaps four, including the newly discovered tubarial salivary glands) pairs of **major salivary glands**: **parotid**, **submandibular**, and **sublingual**, produce about 1 L of saliva per day, ~95% of the daily salivary secretion that they deliver into the oral cavity; as indicated in Chapter 14, the minor salivary glands produce the remaining 5% of the total daily salivary output.

The parotid gland produces **serous secretions**, whereas the submandibular and sublingual glands manufacture **mixed secretions** (a combination of serous and mucous saliva). *Major salivary glands secrete intermittently, whereas minor salivary glands secrete continuously.*

A previously unknown pair of salivary glands, known as the **tubarial salivary glands** located in the posterior aspect of the nasopharynx, in the vicinity of the torus tuberalis, was discovered in 2020. These glands are similar in size to the sublingual glands, and, in histologic sections, they display the presence of mucous acini capped with serous demilunes, indicating that these glands produce a mixed salivary secretion. *If the presence of these glands is confirmed, there will be four pairs, rather than three pairs of major salivary glands.*

All major salivary glands are encapsulated compound tubuloacinar glands except for the parotid glands that are compound acinar glands. The capsule sends septa (trabeculae) into the gland dividing it into lobes and lobules. The glands that produce a watery secretion have terminal *secretory units* that are usually **acinar** (grape-like) in shape, whereas glands that produce a mucous secretion have terminal *secretory units* that are **tubular** in shape. In a gland that produces a mixed secretion, the terminal mucous tubular units frequently have crescent-shaped acini called **serous demilunes** capping them. Although those structures are now believed to be artifacts of fixation, they provide an easily recognizable image of a gland that produces a mixed secretion and are continued to be referenced in this *Atlas and Text*. The cells of the acini are pyramidal in shape, but, in histologic sections, they present a triangular morphology, with a large, round basally located nucleus, and subnuclear basophilia and supranuclear eosinophilia with hematoxylin and eosin (H&E) staining. The cells of the mucous secretory units are mostly taller and pyramidal in shape; in histologic sections, they are somewhat round with a flat, basally located nucleus and pale cytoplasm. Both serous and mucous secretory units are surrounded by a few **myoepithelial cells** that, by contracting slightly, express the secretory product from the secretory unit into the ducts of the gland. These myoepithelial cells share the basement membrane of the secretory units (Fig. 16-1).

The ducts of the major salivary glands are classified by their location and function as well as by their morphology. Those positioned within the lobules are called the intralobular ducts as they directly drain the secretory units and then coalesce to form larger ducts but still within the lobules. Intralobular ducts lead out into larger ducts located outside the lobule called interlobular ducts that lead into even bigger ducts positioned outside or in between the lobes called the interlobar ducts. Eventually, this system of ducts forms the largest of the ducts, called the **terminal ducts**, that deliver saliva into the oral cavity. As this system of ducts transition from the smallest to the largest, their lining epithelia increase in thickness and they are supported by an increasing amount of connective tissue.

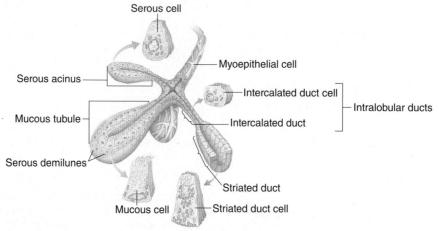

FIGURE 16-1. Graphic representation of major salivary glands.

There are two types of intralobular ducts.

- Intercalated ducts, composed of simple columnar epithelium, are the smallest with a diameter that is smaller than that of the acinus or tubules. They manufacture their own basement membrane that is continuous with that of their terminal secretory unit. They may possess their own myoepithelial cells.

- Striated ducts are composed of simple cuboidal to columnar epithelia. Each **striated duct** receives several intercalated ducts, and, in cross section, the diameter of striated ducts approximates the cross section of their secretory units. Striated ducts are composed of a simple tall cuboidal to simple columnar epithelium and, transmission electron microscopy demonstrated that the basal aspect of these cells displays intricate infoldings of the plasmalemma, forming a complex cytoplasmic compartmentalization, where each compartment houses numerous **mitochondria**. Striated ducts actively resorb sodium ions from and excrete potassium ions into their lumina, thereby modifying the saliva produced by the secretory units. These ducts also release bicarbonates into their lumina. Therefore, the saliva entering the striated ducts, known as the **primary saliva**, becomes modified within the striated duct and is known as **secondary saliva**, upon leaving the striated duct.

The interlobular ducts are positioned outside the lobules, surrounded by slightly more connective tissues on the outside, but the lining epithelium may resemble striated ducts closer to the lobules. The interlobar ducts are larger and possess stratified cuboidal to columnar epithelium and are supported by thicker connective tissue. The terminal ducts have the largest lumina, possess stratified columnar epithelium, and are supported by smooth muscle layers and thick connective tissues.

Parotid Gland

The **parotid gland**, the largest of the three major salivary glands, produces only 30% of the salivary output. It is located superficially and posteriorly to the ramus of the mandible and its principal duct, **parotid duct (Stensen's duct)**, opens into the oral cavity at the parotid papilla. This gland manufactures purely serous saliva (Fig. 16-2). As the individual ages, the parotid gland becomes infiltrated by adipose tissue, so that by age 50 years at least 30% of the gland is occupied by adipocytes.

Submandibular Gland

The **submandibular gland** is approximately one-third the size of the parotid, yet it produces 60% of the salivary output. It is located deep and inferior to the ramus of the

mandible in close association with the mylohyoid muscle. Approximately 90% of the terminal secretory units are serous acini and 10% mucous tubules capped with serous demilunes (Fig. 16-3). The duct system of this gland is very extensive, and its numerous cross-sectional profiles in histologic sections are characteristic of the submandibular gland. The long terminal **submandibular duct (Wharton's duct)** opens in the floor of the mouth, on either side of the lingual frenum, at the **sublingual caruncles**.

Sublingual Gland

The **sublingual gland** is the smallest of the major salivary glands, has an incomplete capsule, and is responsible for only 5% of the total salivary output. It is located on the floor of the mouth, deep to the sublingual fold and produces a mainly mucous secretion. The terminal duct system of this gland is composed of several small **ducts of Bartholin** that open onto the surface of the sublingual fold and some of which can also deliver saliva into the submandibular duct. Most of the terminal

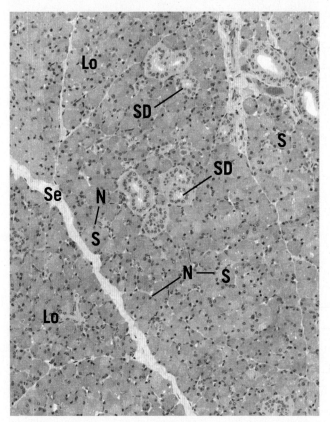

FIGURE 16-2. Low-magnification photomicrograph of a monkey parotid gland. Observe that the gland is subdivided into lobes and **lobules** (Lo) by connective tissue **septa** (Se). Note also the cross-sectional profiles of the terminal **serous secretory units** (S) with their acinar cells whose round **nuclei** (N) are basally located and the presence of **striated ducts** (SD). ×132.

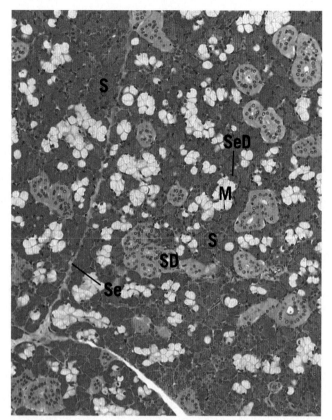

FIGURE 16-3. Low-magnification light micrograph of a monkey submandibular gland. Note that the gland is subdivided into lobules by connective tissue **septa** (Se) derived from the capsule of the gland. Because the submandibular gland produces a mixed secretion, both **serous (S) secretory units** and **mucous** (M) **secretory units** with **serous demilunes** (SeD) are present. The larger, pale structures are **striated ducts** (SD). ×132.

secretory units are mucous tubules, some capped with serous demilunes (Fig. 16-6).

Tubarial Gland

Tubarial glands (Figs. 16-4 and 16-5) are similar in size to and share a characteristic with the sublingual glands. In histologic sections, they display predominantly mucous acini, occasionally capped with serous demilunes, indicating that these glands produce a mostly mucous salivary secretion. *If the constant presence of these glands is confirmed, then there will be four pairs, rather than three pairs of major salivary glands.*

Saliva

Saliva is a **hypotonic** solution composed of 99% water, whose functions include lubrication and cleansing of the oral cavity and mixing with the masticated food to facilitate the ease of deglutition (swallowing). It also controls the oral cavity's bacterial flora by its content of **lysozyme**, **lactoferrin**, **peroxidases**, histidine-rich proteins, and **immunoglobulin A** (**IgA**). Saliva is also responsible for the

initial digestion of carbohydrates by **salivary amylase** and for assisting in the process of **taste** by dissolving food substances. Moreover, saliva acts as a buffer because of its contents of bicarbonates produced by cells of the striated duct.

Pancreas

The **pancreas** is a mixed gland, in that it has both exocrine and endocrine functions (Figs. 16-7 and 16-8). It has a delicate connective tissue **capsule** that provides slender septa that not only subdivide the gland into lobes and lobules but also act as conduits for the blood vessels that enter and leave the gland as well as for the system of ducts that deliver the secretions from the exocrine portion of the gland into the duodenum.

- The **exocrine portion of the pancreas** constitutes the larger component and is a **compound acinar gland** that manufactures a serous bicarbonate-rich secretion as well as enzymes and proenzymes.
  - The exocrine secretion is delivered to the duodenum via a series of ducts that begin as **intercalated ducts** in the center of each acinus (where the ductal cells are called **centroacinar cells**) and join with other intercalated ducts to form larger **intralobular ducts**. A

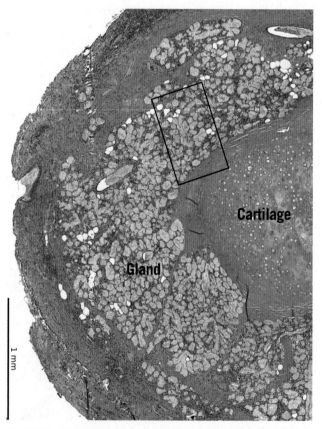

FIGURE 16-4. The low magnification image of a section of the tubarial gland that displays the cartilage of the torus tubarius surrounded by the mixed but mostly mucous tubarial gland. The boxed area is enlarged in Figure 16-5. (Courtesy Dr. Matthijs Valstar.)

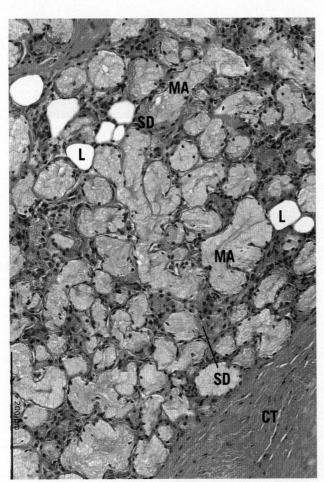

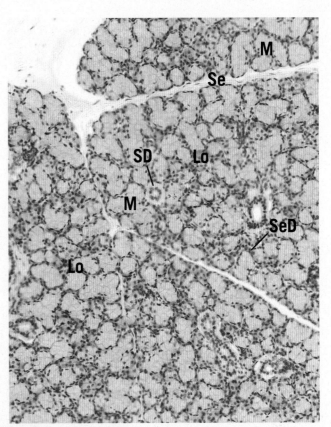

FIGURE 16-5. This photomicrograph is a higher magnification of the boxed area of Figure 16-4. Note the numerous mucous acini (MA) some of which are capped by serous demilunes (SD). The clear areas are lipid cells (L), and the connective tissue (CT) in the lower left contacts the perichondrium of the torus tubarius. (Courtesy Dr. Matthijs Valstar.)

FIGURE 16-6. This low-magnification photomicrograph of the human sublingual gland displays the **septa** (Se) that subdivides the gland into lobes and **lobules** (Lo). Note that the terminal **mucous secretory tubules** (M) are capped by **serous demilunes** (SeD). Observe the striated **duct** (D) near the center of the field. ×132.

number of these ducts join to form larger **interlobular ducts** that merged with similar ducts from other lobules eventually to form the **main pancreatic duct** that delivers the exocrine secretion of the pancreas into the lumen of the **duodenum** at the **major papilla (papilla of Vater)**. The pancreas, unlike the salivary glands, does not possess striated ducts.

• The **endocrine portions of the pancreas**, the 1 to 2 million **pancreatic islets (islets of Langerhans)**, are scattered throughout the exocrine pancreas. Each islet, composed of a richly vascularized spherical cluster of about 2,500 to 3,000 hormone-producing cells is, to a certain extent, isolated from the exocrine pancreas by type III collagen fibers (reticular fibers) that surround each islet.

Vascular Supply of the Pancreas

The **vascular supply** of the pancreas is arranged so that the arterial blood entering the pancreas is diverted into two compartments, one leading only to the exocrine

CLINICAL CONSIDERATIONS 16-1

Bell's Palsy

If a **parotid gland tumor** or the entire parotid gland must be excised, the surgeon must be extremely careful because the facial nerve (cranial nerve VII) forms a plexus within the parotid gland, and five major branches arise from that plexus. These branches serve all the muscles of facial expression and damage to one or more of those branches can paralyze, temporarily—or in certain cases permanently—all the muscles served by the damaged branches, resulting in facial droop, a condition known as **Bell's palsy**. If the condition is temporary in nature, full recovery can be expected in less than 6 months.

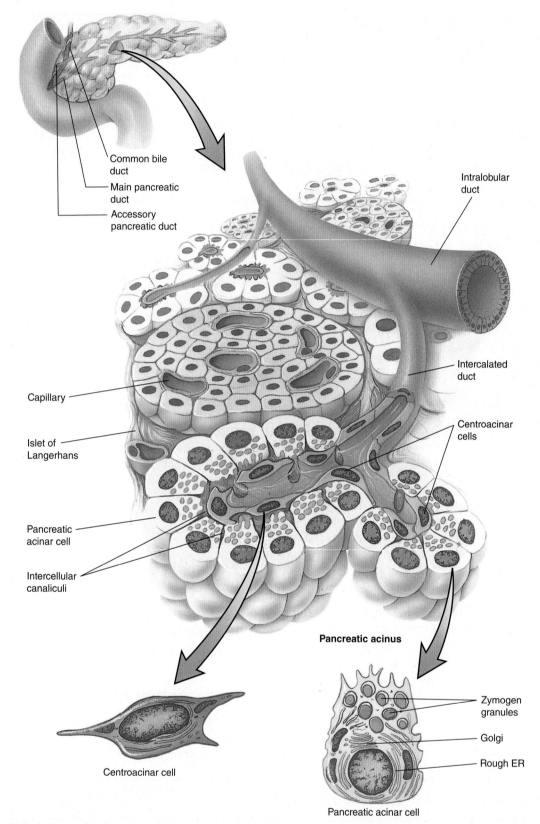

FIGURE 16-7. Schematic diagram of the pancreas illustrating both exocrine and endocrine portions. The **exocrine function** of the pancreas is served by its **acinar cells**, **centroacinar cells**, and **intercalated ducts**. The acinar cells secrete digestive enzymes, and the duct cells supply an alkaline buffer solution. The **endocrine portion** is composed of the **islets of Langerhans**, richly vascularized spherical aggregates of cells encased by reticular fibers. The islets are composed primarily of five types of cells, which can be differentiated from each other only with special stains.

CLINICAL CONSIDERATIONS 16-2

Sialadenitis

Sialadenitis, salivary gland inflammation, is one of the most frequent nonmalignant maladies involving the major salivary glands, usually the parotid gland but occasionally the submandibular or the sublingual gland can be involved.

There are two categories of this condition, **chronic**, which is less painful and often occurs after a meal; and **acute**, which is more painful and is accompanied by a reddish coloration of the skin over the entire area of the gland, which is tender to the touch.

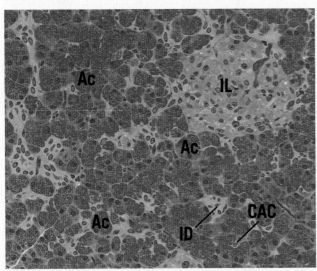

FIGURE 16-8. The exocrine pancreas displays its numerous **acini** (Ac), some with **centroacinar cells** (CAC), the beginning of the **intercalated ducts** (ID), in its center. Note that the acinar cells are well endowed with enzyme and proenzyme containing zymogen granules. The upper right-hand corner exhibits an **islet of Langerhans** (IL), the endocrine component of the pancreas. ×270.

pancreas and the other only to the islets of Langerhans. However, venous blood flow becomes comingled such that blood from the islets of Langerhans, bearing hormones such as somatostatin, enters the exocrine pancreas where it can affect the acinar cells.

Exocrine Pancreas

The **exocrine pancreas** produces ~1.2 L of fluid that is delivered to the **duodenum** via the pancreatic duct. Enzymes (and **proenzymes**) are manufactured by the **acinar cells** (Table 16-1), whereas the **alkaline fluid** is released by cells of the **intercalated ducts**, including the **centroacinar cells**.

The secretion of the enzymes and of the bicarbonate-rich fluid is *intermittent* and *independent of each other*. The release of these products is controlled by the hormones, **cholecystokinin** and **secretin**, released by the diffuse neuroepithelial cells **(DNES cells)** of the epithelial lining of the alimentary tract mucosa as well as by **acetylcholine** released by postganglionic parasympathetic nerve fibers.

- The **bicarbonate-rich fluid** is released by centroacinar cells and intercalated duct cells in response to **secretin** and **acetylcholine**. This alkaline fluid most probably acts as a buffer to neutralize the acidic chyme that enters the duodenum from the pyloric stomach. Both secretin and acetylcholine have to contact their respective receptors on the basal plasma membranes of the cells of these ducts for the alkaline fluid to be released.

- The **enzymes** (and **proenzymes**) are released by the **acinar cells** (see Table 16-1) in response to **cholecystokinin** from the DNES cells and **acetylcholine**. Both cholecystokinin and acetylcholine have to contact their respective receptors on the basal plasma membranes of the acinar cells for the enzymes and proenzymes to be released.

  - **Trypsin inhibitor** is also produced by the acinar cells to protect themselves, as well as the duct system of the pancreas, from inadvertent activity of trypsin.

Endocrine Pancreas

The **endocrine pancreas** is composed of 1 to 2 million **pancreatic islets (of Langerhans)**, scattered spherical aggregates of richly vascularized cords of endocrine cells. The hormones released from the endocrine pancreas are produced by the following cell types (Table 16-2):

- α **(A) cells**, producing **glucagon**;
- β **(B) cells**, manufacturing **insulin**;
- **G cells**, producing **gastrin**;
- δ_1 **(D$_1$) cells**, manufacturing **somatostatin**;
- δ_2 **(D$_2$) cells**, producing **vasoactive intestinal peptide (VIP)**;
- **PP cells**, secreting **pancreatic polypeptide**; and
- ε **cells (epsilon cells)**, secreting **ghrelin**.

Liver

The **liver** is the largest gland of the body (Figs. 16-9 and 16-10). It performs myriad functions, many of which are *not* glandular in nature. It is believed that the parenchymal cells of the liver, known as **hepatocytes**, have a life span of about 5 months, and they are capable of performing each of the ~100 different functions of the liver.

The liver is surrounded by a dense irregular collagenous connective tissue capsule, **Glisson's capsule**.

At the **porta hepatis**, connective tissue elements derived from Glisson's capsule enter the substance of the liver, ferrying **blood vessels** and bile-carrying **hepatic ducts** in and out of the liver and subdividing the liver into **lobes** and **lobules** (see Figs. 16-9 and 16-10). The liver receives all the nutrient-laden blood that leaves the alimentary canal and the spleen via the **portal vein**, forming 75% of its total blood supply. The remaining 25% of its blood supply is derived from the two **hepatic arteries**, direct branches of the celiac trunk of the abdominal aorta that bring oxygenated blood into the liver. Within the hepatic parenchyma, blood is directed through the rich network of **hepatic sinusoids** lined by endothelial cells with large **fenestrae** that lack diaphragms, and they display discontinuities between adjoining cells that, although large, are too small for the passage of blood cells or platelets. Because each hepatocyte is bordered by a vascular **sinusoid**, liver cells can absorb toxic materials and by-products of digestion, which they detoxify and store for future use. Blood is drained from the liver via the **hepatic veins**, tributaries of the inferior vena cava.

Hepatocytes are arranged in radiating **plates of liver cells**, each one cell thick in individuals older than seven years of age, that are arranged such that they form hexagonal lobules (2 mm long and 0.7 mm in diameter). These structures are referred to as **classical (hepatic) lobules** (see Fig. 16-10). Where three **classical lobules** meet, their slender connective tissue elements merge to form **portal areas** that house branches of the hepatic artery, portal vein, bile duct, and lymph vessel. The center of each classical lobule houses a single endothelial-lined **central vein**, which receives blood from the numerous endothelially lined hepatic sinusoids, thus forming the beginning of the blood drainage system of the liver. Central veins lead to **sublobular veins** that merge with other sublobular veins forming larger veins that eventually drain into the **right** and **left hepatic veins** that deliver their blood into the **inferior vena cava**, not at the porta hepatis but at the posterior aspect of the liver.

In addition to the classical (hepatic) lobule, two other conceptual lobulations have been suggested for the liver, **portal lobule**, a triangular structure (in histologic sections) whose three apices are three neighboring

CLINICAL CONSIDERATIONS 16-3

Pancreatic Cancer

Recent investigations of **pancreatic cancer** have disclosed a possible reason why this disease is so resistant to anticancer drugs. It appears that pancreatic cancer cells invade and kill the endothelial cells of adjacent blood vessels, thus preventing blood vessels from delivering anticancer medications to the tumor cells. All pancreatic cells, including pancreatic cancer cells, possess activin receptor-like

kinase 7 (ALK7) receptors on their cell membranes to which activin B, a member of the transforming factor-beta (TGF-β) superfamily, can bind activating the ALK7 receptor. Once activated, ALK7 causes the cancer cells to enter the apoptotic pathway and reduces their ability to migrate. Because pancreatic cancer cells evade this protective mechanism by downregulating the synthesis of ALK7 or activin B, current research is focused on preventing the cancer cells from doing that.

Table 16-1	Enzymes Produced by Pancreatic Acinar Cells*
Enzymes	**Function**
Trypsinogen[†]	As trypsin: converts proenzymes into active enzymes; cleaves dietary proteins present in the chyme
Chymotrypsinogen	As chymotrypsin: cleaves dietary proteins present in the chyme
Carboxypeptidase	Cleaves peptide bonds at the carboxyl terminus of a protein
Aminopeptidase	Cleaves peptide bonds at the amino terminus of a protein
Amylase	Cleaves carbohydrates
Lipase	Digests lipids liberating free fatty acids
DNase (deoxyribonuclease)	Hydrolyzes phosphodiester links of the deoxyphosphate backbone of DNA
RNase (ribonuclease)	Hydrolyzes phosphodiester links of the phosphate backbone of RNA
Elastase	Digests elastic fibers

*Some of these are proenzymes that are activated in the lumen of the duodenum by trypsin.
[†]Trypsinogen and chymotrypsinogen are activated by enterokinases present on the microvilli of the surface absorptive cells forming trypsin and chymotrypsin, respectively.

CLINICAL CONSIDERATIONS 16-4

Gastrinoma and Chronic Pancreatitis

Gastrinoma is a disease in which the **G cells** of the pancreas undergo **excess proliferation** (frequently cancerous), resulting in an **overproduction of the hormone gastrin**. This hormone is responsible for binding to parietal cells of the stomach, causing them to oversecrete hydrochloric acid with a resultant formation of peptic ulcers in the stomach and the duodenum.

Chronic pancreatitis, chronic inflammation of the pancreas, is caused by a plethora of factors, genetic as well as environmental, most frequently excessive alcohol consumption and, to a lesser extent, obstruction of the pancreatic duct. The pathologic features include injury to the acinar cells of the exocrine pancreas caused by the release of a variety of inflammatory pharmaceutical agents by the connective tissue cells. Chronic inflammation induces type I and type III collagen formation with the resultant fibrosis of the organ.

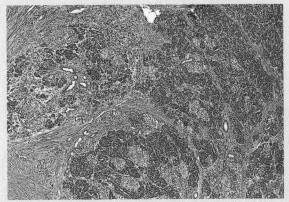

This photomicrograph is of a patient suffering from chronic pancreatitis. Observe that the connective tissue elements are highly exaggerated, the acini are greatly reduced in number, and the islets of Langerhans are very close to each other because of the reduction in acinar population. (Reprinted with permission from Mills SE, et al., eds. *Sternberg's Diagnostic Surgical Pathology*, 6th ed. Philadelphia: Wolters Kluwer, 2015. p. 1585, Figure 35-13.)

	Table 16-2	Hormones Produced by Islets of Langerhans Cells		

Cells	Percent of Total (%)	Hormone	Molecular Weight (Da)	Function
β **cell**	70	Insulin	6,000	Decreases blood glucose level by inducing the uptake, storage, and glycolysis of glucose; stimulates formation of glycerol; hinders lipid digestion by adipocytes
α **cell**	20	Glucagon	3,500	Increases blood glucose level; induces glycogenolysis and gluconeogenesis
δ_1 **cell**	5	Somatostatin	1,640	Inhibits hormone release from other cells of the islet of Langerhans; inhibits enzyme release by acinar cells of the pancreas; reduces smooth muscle activity of the digestive tract and gallbladder
δ_2 **cell**	2	VIP (vasoactive intestinal peptide)	3,800	Stimulates glycogenolysis; reduces smooth muscle activity of the digestive tract; modulates H_2O and ion movements in intestinal epithelial cells
PP cell	1	Pancreatic polypeptide	4,200	Inhibits secretory activity of the exocrine pancreas
G cell	1	Gastrin	2,000	Induces HCl manufacture by parietal cells of the stomach
ε **cell**	1	Ghrelin	3,000	Induces hunger sensations; decreases smooth muscle contraction of the alimentary canal

central veins, and **hepatic acinus (of Rappaport)**, a diamond-shaped structure whose long axis connects two adjacent central veins and short axis connects two adjacent portal areas (see Fig. 16-9). **Portal lobules** were suggested because in a classical lobule blood flows toward the center of the lobule and bile flows to the periphery of the lobule. Whereas in the portal lobule concept, the bile flows to the center of the lobule. **Liver acinus** was devised to describe blood flow and oxygen supply of the hepatic lobule because it reflects pathologic changes in the liver

during hypoxia and toxin-induced alterations. Each acinus is subdivided into three more or less equal zones.

- **Zone 1** is in the vicinity of the short axis of the hepatic acinus between the two portal areas and receives the most oxygen.

- **Zone 3** is in the vicinity of the central vein and receives the least amount of oxygen.

- **Zone 2** is the region between zones 1 and 3 and receives an intermediate amount of oxygen.

CLINICAL CONSIDERATIONS 16-5

Diabetes Mellitus

There are three types of **diabetes mellitus**, type 1, type 2, and gestational diabetes.

Type 1 (insulin-dependent) diabetes is characterized by **polyphagia** (insatiable hunger), **polydipsia** (unquenchable thirst), and **polyuria** (excessive urination). It usually has a sudden onset before twenty years of age, is an autoimmune disorder that is distinguished by damage to and destruction of β cells, resulting in a **low level of plasma insulin**.

Type 2 (non-insulin-dependent) diabetes mellitus commonly occurs in overweight individuals over forty years of age; however, in the past two or three decades, the increase in obesity in young adults and even teenagers has decreased the age at which type 2 diabetes may be acquired. It does not result from low levels of plasma insulin and is **insulin-resistant**, which is a major factor in its pathogenesis. The resistance to insulin is due to decreased binding of insulin to its plasmalemma receptors and defects in postreceptor insulin action. Type 2 diabetes is usually controlled by diet.

Gestational diabetes occurs in less than 10% of pregnancies, and this is less serious for the mother than it is for the fetus. The increase in the mother's blood glucose levels can cause various problems such as breathing difficulties at birth and an increase in the possibility of diabetes and obesity as the child grows older.

Kupffer Cells and Perisinusoidal Stellate Cells

Monocyte-derived macrophages, known as **Kupffer cells**, are interspersed with **endothelial lining cells**, thus participating in the formation of the lining of the sinusoids. Kupffer cells function in removing defunct red blood cells and other undesirable particulate matter from the bloodstream (Fig. 16-11). **Perisinusoidal stellate cells (fat-storing cells; Ito cells)** are believed to function in the accumulation and storage of **vitamin A** and manufacture type III collagen, but, in the case of alcoholic cirrhosis, these cells also manufacture types I and IV collagen fibers, resulting in fibrosis of the liver. These cells also have the capability of dedifferentiating, undergoing mitosis, and forming new hepatocytes. In fact, when up to 75% of a mouse liver is surgically removed, within a short period of time, the perisinusoidal stellate cells regenerate the liver to its previous size. Ito cells are located in the narrow space between the sinusoidal lining cells and the hepatocytes.

Perisinusoidal Space (Space of Disse)

The **perisinusoidal space (space of Disse)** is a narrow, transitional compartment that separates the hepatocytes from the sinusoidal lining cells, thus preventing the hepatocytes from coming into direct contact with blood. Substances manufactured by hepatocytes and meant to enter the bloodstream are released into the perisinusoidal space and pass through the endothelial lining cells to enter the sinusoids. Also, material conveyed by the bloodstream in the sinusoids that are meant for the hepatocytes crosses the sinusoidal lining cells; enters the plasma-containing perisinusoidal space; and, once there, reaches the hepatocytes. Hepatocytes extend numerous microvilli into the perisinusoidal space.

Hepatocytes

Hepatocytes are relatively large cells, some are multinucleated, and possess a rich supply of organelles, especially mitochondria, rough endoplasmic reticulum (rER), smooth ER, peroxisomes, lysosomes, and several Golgi apparatuses. These cells are also well endowed with lipid and glycogen deposits. Hepatocytes form intersecting plates of liver cells that possess two distinct regions, **lateral domains** and **sinusoidal domains** (see Fig. 16-11).

Lateral Domains

When two hepatocytes contact each other, known as their **lateral domain**, they form intricate maze-like networks of intercellular spaces, known as **bile canaliculi**, isolated from the extracellular space by fasciae occludentes. Hepatocytes secrete bile into these bile canaliculi that conduct bile to the **bile ducts** of the **portal area** and into a system of ducts that convey bile to the gallbladder.

Sinusoidal Domains

The surfaces of hepatocytes that border the perisinusoidal space are known as the **sinusoidal domains**. The plasma of the perisinusoidal space contains material released by the hepatocytes to be transported to the blood in the sinusoids and, conversely, material from the blood that is targeted for the hepatocytes. Short, blunt microvilli of hepatocytes project into the perisinusoidal space to increase the surface area of the hepatocytes to facilitate these transfer processes.

Functions of the Liver

The 100 or more functions of the liver may be classified into three categories, namely exocrine functions, endocrine functions, and other functions.

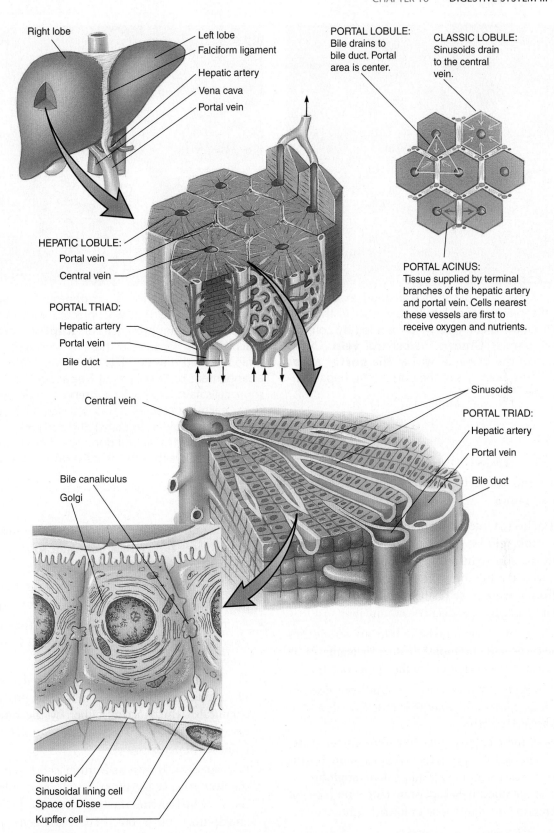

Right lobe

Left lobe
Falciform ligament
Hepatic artery
Vena cava
Portal vein

PORTAL LOBULE:
Bile drains to
bile duct. Portal
area is center.

CLASSIC LOBULE:
Sinusoids drain
to the central
vein.

HEPATIC LOBULE:
Portal vein
Central vein

PORTAL TRIAD:
Hepatic artery
Portal vein
Bile duct

PORTAL ACINUS:
Tissue supplied by terminal
branches of the hepatic artery
and portal vein. Cells nearest
these vessels are first to
receive oxygen and nutrients.

Central vein

Sinusoids

PORTAL TRIAD:
Hepatic artery
Portal vein
Bile duct

Bile canaliculus
Golgi

Sinusoid
Sinusoidal lining cell
Space of Disse
Kupffer cell

FIGURE 16-9. Schematic diagram of the liver, liver lobules, and hepatocytes within liver lobules. **Hepatocytes**, liver cells, deliver endocrine system secretions into the vascular supply, and exocrine secretion, **bile**, into excretory ducts, the **bile ducts**. Each liver cell borders a vascular space, **sinusoid**, on at least one side and other hepatocytes on its remaining sides. Where two hepatocytes adjoin, they delimit a small intercellular space, **bile canaliculus**, into which the bile is delivered. Because sinusoids are lined by endothelial cells (**sinusoidal lining cells**) and macrophages (**Kupffer cells**), hepatocytes do not come into contact with the bloodstream. The **space of Disse** intervenes between hepatocytes and sinusoidal lining cells. This space houses **microvilli** of hepatocytes, occasional fat-storing cells (**Ito cells**), and slender reticular fibers that help form the supporting framework of the liver.

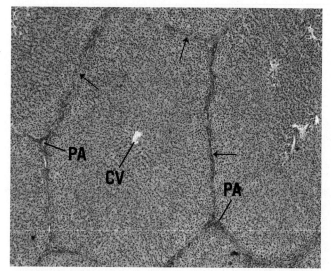

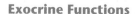

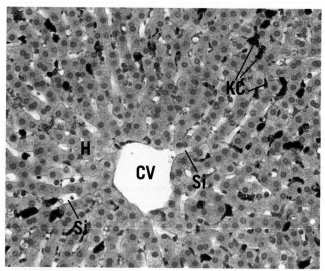

FIGURE 16-10. The pig liver is a good example for viewing the classical liver lobules because, in this animal, each lobule is completely surrounded by connective tissue (*arrows*). Observe the **central vein** (CV) in the middle of the lobule as well as the **portal areas** (PA) that house branches of the portal vein, hepatic artery, and bile ducts. ×56.

FIGURE 16-11. This is a photomicrograph from the liver of a dog that was injected with India ink to demonstrate the presence of **Kupffer cells** (KC), macrophages, located in the liver sinusoids that have phagocytosed tiny droplets of the ink. Note the radial arrangement of the plates of **hepatocytes** (H), where some cells have two nuclei. Observe that, in two dimensions, each hepatocyte displays surfaces bordering the sinusoid (sinusoidal domains) and surfaces that border other hepatocytes (lateral domains). Blood from the **sinusoids** (Si) drains into the **central vein** (CV). ×270.

Exocrine Functions

The liver forms about 1 L of **bile** per day, which is its **exocrine secretion**.

- **Bile** is delivered into a system of conduits: **bile canaliculi**, **cholangioles**, **canals of Hering**, **interlobular bile ducts**, and **right** and **left hepatic ducts**, which then direct the bile into the **common hepatic duct** and, from there, via the **cystic duct** into the **gallbladder**, a storage organ associated with the liver.

- The release of concentrated bile into the duodenum via the cystic and common bile ducts is regulated by hormones of the DNES cells in the alimentary tract.

- Bile is a green, somewhat viscous fluid composed of water, ions, cholesterol, phospholipids, bilirubin glucuronide, and bile acids.
  - One of these components, **bilirubin glucuronide**, is a water-soluble conjugate of nonsoluble **bilirubin**, a toxic breakdown product of **hemoglobin**.
  - It is in the **smooth endoplasmic reticulum (sER)** of the hepatocytes that detoxification of bilirubin occurs.

Endocrine and Other Functions

- The liver synthesizes and releases almost 90% of **plasma proteins** and other plasma components, such as fibrinogen, urea, albumin, prothrombin, and lipoproteins.

- It manufactures proteins that regulate the transfer and metabolism of **iron**.

- It stores lipids and glucose and, if necessary, synthesizes glucose from noncarbohydrate sources, a process known as **gluconeogenesis**.

- The liver manufactures all five classes of lipoproteins (Table 16-3).

- As indicated in Chapter 15, the liver **transports** IgA into the bile and, subsequently, into the lumen of the small intestine.

- The liver is also responsible for the **detoxification** of various drugs, toxins, metabolic by-products, and chemicals, which occurs either by the **microsomal mixed-function oxidase** system of the sER or by **peroxidases** of peroxisomes.

- Macrophages, known as **Kupffer cells**, that reside in the liver, have Fc receptors as well as complement receptors which permit them to recognize, phagocytose, and destroy almost 100% of the pathogens that escape the intestinal lumen and enter the liver.

Gallbladder

The **gallbladder** is a small, pear-shaped organ that receives as much as 1,200 mL of **bile** from the liver every day. The gallbladder not only stores but also concentrates

CLINICAL CONSIDERATIONS 16-6

Kaposi Sarcoma of the Liver

Kaposi sarcoma of the liver is almost solely present in patients with Immunodeficiency diseases and has been observed in as many as a quarter of the patient population who succumbed to AIDS. Additionally, a Kaposi sarcoma–associated herpesvirus has been determined to be a causative factor in this disease. The autopsied livers presented with numerous darkened nodules of a soft consistency, most of which occupied expanded connective tissue of the intrahepatic biliary tract.

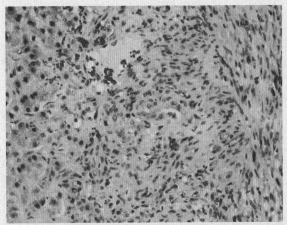

This photomicrograph is of a patient suffering from Kaposi sarcoma of the liver. Observe the presence of relatively normal hepatocytes in the upper left, whereas much of the right-hand side displays the presence of spindle-shaped cells, typical of Kaposi sarcoma cells. An additional typical feature of this disease is the presence of extravasated erythrocytes. (Reprinted with permission from Mills SE, et al., eds. *Sternberg's Diagnostic Surgical Pathology*, 6th ed. Philadelphia: Wolters Kluwer, 2015. p. 1754, Figure 37-25.)

Table 16-3	Classes of Lipoproteins	
Lipoprotein Class	**Density (g/mL)**	**Characteristics and Function**
Chylomicrons	<0.95	Manufactured in the small intestine and released into the lacteals of the lamina propria as relatively large globules (as large as 500 nm in diameter). Composed of ~2% protein, ~90% triglycerides, ~2% cholesterol, and ~6% phospholipids. The protein moiety enables the chylomicron to be miscible with the aqueous plasma.
VLDL	0.95–1.006	Manufactured in the liver and to a much lesser extent in the small intestine and is modified in the bloodstream by the acquisition of additional proteins. These are much smaller (~60 nm in diameter) than chylomicrons. The blood-circulating enzyme lipoprotein lipase cleaves triglycerides from VLDL.
IDL	1.00–1.019	Is formed in the bloodstream as lipoprotein lipase continues to remove triglycerides from VLDL. It is rich in apolipoprotein E and is about 30 nm in diameter.
LDL	1.019–1.063	Is formed in the bloodstream as IDL loses its apolipoprotein E. LDL is ~20 nm in diameter. They have a relatively high cholesterol content, and they are considered the principal causative agents of plaque buildup in blood vessels with ensuing cardiovascular disease resulting in death. LDL appears to block quorum sensing in *Staphylococcus aureus* permitting excessive proliferation of the bacteria.
HDL	1.063–1.210	Is manufactured in the liver, is about 12 nm in diameter, and consists of as much as 50% protein, 40% triglyceride, and 15% cholesterol. They transport cholesterol to the liver and glands synthesizing steroid hormones. HDLs can remove cholesterol from vascular plaques; therefore, high HDL concentration in the blood decreases the possibility of cardiovascular disease.

HDL, high-density lipoprotein; IDL, intermediate-density lipoprotein; LDL, low-density lipoprotein; VLDL, very-low-density lipoprotein.

CLINICAL CONSIDERATIONS 16-7

Hepatitis

Hepatitis is inflammation of the liver and, although it could have various causes such as abuse of alcohol and certain drugs, its most common cause is one of the five types of hepatitis viruses, denoted by the first five letters of the alphabet, A through E.

- **Hepatitis A** is usually spread by poor hygiene (fecal–oral route and contaminated water) as well as by sexual contact. Usually, there are no symptoms, and the patient recovers and does not become a carrier.
- **Hepatitis B**, a more serious condition than hepatitis A, is usually transmitted by body fluids and, in case of users of illicit drugs, by the sharing of needles. Patients can become carriers of the virus and in 10% of the patients the condition may become chronic, leading to cirrhosis and cancer of the liver.
- In the past, **hepatitis C** was transmitted by blood transfusions, but screening has almost completely eradicated that route and now it is transmitted mostly by shared needles among users of illicit drugs. About 75% of people who have the hepatitis C virus will reach the chronic stage, and, of these, 20% to 25% will develop cirrhosis and then liver cancer.
- **Hepatitis D** is also transmitted by the sharing of needles and is always accompanied by hepatitis B. The double infection is a more severe condition.
- **Hepatitis E** is spread by the fecal–oral route and is responsible for epidemics, but mostly in developing countries. Neither chronic nor carrier states are present with this form of the Hepatitis virus.

Universal vaccination is recommended to protect the population from hepatitis B, and this has the added benefit of protection against hepatitis D; it is recommended that travelers to underdeveloped countries where hepatitis A is prevalent be vaccinated against hepatitis A. Vaccines are not currently available against hepatitis C or E.

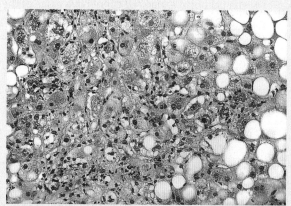

This photomicrograph is of a patient suffering from acute alcohol-induced hepatitis. Observe that the specimen presents some of the earliest histopathologic signs of alcohol-induced hepatitis, namely macrovascular fatty changes, Mallory hyaline, and the infiltration by neutrophils. (Reprinted with permission from Mills SE, et al., eds. *Sternberg's Diagnostic Surgical Pathology*, 5th ed. Philadelphia: Wolters Kluwer Health// Lippincott Williams & Wilkins, 2010. p. 1513.)

bile and, in response to the **cholecystokinin** released by the DNES cells of the alimentary tract and to acetylcholine from postganglionic parasympathetic fibers, forces the bile into the lumen of the duodenum via the cystic and common bile ducts. Bile is a fluid composed of water, electrolytes, cholesterol, phospholipids, and **bile salts** as well as **bilirubin glucuronide**. It emulsifies fats, facilitating the action of the enzyme **pancreatic lipase**. The mucosa of the gallbladder, lined by a simple columnar epithelium, is thrown into highly convoluted folds in the empty gallbladder (Fig. 16-12), but these folds disappear on distention. Occasionally, tubuloalveolar mucous glands are present. The muscular coat of the gallbladder is composed of obliquely oriented smooth muscle layer interspersed with some longitudinally disposed smooth muscle cells.

CLINICAL CONSIDERATIONS 16-8

Jaundice (Icterus)

Jaundice (**icterus**) is characterized by excess bilirubin in the blood and deposition of **bile pigment** in the skin and sclera of the eyes, resulting in a yellowish appearance. It may be hereditary or caused by pathologic conditions such as excess destruction of red blood cells (**hemolytic jaundice**), liver dysfunction, and obstruction of the biliary passages (**obstructive jaundice**).

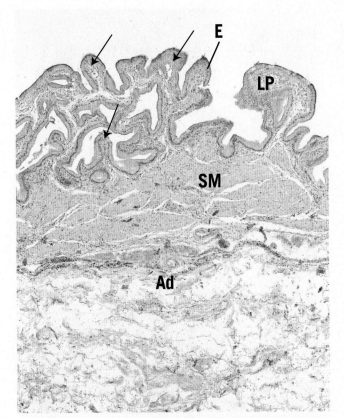

FIGURE 16-12. This very low-magnification photomicrograph of an empty human gallbladder displays its highly folded mucosa (*arrows*). Observe that the **epithelium** (E) is composed of tall columnar cells with basally located nuclei. The **lamina propria** (LP) is a loose connective tissue that is interposed between the epithelium and the **smooth muscle coat** (SM) of this viscus. The connective tissue **adventitia** (Ad) separates relatively easily from Glisson's capsule of the liver. ×56.

CLINICAL CONSIDERATIONS 16-9

Gallstones (Biliary Calculi, Cholelithiasis)

Gallstones (**biliary calculi**) are concretions, usually of fused crystals of **cholesterol** that form in the gallbladder or bile duct. They may accumulate to such an extent that the cystic duct is blocked, thus preventing emptying of the gallbladder, and they may require surgical removal if less invasive methods fail to dissolve or pulverize them. If the obstruction occurs abruptly due to the gallstones, the gallbladder can rapidly become inflamed, a condition known as **chronic cholecystitis**.

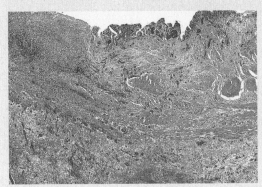

This photomicrograph is from a gallbladder whose cystic duct was obstructed by the presence of gallstones resulting in acute cholecystitis. Observe that much of the luminal surface of the mucosa lacks an epithelial lining and that the lamina propria is edematous. Moreover, the adventitia is thicker than normal. (Reprinted with permission from Mills SE, et al., eds. *Sternberg's Diagnostic Surgical Pathology*, 6th ed. Philadelphia: Wolters Kluwer, 2015. p. 1777, Figure 38-9.)

PLATE 16-1A Salivary Glands

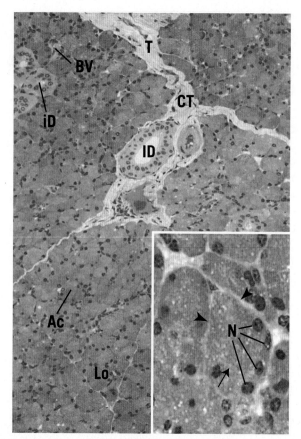

FIGURE 16-1-1. Parotid gland. Monkey. Plastic section. ×132.

The parotid gland is purely serous, with a connective tissue capsule sending **trabeculae** (T) or septa into the substance of the gland, subdividing it into **lobules** (Lo). Slender connective tissue sheets penetrate the lobules, surrounding small **blood vessels** (BV) and **intralobular ducts** (iD). **Interlobular ducts** (ID) are surrounded by increased amounts of **connective tissue** (CT) and large blood vessels. Observe that the **acini** (Ac) are closely packed within each lobule. *Inset.* **Parotid gland. Monkey. Plastic section.** ×540. Note that the round **nuclei** (N) of these serous acini are basally located. The lateral cell membranes (*arrows*) are not clearly visible, nor are the lumina of the acini. Observe the slender sheets of connective tissue (*arrowheads*) investing each acinus.

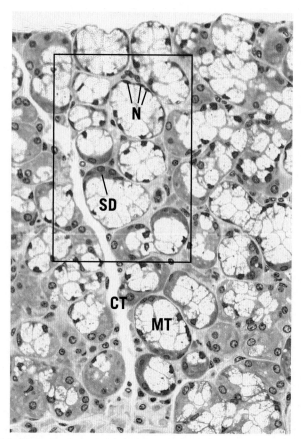

FIGURE 16-1-2. Sublingual gland. Monkey. Plastic section. ×270.

The sublingual gland is a mixed gland in that it produces both serous and mucous secretory products. The **mucous tubules** (MT) possess dark **nuclei** (N) that are flattened against the basal cell membrane. Moreover, the cytoplasm is filled with a frothy-appearing material, representing the viscous secretory product. Many of the mucous tubules are capped by serous cells, forming a crescent-shaped cap, the **serous demilune** (SD). The sublingual gland is subdivided into lobes and lobules by **connective tissue septa** (CT) or trabeculae that act as the supporting network for the nerves, vessels, and ducts of the gland. The *boxed area* is presented at a higher magnification in Figure 16-1-3.

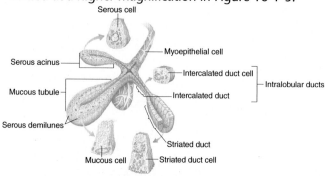

Salivary glands

KEY						
Ac	acinus	**ID**	interlobular duct	**N**	nucleus
BV	blood vessel	**Lo**	lobule	**SD**	serous demilune
CT	connective tissue	**MT**	mucous tubules	**T**	trabeculae
iD	intralobular duct				

PLATE 16-1B   Salivary Glands

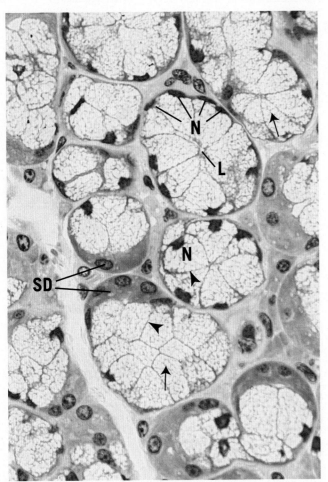

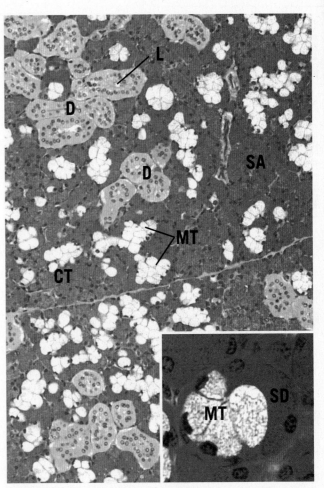

FIGURE 16-1-3. Sublingual gland. Monkey. Plastic section. ×540.

FIGURE 16-1-4. Submandibular gland. Monkey. Plastic section. ×132.

This photomicrograph is a higher magnification of the *boxed area* of Figure 16-1-2. The flattened, dark **nuclei** (N) of the mucous tubules are evident as they appear to be pressed against the basal cell membrane. Observe that much of the cytoplasm is occupied by small, mucin-containing vesicles (*arrows*), that the lateral cell membrane (*arrowheads*) is evident, and that the **lumen** (L) is usually identifiable. **Serous demilunes** (SD) are composed of serous-producing cells whose **nuclei** (N) are round to oval in morphology. Note also that the lateral cell membranes are not distinguishable in serous cells.

The submandibular gland also produces a mixed type of secretion; however, unlike in the sublingual gland, serous acini predominate. **Serous** (SA) and **mucous tubules** (MT) are easily distinguishable from each other, but most mucous units display a cap of serous demilunes. Moreover, the submandibular gland is characterized by an extensive system of **ducts** (D), recognizable by their pale cytoplasm, comparatively large **lumina** (L), and round nuclei. This gland is also subdivided into lobes and lobules by **connective tissue septa** (CT). *Inset.* **Submandibular gland**. **Monkey**. **Plastic section**. ×540. Note the granular appearance of the cells comprising the **serous demilune** (SD) in contrast with the "frothy" appearing cytoplasm of the **mucous tubules** (MT).

KEY					
CT	connective tissue	MT	mucous tubules	SA	serous acini
D	duct	N	nucleus	SD	serous demilune
L	lumen				

PLATE 16-2A Pancreas

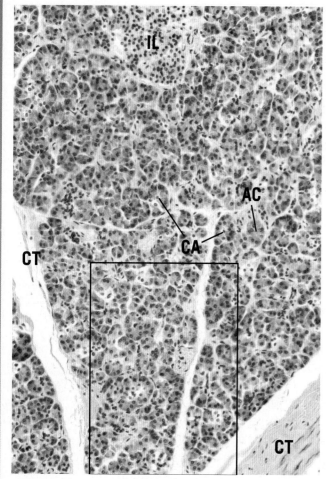

FIGURE 16-2-1. Pancreas. Human. Paraffin section. ×132.

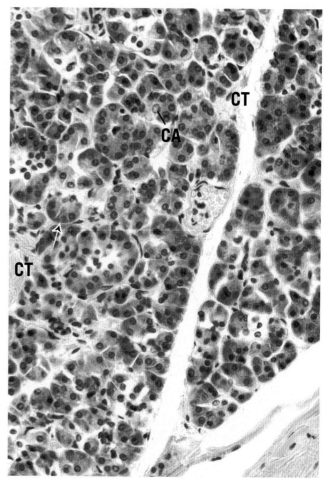

FIGURE 16-2-2. Pancreas. Human. Paraffin section. ×270.

The pancreas is a complex gland because it has both exocrine and endocrine components. The exocrine portion comprises the bulk of the organ as a compound acinar gland, secreting a serous fluid. The gland is subdivided into lobules by **connective tissue septa** (CT). Each **acinus** (Ac) is composed of several pyramid-shaped cells, possessing round nuclei. Pale cells located in the center of the acinus, **centroacinar cells** (CA), form the smallest ducts of the gland. The endocrine portion of the pancreas is composed of small, spherical clumps of cells, **pancreatic islets of Langerhans** (IL), which are richly endowed by capillaries. These pancreatic islets are haphazardly scattered among the serous acini of the pancreas. The *boxed area* is presented at a higher magnification in Figure 16-2-2.

This photomicrograph is a higher magnification of the *boxed area* of Figure 16-2-1. Note that the **connective tissue septa** (CT), although fairly extensive in certain regions, are quite slender in the interlobular areas. The trapezoidal morphologies of individual cells of the serous acini are evident in fortuitous sections (*arrow*). Observe also the **centroacinar cells** (CA), located in the center of acini, which represent the smallest units of the pancreatic duct system.

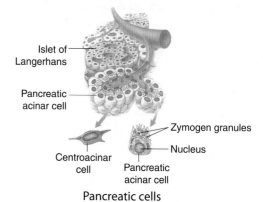

Islet of Langerhans

Pancreatic acinar cell

Zymogen granules

Nucleus

Centroacinar cell

Pancreatic acinar cell

Pancreatic cells

KEY					
Ac	acinus	**CA**	centroacinar cell	**IL**	islets of Langerhans
BV	blood vessel	**CT**	connective tissue septa	**ZG**	zymogen granule

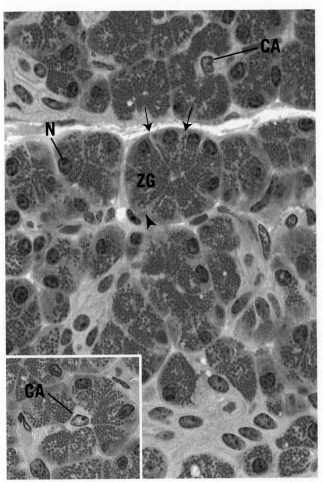

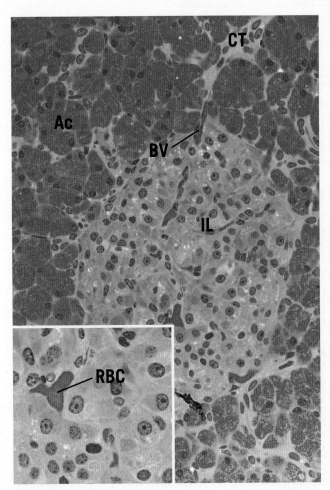

FIGURE 16-2-3. Pancreas. Monkey. Plastic section. ×540.

With the use of plastic sections, the morphology of the pancreatic acinus is well defined. Observe that in fortuitous sections, the acinus resembles a pie, with the individual cells clearly delineated (*arrows*). The **nucleus** (N) of each trapezoid-shaped cell is round and the basal cytoplasm (*arrowhead*) is relatively homogeneous, whereas the apical cytoplasm is packed with **zymogen granules** (ZG). **Centroacinar cells** (CA) may be recognized both by their locations and by the pale appearance of their cytoplasm and euchromatic nuclei. *Inset.* **Pancreas. Monkey. Plastic section.** ×540. Observe the **centroacinar cell** (CA), whose pale cytoplasm and euchromatic nucleus are readily differentiated from the surrounding acinar cells.

FIGURE 16-2-4. Pancreatic Islets (of Langerhans). Monkey. Plastic section. ×270.

The **pancreatic islets of Langerhans** (IL), the endocrine portion of the pancreas, are a more or less spherical configuration of cells randomly scattered throughout the exocrine portion of the gland. As such, each islet is surrounded by serous **acini** (Ac). The islets receive their rich **blood supply** (BV) from the **connective tissue elements** (CT) of the exocrine pancreas. *Inset.* **Pancreatic Islets. Monkey. Plastic section.** ×540. Observe the rich vascularity of the pancreatic islets, as evidenced by the presence of **erythrocyte** (RBC)-engorged blood vessels. Although each islet is composed of A, B, G, PP, epsilon and two types of D cells, they can only be distinguished from each other by special stains. However, it should be noted that, in the human, B cells are the most populous and are usually located in the center of the islet, whereas A cells are generally found at the periphery. This situation is reversed in the monkey.

KEY

Ac	acinus	**CT**	connective tissue septa	**RBC**	erythrocyte
BV	blood vessel	**IL**	islets of Langerhans	**ZG**	zymogen granule
CA	centroacinar cell	**N**	nucleus		

PLATE 16-3A Liver

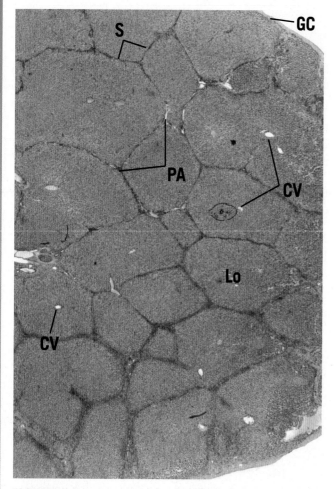

FIGURE 16-3-1. Liver. Pig. Paraffin section. ×14.

Note that the liver is invested by a connective tissue capsule, **Glisson's capsule** (GC), from which, in the pig, **septa** (S) extend to subdivide the parenchyma into more or less hexagonal classical **hepatic lobules** (Lo). Blood vessels, lymph vessels, and bile ducts travel within the connective tissue septa to reach the apices of the hepatic lobules, which are known as the **portal areas** (PA). Bile reaches the portal areas from within the lobules, whereas blood enters the substance of the lobules from the portal areas. Within each lobule, the blood flows through tortuous channels, the liver sinusoids, to enter the **central vein** (CV) in the middle of the hepatic lobule.

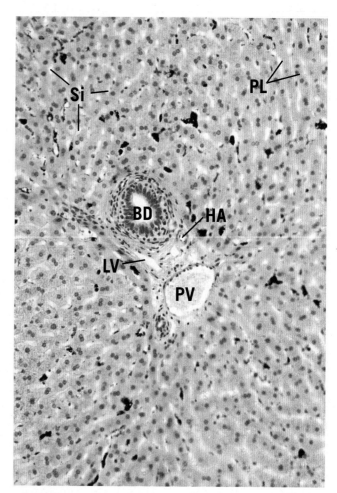

FIGURE 16-3-2. Liver. Dog. Paraffin section. ×132.

The portal area of the liver houses terminal branches of the **hepatic artery** (HA) and **portal vein** (PV). Note that the vein is much larger than the artery and its wall is very thin in comparison to the size of its lumen. Branches of **lymph vessels** (LV) and **bile ducts** (BD) are also present in the portal area. Bile ducts may be recognized by their cuboidal to columnar epithelium. Observe that unlike in the pig, connective tissue septa do not demarcate the boundaries of hepatic lobules, although the various structures of the portal area are invested by connective tissue elements. **Plates of liver cells** (PL) and **sinusoids** (Si) extend from the portal areas.

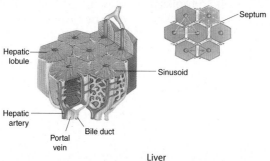

Hepatic lobule

Septum

Sinusoid

Hepatic artery

Bile duct

Portal vein

Liver

KEY					
BD	bile duct	**Lo**	lobule	**PV**	portal vein
CV	central vein	**LV**	lymph vessel	**S**	septa
GC	Glisson's capsule	**PA**	portal area	**Si**	sinusoid
HA	hepatic artery	**PL**	plates of liver cells		

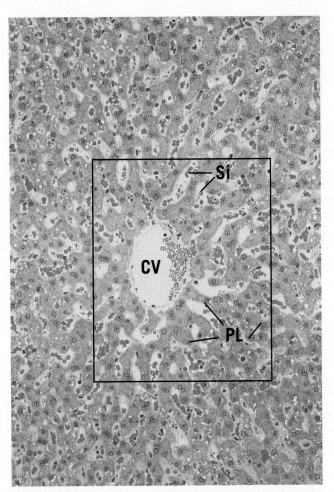

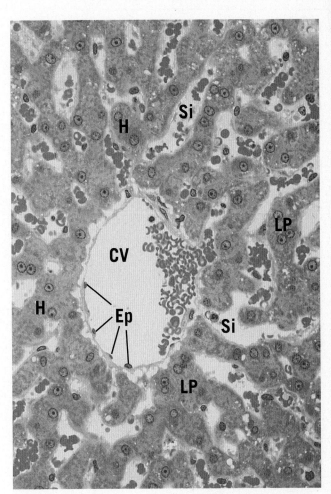

FIGURE 16-3-3. Liver. Monkey. Plastic section. ×132.

The **central vein** (CV) of the liver lobule (a terminal radix of the hepatic vein) collects blood from the **sinusoids** (Si) and delivers it to sublobular veins. The **plates of liver cells** (PL) and hepatic sinusoids appear to radiate, like spokes of a wheel, from the central vein. The *boxed area* is presented at a higher magnification in Figure 16-3-4.

FIGURE 16-3-4. Liver. Monkey. Plastic section. ×270.

This photomicrograph is a higher magnification of the *boxed area* of Figure 16-3-3. Note that the lumen of the **central vein** (CV) is lined by a simple squamous **epithelium** (Ep), which is continuous with the endothelial lining of the hepatic **sinusoids** (Si), tortuous vascular channels that freely communicate with each other. Observe also that the **liver plates** (LP) are composed of **hepatocytes** (H), one to two cell layers thick, and that each plate is bordered by sinusoids.

KEY					
CV	central vein	**H**	hepatocyte	**Si**	Sinusoid
Ep	epithelium	**LP**	liver plates		

PLATE 16-4A Liver

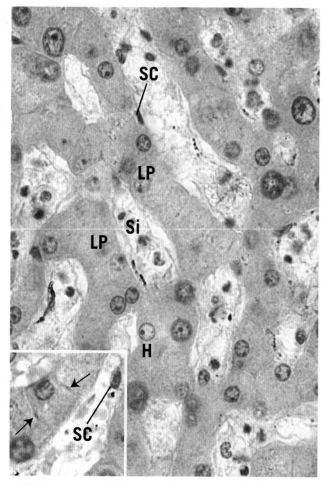

FIGURE 16-4-1. Liver. Monkey. Plastic section. ×540.

This photomicrograph is a high magnification of **liver plates** (LP). Observe that individual **hepatocytes** (H) are polygonal in shape. Each hepatocyte possesses one or two nuclei, although occasionally some have three nuclei. Plates of hepatocytes enclose hepatic **sinusoids** (Si) that are lined by **sinusoidal lining cells** (SC), the endothelium; therefore, hepatocytes do not come into direct contact with the bloodstream. The space between the endothelium and the hepatocytes, the perisinusoidal space (of Disse), is at the limit of resolution of the light microscope. *Inset.* **Liver. Human. Paraffin section**. ×540. The hepatocyte cell membranes are evident in this photomicrograph. Note that in fortuitous sections, small intercellular spaces (*arrows*) are recognizable. These are bile canaliculi through which bile flows to the periphery of the lobule.

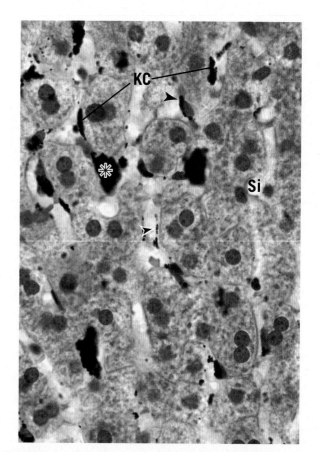

FIGURE 16-4-2. Liver. Paraffin section. ×540.

A system of macrophages known as **Kupffer cells** (KC) is found interspersed among the endothelial lining cells of liver **sinusoids** (Si). These macrophages are larger than the endothelial cells and may be recognized by the presence of phagocytosed material within them. Kupffer cells may be demonstrated by injecting an animal intravenously with India ink, as is the case in this specimen. Observe that some cells appear as large, black smudges because they are filled with phagocytosed ink (*asterisk*), whereas other cells possess only small quantities of the phagocytosed material (*arrowheads*). Note also that much of the sinusoidal lining is devoid of ink, indicating that the endothelial cells are probably not phagocytic.

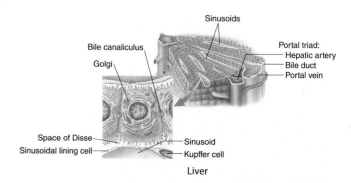

Liver

KEY					
H	hepatocyte	**LP**	liver plate	**Si**	sinusoid
KC	Kupffer cell	**SC**	sinusoidal lining cell		

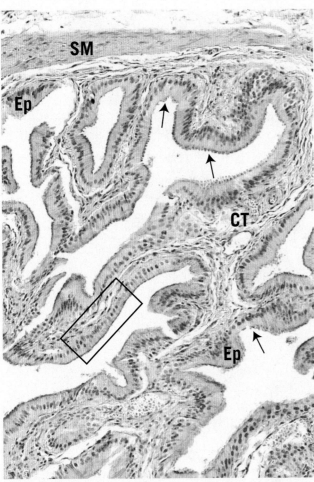

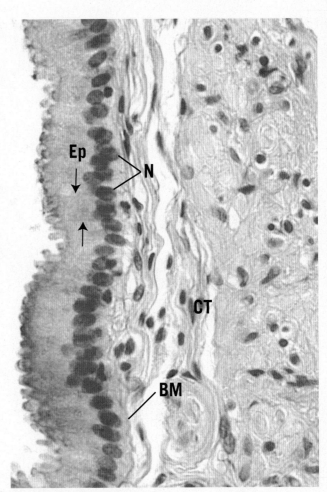

FIGURE 16-4-3. Gallbladder. Human. Paraffin section. ×132.

FIGURE 16-4-4. Gallbladder. Human. Paraffin section. ×540.

The gallbladder is a pear-shaped, hollow organ that functions in storing and concentrating bile. Its histologic structure is relatively simple, but its appearance may be deceiving. The mucosa of an empty gallbladder, as in this photomicrograph, is thrown into numerous folds (*arrows*), providing it with a glandular morphology. However, close observation of the **epithelium** (Ep) demonstrates that all the simple columnar cells of the mucous membrane are identical. A loose **connective tissue** (CT), sometimes referred to as a lamina propria, lies deep to the epithelium. Observe that muscularis mucosae are lacking, and the **smooth muscle** (SM) surrounding the connective tissue is the muscularis externa. The outermost coat of the gallbladder is a serosa or adventitia. A region similar to the *boxed area* is presented in Figure 16-4-4.

This photomicrograph is a higher magnification of a region similar to the *boxed area* of Figure 16-4-3. Note that the **epithelium** (Ep) is composed of identical-appearing tall columnar cells, whose **nuclei** (N) are basally oriented. The lateral cell membranes are evident in certain regions (*arrows*), whereas the apical brush border is usually not visible in H&E-stained specimens. Observe that a relatively thick **basal membrane** (BM) separates the epithelium from the underlying loose **connective tissue** (CT).

KEY					
BM	basement membrane	**Ep**	epithelium	**SM**	smooth muscle
CT	connective tissue	**N**	nucleus		

PLATE 16-5   Salivary Gland, Electron Microscopy

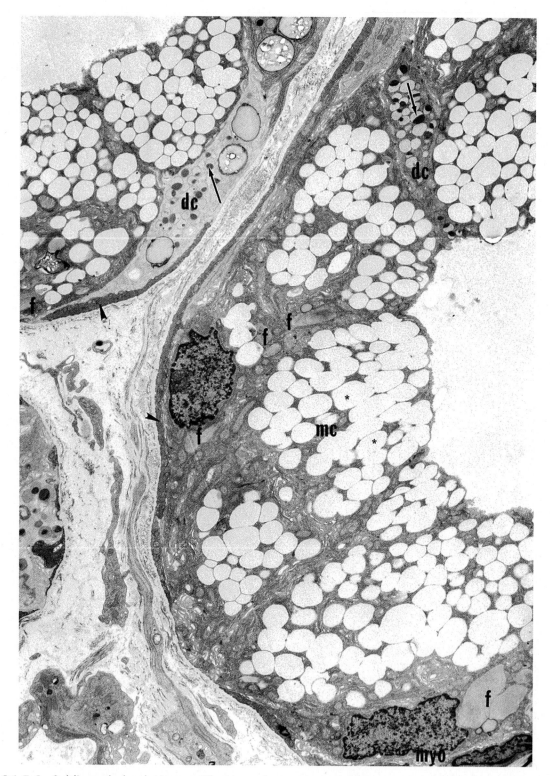

FIGURE 16-5-1. Sublingual gland. Human. Electron microscopy. ×4,050.

The human sublingual gland is composed mostly of mucous acini some of which are capped by serous demilunes. The **mucous cells** (mc) display numerous **filamentous bodies** (f) and secretory granules, which appear to be empty. The **serous cells** (dc) may be recognized by their paler cytoplasm and the presence of secretory granules (*arrows*) housing electron-dense materials. Note also the presence of **myoepithelial cells** (myo), whose processes (*arrowheads*) encircle the acinus. (Courtesy of Dr. A. Riva.)

KEY					
dc	serous cells	**mc**	mucous cells	**myo**	myoepithelial cells
f	filamentous bodies				

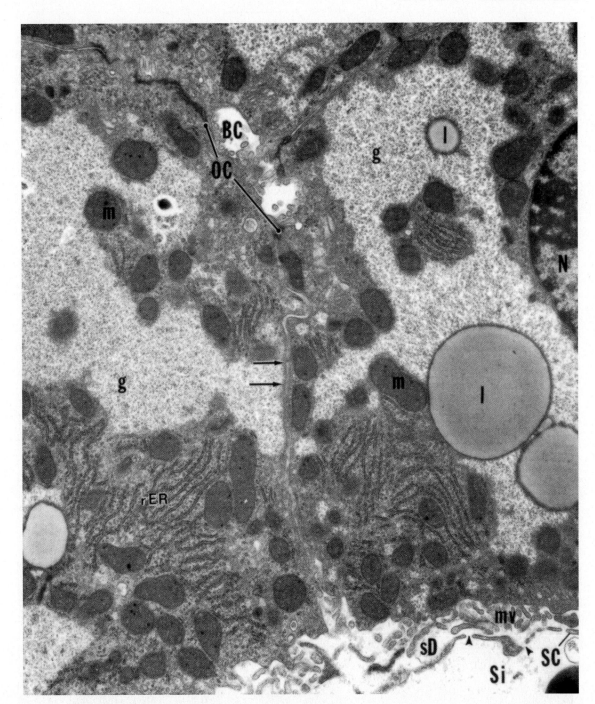

FIGURE 16-6-1. Liver. Mouse. Electron microscopy. ×11,255.

The hepatocytes of this electron micrograph display two of their surfaces, one bordering a **sinusoid** (Si) and the other where two parenchymal cells contact each other (*arrows*). The sinusoidal surface displays **microvilli** (mv) that extend into the **perisinusoidal space of Disse** (sD). They almost contact **sinusoidal lining cells** (SC) that present numerous fenestrae (*arrowheads*). The parenchymal contacts are characterized by the presence of **bile canaliculi** (BC), intercellular spaces that are isolated by the formation of **occluding junctions** (OC). The cytoplasm of hepatocytes houses the normal cellular complements, such as numerous **mitochondria** (m), elements of **rough endoplasmic reticulum** (rER), Golgi apparatus, smooth endoplasmic reticulum, lysosomes, and inclusions such as **glycogen** (g) and **lipid droplets** (l). The **nucleus** (N) of one of the hepatocytes is evident.

KEY					
BC	bile canaliculi	**mv**	microvilli	**SC**	sinusoidal lining cells
g	glycogen	**N**	nucleus	**sD**	perisinusoidal space of
l	lipid droplets	**OC**	occluding junctions		Disse
m	mitochondria	**rER**	rough endoplasmic reticulum	**Si**	sinusoid

PLATE 16-7 Pancreatic Islet of Langerhans, Electron Microscopy

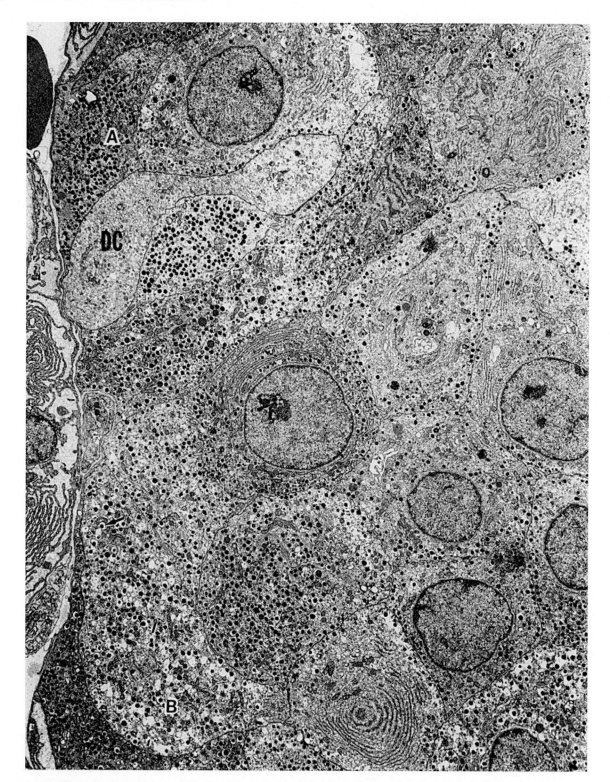

FIGURE 16-7-1. Pancreatic Islets. Rabbit. Electron microscopy. ×3,578.

The pancreatic islets house seven types of parenchymal cells, including, A, B, G, and D cells. **B cells** (B) are the most numerous and may be recognized by the presence of secretory granules whose electron-dense core is surrounded by a clear zone (*arrows*). **A cells** (A), the second most numerous secretory cell, also house many secretory granules; however, these lack an electron-lucent periphery. **D cells** (DC) are the least numerous and are characterized by secretory granules that are much less electron-dense than those of the other two cell types. (From Sato T, et al. Stereological analysis of normal rabbit pancreatic islets. *Am J Anat* 1981;161(1):71–84. Copyright © 1981 Wiley-Liss, Inc. Reprinted by permission of John Wiley & Sons, Inc.)

KEY					
A	A cells	**B**	B cells	**DC**	D cells

Selected Review of Histologic Images

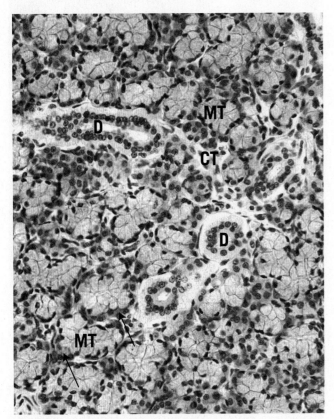

REVIEW FIGURE 16-1-1. Sublingual gland. Human. Paraffin section. ×270.

The sublingual gland produces a mixed, but mostly mucous, saliva as is evidenced by the numerous **mucous tubules** (MT) some with **serous demilunes** (*arrows*). The slender **connective tissue** (CT) elements of the sublingual gland subdivide the gland into lobes and lobules and also convey the **ducts** (D) and the vascular elements of the gland.

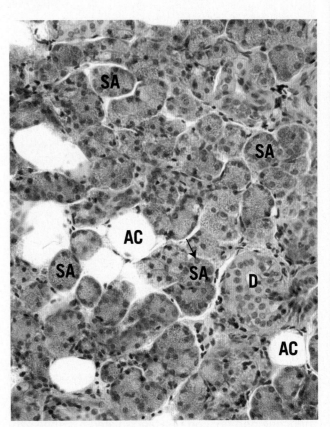

REVIEW FIGURE 16-1-2. Parotid gland. Human. Paraffin section. ×270.

The parotid gland produces a serous saliva as is evidenced by the numerous **serous acini** (SA). The slender connective tissue elements of the parotid gland partitions it into lobes and lobules and also is used by the **ducts** (D), vascular elements, and nerves that serve or just pass through the gland. As the individual ages, the gland displays the presence of **adipose cells** (AC).

KEY					
AC	adipose cell	**D**	duct	**SA**	serous acini
CT	connective tissue	**MT**	mucous tubule		

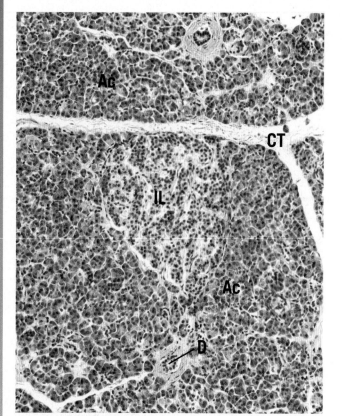

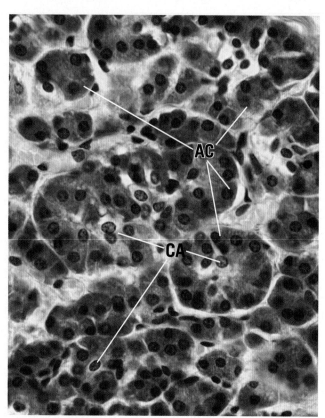

REVIEW FIGURE 16-1-3. Pancreas. Pancreatic Islet of Langerhans. Human. Paraffin section. ×132.

This photomicrograph displays both the exocrine and the endocrine portions of the human pancreas. The **pancreatic islets of Langerhans** (IL) comprise the endocrine portion, and they are isolated from the exocrine pancreas by reticular fibers, which invade the substance of each islet conveying blood vessels into and out of it. The **connective tissue** (CT) of the pancreas not only subdivides it into lobes and lobules but also conveys its vascular supply as well as the system of **ducts** (D) that deliver the exocrine secretions of the acinar cells of the **acini** (Ac) and of the centroacinar cells and intercalated ducts into the duodenum.

REVIEW FIGURE 16-1-4. Pancreas. Human. Paraffin section. ×540.

This is a higher magnification of the exocrine pancreas. Note that the **acinar cells** (AC) possess darker-staining cytoplasm and darker-staining nuclei than do the **centroacinar cells** (CA), which represent the beginning of the excretory duct system of the pancreas. The presence of the centroacinar cells clearly distinguishes the pancreas from the parotid gland whose acini do not possess centroacinar cells.

KEY					
Ac	acinus	**CT**	connective tissue	**IL**	islet of Langerhans
CA	centroacinar cell	**D**	duct		

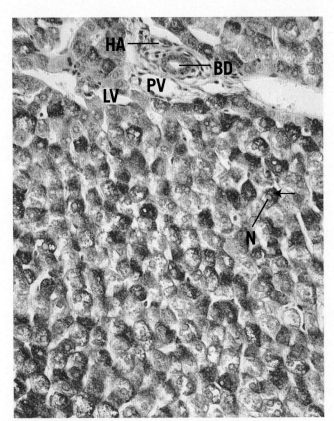

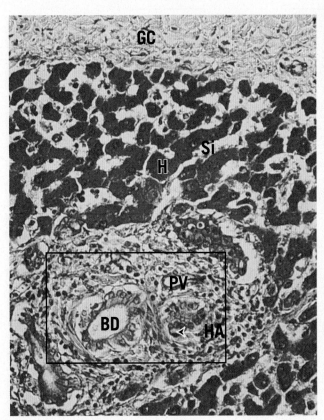

REVIEW FIGURE 16-2-1. Liver. Human. Paraffin section. Best Carmine. Glycogen stain. ×270.

The portal area of the liver houses branches of the **hepatic artery** (HA), **bile ducts** (BD), **lymph vessels** (LV), and **portal vein** (PV). The **nuclei** (N) of the hepatocytes appear pale blue and the **glycogen deposits** (*arrows*) of these cells display a dark reddish color. The hepatocytes near the central vein (not shown) display a much-reduced supply of glycogen.

REVIEW FIGURE 16-2-2. Liver. Human. Paraffin section. Trichrome stain. ×270.

The region enclosed by the rectangle is the portal area and displays branches of the **bile ducts** (BD), **hepatic artery** (HA), and **portal vein** (PV); lymph vessels are not evident in this section. The collagen of the connective tissue elements stains greenish-blue with this stain, as is evident both in the portal area and in **Glisson's capsule** (GC). The plates of **hepatocytes** (H) stain red, and the **sinusoids** (Si) appear to be empty.

KEY					
BD	bile duct	**HA**	hepatic artery	**PV**	portal vein
GC	Glisson's capsule	**LV**	lymph vessel	**Si**	sinusoid
H	hepatocyte	**N**	nucleus		

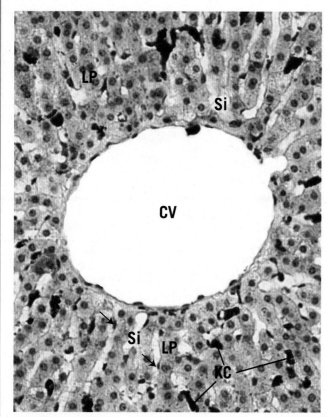

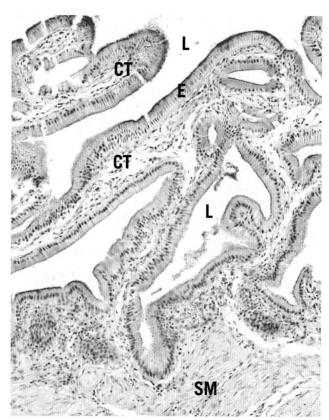

REVIEW FIGURE 16-2-3. Liver. Dog. Paraffin section. Injected with India ink ×270.

This is the area of the **central vein** (CV) of the liver of a dog injected with India ink. The **plates of hepatocytes** (LP) radiate from the central vein, and **liver sinusoids** (Si) deliver their blood into the central vein. Observe that the **Kupffer cells** (KC) phagocytose the India ink and are, therefore, evident as black smudges lining the hepatic sinusoids.

REVIEW FIGURE 16-2-4. Gallbladder. Human. Paraffin section. ×132.

The **lumen** (L) of the empty gallbladder is lined by a mucosa that is highly folded (as in this photomicrograph); however, when the gallbladder is filled with bile, the mucosal folding is greatly reduced. Observe the simple columnar **epithelium** (E) and the underlying **connective tissue** (CT), frequently referred to as the lamina propria. Deep to the mucosa is a thin **smooth muscle** (SM) layer that is responsible for the emptying of the bile into the duodenum.

KEY					
CT	connective tissue	**KC**	Kupffer cell	**Si**	sinusoid
CV	central vein	**L**	lumen	**SM**	smooth muscle layer
E	simple columnar epithelium	**LP**	plate of liver cells		

Summary of Histologic Organization

I. Major Salivary Glands

Three pairs of **major salivary glands** are associated with the oral cavity. These are the **parotid, submandibular,** and **sublingual glands.** Recently, a possible fourth pair, the **tubarial salivary glands,** has been proposed. The secretory products are delivered first to the **intercalated ducts** and then to the **striated ducts,** which are collectively categorized as **intralobular ducts.** Saliva from each lobule is delivered to the system of ducts of increasing size; the **interlobular ducts,** the **interlobar ducts,** then finally the **terminal ducts** delivering saliva into the oral cavity.

A. Parotid Gland

The **parotid gland** is a purely serous **compound acinar gland** whose **capsule** sends **septa** (frequently containing adipose cells) into the substance of the gland, dividing it into **lobes** and **lobules. Serous acini,** surrounded by **myoepithelial cells,** deliver their secretions into **intercalated ducts.**

B. Submandibular Gland

This compound **tubuloacinar gland** is mostly **serous,** although it contains enough **mucous units,** capped by **serous demilunes,** to manufacture a mixed secretion. **Acini** are surrounded by **myoepithelial cells.** The **capsule** sends **septa** into the substance of the gland, subdividing it into **lobes** and **lobules.** The **duct** system is extensive.

C. Sublingual Gland

The **sublingual gland** is a **compound tubuloacinar gland** whose capsule is not very definite. The gland produces a **mixed** secretion, possessing mostly **mucous tubules** capped by **serous demilunes** and surrounded by **myoepithelial cells.** The **intralobular duct** system is not very extensive.

II. Pancreas

The **exocrine pancreas** is a **compound acinar serous gland** whose connective tissue **capsule** sends **septa** to divide the parenchyma into lobules. **Acini** present **centroacinar cells,** the beginning of the ducts that empty into **intercalated ducts,** which lead to **intralobular,** then **interlobular ducts.** The **main duct** receives secretory products from the interlobular ducts. There are no striated ducts in the pancreas. The **endocrine pancreas** with its **pancreatic islets of Langerhans** (composed of A, B, G, PP, epsilon, and two types of **D cells**) is scattered among the serous acini.

III. Liver

A. Capsule

Glisson's capsule invests the liver and sends **septa** into the substance of the liver at the **porta hepatis** to subdivide the parenchyma into lobules.

B. Lobules

1. Classical Hepatic Lobule

Classical hepatic lobules are hexagonal (in histological sections) with **portal areas (triads)** at the periphery and a **central vein** in the center. **Plates** (trabeculae) of liver cells anastomose. **Sinusoids** are lined by endothelial cells and **Kupffer cells** (macrophages). Within the **perisinusoidal space (of Disse),** fat-accumulating hepatic stellate cells (perisinusoidal cells or Ito cells) may be noted. **Portal areas** housing **bile ducts, lymph vessels,** and branches of the **hepatic artery** and the **portal vein** are surrounded by **terminal plates** composed of **hepatocytes.** Bile passes peripherally within **bile canaliculi,** intercellular spaces between liver cells, to enter **bile ductules,** then **canals of Hering** (and **cholangioles**), to be delivered to **bile ducts** at the portal areas.

2. Portal Lobule

The apices of triangular cross sections of **portal lobules** are **central veins.** Thus, **portal areas** form the centers of these lobules. The portal lobule is based on bile flow.

3. Hepatic Acinus (Acinus of Rappaport)

The **hepatic acinus** in the tissue section is a diamond-shaped area of the liver whose long axis is the straight line between neighboring **central veins** and whose short axis is the intersecting line between neighboring portal areas. The liver acinus is based on **blood flow** and is subdivided into **zones 1, 2,** and **3.**

IV. Gallbladder

The **gallbladder** is connected to the liver via its **cystic duct,** which joins the **common hepatic duct.**

A. Epithelium

The gallbladder is lined by a **simple columnar epithelium.**

B. Lamina Propria

The **lamina propria** is thrown into intricate folds that disappear in the distended gallbladder.

C. Muscularis Externa

The **muscularis externa** is composed of an obliquely oriented **smooth muscle** layer.

D. Serosa

Adventitia attaches the gallbladder to the capsule of the liver, whereas the **serosa** covers the remaining surface.

Chapter Review Questions

16-1. The release of a bicarbonate-rich fluid from the pancreas requires which of the following substances?

A. Acetylcholine and cholecystokinin

B. Acetylcholine and secretin

C. Cholecystokinin and secretin

D. Cholecystokinin and somatostatin

16-2. Alpha cells of the islets of Langerhans release a hormone that:

A. decreases blood glucose levels.

B. increases blood glucose levels.

C. inhibits hormone release from other islet cells.

D. inhibits secretions from the exocrine pancreas.

E. stimulates glycogenolysis in the liver.

16-3. Hepatitis D is almost always accompanied by which of the following?

A. Hepatitis E

B. Hepatitis C

C. Hepatitis B

D. Hepatitis A

16-4. Bell's palsy is a possible complication during surgery involving which of the following glands?

A. Liver

B. Pancreas

C. Submandibular gland

D. Sublingual gland

E. Parotid gland

16-5. In case of liver damage, new hepatocytes are formed by which of the following cells?

A. Hepatocytes

B. Kupffer cells

C. Cells of the bile duct

D. Perisinusoidal stellate cells

E. Bile canaliculi

CHAPTER

17

URINARY SYSTEM

CHAPTER OUTLINE

The two kidneys, two ureters, the urinary bladder, and the urethra constitute the urinary system. Much of the ensuing discussion involves the **kidneys**, whose principal functions are the formation of urine; filtration of blood; regulation of blood pressure and fluid volume of the body; control of acid–base balance; formation and release of certain hormones; and conversion of vitamin D_3 to its more active form.

The functional unit of the kidney is the **uriniferous tubule** (Fig. 17-1 and Table 17-1), consisting of the **nephron** and the **collecting tubule**, each of which is derived from a different embryologic primordium.

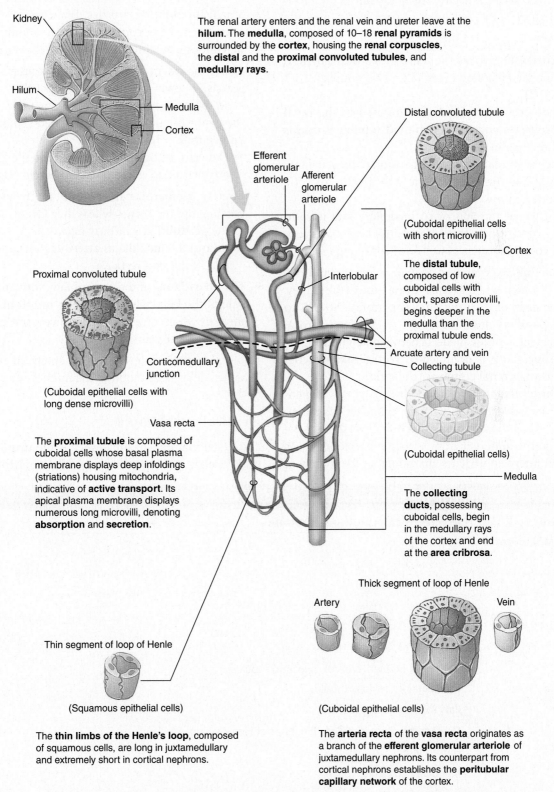

The renal artery enters and the renal vein and ureter leave at the **hilum**. The **medulla**, composed of 10–18 **renal pyramids** is surrounded by the **cortex**, housing the **renal corpuscles**, the **distal** and the **proximal convoluted tubules**, and **medullary rays**.

Distal convoluted tubule

(Cuboidal epithelial cells with short microvilli)

The **distal tubule**, composed of low cuboidal cells with short, sparse microvilli, begins deeper in the medulla than the proximal tubule ends.

Efferent glomerular arteriole

Afferent glomerular arteriole

Interlobular

Proximal convoluted tubule

(Cuboidal epithelial cells with long dense microvilli)

Corticomedullary junction

Arcuate artery and vein

Collecting tubule

(Cuboidal epithelial cells)

Vasa recta

The **proximal tubule** is composed of cuboidal cells whose basal plasma membrane displays deep infoldings (striations) housing mitochondria, indicative of **active transport**. Its apical plasma membrane displays numerous long microvilli, denoting **absorption** and **secretion**.

The **collecting ducts**, possessing cuboidal cells, begin in the medullary rays of the cortex and end at the **area cribrosa**.

Thick segment of loop of Henle

Artery   Vein

Thin segment of loop of Henle

(Squamous epithelial cells)

(Cuboidal epithelial cells)

The **thin limbs of the Henle's loop**, composed of squamous cells, are long in juxtamedullary and extremely short in cortical nephrons.

The **arteria recta** of the **vasa recta** originates as a branch of the **efferent glomerular arteriole** of juxtamedullary nephrons. Its counterpart from cortical nephrons establishes the **peritubular capillary network** of the cortex.

FIGURE 17-1. Schematic diagram of the kidney and its functional unit, the uriniferous tubule.

Kidney

The **kidneys**, bean-shaped organs, possess a lateral convex and a medial concave border. The depression in the concave border, named the **hilum**, houses the renal pelvis and is the location where arteries and nerves enter and the ureter and veins leave the kidney (see Fig. 17-1). Each kidney has a connective tissue **capsule**.

The kidney is divided into a **cortex** and a **medulla** (Fig. 17-2).

- The **cortex** has two components, the cortical labyrinth and the medullary rays (see Table 17-1 and Figs. 17-1 and 17-2).
  - The **cortical labyrinth** is composed of the **renal corpuscles** and the **convoluted tubular portions of the nephron**.
  - Each **medullary ray** is an extension of the renal medulla into the cortex, where it forms the core of a kidney **lobule**.
    - Each of the 500 or so medullary rays is composed of pars recta of proximal and distal convoluted tubules as well as of collecting tubules.
- The **medulla** is composed of 10 to 18 **renal pyramids**, each of which is said to constitute a **lobe** of the kidney.
  - The apex of each pyramid is perforated by 15 to 20 **papillary ducts** (of Bellini) at the **area cribrosa**.
  - The region of the medulla between neighboring renal pyramids is occupied by cortical-like material known as **renal columns** (of Bertin).

The histophysiology of the kidney is greatly dependent on its vascular supply. Direct branches of the abdominal aorta, the two **renal arteries** deliver 20% of the total blood volume per minute to the two kidneys. As the renal artery approaches the hilum of the kidney, it subdivides into several major branches. Each branch divides to give rise to two or more **interlobar arteries** (see Fig. 17-1).

- **Interlobar arteries** proceed in the renal columns between neighboring pyramids toward the cortex and, at the corticomedullary junction, give rise to **arcuate arteries** that follow the base of the pyramid.
- Small, **interlobular arteries**, branches of the arcuate arteries, enter the cortical labyrinth, equidistant from neighboring medullary rays, to reach the **renal capsule**.
- Along the extent of the interlobular arteries, smaller vessels, known as **afferent glomerular arterioles**, arise, become enveloped by **Bowman's capsule** of the nephron, and form a fenestrated capillary plexus known as the **glomerulus**.
  - Collectively, Bowman's capsule and the glomerulus are referred to as the **renal corpuscle** (Fig. 17-3).
- **Efferent glomerular arterioles** drain the glomerulus, passing into the cortex, where they form:
  - the **peritubular capillary network**,
  - or into the medulla as **arteriolae rectae spuriae**, a part of the vasa recta.
- The interstitium of the cortical labyrinth and the capsule of the kidney are drained by **interlobular veins**, most of which enter the **arcuate veins**, tributaries of the **interlobar veins**.
- Blood from the interlobar veins enters the **renal vein**, which delivers its blood to the inferior vena cava.

Uriniferous Tubule

The functional unit of the kidney is the **uriniferous tubule** (see Fig. 17-1), consisting of the **nephron** and the

Location	Region of the Uriniferous Tubule
Cortical labyrinth	Renal corpuscle
	Proximal convoluted tubule
	Distal convoluted tubule
	Connecting tubule/arched collecting tubule
Medullary ray	Pars recta of proximal tubule
	Pars recta of the distal tubule
	Collecting tubules (cortical collecting tubules)
Medulla	Pars recta of proximal tubules
	Pars recta of distal tubules
	Descending and ascending thin limbs of Henle's loop
	Henle's loop
	Medullary collecting tubules
	Papillary ducts

Table 17-1 Locations of the Various Regions of the Uriniferous Tubule

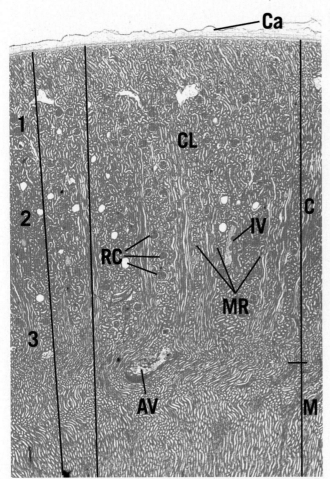

FIGURE 17-2. Kidney cortex and medulla. Human. Paraffin section. ×14.

The kidney cortex and part of the medulla are presented at a low magnification to provide an insight into the cortical architecture. The **capsule** (Ca) appears as a thin, light line at the top of the photomicrograph. The darker area below it, occupying the top half of the photomicrograph, is the **cortex** (C); the lower lighter region is the **medulla** (M). Note that longitudinal rays of the medulla appear to invade the cortex, which are known as **medullary rays** (MR). The tissue between medullary rays appears convoluted and is referred to as the **cortical labyrinth** (CL). It is occupied by dense, round structures, the **renal corpuscles** (RC). These are the first part of the nephrons, and their location in the cortex is indicative of their time of development as well as of their function. They are referred to as **superficial** (1), **midcortical** (2), or **juxtamedullary nephrons** (3). Each medullary ray and one-half of the cortical labyrinth on either side of it constitutes a lobule of the kidney. The lobule extends into the medulla, but its borders are undefinable histologically (approximated by vertical lines). The large vessels at the corticomedullary junction are **arcuate vessels** (AV); those in the cortical labyrinth are **interlobular vessels** (IV).

collecting tubule, each of which is derived from a different embryologic primordium, the metanephric blastema and ureteric bud, respectively.

Nephron

There are three types of nephrons, classified by the location of their renal corpuscles in the kidney cortex:

- **juxtamedullary nephrons**, with renal corpuscles positioned near the medulla;
- **midcortical (intermediate) nephrons**, whose renal corpuscles are located in the **midcortical region**; and
- **cortical (subcapsular) nephrons**, located just beneath the capsule.

The lengths of the three types of nephrons have similar total lengths of ~40 mm; however, the lengths of their thin limbs of Henle's loop positioned within the medulla differ. Being positioned closest to the medulla, juxtamedullary nephrons possess the longest Henle's loops, extending into the medulla. These long thin limbs of Henle's loop assist in the establishment of a concentration gradient in the renal medulla, permitting the formation of hypertonic urine (a process that is described below). Therefore, the juxtamedullary nephron will be described in detail and, for the sake of simplicity, will be referred to as "the nephron."

Bowman's Capsule and the Glomerulus (Renal Corpuscle)

The nephron begins at **Bowman's capsule**, a distended, blindly ending invaginated region of the tubule; it is at the region of the invagination, the **vascular pole of Bowman's capsule**, that the afferent glomerular arteriole enters and the efferent glomerular arteriole leaves Bowman's capsule.

- The outer layer of this capsule, known as the **parietal layer**, is composed of a simple squamous epithelium (see Figs. 17-2 and 17-3). The space between the parietal and visceral layers is known as **Bowman's space (urinary space)**.
- The simple squamous epithelium of the inner, **visceral layer** consists of modified cells, known as **podocytes**, which have a number of larger and smaller processes.
  - The larger of these, the **primary (major) processes** form secondary processes, known as **pedicels**, which wrap around the glomerular capillaries and interdigitate with pedicels of neighboring podocyte.
  - The spaces between adjoining pedicels, known as **filtration slits**, are bridged by thin **slit diaphragms** that extend from one pedicel to the

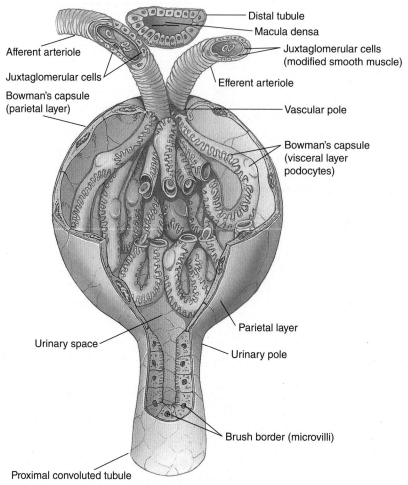

FIGURE 17-3. Schematic diagram of the renal corpuscle. Note the relationships among the afferent and efferent arterioles (glomerular arterioles) and the capillary bed, the glomerulus. The parietal layer of **Bowman's capsule** is composed of simple squamous epithelium, whereas its visceral layer is modified to form podocytes. The ultrafiltrate enters **Bowman's (urinary) space** and leaves the renal corpuscle at its urinary pole, via the proximal convoluted tubule. The **afferent glomerular arteriole** enters and the **efferent glomerular arteriole** leaves the renal corpuscle at its **vascular pole**, the former supplying and the latter draining the glomerulus. The **macula densa** component of the distal tubule comes in close proximity to the juxtaglomerular cells of the afferent (and efferent) glomerular arterioles.

next (Fig. 17-3). These slit diaphragms are composed of the extracellular portions of two flexible transmembrane proteins of each adjacent pedicel, whose flexibility, as well as the presence of actin filaments within the pedicels, permits slight movement of the pedicels to adjust, as necessary, the width of the filtration slits.

- **Glomerular capillaries** are fenestrated with large pores (60 to 90 nm in diameter) lacking diaphragms. The endothelial cell membranes possess aquaporin-1 channels designed for the rapid passage of water through them.
  - Blood from the afferent arterioles entering the glomeruli, under high vascular pressure (approximately **60 mm Hg**) force ~10% of its fluid volume, known as **ultrafiltrate** into Bowman's spaces.

- Vascular pressure is opposed by two forces, the **colloid osmotic pressure** of the blood (approximately **32 mm Hg**) and the pressure exerted by the ultrafiltrate present in Bowman's space, known as the **oncotic pressure** (about **18 mm Hg**).
- Therefore, the average **net filtration force**, expressing ultrafiltrate from the blood into Bowman's space, is relatively high, about **10 mm Hg**.

- A thick **glomerular basal lamina** (Table 17-2), manufactured by the podocytes and the endothelial cells of the glomerular capillary, is interposed between them. Together, the glomerular endothelium, the fused basal laminae, and the slit diaphragm (between adjacent pedicels) constitute the **filtration barrier** permitting only the passage of water, ions, and small molecules from the capillary into Bowman's space.

- The presence of the polyanionic **heparan sulfate** in the **lamina rara** of the basal lamina impedes the passage of large and negatively charged proteins through the barrier.
- Moreover, type IV collagen of the **lamina densa** acts as a molecular sieve and traps proteins larger than 69,000 Da (whose molecular radius is larger than 4 nm). It should be noted that type IV collagen of the lamina densa in most regions of the body is composed of α_1 and α_2 chains, whereas in the renal corpuscle it consists of α_3, α_4, and α_5 chains making it able to vary the pore size of the basal lamina. With the continued formation of the ultrafiltrate the filtered material accumulates in the basal lamina; therefore, **intraglomerular mesangial cells** phagocytose the lamina densa, which then is renewed by the combined actions of the podocytes and endothelial cells, in order to maintain the efficiency of the filtering system.

- Interstitial connective tissue is replaced by two types of smooth muscle cell derivatives known as **extraglomerular mesangial cells** and **intraglomerular mesangial cells** (Table 17-3). Intraglomerular mesangial cells not only act as smooth muscle cells controlling the blood flow through the glomerulus but also function in phagocytosing the fused basal lamina of the glomerular capillaries and podocytes.

- The ultrafiltrate that entered Bowman's space (see Figs. 17-3 to 17-5) is drained from there by the **neck of the proximal tubule**. The **simple cuboidal epithelium** of the proximal tubule adjoins the simple squamous epithelium of the parietal layer of Bowman's capsule at the **urinary pole of Bowman's capsule**.

Proximal Tubule

The **proximal tubule** is composed of two regions, the **proximal convoluted tubule** that forms loops in the vicinity of the renal corpuscle and the much shorter, **pars recta of the proximal tubule** (also known as the **descending thick limb of Henle's loop**) that descends from the cortex part way into the medulla (see Figs. 17-1 and 17-3).

- The cells of the proximal convoluted tubule possess an extensive **brush border (microvilli)** on their luminal surface. Their lateral and basal plasma membranes are considerably convoluted, and the lateral membranes form numerous interdigitations with membranes of

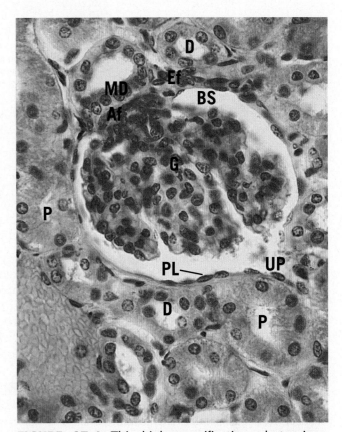

FIGURE 17-4. This high-magnification photomicrograph of the human kidney cortex displays the **afferent** (Af) and **efferent** (Ef) glomerular arterioles in the vicinity of the **macula densa** (MD) of the renal corpuscle. Note the simple squamous epithelium of the **parietal layer** (PL) of Bowman's capsule, **Bowman's space** (BS), and the capillary network, the **glomerulus** (G), that is invested by the podocytes, the visceral layer of Bowman's capsule. Observe the **proximal** (P) and **distal** (D) **convoluted tubules** surrounding the renal corpuscle. Note also the vascular pole of Bowman's capsule (at the macula densa) and the **urinary pole** (UP) at the opposite pole of Bowman's capsule. ×540.

Table 17-2	Components, Location, and Function of the Glomerular Basement Membrane		
Region of the Basement Membrane	**Location**	**Components**	**Function**
Lamina rara externa	Adjacent to the podocyte	Laminin, fibronectin, entactin, and very rich in heparan sulfate	Retards movement of negatively charged molecules
Lamina densa	Between the two laminae rarae	Type IV collagen	Filters plasma to form an ultrafiltrate
Lamina rara interna	Adjacent to the capillary endothelium	Laminin, fibronectin, entactin, and very rich in heparan sulfate	Retards movement of negatively charged molecules

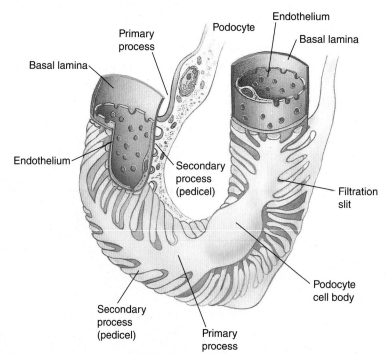

FIGURE 17-5. This schematic diagram displays a podocyte (cells of the visceral layer of Bowman's capsule) whose primary processes follow the longitudinal axis of the glomerular capillary, whereas its pedicels wrap around the circumference of the glomerular capillary. The fenestrated capillaries constituting the glomerulus are invested by **pedicels** arising from the **primary processes** of podocytes. Filtration slits between adjoining pedicels are bridged by thin diaphragms that, in association with the fused **basal laminae** of the capillary endothelium and podocyte, contribute to the formation of the **filtration barrier**. Observe that the capillary is fenestrated and a fused basal lamina, manufactured by both the capillary and the podocyte, is interposed between the capillary and the podocyte.

Table 17-3	Functions of Intraglomerular Mesangial Cells
Phagocytosis of glomerular basement membrane and molecules trapped in it (69,000 Da or greater)	
Physically support podocytes and their primary and secondary processes	
Secretion of cytokines (e.g., PDGF, IL-1) to facilitate repair of damaged glomerular components	
Contractile elements assist in reducing the luminal diameter of glomerular capillaries to increase the filtration rate	

IL-1, interleukin-1; PDGF, platelet-derived growth factor.

adjoining cells. The exaggerated folding of the basal plasmalemma partitions the cytoplasm into regions rich in mitochondria and provides a striated appearance when viewed with a light microscope.

- The cells of the straight portion, or **pars recta**, of the proximal tubules are histologically similar to those of the convoluted portion; however, their brush borders become shorter at the distal terminus of the proximal tubule where it joins the descending thin limb of Henle's loop.

In a healthy individual, the **proximal tubule** resorbs ~65% to 80% of the water, sodium, and chloride, and 100% of the proteins, amino acids, and glucose from the ultrafiltrate. The proximal tubule also secretes organic acids, bases, and other substances into the ultrafiltrate.

- The movement of sodium is via an active transport mechanism utilizing a **sodium-potassium-ATPase** pump in the basal plasmalemma, with chloride and water following passively. Because salt and water are resorbed in equimolar concentrations, the **osmolarity** of the ultrafiltrate is *not* altered in the proximal tubule but remains the same as that of blood.

- Glucose from the ultrafiltrate enters the apical aspect of the cells of the proximal tubule via **glucose transporters** and sodium and potassium enter via **Na⁺K⁺-ATPase pumps** (to be transported out of the cell via the aforementioned basally located sodium-potassium-ATPase pumps).

- The endocytosed proteins are degraded into amino acids that are also released at the basal plasmalemmae into the renal interstitium for distribution by the vascular system.

The resorbed materials are eventually returned into the **peritubular capillary network** of the cortical labyrinth for distribution to the remainder of the body.

CLINICAL CONSIDERATIONS 17-1

Glomerular Diseases

Acute glomerulonephritis is usually the result of a localized beta streptococcal infection in a region of the body other than the kidney (e.g., strep throat). Plasma cells secrete antibodies that complex with streptococcal antigens, forming an insoluble antigen–antibody complex that is filtered by the basal lamina between the podocytes and the endothelial cells of the glomerulus. As the immune complex builds up in the glomerular basal lamina, the epithelial cells and mesangial cells proliferate. Additionally, leukocytes accumulate in the glomerulus, congesting and blocking it. Moreover, pharmacologic agents released at the site of damage cause the glomerulus to become leaky, and proteins, platelets, and erythrocytes may enter the glomerular filtrate. Usually, after the acute inflammation abates, the glomeruli repair themselves and the normal kidney function returns. Occasionally, however, the damage is extensive and kidney function becomes permanently impaired.

In **diabetic glomerulosclerosis, diabetes mellitus** causes vascular pathologies that involve blood vessels throughout the body, including those of the glomerular capillary network, where synthesis of the basement membrane components increases to such an extent that it interferes with normal filtration. Additionally, hypercellularity of the mesangial cell population also interferes with the function of the normal filtration barrier and sclerosis ensues. Electron micrography demonstrates that the lamina densa of the glomerular basal membrane may increase as much as 10-fold, which becomes engorged with various plasma proteins. In the United States, ~35% of patients with end-stage renal disease suffer from diabetic glomerulosclerosis caused by both type 1 and type 2 diabetes mellitus.

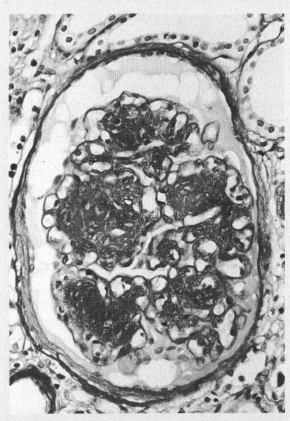

This figure is from the kidney of a patient with end-stage renal disease as a result of diabetes mellitus. Note that the glomerular capillaries are engorged with blood, the intraglomerular cell population is increased, and the glomerular basement membrane displays evidence of being thickened. (Reprinted with permission from Rubin R, et al., eds. *Rubin's Pathology: Clinicopathologic Foundations of Medicine*, 5th ed. Philadelphia: Wolters Kluwer Health/Lippincott Williams & Wilkins, 2008. Figure 16-26.)

Thin Limbs of Henle's Loop

The thin limbs of Henle's loop have three components, named after the flow of the fluid in their lumina: the descending thin limb, Henle's loop, and the ascending thin limb.

- The **descending thin limb** of juxtaglomerular nephrons extends to the apex of the medullary pyramid (those of midcortical and cortical nephrons extend only part way into the medulla and will not be discussed).

- The **descending thin limb of Henle's loop** is completely permeable to water, fairly permeable to urea but only somewhat permeable to salts, hence the ultrafiltrate in the lumen will attempt to equilibrate its osmolarity with the renal interstitium in its vicinity.

CLINICAL CONSIDERATIONS 17-2

Tubular Necrosis

Tubular necrosis may result in **acute renal failure**. Cells of the renal tubules die either from injury from exposure to toxic chemicals, such as mercury or carbon tetrachloride, or because of severe cardiovascular shock that reduces blood flow to the kidneys. The dead cells become sloughed off and occlude the lumina of their tubules. If the basal laminae remain intact, epithelial cell division may be able to repair the damage in less than 3 weeks.

- **Henle's loop** is near the apex of the medullary pyramid, and it connects the descending and ascending thin limbs in a hairpin-like loop.

- The **ascending thin limb of Henle's loop** parallels the descending thin limb as the cortical-ward continuation of Henle's loop.

  - The **ascending thin limb of Henle's loop** is mostly impermeable to water but is relatively permeable to salts and urea; thus, the movement of water is impeded, but that of sodium, chloride, and urea is not.

The ultrafiltrate will maintain the same osmolarity as the renal interstitium in its immediate surroundings as the concentration gradient decreases approaching the cortex. Because of the conditions of the renal interstitium, *sodium and chloride will leave* and *urea will enter* the lumen of the ascending thin limb of Henle's loop.

The ascending thin limb of the nephron continues onto the next region, the pars recta of the distal tubule, also known as the thick limb of ascending Henle's loop.

Distal Tubule

The **distal tubule** has two regions, the short **pars recta of the distal tubule**, also known as the **ascending thick limb of Henle's loop**, and the much longer **distal convoluted tubule**. The distal convoluted tubule is shorter than the proximal convoluted tubule; therefore, in any histologic section of the renal cortex, there are fewer profiles of it surrounding the renal corpuscle. The cells of the distal convoluted tubule resemble those of the pars recta of the distal tubule.

- The **ascending thick limb of Henle's loop**, also known as the **pars recta of the distal tubule**, is composed of simple cuboidal cells that resemble the cells of the proximal tubule, except that they are shorter and their luminal surfaces do not possess as extensive microvilli. The pars recta of the distal tubule begins *deeper in the medulla* than the end of the pars recta of the proximal tubule. This segment of the nephron is impermeable to water and urea but possesses $Na^+/K^+/2Cl^-$ cotransporters on the *luminal (apical) surface* of the cells that *actively* pump sodium, potassium, and chloride ions from its lumen into the cell. The Na^+/K^+-ATPase pumps, located on the basal cell membrane:

  - transfer sodium out of the cell into the renal interstitium (and chloride follows to maintain electrical equilibrium);

  - deliver potassium ions from the renal interstitium into the cell and sodium and chloride ions in the opposite direction, that is from the cell into the renal interstitium.

- As the ultrafiltrate ascends in the ascending thick limb of Henle's loop, the actions of the various ion pumps of these cells establish a gradient of ions concentration in the renal interstitium, where the highest concentration is deep in the medulla and the lowest concentration is at the corticomedullary junction.

  - The pars recta of the distal tubule ascends into the cortex to contact the afferent and efferent glomerular arterioles *of its own renal corpuscle.*

- Cells of the distal tubule that contact the afferent (and efferent) glomerular arteriole at the vascular pole are modified, in that they are tall cuboidal cells whose nuclei are close to one another. This region is referred to as the **macula densa** of the distal tubule and forms only a part of the circumference of the distal tubule.

  - The tall, narrow macula densa cells with apically positioned nuclei appear close to each other, forming a dense spot, hence the name macula densa (dense spot).

  - The apical cell membranes have numerous microvilli and a single nonmotile **primary cilium** (that most probably monitors fluid flow and fluid NaCl content of the ultrafiltrate), all projecting into the lumen of the distal tubule.

  - Because pars recta of the distal tubule is impermeable to water, the ultrafiltrate is **hypoosmotic** by the time it reaches the macula densa region.

  - Cells of the macula densa communicate with their basally located neighbors, the **juxtaglomerular (JG) cells** (modified smooth muscle cells) of the afferent (and sporadically, efferent) glomerular arterioles, and **extraglomerular mesangial (lacis) cells**. These three cell types form the **juxtaglomerular (JG) apparatus**, which functions as a unit to monitor the osmolarity and volume of the ultrafiltrate (Table 17-4).

  - If either the concentration of sodium is too low or the volume of the ultrafiltrate is too high, the **macula densa cells**, via gap junctions (but also by the release of prostaglandin), instruct the **juxtaglomerular cells** to release their stored proteolytic enzyme, **renin**, into the bloodstream and instruct the smooth muscle cells of the afferent glomerular arterioles to relax, thereby increasing blood flow into the glomerular capillary network.

  - **Renin** cleaves two amino acids from the circulating protein/hormone precursor **angiotensinogen**, changing it to **angiotensin I**, which, in turn, is cleaved by converting enzyme located on the luminal surfaces of capillaries (especially in the lungs), forming **angiotensin II**. This powerful vasoconstrictor also prompts the release of the mineralocorticoid **aldosterone** from the suprarenal cortex and **antidiuretic hormone (ADH)** from the pars nervosa of the pituitary gland. **ADH** affects the next segment of the uriniferous tubule, the collecting tubule.

- **Aldosterone** binds to aldosterone receptors on cells of the distal convoluted tubules, prompting them to resorb sodium (and chloride) from and secrete hydrogen, potassium, and ammonium ions into the ultrafiltrate. The addition of sodium to the extracellular compartment causes the retention of fluid with the subsequent elevation in blood pressure.

Concentration of Urine in the Nephron (Countercurrent Multiplier System)

The concentration of urine occurs only in juxtamedullary nephrons, whose long thin limbs of Henle's loop function in the establishment of an **osmotic concentration gradient**. This gradient gradually increases from about 300 mOsm/L in the interstitium of the outer medulla to as much as 1,200 mOsm/L at the renal papilla.

- The luminally located $Na^+/K^+/2Cl^-$ cotransporters in conjunction with the basally located $Na+/K+$ ATPase pumps of the ascending thick limb of Henle's loop transfer chloride and sodium ions from the lumen into the renal interstitium.
- Water is not permitted to leave the ascending thick limb; hence, the salt concentration of the renal interstitium increases.
- Because the supply of sodium and chloride inside the ascending thick limb decreases as the ultrafiltrate proceeds toward the cortex (because it is constantly being removed from the lumen), less and less sodium and chloride are available for transport; consequently, the interstitial salt concentration decreases closer to the cortex.
- The osmotic concentration gradient of the inner medulla, deep to the junction of the thin and thick ascending limbs of Henle's loop, is controlled by **urea** concentration rather than that of sodium and chloride.
- As the ultrafiltrate passes down the descending thin limb of Henle's loop, it reacts to the increasing gradient of osmotic concentration in the interstitium.
- Water leaves and a limited amount of salts enter the lumen, **reducing the volume** and **increasing the salt concentration** of the ultrafiltrate (which becomes **hypertonic**).
- In the **ascending thin limb of Henle's loop**, water is conserved but salts are permitted to leave the ultrafiltrate, decreasing its osmolarity and contributing to the maintenance of the osmotic concentration gradient.

Function of the Vasa Recta (Countercurrent Exchange System)

The **vasa recta** assists in the maintenance of the osmotic concentration gradient of the renal medulla because these capillary loops are completely permeable to salts and water. Thus, as the blood descends in the arteria recta, it becomes hyperosmotic, but as it ascends in the vena recta, its osmolarity returns to normal.

It is also important to realize that the arteria recta carries a smaller volume than the vena recta, permitting the removal of the fluid and salts transported into the renal interstitium by the various components of the uriniferous tubules.

Collecting Tubules

Collecting tubules are not part of nephrons; they have different embryologic origins. Collecting tubules, composed of a simple cuboidal to columnar epithelium whose lateral cell membranes are evident with the light microscope, begin at the terminal ends of distal convoluted tubules as either **connecting tubules** or **arched collecting tubules**. Several distal convoluted tubules join each **collecting tubule**, delivering ultrafiltrate from their particular nephron. Each collecting tubule has two regions: the **cortical collecting tubule** which descends from the medullary rays of the cortex to enter the renal pyramids of the medulla, and the **medullary collecting tubule** once it enters the medulla. Several medullary collecting tubules merge to form larger conduits known as the **papillary ducts of Bellini** (Fig. 17-6), which terminate as open structures at the area cribrosa and deliver the urine into a **minor calyx**.

The cells of the collecting tubule are of two types: the lightly staining principal cells and darker-staining intercalated cells.

- **Principal cells** (also known as **light cells**) possess a single, nonmotile, apically situated primary cilium that probably functions as a mechanosensor that monitors fluid flow along the lumen of the tubule. These cells possess **ADH-sensitive (antidiuretic hormone-sensitive) aquaporin-2 channels** that permit the cell to be permeable to water.
- **Intercalated cells** (also known as **dark cells**) are fewer in number and are of two types, α and β: **Type α dark cells** secrete H^+ into the tubular lumen and **type β dark cells** resorb H^+ and secrete HCO_3^-; therefore, the former acidify urine whereas the latter function in making the urine less acidic.

The ultrafiltrate that enters the collecting tubule is **hypoosmotic**. As it passes down the collecting tubule, *it is subject to the increasing osmotic gradient of the renal interstitium.*

- **Antidiuretic hormone (ADH)** released from the pars nervosa of the pituitary gland binds to G protein–associated V_2 **receptors** in the basal cell membranes of the **principal cells** of the collecting tubule. The binding causes the *insertion* of **aquaporin channels** (AQP2, AQP3, and AQP4) into the *luminal cell membrane* of these cells.

- Water from the lumen of the collecting tubule can now enter the cell and immediately leave the cell (to enter the renal interstitium) at the *basal cell membrane* via aquaporin channels (APQ3 and APQ4) that are always present in the basal membrane (irrespective of the presence of ADH), thereby reducing the volume but increasing the concentration of the urine.

- In the absence of ADH, the cells of the collecting tubule are impermeable to water, and the urine remains **hypotonic**.

CLINICAL CONSIDERATIONS 17-3

Diabetes Insipidus

Diabetes insipidus occurs because of damage to the cells of the hypothalamus that manufacture ADH. The low levels of ADH interfere with the ability of the collecting tubules of the kidney to concentrate urine. The excess fluid loss in the formation of copious quantities of dilute urine results in **polydipsia** (excessive thirst) and dehydration.

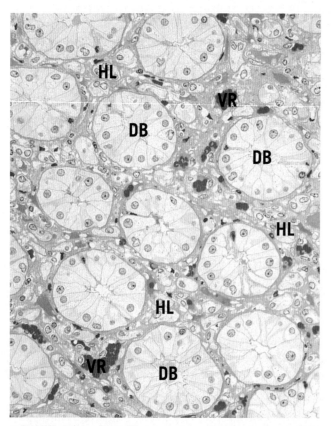

FIGURE 17-6. The lower region of the renal medulla of a monkey presents cross sections of the large papillary **ducts of Bellini** (DB). Note also the presence of the blood-filled **vasa recta** (VR) as well as the cross sections of the thin limbs of **Henle's loop** (HL). ×270.

CLINICAL CONSIDERATIONS 17-4

Kidney Disorders

Urate nephropathy is the deposition of uric acid crystals in the kidney tubules or the renal interstitium as a result of elevated levels of uric acid in the blood. In most cases, this condition is due to the patient suffering from primary gout; however, high uric acid blood levels also occur in cases of chemotherapy in cancer treatment as well as in patients who have reduced excretions of uric acid, such as in cases of lead poisoning. Although in most patients, urate nephropathy is not life-threatening, it may result in acute renal failure with fatal consequences.

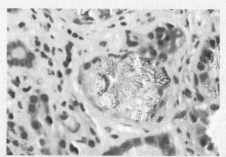

This figure is from the kidney of a patient demonstrating the deposition of uric acid crystals in the collecting tubule, indicating that the individual is suffering from urate nephropathy. (Reprinted with permission from Strayer DS, et al., eds. *Rubin's Pathology: Mechanisms of Human Disease*, 8th ed. Philadelphia: Wolters Kluwer, 2020. Figure 22-81B.)

Kidney stones usually form because of the condition known as **hyperparathyroidism**, in which the formation of excess parathyroid hormone (PTH) by the parathyroid glands results in an increased level of osteoclastic activity. The resorption of bone, as well as the increased absorption of calcium and phosphates from the gastrointestinal tract, eventuates higher than normal blood calcium levels. As the kidneys excrete higher than normal concentrations of calcium and phosphates, their presence in the urine, especially under alkaline conditions, causes their precipitation in the kidney tubules. Continued accretion of these ions onto the crystal surface causes an increase in the size of the crystals, and they become known as kidney stones.

Cancers of the kidney are usually solid tumors, whereas cysts of the kidney are usually benign. The most common symptom of kidney cancer is **blood in the urine**, although the amount of blood may be undetectable without a microscopic examination of the urine. Usually, kidney cancers are accompanied by pain and fever, but frequently they are discovered by abdominal palpation during routine physicals when the physician detects a lump in the region of the kidney. Because kidney cancers spread early and usually to the lung, the prognosis is poor.

CLINICAL CONSIDERATIONS 17-5

Odor and Color of Urine

The **odor and color of urine may** provide clues to the individual's disease state. Normal urine is either colorless or has a yellow color if the urine is concentrated. Similarly, dilute urine has very little odor, whereas concentrated urine has a pungent smell. If the color of urine is reddish, the individual may have porphyria or fresh blood in the urine; if the color is brown, the possibility is that breakdown by-products of damaged muscle or breakdown by-products of hemoglobin are in the urine. Black discoloration could be caused by the presence of melanin pigment in the urine, whereas cloudy urine could be an indication of the presence of acidic crystals or the presence of pus derived from urinary tract infection. Additionally, certain medications can discolor the urine, and the patient should be warned about the color change. Changes in the odor of urine can be caused by diabetes that is not being controlled (a sweet odor); fetid odor could indicate the presence of a urinary tract infection; and a musty odor of urine in a young patient may suggest phenylketonuria.

Table 17-4	Renin–Angiotensin–Aldosterone System	
High Ultrafiltrate Level in Pars Recta of Distal Tubule at the Macula Densa	**Low Sodium Level in Pars Recta of Distal Tubule at the Macula Densa**	
Juxtaglomerular cells release renin, and smooth muscle cells of the afferent glomerular arterioles relax.		
Renin cleaves angiotensinogen to form angiotensin I.		
Angiotensin-converting enzyme cleaves angiotensin I to form angiotensin II		
Angiotensin II increases systemic vascular resistance, including that of the efferent glomerular arteriole.	Angiotensin II causes the release of aldosterone from the suprarenal cortex.	
Glomerular filtration rate is increased.	Aldosterone prompts additional resorption of sodium and chloride from the ultrafiltrate located in the distal convoluted tubule.	
Volume of ultrafiltrate is decreased at the collecting tubules.	More sodium is available to enter the bloodstream.	

Extrarenal Excretory Passages

The **extrarenal excretory passages** consist of the ureters, urinary bladder, and urethra. The ureters and bladder are also lined by transitional epithelia.

- The **ureters** possess a fibroelastic lamina propria and two to three layers of smooth muscle, arranged as inner longitudinal, middle circular, and outer longitudinal layers. The third muscle layer, the **outer longitudinal layer**, usually appears only in the lower one-third of the ureter.

- The **transitional epithelial lining** of the **bladder** and the other urinary passages offers an impermeable barrier to urine.
  - To be able to perform its function, the plasma membrane of the surfacemost cells is thicker than the average plasma membrane and is composed of a lattice structure consisting of hexagonally arrayed elements.
  - Furthermore, because cells of the transitional epithelium must line an ever-larger surface as the urinary bladder distends, the plasma membrane is folded in a mosaic-like fashion.
  - Folding occurs at the **interplaque regions**, whereas the thickened **plaque regions** present **vesicular profiles**, which probably become unfolded as urine accumulates in the bladder.

The subepithelial connective tissue of the bladder is composed, according to most authors, of a lamina propria and a submucosa. The three smooth muscle layers are extensively interlaced, making them indistinguishable in some areas (Fig. 17-7).

The **urethra** of the male differs from that of the female not only in its length but also in its function and epithelial lining. The lamina propria of both sexes contain mucous **glands of Littré** and **intraepithelial glands**, which lubricate the lining of the urethra, facilitating the passage of urine to the outside. The urethra is described in Chapter 18, "Female Reproductive System," and Chapter 19, "Male Reproductive System."

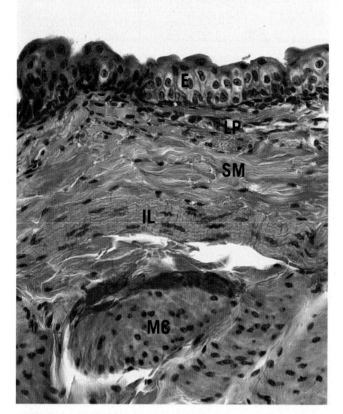

FIGURE 17-7. The human bladder is lined by a transitional **epithelium** (E) overlying a fibroelastic connective tissue **lamina propria** (LP) deep to which is the **submucosa** (SM). The muscularis of the bladder is composed of an **inner longitudinal** (IL), **middle circular** (MC), and outer longitudinal smooth muscle layers (not shown). ×132.

CLINICAL CONSIDERATIONS 17-6

Bladder Cancer

Annually, there are more than 50,000 new cases of transitional epithelial cell **carcinomas of the bladder** in the United States. Interestingly, almost 65% of the affected individuals are male, and about half of these patients smoke cigarettes. The most prominent symptom of bladder cancer is blood in the urine (hematuria), followed by burning sensation and pain on urination, as well as an increased frequency of the urge to urinate. Although these symptoms are frequently confused with cystitis, the condition becomes suspicious once the antibiotics fail to alleviate the problem and cytology of the urine demonstrates the presence of cancerous transitional cells. If caught early, before the carcinoma invades the deeper tissues, the survival rate is as great as 95%; however, if the tumor is a rapidly dividing one that invades the muscular layers of the bladder and reaches the lymph nodes, the 5-year survival rate drops to less than 45%.

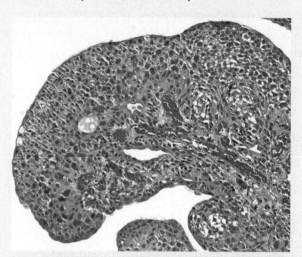

This figure is from a urinary bladder with high-grade papillary urothelial carcinoma. Note that the transitional epithelium is disorganized and the individual epithelial cells display dense, pleomorphic nuclei. (Reprinted with permission from Rubin R, et al., eds. *Rubin's Pathology: Clinicopathologic Foundations of Medicine*, 5th ed. Philadelphia: Wolters Kluwer Health/Lippincott Williams & Wilkins, 2008. p. 757.)

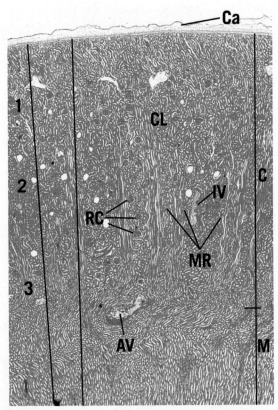

FIGURE 17-1-1. Kidney cortex and medulla. Human. Paraffin section. ×14.

The kidney cortex and part of the medulla are presented at a low magnification to provide an insight into the cortical architecture. The **capsule** (Ca) appears as a thin, light line at the top of the photomicrograph. The darker area below it, occupying the top half of the photomicrograph, is the **cortex** (C); the lower lighter region is the **medulla** (M). Note that longitudinal rays of the medulla appear to invade the cortex; these are known as **medullary rays** (MR). The tissue between medullary rays appears convoluted and is referred to as the **cortical labyrinth** (CL). It is occupied by dense, round structures, the **renal corpuscles** (RC), composed of Bowman's capsules and glomeruli. These are the first part of the nephrons, and their location in the cortex is indicative of their time of development as well as of their function. They are referred to as **cortical (subcapsular)** (1), **midcortical** (2), or **juxtamedullary nephrons** (3). Each medullary ray and one-half of the cortical labyrinth on either side of it constitutes a lobule of the kidney. The lobule extends into the medulla, but its borders are undefinable histologically (approximated by vertical lines). The large vessels at the corticomedullary junction are **arcuate vessels** (AV); those in the cortical labyrinth are **interlobular vessels** (IV).

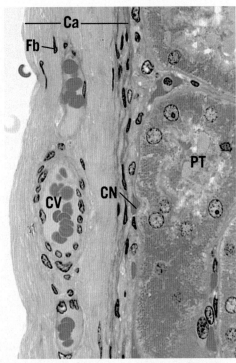

FIGURE 17-1-2. Kidney capsule. Monkey. Plastic section. ×540.

The kidney is invested by a **capsule** (Ca) composed of dense collagenous connective tissue. The two layers of the capsule are evident, in that the **outer layer** is paler and houses occasional **fibroblasts** (Fb); the **inner layer** is thinner, darker in color and instead of fibroblasts it has **myofibroblasts** whose nuclei are plumper than those of fibroblasts. Although this structure is not highly vascular, it does possess some **capsular vessels** (CV). Observe the numerous red blood cells in the lumina of these vessels. The deeper aspect of the capsule possesses a rich **capillary network** (CN) that is supplied by the terminal branches of the interlobular arteries and is drained by the stellate veins, tributaries of the interlobular veins. Note the cross sections of the **proximal convoluted tubules** (PT).

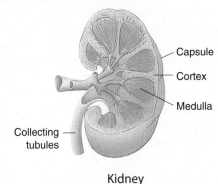

Kidney

KEY					
AV	arcuate vessel	CV	capsular vessel	PT	proximal convoluted
C	cortex	Fb	fibroblast		tubule
Ca	capsule	IV	interlobular vessel	RC	renal corpuscle
CL	cortical labyrinth	M	medulla		
CN	capillary network	MR	medullary ray		

PLATE 17-1A   Kidney, Survey and General Morphology

PLATE 17-1B   Kidney Cortex and Its Vascular Supply

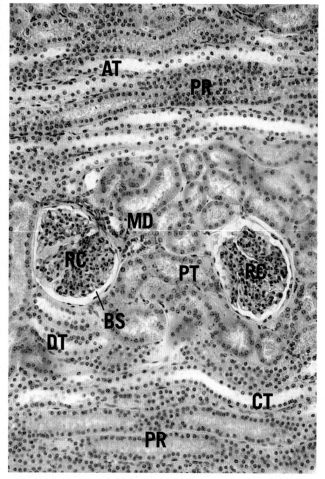

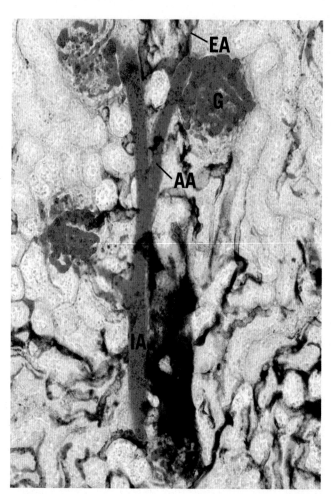

FIGURE 17-1-3. Kidney cortex. Human. Paraffin section. ×132.

FIGURE 17-1-4. Colored colloidin-injected kidney. Paraffin section. ×132.

The various components of the cortical labyrinth and portions of two medullary rays are evident. The orientation of this photomicrograph is perpendicular to that of Figure 17-1-1. Note that two **renal corpuscles** (RC) in the center of the photomicrograph display a slight shrinkage artifact and thus clearly demonstrate **Bowman's space** (BS). The renal corpuscles are surrounded by cross sections of **proximal convoluted tubules** (PT), **distal convoluted tubules** (DT), and **macula densa** (MD). Because the proximal convoluted tubule is much longer than the convoluted portion of the distal tubule, the proximal convoluted tubule profiles around a renal corpuscle outnumber the distal convoluted tubule profiles by approximately 7 to 1. The medullary rays contain the **pars recta** (PR) of the **proximal tubule**, the **ascending thick limbs of Henle's loop** (AT), and **collecting tubules** (CT).

This specimen was prepared by injecting the renal artery with colored colloidin, and a thick section was taken to demonstrate the vascular supply of the renal corpuscle. Each renal corpuscle contains tufts of capillaries, the **glomerulus** (G), which is supplied by the **afferent glomerular arteriole** (AA) and drained by the **efferent glomerular arteriole** (EA). Note that the outer diameter of the AA is greater than that of the efferent glomerular arteriole; however, the diameters of the two lumina are about equal. It is important to realize that the glomerulus is an arterial capillary network; therefore, the pressure within these vessels is greater than that of normal capillary beds. This results in more effective filtration pressure. The large vessel in the middle is an **interlobular artery** (IA), and it is the parent vessel of the afferent glomerular arterioles.

KEY					
AA	afferent arteriole	**DT**	distal convoluted tubule	**PT**	proximal convoluted
AT	ascending thick limb of	**EA**	efferent arteriole		tubule
	Henle's loop	**G**	glomerulus	**RC**	renal corpuscle
BS	Bowman's space	**IA**	interlobular artery		
CT	collecting tubule	**PR**	pars recta		

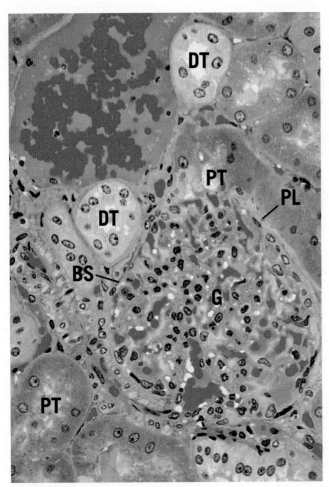

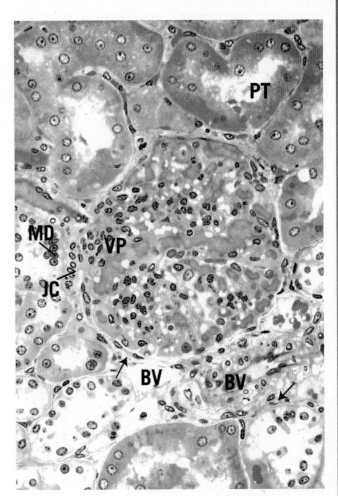

FIGURE 17-2-1. Kidney cortical labyrinth. Monkey. Plastic section. ×270.

The center of this photomicrograph is occupied by a renal corpuscle. The urinary pole is evident as the short neck empties into the convoluted portion of the **proximal tubule** (PT). The renal corpuscle is composed of the **glomerulus** (G), tufts of capillaries, the visceral layer of Bowman's capsule (podocytes) that is intimately associated with the glomerulus, **Bowman's space** (BS), into which the ultrafiltrate is expressed from the capillaries, and the **parietal layer** (PL) of Bowman's capsule, consisting of a simple squamous epithelium. Additionally, mesangial cells are also present in the renal corpuscle. Most of the tubular profiles surrounding the renal corpuscle are transverse sections of the darker-staining **proximal tubules** (PT), which outnumber the cross sections of the lighter-staining **distal tubules** (DT).

FIGURE 17-2-2. Kidney cortical labyrinth. Monkey. Plastic section. ×270.

The renal corpuscle in the center of the photomicrograph displays all of the characteristics identified in Figure 17-2-1, except that instead of the urinary pole, the **vascular pole** (VP) is presented. That is the region where the afferent and efferent glomerular arterioles enter and leave the renal corpuscle, respectively. Some of the smooth muscle cells of the afferent (and sometimes efferent) glomerular arterioles are modified in that they contain vesicles housing renin. These modified cells are known as **juxtaglomerular cells** (JC). They are closely associated with the **macula densa** (MD) region of the distal tubule. Again, note that most of the cross-sectional profiles of tubules surrounding the renal corpuscle belong to the convoluted portion of the **proximal tubules** (PT), whereas only one or two are distal tubules. Observe the rich **vascularity** (BV) of the renal cortex as well as the scant amount of connective tissue elements (*arrows*) associated with these vessels.

KEY					
BS	Bowman's space	**G**	glomerulus	**PL**	parietal layer
BV	blood vessel	**JC**	juxtaglomerular cell	**PT**	proximal tubule
DT	distal tubule	**MD**	macula densa	**VP**	vascular pole

PLATE 17-2B Renal Cortex

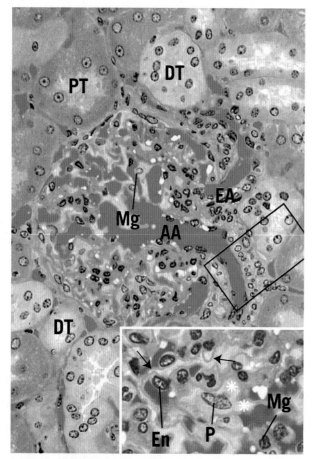

FIGURE 17-2-3. Kidney cortical labyrinth. Monkey. Plastic section. ×270.

The vascular pole of this renal corpuscle is clearly represented. It is in this region that the **afferent glomerular arteriole** (**AA**) enters the renal corpuscle and the **efferent glomerular arteriole** (EA) leaves, draining the glomerulus. Observe that these two vessels and their capillaries are supported by **mesangial cells** (Mg). Note that although the outer diameter of the afferent glomerular arteriole is greater than that of the efferent glomerular arteriole, their luminal diameters are approximately the same. The renal corpuscle is surrounded by cross-sectional profiles of **distal** (DT) and **proximal** (PT) **tubules**. The *boxed area* is presented at a higher magnification in Figure 17-2-4. *Inset.* **Glomerulus. Kidney. Monkey. Plastic section.** ×720. The glomerulus is composed of capillaries whose **endothelial cell** (En) nuclei bulge into the lumen. The endothelial cells are separated from **podocytes** (P), modified cells forming the visceral layer of Bowman's capsule, by a thick basal lamina (*arrows*). **Mesangial cells** (Mg) form both supporting and phagocytic elements of the renal corpuscle. Note that major processes (white *asterisks*) of the podocytes are also distinguishable in this photomicrograph.

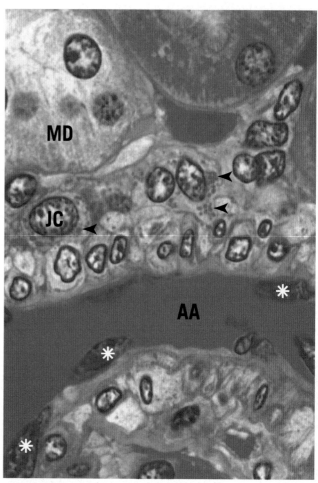

FIGURE 17-2-4. Juxtaglomerular apparatus. Kidney. Monkey. Plastic section. ×1,325.

The *boxed area* of Figure 17-2-3 is magnified to present the juxtaglomerular apparatus. This is composed of the **macula densa** (MD) region of the distal tubule and apparent **juxtaglomerular cells** (JC), modified smooth muscle cells of the **afferent glomerular arteriole** (AA). Observe the granules (*arrowheads*) in the juxtaglomerular cells, which house the enzyme renin. Note the nuclei (*asterisks*) of the endothelial cells lining the AA.

KEY					
AA	afferent arteriole	**En**	endothelial cell	**Mg**	mesangial cell
DT	distal tubule	**JC**	juxtaglomerular cell	**P**	podocyte
EA	efferent arteriole	**MD**	macula densa	**PT**	proximal tubule

PLATE 17-3 Glomerulus, Scanning Electron Microscopy

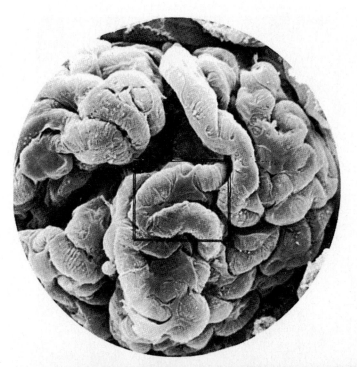

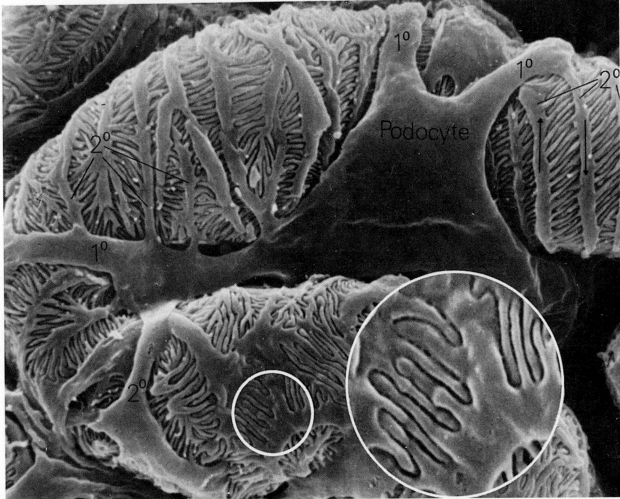

FIGURE 17-3-1. Scanning electron micrograph of a glomerulus, displaying the primary and secondary processes and pedicels of podocytes. **Top**, ×700; **bottom**, ×4,000; and *inset*, ×6,000. (Reprinted with permission from Ross MH, et al. *Histology: A Text and Atlas*, 2nd ed. Baltimore: Williams & Wilkins, 1989. p. 536.)

PLATE 17-4 Renal Corpuscle, Electron Microscopy

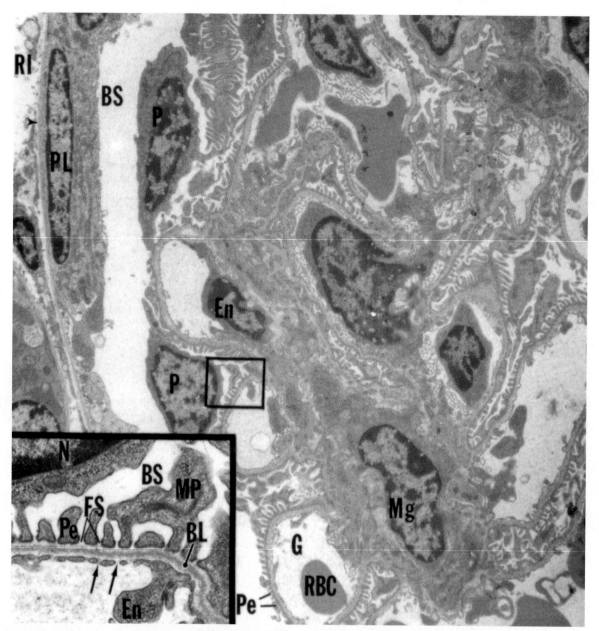

FIGURE 17-4-1. Kidney cortex. Renal corpuscle. Mouse. Electron microscopy. ×3,780.

Various components of the renal corpuscle are displayed in this electron micrograph. Note the basal lamina (*arrowhead*) separating the simple squamous cells of the **parietal layer** (PL) of Bowman's capsule from the **renal interstitium** (RI). **Bowman's space** (BS) and the **podocytes** (P) are shown to advantage, as are the **glomeruli** (G) and surrounding **pedicels** (Pe). **Mesangial cells** (Mg) occupy the space between capillary loops, and several **red blood cells** (RBC) and **endothelial lining** (En) are also evident. *Inset*. **Podocyte and glomerulus.** **Mouse. Electron microscopy**. ×6,300. This is a higher magnification of the *boxed area*, presenting a portion of a podocyte. Observe its **nucleus** (N), **major process** (MP), and **pedicels** (Pe). Note that the pedicels lie on a **basal lamina** (BL) that is composed of a lamina rara externa, lamina densa, and lamina rara interna. Observe the fenestrations (*arrows*) in the **endothelial lining** (En) of the glomerulus. The spaces between the pedicels, known as **filtration slits** (FS), lead into **Bowman's space** (BS).

KEY					
BL	basal lamina	**Mg**	mesangial cells	**Pe**	pedicels
BS	Bowman's space	**MP**	major process	**PL**	parietal layer
En	endothelial lining	**N**	nucleus	**RBC**	red blood cells
FS	filtration slits	**P**	podocytes	**RI**	renal interstitium
G	glomeruli				

PLATE 17-5A Renal Medulla

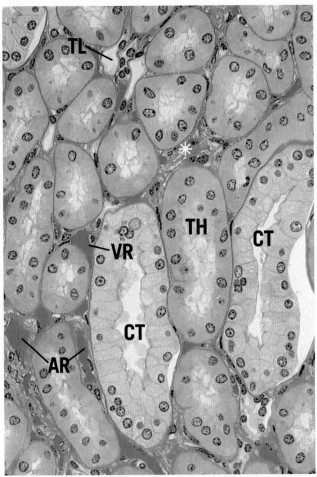

FIGURE 17-5-1. Renal medulla. Monkey. Plastic section. ×270.

This photomicrograph of the renal medulla demonstrates the arrangement of the various tubular and vascular structures. The formed connective tissue elements among the tubules and vessels are sparse and constitute mainly fibroblasts, macrophages, and fibers (white *asterisks*). The major tubular elements are the **collecting tubules** (CT), recognizable by the conspicuous lateral plasma membranes of their tall cuboidal (or low columnar) cells, **thick limbs of Henle's loop** (TH), and occasional **thin limbs of Henle's loop** (TL). Many vascular elements are noted; these are the vasa recta spuria, whose thicker-walled descending limbs are the **arteriolae rectae spuriae** (AR) and thinner-walled ascending limbs are the **venulae rectae spuriae** (VR).

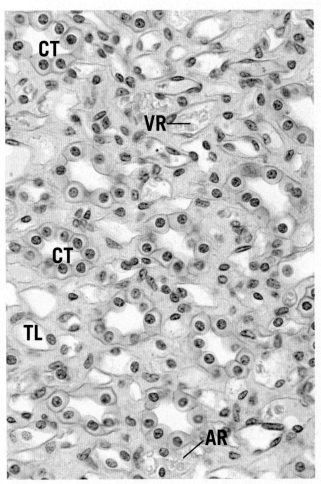

FIGURE 17-5-2. Renal papilla. x.s. Human. Paraffin section. ×270.

The most conspicuous tubular elements of the renal papilla are the **collecting tubules** (CT), with their cuboidal cells, whose lateral plasma membranes are evident. The numerous thin-walled structures are the **thin limbs of Henle's loop** (TL), as well as the **arteriolae rectae spuriae** (AR) and **venulae rectae spuriae** (VR) that may be identified by the presence of blood in their lumina. The formed connective tissue elements may be discerned in the interstitium among the various tubules of the kidney. An occasional **thick limb of Henle's loop** (TH) may also be observed.

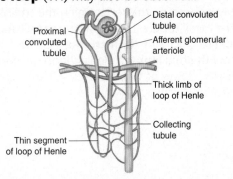

Uriniferous tubule

KEY					
AR	arteriolae rectae spuriae	**TH**	thick limb of Henle's loop	**VR**	venulae rectae spuriae
CT	collecting tubule	**TL**	thin limb of Henle's loop		

PLATE 17-5B   Renal Medulla

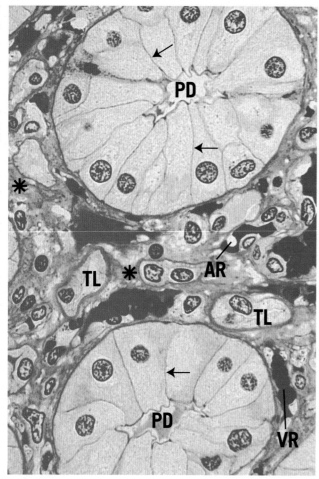

FIGURE 17-5-3. Renal papilla. x.s. Monkey. Plastic section. ×540.

In the deeper aspect of the medulla, collecting tubules merge with each other, forming larger and larger structures. The largest of these ducts are known as **papillary ducts** (PD), or ducts of Bellini, which may be recognized by their tall, pale columnar cells and their easily discernible lateral plasma membranes (*arrows*). These ducts open at the apex of the renal papilla, in the region known as the area cribrosa. The **thin limbs of Henle's loop** (TL) are evident. These structures form the hairpin-like loops of Henle in this region, where the ascending thin limbs recur to ascend in the medulla, eventually to become thicker, forming the straight portion of the distal tubule. Note that the **arteriolae rectae spuriae** (AR) and the **venulae rectae spuriae** (VR) follow the thin limbs of Henle's loop deep into the renal papilla. Some of the connective tissue elements are marked by *asterisks*.

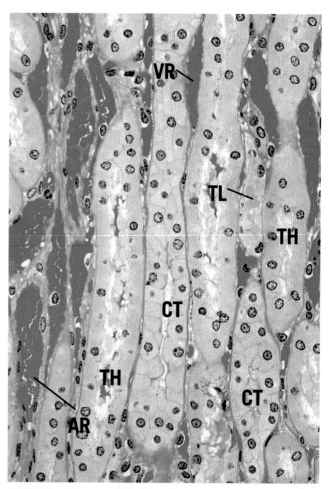

FIGURE 17-5-4. Renal medulla. l.s. Monkey. Plastic section. ×270.

This photomicrograph is similar to Figure 17-5-1, except that it is a longitudinal rather than a transverse section of the renal medulla. The center is occupied by a **collecting tubule** (CT), as is distinguished by the tall cuboidal cells whose lateral plasma membranes are evident. The collecting tubule is flanked by **thick limbs of Henle's loop** (TH). The vasa recta are filled with blood, and the thickness of their walls identifies whether they are **arteriolae rectae spuriae** (AR) or **venulae rectae spuriae** (VR). A **thin limb of Henle's loop** (TL) is also identifiable.

KEY					
AR	arteriolae rectae spuriae	**PD**	papillary duct	**TL**	thin limb of Henle's loop
CT	collecting tubule	**TH**	thick limb of Henle's loop	**VR**	venulae rectae spuriae

PLATE 17-6A Ureter

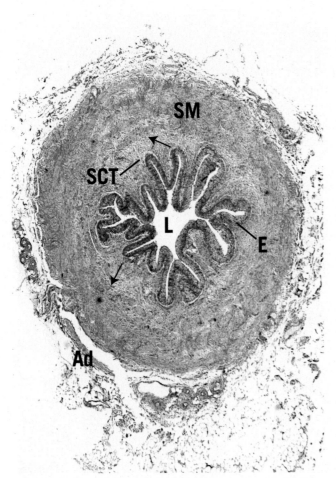

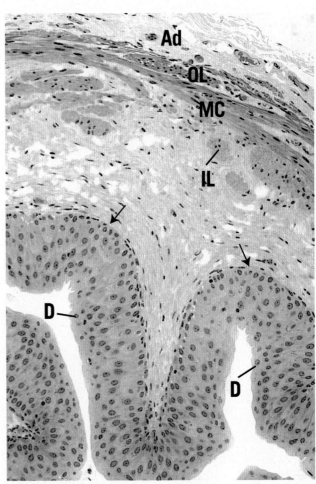

FIGURE 17-6-1. Ureter. x.s. Human. Paraffin section. ×14.

This low-power photomicrograph of the ureter displays its stellate-shaped **lumen** (L) and thick lining **epithelium** (E). The interface between the **subepithelial connective tissue** (SCT) and the **smooth muscle coat** (SM) is indicated by *arrows*. The muscle coat is surrounded by a fibrous **adventitia** (Ad), which houses the numerous vascular channels and nerve fibers that travel with the ureter. Thus, the wall of the ureter consists of the mucosa (epithelium and underlying connective tissue), muscularis, and adventitia.

FIGURE 17-6-2. Ureter. x.s. Monkey. Plastic section. ×132.

The mucosa is highly convoluted and consists of a thick, transitional epithelium whose free surface possesses characteristic **dome-shaped cells** (D). The basal cell layer sits on a basal lamina (*arrows*), which separates the epithelium from the underlying fibrous connective tissue. The **muscularis** consists of three layers of smooth muscle: **inner longitudinal** (IL), **middle circular** (MC), and **outer longitudinal** (OL). These three layers are not always present, for the outer longitudinal layer is found only in the inferior one-third of the ureter, that is, the portion nearest the urinary bladder. The **adventitia** (Ad) is composed of fibrous connective tissue that anchors the ureter to the posterior body wall and adjacent structures.

KEY

Ad	adventitia	**L**	lumen	**SCT**	subepithelial connective tissue
D	dome-shaped cell	**MC**	middle circular muscularis		
E	epithelium	**OL**	outer longitudinal muscularis	**SM**	smooth muscle coat
IL	inner longitudinal muscularis				

PLATE 17-6B   Urinary Bladder

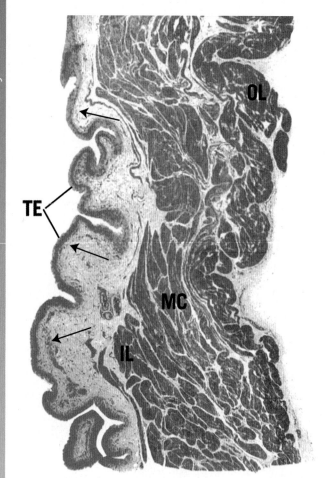

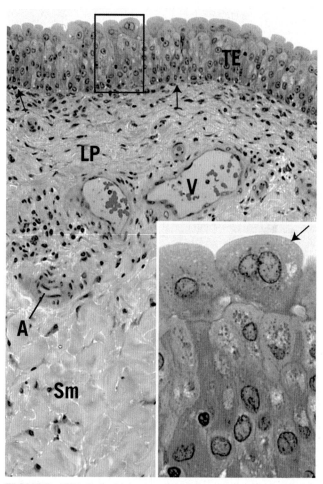

FIGURE 17-6-3. Urinary bladder. Monkey. Plastic section. ×14.

The urinary bladder stores urine until it is ready to be voided. Because the volume of the bladder changes with the amount of urine it contains, its mucosa may or may not display folds. This particular specimen is not distended, hence the numerous folds (*arrows*). Moreover, the **transitional epithelium** (TE) of this preparation is also thick, whereas in the distended phase, the epithelium would be much thinner. Note also that the thick **muscularis** is composed of three layers of smooth muscle: **inner longitudinal** (IL), **middle circular** (MC), and **outer longitudinal** (OL). The muscle layers are surrounded either by an adventitia composed of loose connective tissue—as is the case in this photomicrograph—or by a serosa, depending on the region of the bladder being examined.

FIGURE 17-6-4. Urinary bladder. Monkey. Plastic section. ×132.

The bladder is lined by **transitional epithelium** (TE), whose typical surface dome-shaped cells are shown to advantage. Some of these cells are binucleated. The epithelium is separated from the underlying connective tissue by a basal lamina (*arrows*). This subepithelial connective tissue is frequently said to be divided into a **lamina propria** (LP) and a **submucosa** (Sm). The vascularity of this region is demonstrated by the numerous **venules** (V) and **arterioles** (A). These vessels possess smaller tributaries and branches that supply the regions closer to the epithelium. *Inset.* **Transitional epithelium. Monkey. Plastic section.** ×540. The *boxed region* of the transitional epithelium is presented at a higher magnification to demonstrate the large, dome-shaped cells (*arrow*) at the free surface. These cells are characteristic of the empty bladder. When that structure is distended with urine, the dome-shaped cells assume a flattened morphology and the entire epithelium becomes thinner (being reduced from five to seven to only three cell layers thick). Note that occasional cells may be binucleated.

KEY					
A	arteriole	**MC**	middle circular muscularis	**Sm**	submucosa
IL	inner longitudinal muscularis	**OL**	outer longitudinal muscularis	**TE**	transitional epithelium
LP	lamina propria			**V**	venule

Selected Review of Histologic Images

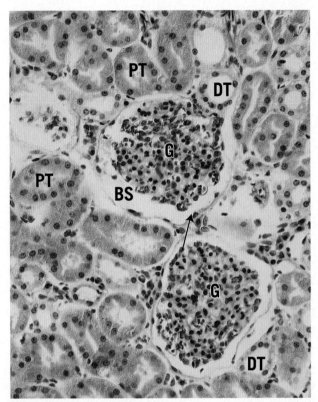

REVIEW FIGURE 17-1-1. Kidney cortex. Human. Paraffin section. ×270.

Two renal corpuscles and cross sections of their associated **distal convoluted tubules** (DT) and **proximal convoluted tubules** (PT) are clearly evident. Note that the **glomerulus** (G), **Bowman's space**, also known as urinary space (BS), and the parietal layer (*arrow*) of Bowman's capsule are also labeled.

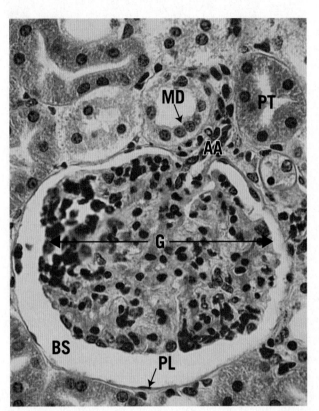

REVIEW FIGURE 17-1-2. Kidney cortex. Human. Paraffin section. ×540.

This high-magnification photomicrograph of a renal corpuscle demonstrates that the **afferent glomerular arteriole** (AA) is closely associated with the **macula densa** (MD) of the distal tubule. The **glomerulus** (G) occupies most of the renal corpuscle, whose **parietal layer** (PL), composed of simple squamous epithelium, encloses **Bowman's space** (BS). One of the cross sections of the **proximal convoluted tubule** (PT) is also labeled.

KEY					
AA	afferent glomerular arteriole	**DT**	distal convoluted tubule	**PL**	parietal layer
		G	glomerulus	**PT**	proximal convoluted tubule
BS	Bowman's space	**MD**	macula densa		

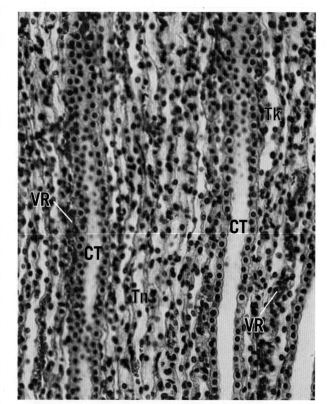

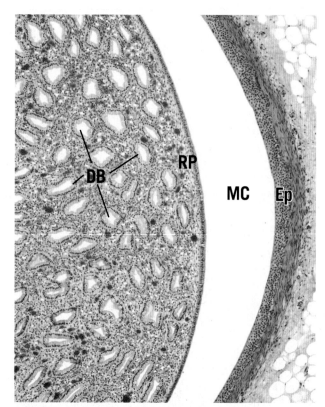

REVIEW FIGURE 17-1-3. Kidney medulla. Human. Paraffin section. l.s. ×270.

This longitudinal section of the renal medulla displays the **collecting tubules** (CT) to advantage. Their simple cuboidal epithelia possess round centrally placed nuclei and conspicuous lateral cell membranes. The **thin limbs** (Tn) and **thick limbs** (Tk) **of Henle's loop** are recognizable because the cells composing them are of different thicknesses. These are also distinguishable from the **vasa recta** (VR) whose lumina contain blood cells.

REVIEW FIGURE 17-1-4. Renal papilla. Human. Paraffin section. ×56.

This low-magnification photomicrograph is of the apex of one of the renal pyramids, a region known as the **renal papilla** (RP). The **ducts of Bellini** (DB) empty their contents into the **minor calyx** (MC) whose **transitional epithelium** (Ep) reflects onto the surface of the renal papilla.

KEY					
CT	collecting tubule	**MC**	minor calyx	**Tk**	thick limb of Henle's loop
DB	ducts of Bellini	**RP**	renal papilla	**VR**	vasa recta
Ep	transitional epithelium	**Tn**	thin limb of Henle's loop		

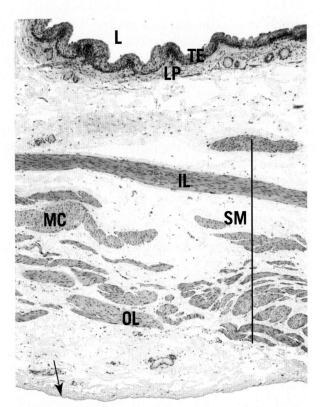

REVIEW FIGURE 17-2-1. Urinary bladder. Human. Paraffin section. ×56.

The urinary bladder receives urine from the two ureters and stores it in its **lumen** (L) until it is emptied. The mucosa of the bladder is highly folded when empty, but as urine accumulates the mucosa becomes smoother. The urinary bladder is lined by a **transitional epithelium** (TE) deep to which is the **lamina propria** (LP) that possesses mucous glands of Littré in the vicinity of the urethral opening. The **smooth muscle** (SM) coat of the urinary bladder is arranged in three layers, **inner longitudinal** (IL), **middle circular** (MC), and **outer longitudinal** (OL). Parts of the bladder are covered by serosa (*arrow*) and parts by an adventitia.

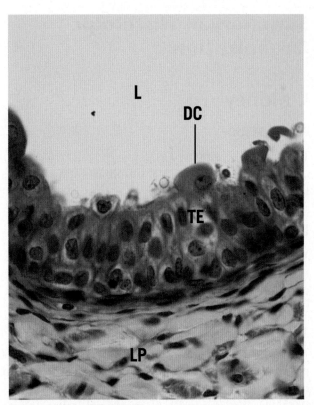

REVIEW FIGURE 17-2-2. Urinary bladder. Human. Paraffin section. ×540.

The **lumen** (L) of the urinary bladder is lined by a **transitional epithelium** (TE) that is recognizable by the presence of **dome-shaped cells** (DC) at its luminal surface. Deep to the transitional epithelium is the **lamina propria** (LP) that is separated from the epithelium by a basement membrane.

KEY					
DC	dome-shaped cell	**LP**	lamina propria	**SM**	smooth muscle
IL	inner longitudinal layer	**MC**	middle circular layer	**TE**	transitional epithelium
L	lumen	**OL**	outer longitudinal layer		

Summary of Histologic Organization

I. Kidney

A. Capsule

The **capsule** is composed of dense, irregular collagenous connective tissue. Occasional **fibroblasts** and blood vessels may be seen.

B. Cortex

The **cortex** consists of parts of **nephrons** and **collecting tubules** arranged in **cortical labyrinths** and **medullary rays**. Additionally, blood vessels and associated connective tissue (**renal interstitium**) are present.

1. Cortical Labyrinth

The **cortical labyrinth** is composed of **renal corpuscles**, **proximal convoluted tubules**, **distal convoluted tubules**, and the **macula densa** region of **distal tubules**. Renal corpuscles consist of **mesangial cells**, **parietal** (simple squamous) and **visceral** (modified to **podocytes**) **layers** of Bowman's capsule, and an associated capillary bed, the **glomerulus**, as well as the intervening **Bowman's space**, which receives the ultrafiltrate. The **afferent** and **efferent glomerular arterioles** supply and drain the glomerulus, respectively, at its vascular pole. **Bowman's space** is drained at the **urinary pole** into the **proximal convoluted tubule**, composed of eosinophilic simple cuboidal epithelium with a brush border. The **distal convoluted tubule** profiles are fewer in number and may be recognized by the pale cuboidal epithelial cells. The **macula densa** region of the distal tubule is associated with the **juxtaglomerular** (modified smooth muscle) **cells** of the afferent (and sometimes efferent) glomerular arterioles and **extraglomerular** and **intraglomerular mesangial cells**, forming the juxtaglomerular apparatus.

2. Medullary Rays

Medullary rays are continuations of medullary tissue extending into the cortex. They are composed mostly of **collecting tubules, pars recta of proximal tubules, ascending thick limbs of Henle's loop**, and blood vessels.

C. Medulla

The **medulla** is composed of **renal pyramids** that are bordered by **cortical columns**. The renal pyramids consist of (1) **collecting tubules** whose simple cuboidal epithelium displays clearly defined lateral cell membranes; (2) **thick descending limbs of Henle's loop**, whose cells resemble those of the proximal tubule; (3) **thin limbs of Henle's loop**, resembling capillaries but containing no blood; and (4) **ascending thick limbs of Henle's loop**, whose cells are similar to those of the distal tubule. Additionally, numerous blood vessels, the **vasa recta**, are present, as well as slight connective tissue elements, the **renal interstitium**. The apex of the renal pyramid is the **renal papilla**, whose perforated tip is the **area cribrosa**, where the large **collecting ducts (of Bellini)** open to deliver the urine into the **minor calyx**.

D. Renal Pelvis

The **renal pelvis**, subdivided into the **minor** and **major calyces**, constitutes the beginning of the main excretory duct of the kidney. The **transitional epithelium** of the minor calyx is reflected onto the renal papilla. The calyces are lined by transitional epithelium. The subepithelial connective tissue of both is loosely arranged and abuts the **muscularis**, composed of **inner longitudinal** and **outer circular** layers of **smooth muscle**. An **adventitia** of loose connective tissue surrounds the muscularis.

II. Extrarenal Passages

A. Ureter

The **ureter** possesses a stellate-shaped lumen that is lined by **transitional epithelium**. The subepithelial connective tissue (sometimes said to be subdivided into **lamina propria** and **submucosa**) is composed of fibroelastic connective tissue. The **muscularis** is again composed of **inner longitudinal** and **outer circular** layers of **smooth muscle**, although in its lower portion near the bladder a third, **outermost longitudinal** layer of **smooth muscle** is present. The muscularis is surrounded by a fibroelastic **adventitia**.

B. Bladder

The **urinary bladder** resembles the ureter except that it is a much larger structure and does not possess a stellate lumen, although the mucosa of the empty bladder is thrown into folds. The **lamina propria** is fibroelastic in character and may contain occasional **mucous glands** at the internal orifice of the urethra. The **muscularis** is composed of three indefinite layers of smooth muscle: **inner longitudinal, middle circular**, and **outer longitudinal**. The circular muscle coat forms the **internal sphincter** at the neck of the bladder. An **adventitia** or **serosa** surrounds the bladder. The urethra is described in Chapter 18, "Female Reproductive System," and Chapter 19, "Male Reproductive System."

Chapter Review Questions

17-1. Which of the following infections is the most common cause of acute glomerulonephritis?

  A. Nisserial

  B. Treponemal

  C. Chlamydial

  D. Streptococcal

  E. Trichonomial

17-2. Diabetes insipidus is a disease caused by low levels of which of the following substances?

  A. ADH

  B. Renin

  C. Prostaglandin

  D. Angiotensinogen

  E. Insulin

17-3. Which of the following regions of the uriniferous tubules conserve most of the water?

  A. Glomerulus

  B. Proximal tubule

  C. Thick limb of Henle's loop

  D. Distal tubule

  E. Collecting tubule

17-4. Which condition would trigger the secretion of renin?

  A. Low blood pressure

  B. Reduced ADH

  C. Increased aldosterone

  D. Bladder infection

17-5. Hyperparathyroidism is responsible for which of the following kidney disorders?

  A. Bladder cancer

  B. Acute glomerulonephritis

  C. Kidney stones

  D. Cancer of the kidney

  E. Glomerulosclerosis

CHAPTER

18 FEMALE REPRODUCTIVE SYSTEM

The female reproductive system (Fig. 18-1) is composed of the ovaries, genital ducts, external genitalia, and the mammary glands, although, in a strict sense, the mammary glands are not considered to be genital organs.

The reproductive system functions in the propagation of the species and is under the control of a complex interplay of hormonal, neural, and, at least in the humans, psychological factors.

Ovary

Each of the two **ovaries** is a small, almond-shaped structure whose thick connective tissue capsule, the **tunica albuginea**, is covered by a **simple squamous** to **cuboidal mesothelium** known as the **germinal epithelium** (a modified mesothelium). Unlike in the testis, the germinal epithelium of the ovary is a misnomer because no germ cells comprise this structure. The ovary is loosely organized into two layers, the outer **cortex** rich in ovarian follicles and the inner medulla, a highly vascular connective tissue stroma (Figs. 18-2 and 18-3).

- The **cortex**, located just deep to the tunica albuginea, houses **ovarian follicles**, each composed of a **primary oocyte** (egg, ovum) surrounded by supporting cells known as **follicular cells** when they are flat and **granulosa cells** when they become cuboidal.
  - During embryonic development, the female germ cells **oogonia** undergo a series of mitosis to form numerous **primary oocytes**, each enveloped by follicular cells, together comprising a **primordial follicle** (Fig. 18-4).
  - Primary oocytes enter **meiosis I** in the developing embryo, but the process is arrested at **prophase I** under the influence of **oocyte maturation inhibitor**, secreted by the follicular cells until puberty.

- At puberty, a handful of follicles undergo maturation each month, driven initially by local factors and later by **follicle-stimulating hormone (FSH)** released by the anterior pituitary. The follicles enlarge as **primary oocytes** grow, flat **follicular cells** transform to cuboidal **granulosa cells**, and become encapsulated by the ovarian **stroma** (connective tissue).
- Near ovulation, the granulosa cells release **meiosis-inducing substance**, which, in conjunction with a surge of **luteinizing hormone (LH)** released by the **anterior pituitary**, causes the completion of meiosis I, resulting in the transformation of the primary oocyte into a **secondary oocyte**, which immediately enters **meiosis II** but becomes arrested at **metaphase II** at the time of ovulation.
- The **medulla** is a highly vascularized loose connective tissue stroma rich in fibroblasts and estrogen-secreting **interstitial cells**.
  - Additionally, occasional **hilar cells** are present in the medulla; these cells resemble interstitial cells of the testis, and they manufacture a small amount of androgens.

Ovarian Follicles

By 3 months in development, female fetuses have 4 to 5 million primary oocytes from mitosis and differentiation of oogonia. After this developmental time point, no

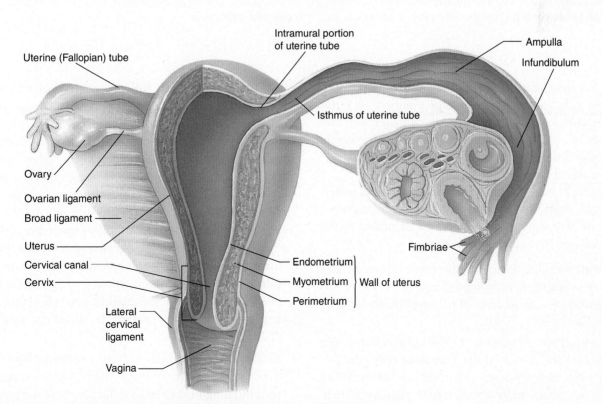

FIGURE 18-1. Female reproductive organs, the ovaries and genital ducts.

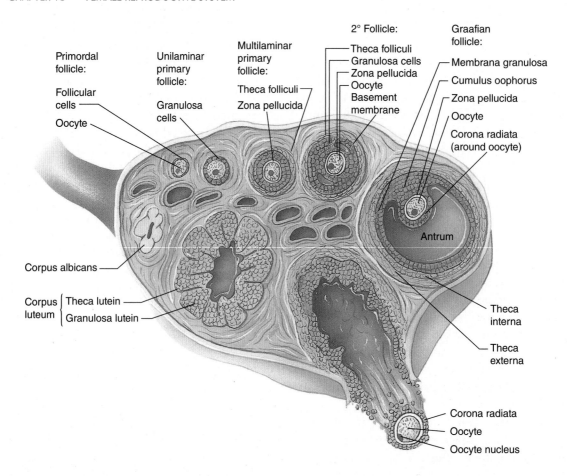

FIGURE 18-2. Illustration of the ovary. Each follicle houses a **primary oocyte** arrested in the prophase of the first meiotic division. The most developed Graafian follicle releases its oocyte during ovulation. As that primary oocyte is being released, it finishes its first meiotic division, becomes a **secondary oocyte**, and is arrested in the **metaphase** stage of the second meiotic division. Subsequent to ovulation, the Graafian follicle differentiates into the **corpus luteum**, which will eventually degenerate into the **corpus albicans**.

more oogonia are in reserve and the formed primary oocytes in follicles degenerate in large numbers. At birth, female fetuses are said to possess approximately 400,000 follicles in two ovaries, which continue to degenerate over time. Ultimately, only about 400 to 500 oocytes ever mature and are ovulated in a woman's lifetime.

Starting at puberty, follicles pass through various maturational stages that are histologically distinguishable; therefore, five types of follicles can be identified in the ovaries during reproductive active age.

- The **primordial follicle** is the most immature and nongrowing form, composed of a **primary oocyte** surrounded by a single layer of flattened **follicular cells** (see Fig. 18-4).

- As maturation progresses, the follicular cells become cuboidal and are called the **granulosa cells**. The primary oocyte surrounded by a single layer of granulosa cells is referred to as a **unilaminar primary follicle** (see Fig. 18-5, *inset*).

- **Multilaminar primary follicles** display a primary oocyte surrounded by several layers of granulosa cells (see Fig. 18-5). The growing primary oocyte secretes an acellular capsule called **zona pellucida**, between its cell membrane and the granulosa cells. Immediately external to the granulosa cells, the ovarian stromal cells, induced by FSH, become plump as they start to secrete **androgens**, and form a loosely organized layer known as **theca interna**. Androgens manufactured by the theca interna cells are transferred across the basement membrane for the granulosa cells to convert to **estrogens**. Typical ovarian stromal cells outside the theca interna become oriented in a spherical fashion and form an ill-defined capsule, the **theca externa** (Table 18-1).

- As the follicle continues to grow, a **secondary follicle** is characterized by follicular fluid (**liquor folliculi**) accumulating in the extracellular spaces of the granulosa cells (see Fig. 18-6). The fluid is secreted by the

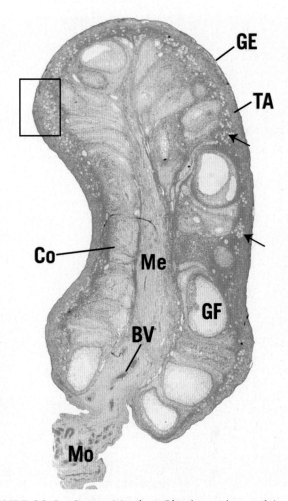

FIGURE 18-3. Ovary. Monkey. Plastic section. ×14.

The ovary is subdivided into a **medulla** (Me) and a **cortex** (Co). The medulla houses large **blood vessels** (BV) from which the cortical vascular supply is derived. The cortex of the ovary contains numerous ovarian follicles, most of which are very small (*arrows*); a few maturing follicles have reached the **Graafian follicle** (GF) stage. The thick, fibrous connective tissue capsule, **tunica albuginea** (TA), is shown to advantage; the **germinal epithelium** (GE) is evident occasionally. Observe that the **mesovarium** (Mo) not only suspends the ovary but also conveys the vascular supply to the medulla. A region similar to the *boxed area* is presented at a higher magnification in Figure 18-4.

granulosa cells and contains various hormones, such as **inhibin**, **activin**, **progesterone**, **estrogen**, and **folliculostatin**, which assist in the feedback regulation of FSH release. Moreover, as estrogen reaches a threshold level, it causes a surge of LH release. At this stage, the zona pellucida is thick and prominent. A clearly distinguishable basement membrane separates granulosa cells from theca interna, which in turn is loosely surrounded by the theca externa.

- The most mature form, **Graafian follicle** (also referred to as the **mature follicle**), is characterized by

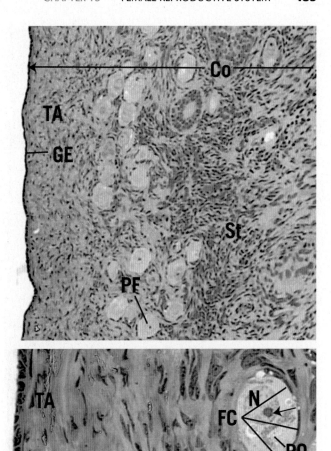

FIGURE 18-4. Ovary. Monkey. Plastic section. ×132.

This photomicrograph is a higher magnification of a region similar to the *boxed area* of Figure 18-3. Observe that the **germinal epithelium** (GE) covers the collagenous capsule, the **tunica albuginea** (TA). This region of the **cortex** (Co) houses numerous **primordial follicles** (PF). Observe that the connective tissue of the ovary is highly cellular and is referred to as the **stroma** (St). *Inset.* **Ovary. Cortex. Monkey. Plastic section.** ×540. The primordial follicle is composed of a **primary oocyte** (PO), whose **nucleus** (N) and *nucleolus* (*arrow*) are evident. Observe the single layer of flat **follicular cells** (FC) surrounding the primary oocyte. The **tunica albuginea** (TA) and the **germinal epithelium** (GE) are also shown to advantage in this photomicrograph.

its large size (as much as 2.5 cm in diameter near the time of ovulation), a large singular antrum filled with liquor folliculi, and lined by the granulosa cells, the **membrana granulosa** (Fig. 18-7).

- The primary oocyte and its zona pellucida are surrounded by several layers of granulosa cells forming the **corona radiata**, and this complex jutting into the antrum is collectively called the **cumulus oophorus**.
- The membrana granulosa is separated from the theca interna by the basement membrane.

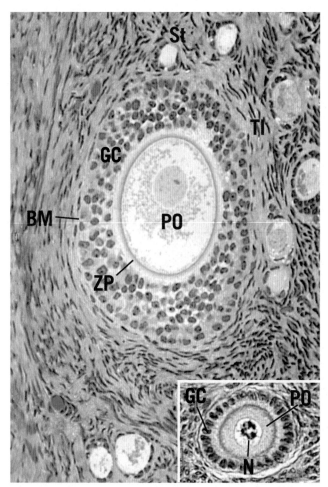

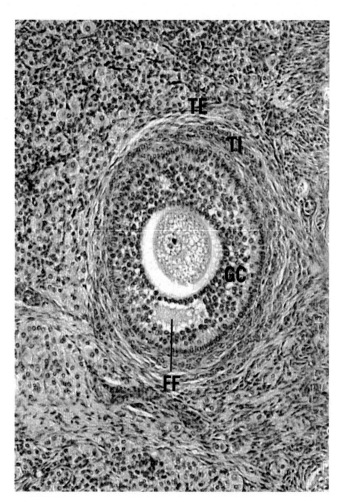

FIGURE 18-5. Primary follicles. Monkey. Plastic section. ×270.

FIGURE 18-6. Secondary follicles. Rabbit. Paraffin section. ×132.

Primary follicles differ from primordial follicles not only in size but also in morphology and number of follicular cells. The unilaminar primary follicle of the *inset* (×270) displays a single layer of cuboidal **granulosa cells** (GC) that surround the relatively small **primary oocyte** (PO), whose **nucleus** (N) is evident. The multilaminar primary follicle displays a **primary oocyte** (PO) that has increased in size. The **granulosa cells** (GC) now form a stratified layer around the oocyte, being separated from it by the intervening **zona pellucida** (ZP). The **stroma** (St) is being reorganized around the follicle to form the **theca interna** (TI). Note the presence of a **basement membrane** (BM) between the follicular cells and the theca interna.

- The theca externa merges imperceptibly with the surrounding ovarian stroma.

The entire follicular maturation process spans several months, with 10 to 20 primordial follicles entering maturation and grow under the influence of FSH each month. Therefore, several Graafian follicles may develop each month, but interestingly, one (or occasionally two) of the Graafian follicles begins to overtake and exceed the development of the other Graafian follicles and becomes

Secondary follicles are similar to primary multilaminar follicles, the major difference being their larger size. Moreover, the stratification of the **granulosa cells** (GC) has increased, displaying more layers, and more importantly, a **follicular fluid** (FF) begins to appear in the intercellular spaces, which coalesces into several Call–Exner bodies. Note also that the stroma immediately surrounding the follicular cells is rearranged to form a cellular **theca interna** (TI) and a more fibrous **theca externa** (TE).

known as the **dominant (Graafian) follicle**, which is no longer FSH dependent.

- The dominant follicle begins to manufacture and release the hormone **inhibin** that prevents the anterior pituitary from releasing FSH. The lack of FSH results in the atrophy of many FSH-dependent follicles, whereas the dominant follicle proceeds to ovulation. As the FSH-dependent follicles degenerate, they become **atretic follicles** and eventually undergo fibrosis and become scar-like temporary structures known as **corpora fibrosum** that resemble corpus albicans but are considerably smaller in size.

Table 18-1	Characteristics of Ovarian Follicles				
Stage of Follicle	**Primary Oocyte Diameter**	**Follicular/Granulosa Cells**	**Hormone Dependency for Growth**	**Theca Folliculi**
Primordial	25 μm	Single layer, squamous	Local factors	Not present
Unilaminar primary	100–120 μm	Single layer, cuboidal	Local factors	Not present
Multilaminar primary	150 μm	Several layers, cuboidal	Local factors	Present
Secondary	200 μm	Several layers, cuboidal with some follicular fluid in the extracellular spaces	Follicle-stimulating hormone (FSH)	Present
Graafian	>200 μm	Membrana granulosa; cumulus oophorus; corona radiata; antrum filled with liquor folliculi	FSH	Present
Dominant Graafian	up to 2.5 cm	Same as in Graafian follicle	Luteinizing hormone (for ovulation) Not FSH dependent	Present

- The dominant follicle, mostly because of the surge in **luteinizing hormone (LH)**, ruptures, thus releasing the secondary oocyte with its corona radiata into the peritoneum.

- The **LH surge** not only induces completion of meiosis I and initiation of meiosis II in the oocyte of the Graafian follicle, but it also results in resumption of meiosis I in the primary oocyte in other maturing follicles.

- Additionally, LH induces the development of the **corpus luteum** from the **theca interna** and **membrana granulosa** of the Graafian follicle.

Corpus Luteum and Corpus Albicans

Once the Graafian follicle expels its oocyte at ovulation, it becomes transformed into the **corpus hemorrhagicum**, an irregular spherical structure composed of granulosa and theca cells thrown into folds and blood in the center (Fig. 18-8). Within a couple of days, the corpus hemorrhagicum is transformed into the **corpus luteum**, a yellow glandular structure as the granulosa and theca cells transform into granulosa lutein and theca lutein cells, respectively (Figs. 18-9 and 18-10). Corpus luteum secretes **progesterone**, a hormone that suppresses LH release by inhibiting gonadotropin-releasing hormone (GnRH) and facilitates the thickening of the uterine endometrium and stimulates uterine glandular secretions. Additionally, **estrogen** (inhibitor of FSH) and **relaxin** (which causes the fibrocartilage of the pubic symphysis to become more pliable) are also released by the corpus luteum.

If pregnancy does not occur, the corpus luteum **atrophies** within 10 to 14 days, a process known as **luteolysis**, and the absence of estrogen and progesterone will once again permit the release of FSH and LH from the adenohypophysis. In this case, the corpus luteum is known as the **corpus luteum of menstruation** and will degenerate into the **corpus albicans**, a form of collagenous connective tissue scar (Fig. 18-11). If pregnancy occurs, the embryo implanting into the endometrium starts to release **human chorionic gonadotropin (hCG)** ~7 days after ovulation, which stimulates the corpus luteum to persist and grow into **corpus luteum of pregnancy** (Fig. 18-12). The corpus luteum of pregnancy can grow quite large, almost half the size of the ovary itself, and continues to secrete progesterone and estrogen until ~5 months of pregnancy, degenerating only after the **placenta** can produce a sufficient amount of these hormones on their own.

Genital Ducts

The genital ducts are composed of the two oviducts and the single uterus.

Oviduct

Each **oviduct (uterine tube, fallopian tube)** is a short muscular tube leading from the vicinity of the ovary to the uterine lumen (Figs. 18-13 and 18-14). The oviduct is subdivided into four regions:

- the **infundibulum** (whose **fimbriae** approximate the ovary),

- **ampulla**, funnel-like and longest segment in which most fertilization occurs,

- **isthmus**, and the

- **intramural portion**, which pierces the wall of the uterus.

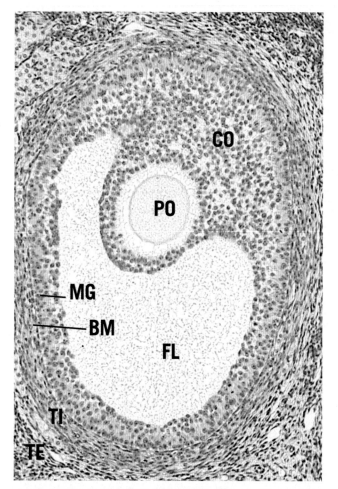

FIGURE 18-7. Graafian follicle. Paraffin section. ×132.

The Graafian follicle is the most mature of all ovarian follicles and is ready to release its primary oocyte in the process of ovulation. The **follicular fluid** (FL) fills a single chamber, the antrum, which is surrounded by a wall of granulosa cells known as the **membrana granulosa** (MG). Some of the granulosa cells, which surround the **primary oocyte** (PO), jut into the antrum as the **cumulus oophorus** (CO). Observe the **basement membrane** (BM), which separates the granulosa cells from the **theca interna** (TI). The fibrous **theca externa** (TE) merges almost imperceptibly with the surrounding stroma.

The mucosa of the oviduct, composed of a ciliated simple columnar epithelium and vascular lamina propria (see Fig. 18-14), is extensively folded in the infundibulum and ampulla, but the folding is reduced in the isthmus and intramural portions. The simple columnar epithelium is composed of two types of cells (Fig. 18-15):

- **ciliated columnar cells**, whose cilia beat toward the uterus to transport the ovulated ovum into the uterus and

- **peg cells**, which are also columnar but have no cilia. Their apical region is expanded and houses the secretory products,

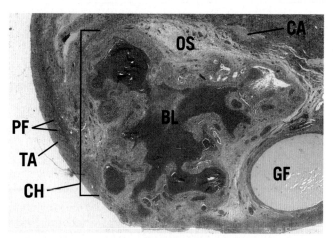

FIGURE 18-8. Corpus hemorrhagicum. Human. Paraffin section. ×8. After ovulation, the remaining granulosa and theca cells of the Graafian follicle collapse into folds and form the **corpus hemorrhagicum** (CH) containing **blood** (BL) in the center. The granulosa and theca cells soon transform into granulosa lutein and theca lutein cells and transform corpus hemorrhagicum to a corpus luteum, a temporary endocrine structure. Observe the ovarian histology in the vicinity, displaying **tunica albuginea** (TA), numerous **primordial follicles** (PF) in the cortex, a **Graafian follicle** (GF), **corpus albicans** (CA), and the ovarian **stroma** (OS).

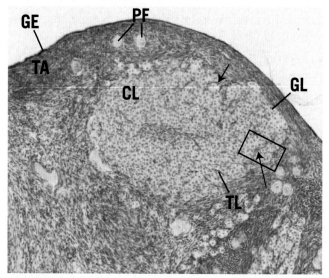

FIGURE 18-9. Cat ovary, Corpus luteum. Paraffin section. ×124.

Corpus luteum (CL) is an endocrine structure comprised of enlarged and vesicular granulosa cells, now referred to as **granulosa lutein cells** (GL), which constitute the most cell population forming the folds; the spaces between the folds are occupied by connective tissue elements, blood vessels, and cells of the theca interna (*arrows*). These theca interna cells also enlarge, become glandular, and are referred to as the **theca lutein cells** (TL). Note the **primordial follicles** (PF) in the vicinity and the **tunica albuginea** (TA) lined by the **germinal epithelium** (GE).

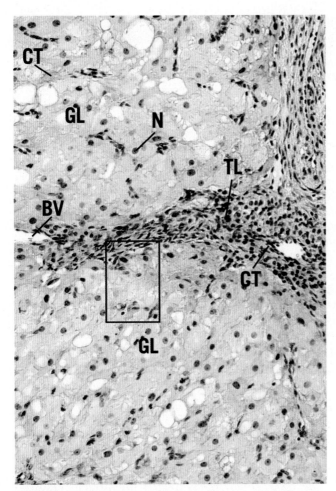

FIGURE 18-10. Corpus luteum. Human. Paraffin section. ×132.

This photomicrograph is a higher magnification of a region similar to the *boxed area* of Figure 18-9. The **granulosa lutein cells** (GL) of the corpus luteum are easily distinguished from the **connective tissue** (CT) elements, because the former display round **nuclei** (N), mostly in the center of large round cells. The center of the field is occupied by a fold, housing **theca lutein cells** (TL) amid numerous **connective tissue** (CT) and **vascular** (BV) elements.

- **factors for the capacitation** of spermatozoa and a
- **nutrient-rich medium** that nourishes the spermatozoa as well as the fertilized ovum traveling toward the uterus.

The mucosa is surrounded by a smooth muscle coat composed of poorly defined inner circular and outer longitudinal layers that are thinner distally but become thicker closer to the uterus. Via peristaltic action, the muscle layer assists the cilia to propel the oocyte or fertilized egg to the uterus. The muscular coat of the oviduct is covered by serosa, whereas its intramural portion is embedded in the uterus and is surrounded by uterine connective tissue.

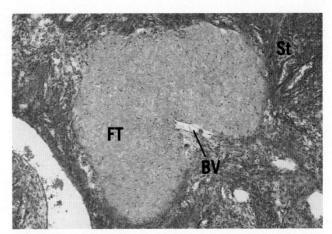

FIGURE 18-11. Corpus albicans. Cat ovary. Paraffin section ×84.

As the corpus luteum involutes, its cellular elements degenerate and undergo autolysis. The corpus luteum becomes invaded by macrophages that phagocytose the dead cells, leaving behind relatively acellular **fibrous tissue** (FT). The previously rich **vascular supply** (BV) also regresses, and the entire corpus albicans appears pale in comparison to the relatively dark ovarian **stroma** (St). The corpus albicans will regress until it becomes a small scar.

Uterus

The **uterus**, a pear-shaped organ, has three regions, a **fundus**, **body**, and **cervix**. During pregnancy, it houses and supports the developing embryo and fetus. The uterine wall is composed of three layers: a spongy mucosal layer forming the **endometrium**, a thick smooth muscle layer called the **myometrium**, and serosa or adventitia comprising **perimetrium** (Fig. 18-16).

The **endometrium** is comprised of the simple columnar epithelial lining and the lamina propria composed of cellular loose connective tissue, richly endowed with **endometrial glands (uterine glands)** and vasculature. The endometrium is subdivided into two layers, each with its own blood supply (Table 18-2).

- The deeper **basal layer (stratum basale)** abutting the myometrium is served by short **straight arteries** and is occupied by the base of the uterine glands. This layer remains intact during menstruation.
- The superficial **functional layer (stratum functionale)** is served by the **helicine (coiled) arteries** and undergoes hormonally modulated cyclic changes of shedding, regrowing, thickening, and shedding again.

Ovarian and Menstrual Cycles

Between menarche and menopause, the cyclical hormonal fluctuations from the pituitary and the ovaries

Table 18-2	Phases of the Menstrual Cycle		
Phases of the Cycle	**Length (d)**	**Hormone Involved**	**Endometrial Characteristics**
Menstrual	3–5	Reduced levels of estrogens and progesterone	Helical arteries are shut down, resulting in necrosis and sloughing of functionalis layer of the endometrium; epithelial cells in the base of the uterine glands (located in the basal layer of the endometrium) start to reepithelialize the uterine endometrium.
Proliferative	10	Dependent on the increased blood levels of FSH from the pituitary and estrogens from the ovaries; at the end of the proliferative phase, estrogen, FSH, and luteinizing hormone (LH) blood levels peak.	The denuded surface of the endometrium becomes reepithelialized, the functionalis layer becomes thickened (~3 mm thick), and its helical arteries are reestablished and begin to become coiled; uterine glands are not yet coiled.
Secretory	14	Estrogen levels rise in the blood and progesterone blood levels peak from the corpus luteum; FSH and LH blood levels are decreased.	Helical arteries and uterine glands of the functionalis become highly coiled; the functionalis reaches its full thickness (~5 mm thick); the uterine glands are filled with their secretory products; cells of the stroma undergo decidual reaction and accumulate glycogen and lipids that provide nutrients for the blastocyst embedding itself in the endometrium.

result in the cyclical thickening then shedding of the endometrial stratum functionale, a process known as the **menses**. The ovarian hormonal fluctuations resulting from the growing follicles and corpus luteum are known as the ovarian cycle, and the endometrial changes that occur in response are known as the menstrual cycle. The two cycles loosely coincide (Fig. 18-17).

- In response to **FSH**, the growing ovarian follicles (**ovarian follicular phase**) release **estrogen**, which promotes **uterine proliferative phase** marked by the reestablishment and thickening of the stratum functionale, namely, the renewal, subsequent to the menstrual phase, of the following structures: epithelial lining, connective tissue, glands, and blood vessels (**helicine arteries**) (Fig. 18-18; also see Fig. 18-16). The ovarian follicular and uterine proliferative phases coincide for approximately 14 days beginning from the first day of menstruation.

- The **LH** surge at day 14 in the menstrual cycle triggers ovulation and subsequent formation of corpus luteum in the ovary (**ovarian luteal phase**) which releases **progesterone** in addition to **estrogen**. These two hormones facilitate the **uterine secretory phase** for the next 14 days, which can be histologically and physiologically subcategorized into early (days 14 to 21; Fig. 18-19) and late (days 21 to 28; Fig. 18-20) secretory phases, both characterized by the further thickening of the endometrium. **Progesterone** in particular is responsible for coiling of the endometrial glands, accumulation of glandular secretions, and additional coiling and lengthening of the **helicine arteries**.

- In the absence of pregnancy, the corpus luteum degenerates and, as a consequence, progesterone secretion diminishes, thereby initiating the **menstrual phase** (Figs. 18-21 and 18-22). Moreover, the decrease in progesterone levels triggers intermittent **vasoconstriction** of the helicine arteries, with subsequent necrosis of the vessel and the endometrial tissue of the functional layer.

- During relaxation (between events of vasoconstriction), the helicine arteries rupture, and the rapid blood flow dislodges the blood-filled necrotic functional layer, which becomes sloughed as the **hemorrhagic discharge** so that only the basal layer of the endometrium remains as the lining of the uterus.

Because the basal layer is supplied by the straight arteries, it is unaffected by the cyclic endocrine changes and serves as a reservoir of endometrial tissue from which the functional layer can regrow. Interestingly, the endometrium of the inferior aspect of the uterus is composed almost exclusively of a thin basal layer; thus, implantation of an embryo in the region close to the cervix can pose complications of the placental tissue invading through the thin endometrium and into the myometrium (placenta accreta) or even through it (placenta percreta).

Myometrium is the thickest layer of the uterus and is comprised of smooth muscle tissue. During pregnancy, the smooth muscle cells of the myometrium undergo both **hypertrophy** and **hyperplasia**, increasing the thickness of the muscle wall of the uterus. The smooth muscle cells increase from the 50-μm length of the nonpregnant uterus to as much as 500 μm in the gravid uterus.

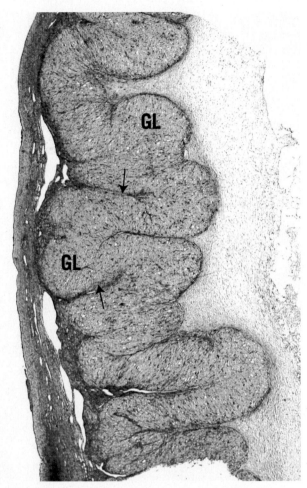

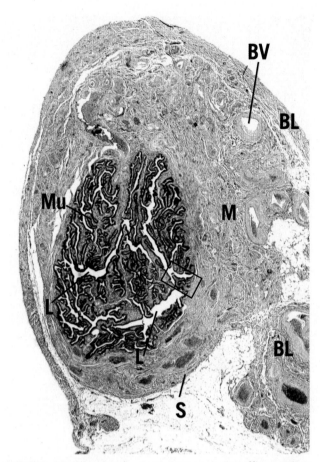

FIGURE 18-13. Oviduct. x.s. Human. Paraffin section. ×14.

FIGURE 18-12. Corpus luteum of pregnancy. Human. Paraffin section. ×14.

In case of successful fertilization, and in response to hCG released by the implanting conceptus, the corpus luteum grows larger, taking up much of the ovary and persists until ~5 months in pregnancy. This enlarged endocrine structure, releasing progesterone and estrogen, is called the corpus luteum of pregnancy. Note the large cellular folds comprised mostly of **granulosa lutein cells** (GL) with theca lutein cells in the folds (*arrows*). The remnants of the antrum are filled with fibrin and serous exudate that will be replaced by connective tissue elements.

- Additionally, these smooth muscle cells acquire **gap junctions** that facilitate their coordinated contractile actions.

- At parturition, **oxytocin**, and **prostaglandins** cause the uterine muscles to undergo rhythmic contractions that assist in expelling the fetus.

- Subsequent to delivery, the lack of estrogen is responsible for **the apoptosis** of many of the smooth muscle cells with a consequent reduction in the thickness of the myometrium.

Cervix of the Uterus

The **cervix** is the narrow inferior aspect of the uterus that partially protrudes into the vagina. The lumen of the cervix

The oviduct, also referred to as the fallopian or uterine tube, extends from the ovary to the uterine cavity. It is suspended from the body wall by the **broad ligament** (BL), which conveys a rich **vascular supply** (BV) to the **serosa** (S) of the oviduct. The thick **muscularis** (M) is composed of ill-defined inner circular and outer longitudinal muscle layers. The **mucosa** (Mu) is thrown into longitudinal folds, which are so highly exaggerated in the infundibulum and ampulla that they subdivide the **lumen** (L) into labyrinthine spaces. A region similar to the *boxed area* is presented at a higher magnification in Figure 18-14.

(**cervical canal**) serves as a narrow conduit between the uterine cavity (superiorly) and the vaginal canal inferiorly (Fig. 18-23). The opening of the cervical canal into the uterine cavity is known as the **internal os**, and its opening into the vaginal canal is known as the **external os**.

- The lining of the cervical canal is continuous with the endometrial lining at the internal os, and it is comprised of **simple columnar epithelium**, whose cells secrete a mucous substance (Fig. 18-24).

- The inferior portion of the cervix protruding into the vagina is lined by a **stratified squamous nonkeratinized epithelium** that is continuous with the vaginal epithelium (Fig. 18-25).

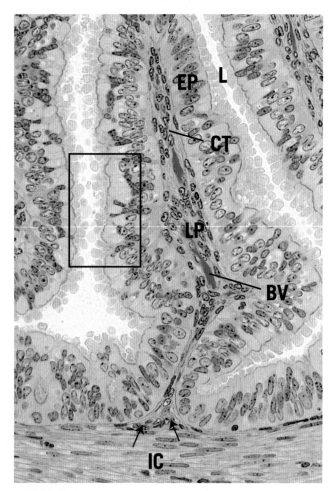

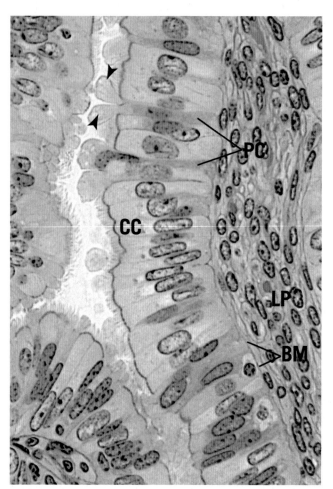

FIGURE 18-14. Oviduct. x.s. Monkey. Plastic section. ×270.

FIGURE 18-15. Oviduct. x.s. Monkey. Plastic section. ×540.

This photomicrograph is a higher magnification of the *boxed area* of Figure 18-13. Observe the **inner circular muscle** (IC) layer of the muscularis. The **lamina propria** (LP) is very narrow in this region (*arrows*) but presents longitudinal epithelium-lined folds. The core of these folds is composed of **vascular** (BV), loose, but highly cellular **connective tissue** (CT). The simple columnar **epithelium** (EP) lines the labyrinthine **lumen** (L) of the oviduct. A region similar to the *boxed area* is presented at a higher magnification in Figure 18-15.

This photomicrograph is a higher magnification of a region similar to the *boxed area* of Figure 18-14. The **lamina propria** (LP) is a highly cellular, loose connective tissue that is richly vascularized. The **basal membrane** (BM) separating the connective tissue from the epithelial lining is evident. Note that the epithelium is composed of two different cell types, a thinner **peg cell** (PC), which bears no cilia but whose apical extent bulges above the ciliated cells. These bulges (*arrowheads*) contain nutritive materials that nourish gametes. The second cell type of the oviduct epithelium is a **ciliated cell** (CC), whose cilia move in unison with those of neighboring cells, propelling the nutrient material toward the uterine lumen.

- Therefore, there is an abrupt transition of epithelial lining at the external os.

- The **wall of the cervix** is thick and is composed of a dense irregular fibroelastic connective tissue housing some smooth muscle cells and branched cervical glands.

- The **cervical glands** produce a serous secretion that lubricates the vagina.
  - After fertilization, these glands produce thick, viscous mucus that impedes the entry of additional spermatozoa and microorganisms into the uterine lumen.

- The thick cervical wall becomes thinner and less rigid at parturition owing to the effects of the hormone oxytocin.

Fertilization and Implantation

The union of the haploid sperm pronucleus with the pronucleus of the haploid ovum is known as **fertilization**, whereby a new diploid cell, the **zygote**, is formed. Fertilization usually occurs in the **ampulla** of the oviduct.

- As the zygote travels along the oviduct, it undergoes mitotic cell division, known as **cleavage**, to form a solid cluster of cells, known as the **morula**. By the fifth day after fertilization, the morula enters the lumen of the uterus.

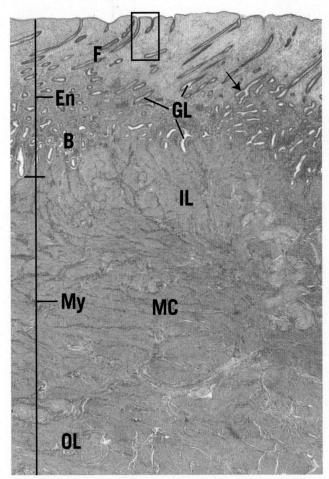

FIGURE 18-16. Uterus. Proliferative phase. Human. Paraffin section. ×14.

The uterus is a thick-walled organ whose wall consists of three layers. The external serosa (or in certain regions, adventitia) is unremarkable and is not presented in this photomicrograph. The thick **myometrium** (My) is composed of smooth muscle, subdivided into three poorly delineated layers: **outer longitudinal** (OL), **middle circular** (MC), and **inner longitudinal** (IL). The **endometrium** (En) is subdivided into a **basal layer** (B) and a **functional layer** (F). The functional layer varies in thickness and constitution and passes through a sequence of phases during the menstrual cycle. Note that the functional layer is in the proliferative phase of the menstrual cycle and that the forming **glands** (GL) are straight. The deeper aspects of some of these glands display branching (*arrow*). The *boxed area* is presented at a higher magnification in Figure 18-18.

- Once in the uterus, the cells of the morula rearrange themselves into a fluid-filled structure, the **blastocyst**, with a small cluster of cells, the **inner cell mass (embryoblasts)** responsible for the formation of the embryo pooled to one side.

- Approximately 5 to 7 days after fertilization, the cells at the periphery of the blastocyst, the **trophoblasts**, proliferate and initiate the process of **implantation** into the endometrium. By the fourteenth day postfertilization, the entire blastocyst is embedded in the endometrium and implantation is complete.

- As the trophoblasts proliferate, they form an inner cellular layer, the **cytotrophoblasts**, and an outer layer, the **syncytiotrophoblasts**.

Placenta

The placenta, a chimeric organ derived from both maternal and fetal tissues, is a highly vascular structure that permits the exchange of various materials between the maternal and fetal circulatory systems (Figs. 18-26 through 18-28). It is important to note that the exchanges of materials occur without the commingling of the maternal and fetal bloods.

Fetal Component

The syncytiotrophoblasts and cytotrophoblasts constitute the fetal component of the placenta. Cytotrophoblasts divide and give rise to additional syncytiotrophoblasts, which

- secrete **hCG** that ensures retention of the **corpus luteum** and sustained supply of **progesterone**.

- initiate the formation of extracellular spaces called **lacunae**.

- collaborate with maternal vasculature and endometrial glands to fill lacunae with maternal blood and uterine secretions.

The fetal tissue forms the **chorion**, the precursor of the **chorionic plate**, the structure that gives rise to the **chorionic villi**, numerous finger-like projections that jut into the lacunae. These projections are initially slender and are known as **primary villi** comprised of outer syncytiotrophoblasts and inner cytotrophoblasts. Once fetal mesenchymal cells and capillary networks form in the center of the villus, the more substantial villi, known as **secondary villi** are characterized by a decreased population of cytotrophoblasts as these cells become incorporated into the syncytiotrophoblasts.

- The fetal capillary beds are located adjacent to the syncytiotrophoblasts and lie in close proximity to the maternal blood in the lacunae.

- Oxygen and nutrients in the maternal blood diffuse through the villi to reach the fetal capillaries.

- Carbon dioxide and waste products in the fetal blood also diffuse through the villi to reach the maternal blood in the lacunae.

- The exchange of gases and material occurs by passing through the **placental barrier** whose components are listed in Table 18-3.

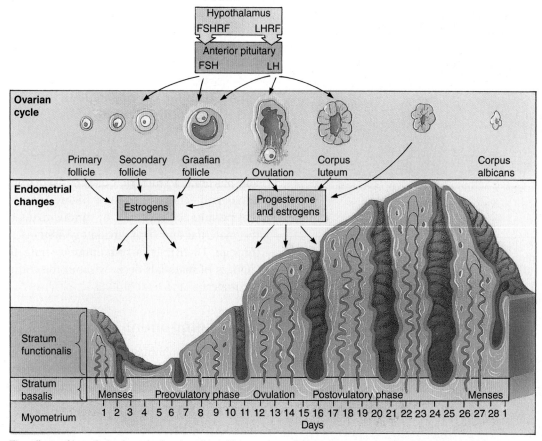

The effects of hypothalamic and adenohypohyseal hormones on the ovarian cortex and uterine endometrium.

FIGURE 18-17. The schematic diagram of the ovarian and menstrual (endometrial) cycles, which, on average, spans ~28 days. It should be noted, however, that the duration of the cycles can vary considerably between 21 days to 40 or more days. The first day of the beginning of menstruation is considered day 1 of a cycle with menstruation lasting approximately 3 to 5 days, a time period known as the menstrual phase. Day 1 also marks the beginning of the ovarian follicular phase marked by the growth of follicles (follicular phase; days 1 to 14) which begin to release estrogen and the increasing level of estrogen promotes stratum functionale to regrow during the proliferative phase spanning days 5 to 14. When estrogen reaches a threshold at around the midpoint in the cycle, an LH surge from the pituitary triggers ovulation. Once the oocyte complex has been released, the remnant of the dominant Graafian follicle becomes a corpus luteum and begins to release progesterone in addition to estrogen, beginning the Luteal phase that spans between days 14 to 28. In response to progesterone, in particular, the endometrium enters the secretory phase in which the uterine glands continue to lengthen and secrete nutrient-rich products. The quickly lengthening glands start to coil between days 14 and 21, sometimes referred to as the early secretory phase. In case of successful fertilization, the conceptus would begin to implant on approximately day 20 to 21 of the cycle, and the uterine glandular secretions providing the nutritious and favorable environment for the conceptus at this critical time. The uterine glands coil even further and increase secretions to support the potentially implanting conceptus between days 21 to 28, which is known as the late secretory phase. At this time, the stratum functionale is in its greatest thickness. In the absence of pregnancy, the corpus luteum regresses and the resulting decrease in progesterone and estrogen causes vasoconstriction of spiral arteries, which subsequently results in shedding of the stratum functionale, thus marking the end of one menstrual cycle and the beginning of the next.

Table 18-3	Components of the Placental Barrier
Endothelial cells of the fetal capillary	
Basal lamina of the fetal endothelium	
Connective tissue of the secondary villus	
Basal lamina of the cytotrophoblasts	
Cytotrophoblasts	
Syncytiotrophoblasts	

Maternal Component

The maternal component of the placenta is the **endometrium** that becomes modified to form the **decidua** (modified endometrial mucosa) in response to the invasion of the syncytiotrophoblasts. Three regions of decidua form during pregnancy:

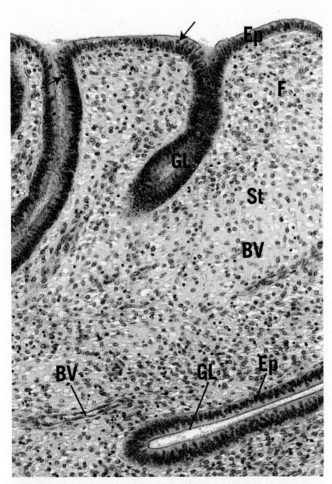

FIGURE 18-18. Uterus. Proliferative phase. Human. Paraffin section. ×132.

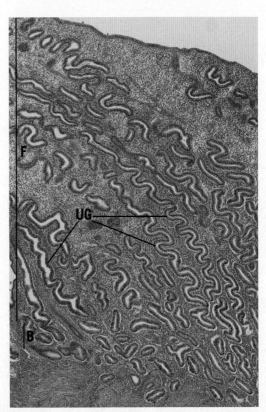

FIGURE 18-19. Endometrium. Early secretory phase. Human. Paraffin Section. ×37.

Note the coiled appearance of the rapidly lengthening **uterine glands** (UG) and the thickened **stroma functionale** (F). The **basal layer** (B) of the endometrium remains unchanged; however; it appears much thinner compared to the thickened functional layer.

This photomicrograph is a higher magnification of the *boxed area* of Figure 18-16. Note that the **functional layer** (F) of the endometrium is lined by a simple columnar **epithelium** (Ep) that is displaying mitotic activity (*arrows*). The forming **glands** (GL) also consist of a simple columnar **epithelium** (Ep) whose cells are actively dividing. The **stroma** (St) is highly cellular, as evidenced by the numerous connective tissue cell nuclei visible in this field. Note also the rich **vascular supply** (BV) of the endometrial stroma.

- **decidua basalis**, the richly vascularized maternal portion of the placenta, that forms lacunae and induces the trophoblasts to form the chorionic villi;

- **decidua capsularis**, the tissue separating the lumen of the uterus from the embryo and will be known as the **chorion laeve**; and

- **decidua parietalis**, the endometrial tissue between the uterine lumen and the myometrium.

In addition to its role in the delivery of nutrients and oxygen to the fetus and exchanging it for fetal waste products, the placenta manufactures hormones and factors necessary for the maintenance of pregnancy and the delivery of the fetus (Table 18-4).

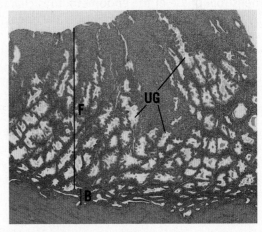

FIGURE 18-20. Endometrium. Late secretory phase. Human. Paraffin Section. ×28.

The **stratum functionale** (F) is in its thickest form during this phase of the menstrual cycle. Note the much more dramatic coiling of the **uterine glands** (UG) as well as their dilated lumina. The glandular cells also appear to fold into the lumina as well, which confer the glands a sessile appearance rather than a smooth coiled appearance. The **basal layer** (B) appears much thinner in comparison although it remains unchanged throughout the cycle.

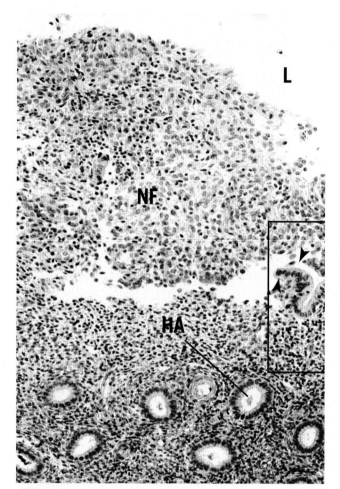

FIGURE 18-21. Endometrium. Menstrual phase. Human. Paraffin section. ×132.

The menstrual phase of the endometrium is characterized by periodic constriction and sequential opening of **helical arteries** (HA), resulting in ischemia with subsequent necrosis of the functional layer. Owing to these spasmodic contractions, sudden spurts of arterial blood detach **necrotic fragments** (NF) of the superficial layers of the endometrium that are then discharged as menstrual flow. The endometrial stroma becomes engorged with blood, increasing the degree of ischemia, and eventually the entire functional layer is sloughed off. Observe the lack of intact epithelium (*arrowheads*) lining the **lumen** (L). The *boxed area* is presented at a higher magnification in Figure 18-22.

Vagina

The **vagina**, an 8- to 9-cm long muscular sheath, extending from the cervix of the uterus to the vestibule, is adapted for the reception of the penis during copulation and the passage of the fetus from the uterus during birth. The wall of the vagina is composed of three layers: the mucosa, muscularis, and the adventitia (Figs. 18-29 and 18-30).

- The **mucosa** consists of a nonkeratinized stratified squamous epithelium and lamina propria comprised

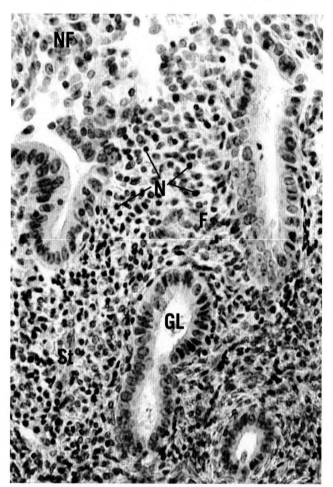

FIGURE 18-22. Endometrium Menstrual phase. Human. Paraffin section. ×270.

This photomicrograph is a higher magnification of the *boxed area* of Figure 18-21. Observe that some of the endometrial **glands** (GL) are torn and a **necrotic fragment** (NF) has been detached from the **functional layer** (F) of the endometrium. The **stroma** (St) is infiltrated by leukocytes, whose dense **nuclei** (N) mask most of the endometrial cells. Note that some of the endometrial cells are still enlarged, indicative of the decidual reaction.

of a loose, fibroelastic connective tissue without any glands.

- Frequently, in a virgin, the external orifice of the vagina is partially occluded by the **hymen**, a thin, somewhat vascular connective tissue membrane, covered on both sides by stratified squamous epithelium.

- The **muscularis** is composed of a mostly longitudinally disposed smooth muscle layer interspersed with some circularly arranged fibers. At its external orifice, the muscularis of the vagina possesses a sphincter, composed of circularly arrayed smooth muscle fibers.

- The **adventitia** is a dense fibroelastic connective tissue that affixes the vagina to the surrounding pelvic connective tissue.

Table 18-4	Principal Hormones and Factors Produced by the Various Components of the Placenta	
Syncytiotrophoblasts	**Cytotrophoblasts**	**Decidua Cells**
Estrogens	Gonadotropin-releasing hormone	Insulin-like growth factor binding proteins
Progesterone	Corticotropin-releasing hormone	Relaxin
Chorionic gonadotropin	Thyrotropin-releasing hormone	Prolactin
Chorionic somatotropin	Growth hormone–releasing hormone	Prostaglandins
Placental growth hormone	Inhibin	
Leptin	Activin	
	Leptin	
	Insulin-like growth factors I and II	

CLINICAL CONSIDERATIONS 18-1

Gonorrhea and Pelvic Inflammatory Disease

Gonorrhea is a sexually transmitted bacterial infection caused by the gram-negative diplococcus *Neisseria gonorrhoeae*. In the United States, over a million cases of gonorrhea occur annually. Frequently, this sexually transmitted disease (STD) is responsible for pelvic inflammatory disease (PID) and acute salpingitis.

Pelvic inflammatory disease (**PID**) is an infection of the cervix, uterus, fallopian tubes, and/or ovary, usually a sequel to microbial infection. Individuals suffering from PID exhibit tenderness and pain in the lower abdominal region, fever, unpleasant-smelling vaginal discharge, and episodes of abnormal bleeding.

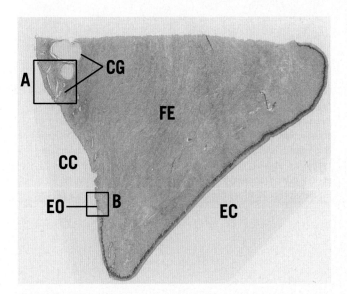

FIGURE 18-23. Cervix. Human. Paraffin Section. ×5

The survey of the cervix at a low magnification demonstrates the **cervical canal** (CC) lined by a much thinner epithelium which abruptly changes to a thicker epithelium at the **external os** (EO). Observe several **cervical glands** (CG) more prominently associated with the lining of the cervical canal. The thicker epithelium-lined region of the cervix protrudes out into the vaginal lumen and is called the **ectocervix** (EC). Note the thickest bulk of the cervix is comprised of **fibroelastic** (FE) connective tissue. The *boxed areas* are presented at higher magnifications in Figures 18-24 and 18-25.

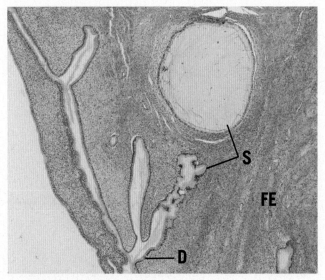

FIGURE 18-24. Cervix. Human. Paraffin Section. ×38.

This is a higher magnification of the cervical canal (*boxed area A* in Fig. 18-23) lined by a simple columnar epithelium. Observe the cervical glands whose **ducts** (D) communicate with the lumen and the **secretory** (S) units within the **fibroelastic** (FE) stroma.

External Genitalia

The **external genitalia**, composed of **labia majora**, **labia minora**, **clitoris**, and **vestibular glands**, are also collectively referred to as the **vulva**. These structures are richly innervated and function during sexual arousal and copulation.

CLINICAL CONSIDERATIONS 18-2

Adenomyosis

Adenomyosis is a common condition in which the endometrial glands invade the myometrium and cause the uterus to enlarge, occasionally becoming two or three times its normal dimensions. In most women, adenomyosis has no symptoms, and it is only on gynecologic examination that the condition is discovered. When it becomes symptomatic, the woman is usually between age 35 and 50 years, she may experience pain during intercourse, and she notices an increase in menstrual flow as well as bleeding between periods. Although the condition is benign, if the symptoms are severe and uncontrollable, hysterectomy may be indicated.

Endometrial Disorders

Endometriosis is distinguished by the presence of ectopic endometrial tissue dispersed to various sites along the peritoneal cavity. Occasionally, the tissues may migrate to extraperitoneal areas, including the eyes and brain. The etiology of this disease is not known. In some cases, the lesions of endometriosis involve small cysts attached separately or in small clumps on the visceral or parietal peritoneum.

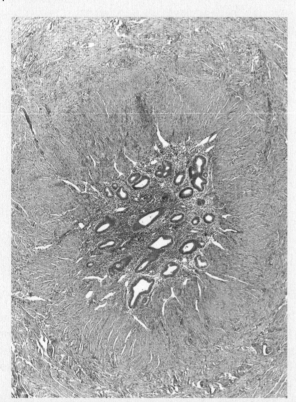

This photomicrograph is from the fallopian tube of a patient with endometriosis. Observe that uterine glands and stroma occupy the lumen of the oviduct. (Reprinted with permission from Mills SE, et al., eds. *Sternberg's Diagnostic Surgical Pathology*, 5th ed. Philadelphia: Wolters Kluwer Health//Lippincott Williams & Wilkins, 2010. p. 2377.)

Endometrial carcinoma is a malignancy of the uterine endometrium usually occurring in postmenopausal women. The most common type of endometrial cancer is adenocarcinoma. Because the cancer cells do not invade the cervix during the early stages, Pap smears are not very effective in diagnosing this disease until it has entered its later stages. The major symptom of endometrial cancer is abnormal uterine bleeding.

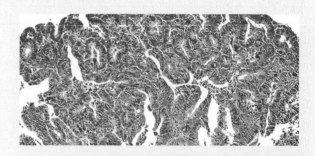

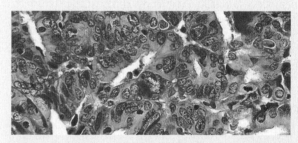

This photomicrograph is from the uterus of a patient with grade 1 carcinoma of the endometrium. **Top**: Observe that the uterine glands are very crowded with a scant amount of connective tissue between the glands. **Bottom**: The cells of the gland are interspersed with malignant cells displaying cytologic atypia. (Reprinted with permission from Mills SE, et al., eds. *Sternberg's Diagnostic Surgical Pathology*, 6th ed. Philadelphia: Wolters Kluwer, 2015. p. 2461, Figure 53-27.)

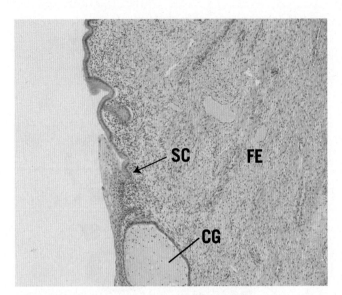

FIGURE 18-25. Cervix. Human. Paraffin Section. ×66.

This is a higher magnification of the external os (*boxed area B* in Fig. 18-23) in which an abrupt transition from simple columnar to nonkeratinized stratified squamous epithelia (*arrow*) is noted. Also known as the **squamo-columnar** (SC) junction, this site and the surface of the **ectocervix** (EC) are scraped for cytologic observation during Pap smear. Note the dilated **cervical gland** (CG) under the epithelium and the fibroelastic stroma.

Mammary Gland

The **mammary glands**, highly modified **sweat glands**, are identical in males and females until the onset of puberty, when, under the hormonal influences (primarily estrogen), the breasts develop. Technically, the mammary glands are not considered to belong in the reproductive system, but historically they have been discussed along with the female reproductive system and this *Text and Atlas* follows that tradition.

In the mature breast, the mammary gland is composed of numerous individual compound glands, each of which is considered a lobe, where each lobe is drained by a **lactiferous duct** that delivers **milk**, the secretion of the mammary glands, onto the surface of the nipple. The pigmented region of the skin surrounding the nipple, known as the **areola**, is richly endowed by sweat, sebaceous, and areolar glands (Figs. 18-31 and 18-32).

- Normally, mammary glands are inactive unless pregnancy ensues. Inactive mammary glands are characterized by small secretory units both in size and number, with relatively more prominent ducts in comparison.

- During pregnancy, several hormones interact to promote proliferation of the cells of the **terminal interalveolar ducts**, which differentiate into cuboidal

Placental structure

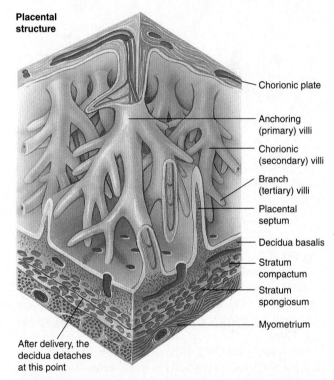

- Chorionic plate
- Anchoring (primary) villi
- Chorionic (secondary) villi
- Branch (tertiary) villi
- Placental septum
- Decidua basalis
- Stratum compactum
- Stratum spongiosum
- Myometrium

After delivery, the decidua detaches at this point

FIGURE 18-26. The human placenta is composed of a **maternally derived** and a **fetally derived** region. It is constructed in such a fashion that the mother's blood does **not** come in contact with the blood of the fetus, yet it permits the exchange of nutrients, gases, and waste products between them. The maternal portion of the placenta is composed of the **decidua basalis**, whereas the fetal portion consists of the **chorionic plate** and its extensions. There are three types of villi arising from the **chorionic plate** and its extensions. There are three types of villi arising from the chorionic plate: those that contact the decidua basalis (**anchoring** or **primary villi**), those that arise directly from the chorionic plate but do not contact the decidua basalis (**chorionic** or **secondary villi**), and branches arising from the secondary villi (**branch** or **tertiary villi**).

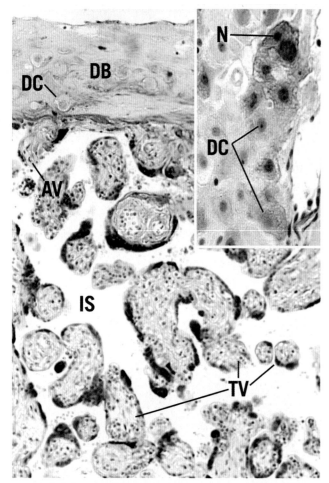

FIGURE 18-27. Placenta. Human. Paraffin section. ×132.

The human placenta is intimately associated with the uterine endometrium. At this junction, the **decidua basalis** (DB) is rich in clumps of large, round to polygonal **decidual cells** (DC), whose distended cytoplasm is filled with lipid and glycogen. **Anchoring chorionic villi** (AV) are attached to the decidua basalis; other villi are blindly ending in the **intervillous space** (IS). These are the most numerous and are referred to as **terminal villi** (TV), most of which are cut in cross or oblique sections. These villi are freely branching and, in the mature placenta, are smaller in diameter than in the immature placenta. *Inset.* **Placenta. Human. Paraffin section.** ×270. Note that the **decidual cells** (DC) are round to polygonal in shape. Their **nuclei** (N) are more or less centrally located, and their cytoplasm appears vacuolated owing to the extraction of glycogen and lipids during histologic preparation.

secretory cells forming spherical units called **alveoli** (Figs. 18-33 and 18-34).

- The hormones involved in promoting this process are **progesterone, estrogen,** and **human chorionic mammotropin** from the placenta and **lactogenic hormone (prolactin)** from the **acidophils** of the adenohypophysis.

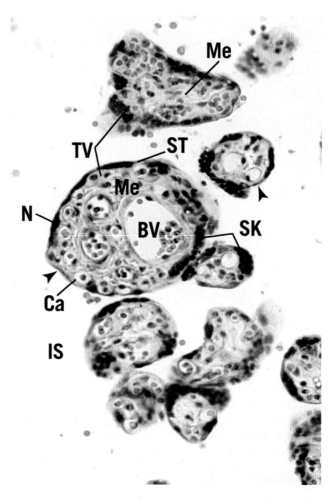

FIGURE 18-28. Placenta. Human. Paraffin section. ×270.

Cross sections of **terminal villi** (TV) in a mature placenta are surrounded by the **intervillous space** (IS) that, in the functional placenta, is filled with maternal blood. Hence, the cells of the villus act as a placental barrier. This barrier is greatly reduced in the mature placenta, as presented in this photomicrograph. The external layer of the terminal villus is composed of **syncytial trophoblasts** (ST), whose numerous **nuclei** (N) are frequently clustered together as **syncytial knots** (SK). The core of the villus houses numerous fetal **capillaries** (Ca) that are located usually in regions of the villus void of syncytial nuclei (*arrowheads*). Larger fetal **blood vessels** (BV) are also found in the core, surrounded by **mesoderm** (Me). The cytotrophoblasts and phagocytic Hofbauer cells of the immature placenta mostly disappear by the end of the pregnancy.

- Shortly after giving birth, the mammary glands begin to lactate, which is aided by the contraction of the **myoepithelial cells** surrounding the alveoli and terminal interalveolar ducts in response to **oxytocin** released from the neurohypophysis (in response to suckling), forcing milk out of the breast (**milk ejection reflex**) (see Fig. 18-34).

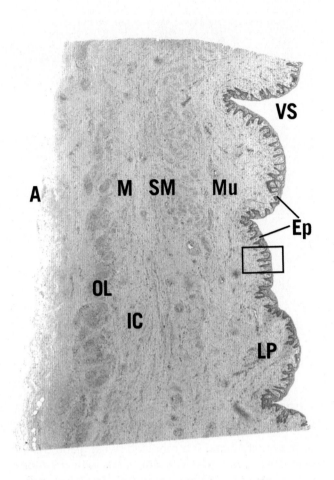

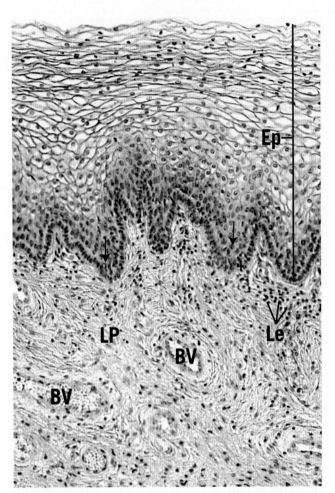

FIGURE 18-29. Vagina. l.s. Monkey. Plastic section. ×14.

The vagina is a fibromuscular tube, whose **vaginal space** (VS) is mostly obliterated because its walls are normally in contact with each other. This wall is composed of four layers: **mucosa** (Mu), s**ubmucosa** (SM), **muscularis** (M), and **adventitia** (A). The mucosa consists of an **epithelium** (Ep) and underlying **lamina propria** (LP). Deep to the mucosa is the submucosa, whose numerous large blood vessels impart to it an erectile tissue appearance. The smooth muscle of the muscularis is arranged in two layers, an **inner circular** (IC) and a thicker **outer longitudinal** (OL). A region similar to the *boxed area* is presented at a higher magnification in Figure 18-30.

FIGURE 18-30. Vagina. l.s. Human. Paraffin section. ×132.

This photomicrograph is a higher magnification of a region similar to the *boxed area* in Figure 18-29. The stratified squamous nonkeratinized **epithelium** (Ep) of the vagina is characterized by the empty appearance of the cells, constituting most of its thickness. This is owing to the extraction lipids and glycogen during histologic preparation. Observe that the cells in the deeper aspect of the epithelium possess fewer inclusions; therefore, their cytoplasm appears normal. Note also that the **lamina propria** (LP) is richly **vascularized** (BV) and always possesses numerous **leukocytes** (Le) (*arrows*). Finally, note the absence of glands and muscularis mucosae.

- **Milk** is composed of water, proteins, lipids, and lactose.
- However, milk secreted during the first few days is called **colostrum** with different composition, in that

it is rich in vitamins, minerals, **lymphoid cells**, and proteins, especially **immunoglobulin A**, providing antibodies and immunologic support for the neonate for the first few months of life.

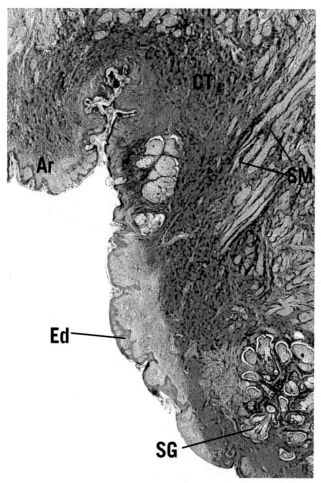

FIGURE 18-31. Mammary gland. Nipple. Human. Paraffin section. ×14.

The large, conical nipple of the breast is covered by a thin **epidermis** (Ed), composed of stratified squamous keratinized epithelium. Although the nipple possesses neither hair nor sweat glands, it is richly endowed with **sebaceous glands** (SG). The dense irregular **connective tissue** (CT) core displays numerous longitudinally positioned lactiferous ducts that pierce the tip of the nipple to convey milk to the outside. The lactiferous ducts are surrounded by an extensive network of **smooth muscle fibers** (SM) that are responsible for the erection of the nipple, elevating it to facilitate the suckling process. The region immediately surrounding the nipple is known as the **areola** (Ar).

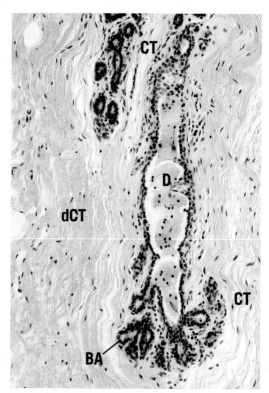

FIGURE 18-32. Mammary gland. Inactive. Human. Paraffin section. ×132.

The mammary gland is a modified sweat gland that, in the inactive stage, presents **ducts** (D) with occasional **buds of alveoli** (BA) branching from the blind ends of the duct. The remainder of the breast is composed of **dense collagenous connective tissue** (dCT) interspersed with lobules of fat. However, in the immediate vicinity of the ducts and buds of alveoli, the **connective tissue** (CT) is more loosely arranged. It is believed that this looser connective tissue is derived from the papillary layer of the dermis.

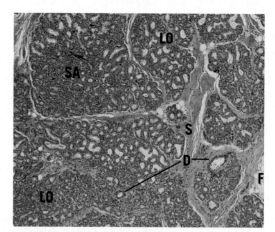

FIGURE 18-33. Mammary gland. Active. Human. Paraffin section. ×69.

Mammary glands become active during pregnancy, and it is marked by the elaboration of the **secretory alveoli** (SA) and their **ducts** (D). As the pregnancy progresses, the **fatty** (F) tissues are almost entirely replaced by the glandular tissues. Observe the **lobules** (LO) of glands separated by the connective tissue **septa** (S).

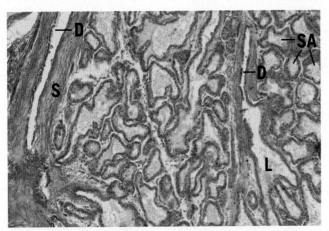

FIGURE 18-34. Mammary gland. Lactating. Human. Paraffin section. ×104.

After parturition, the lactating mammary glands are characterized by some lobules with dilated secretory alveoli, engorged with milk in the lumen, and some lobules that resemble active mammary glands in Figure 18-33, suggesting that not all lobules are lactating at the same time thus allowing some units to rest between intense production and secretion of milk. The lactating lobule in this photomicrograph demonstrates the enlarged **lumen** (L) of the **secretory alveoli** (SA) and the **ducts** (D) in the lobular **septa** (S).

CLINICAL CONSIDERATIONS 18-4

Hydatidiform Mole

Also known as molar pregnancy, **hydatidiform mole** results from abnormal fertilization or fertilization involving gametes with chromosomal anomalies. Complete moles may result from the fertilization of an anucleate oocyte with two sperms (dispermy) or a single sperm with duplicate haploid chromosomes. A complete mole is characterized by fast-growing edematous chorionic villi of the placental tissues and no fetal tissues. Partial moles are often triploid, resulting from fertilization of a haploid ovum with two sperms or a single sperm with duplicate haploid chromosomes. Partial moles are also characterized by fast-growing, edematous placental tissues, but in addition, fetal tissues are present. Patients test positive for pregnancy; however, they experience faster than expected swelling of the abdomen and present with severe nausea and vomiting, and sometimes a vaginal discharge of grape-like clusters of tissue. Lack of a heartbeat and observation of echogenic mass on sonography described as "snowstorm pattern" is diagnostic of hydatidiform mole. Prognosis of molar pregnancy is good with early diagnosis and appropriate treatment; however, 20% of complete moles can become malignant choriocarcinoma.

CLINICAL CONSIDERATIONS 18-5

Paget's Disease of the Nipple

Paget's disease of the nipple usually occurs in elderly women and is associated with breast cancer of ductal origin. Initially, the disease manifests as a scaly or crusty nipple frequently accompanied by a fluid discharge from the nipple. Usually, the patient has no other symptoms and frequently neglects the condition.

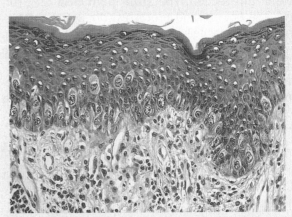

This photomicrograph is from the nipple of a female patient with Paget's disease of the nipple. Note the large Paget cells throughout the basal aspect of the stratified squamous keratinized epithelium, with their light pink cytoplasm, vesicular-appearing nuclei, and large nucleoli. (Reprinted with permission from Mills SE, et al., eds. *Sternberg's Diagnostic Surgical Pathology*, 6th ed. Philadelphia: Wolters Kluwer, 2015. p. 324, Figure 9-11.)

PLATE 18-1   Ovary and Corpus Luteum

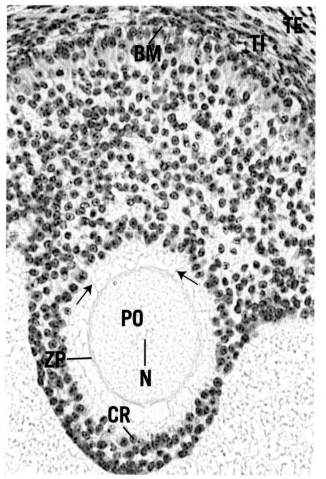

FIGURE 18-1-1. Graafian follicle. Cumulus oophorus. Paraffin section. ×270.

This photomicrograph is a higher magnification of Figure 18-7. Observe that the cumulus oophorus houses the **primary oocyte** (PO), whose **nucleus** (N) is just visible in this section. The **zona pellucida** (ZP) surrounds the oocyte, and processes (*arrows*) of the surrounding follicular cells extend into this acellular region. The single layer of follicular cells appears to radiate as a crown at the periphery of the primary oocyte and is referred to as the **corona radiata** (CR). Note the **basement membrane** (BM), as well as the **theca interna** (TI) and the **theca externa** (TE).

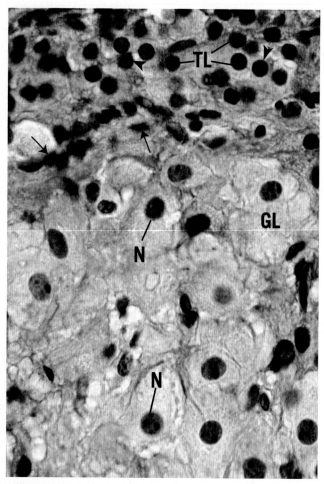

FIGURE 18-1-2. Corpus luteum. Human. Paraffin section. ×540.

This photomicrograph is similar to the *boxed area* of Figure 18-10. Observe the large **granulosa lutein cells** (GL), whose cytoplasm appears vesicular, representing the spaces occupied by lipids in the living tissue. Note that the **nuclei** (N) of these cells are farther away from each other than the nuclei of the smaller **theca lutein cells** (TL), which also appear to be darker staining (*arrowheads*). The flattened nuclei (*arrows*) belong to various connective tissue cells.

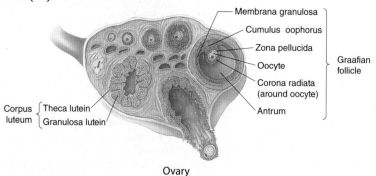

Ovary

KEY						
BM	basement membrane	**N**	nucleus	**TI**	theca interna
CR	corona radiata	**PO**	primary oocyte	**TL**	theca lutein cells
GL	granulosa lutein cells	**TE**	theca externa	**ZP**	zona pellucida

PLATE 18-2 Ovary and Oviduct

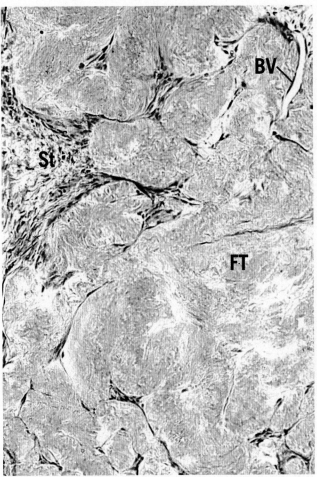

FIGURE 18-2-1. Corpus albicans. Human. Paraffin section. ×132.

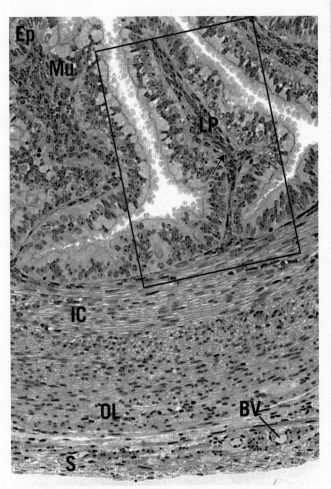

FIGURE 18-2-2. Oviduct. x.s. Monkey. Plastic section. ×132.

As the corpus luteum involutes, its cellular elements degenerate and undergo autolysis. The corpus luteum becomes invaded by macrophages that phagocytose the dead cells, leaving behind relatively acellular **fibrous tissue** (FT). The previously rich **vascular supply** (BV) also regressed, and the entire corpus albicans appears pale in comparison to the relatively dark staining of the surrounding ovarian **stroma** (St). The corpus albicans will regress until it becomes a small scar on the surface of the ovary.

This photomicrograph is a higher magnification of a region similar to Figure 18-13. The entire thickness of the wall of the oviduct displays its **vascular** (BV) **serosa** (S) that envelops the thick muscularis, whose **outer longitudinal** (OL) and **inner circular** (IC) layers are not very well delineated. The **mucosa** (Mu) is highly folded and is lined by a simple columnar **epithelium** (Ep). The loose connective tissue of the **lamina propria** (LP) is richly vascularized (*arrow*). The *boxed area* is presented in a higher magnification in Figure 18-3-1.

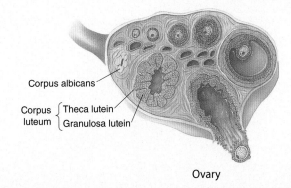

Corpus albicans

Corpus luteum { Theca lutein / Granulosa lutein

Ovary

KEY					
BV	blood vessels	**IC**	inner circular layer	**OL**	outer longitudinal layer
Ep	epithelium	**LP**	lamina propria	**S**	serosa
FT	fibrous tissue	**Mu**	mucosa	**St**	stroma

PLATE 18-3 Oviduct, Electron Microscopy

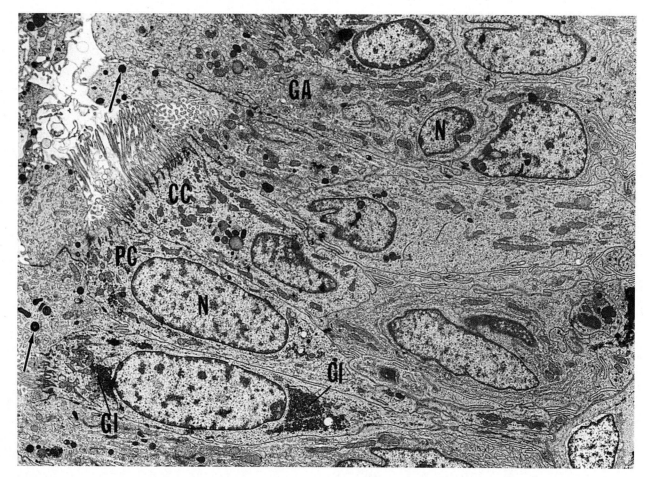

FIGURE 18-3-1. Oviduct epithelium. Human. Electron microscopy. ×4,553.

The human oviduct at midcycle (day 14) presents two types of epithelial cells, the **peg cell** (PC) and the **ciliated cell** (CC). The former are secretory cells, as indicated by their extensive **Golgi apparatus** (GA) situated in the region of the cell apical to the **nucleus** (N). Observe the electron-dense secretory products (*arrows*) in the expanded, apical free ends of these cells. Note also that some ciliated cells display large accumulations of **glycogen** (Gl) at either pole of the nucleus. (From Verhage HG, et al. Cyclic changes in ciliation, secretion and cell height of the oviductal epithelium in women. *Am J Anat* 1979;156(4):505–521. Copyright © 1979 Wiley-Liss, Inc. Reprinted by permission of John Wiley & Sons, Inc.)

KEY					
CC	ciliated cell	**Gl**	glycogen	**PC**	peg cell
GA	Golgi apparatus	**N**	nucleus		

PLATE 18-4 Uterus

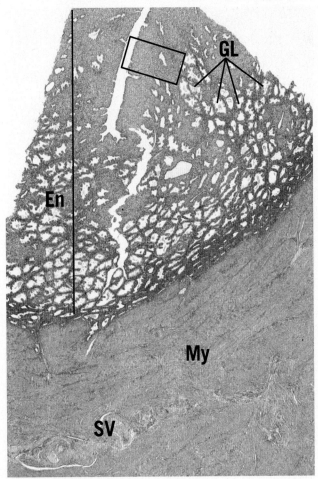

FIGURE 18-4-1. Uterus. Luteal phase. Human. Paraffin section. ×14.

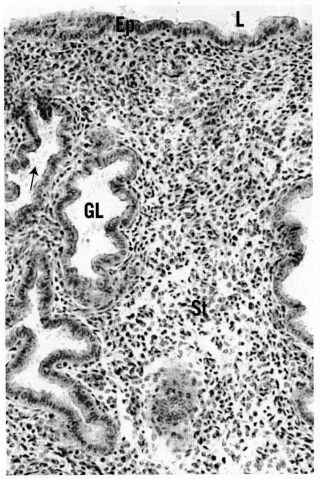

FIGURE 18-4-2. Uterus. Early luteal phase. Human. Paraffin section. ×132.

The **myometrium** (My) of the uterus remains constant during the various endometrial phases. Observe its three layers, noting especially that the middle circular layer of smooth muscle is richly vascularized and is therefore frequently referred to as the **stratum vasculare** (SV). The **endometrium** (En) is richly endowed with **glands** (GL) that become highly tortuous in anticipation of the blastocyst that will be nourished by secretions of these glands subsequent to implantation. A region similar to the *boxed area* is presented at a higher magnification in Figure 18-4-2.

This photomicrograph is a higher magnification of a region similar to the *boxed area* of Figure 18-4-1. The functional layer of the endometrium is covered by a simple columnar **epithelium** (Ep), separating the endometrial **stroma** (St) from the uterine **lumen** (L). Note that the **glands** (GL), also composed of simple columnar epithelium, are more abundant than those in the follicular phase. Observe also that these glands appear more tortuous and are dilated and their lumina contain a slight amount of secretory product (*arrow*).

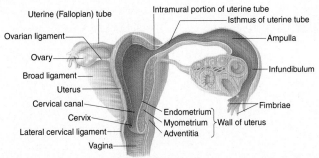

Female reproductive system

KEY					
En	endometrium	**L**	lumen	**St**	stroma
Ep	epithelium	**My**	myometrium	**SV**	stratum vasculare
GL	gland				

PLATE 18-5 Uterus

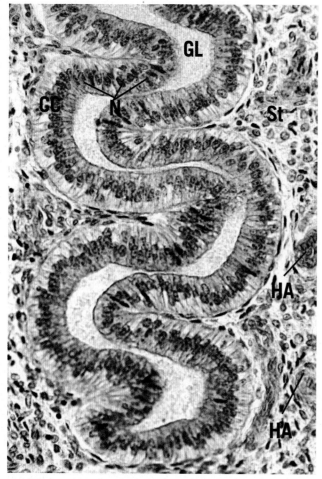

FIGURE 18-5-1. Uterus. Midluteal phase. Human. Paraffin section. ×270.

During the midluteal phase, the **endometrial glands** (GL) become quite tortuous and corkscrew-shaped, and the simple **columnar cells** (CC) accumulate glycogen (*arrow*). Observe that during this phase of the endometrium, the glycogen is basally located, displacing the **nucleus** (N) toward the center of the cell. Note also that the **stroma** (St) is undergoing a decidual reaction in that some of the connective tissue cells enlarge as they become engorged with lipid and glycogen. A **helical artery** (HA) is evident as several cross sections.

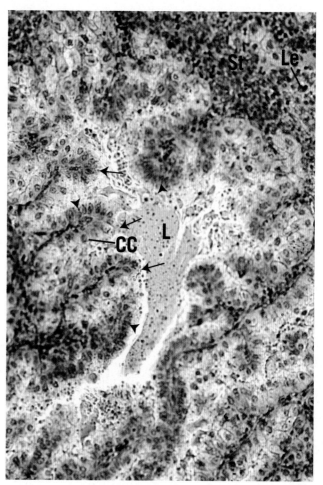

FIGURE 18-5-2. Uterus. Late luteal phase. Human. Paraffin section. ×132.

During the late luteal phase of the endometrium, the glands assume a characteristic ladder (or sawtooth) shape (*arrows*). The simple **columnar epithelial cells** (CC) appear pale and, interestingly, the position of the glycogen is now apical (*arrowheads*) rather than basal. The apical location of the glycogen imparts a ragged, torn appearance to the free surface of these cells. Note that the lumina (L) of the glands are filled with a glycogen-rich, viscous fluid. Observe also that the **stroma** (St) is infiltrated by numerous **leukocytes** (Le).

KEY					
CC	columnar cell	**L**	lumen	**N**	nucleus
GL	gland	**Le**	leukocyte	**St**	stroma
HA	helical artery				

PLATE 18-6   Mammary Gland

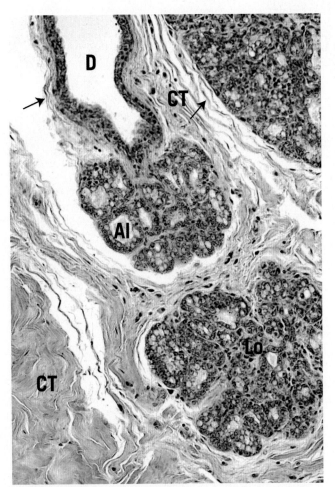

FIGURE 18-6-1. Mammary gland. Lactating. Human. Paraffin section. ×132.

During pregnancy, the **ducts** (D) of the mammary gland undergo major development, in that the buds of alveoli proliferate to form **lobules** (Lo) composed of numerous **alveoli** (Al). The interlobular **connective tissue** (CT) becomes reduced to thin sheets in regions; elsewhere, it maintains its previous character to support the increased weight of the breast. Observe that the connective tissue in the immediate vicinity of the ducts and lobules (*arrows*) retains its loose consistency.

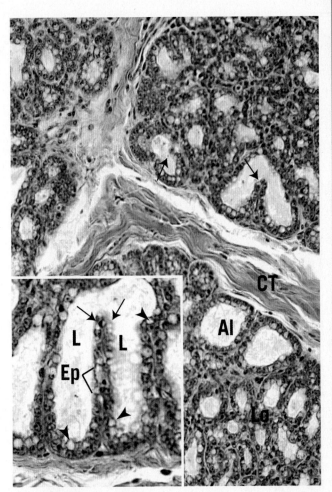

FIGURE 18-6-2. Mammary gland. Lactating. Human. Paraffin section. ×132.

The lactating mammary gland presents numerous **lobules** (Lo) of **alveoli** (Al) that are tightly packed so that the **connective tissue** (CT) elements are greatly compressed. This photomicrograph clearly illustrates the crowded nature of this tissue. Although this tissue bears a superficial resemblance to the histology of the thyroid gland, the presence of ducts and branching alveoli (*arrows*), as well as the lack of colloid material, should assist in distinguishing this tissue as the active mammary gland. *Inset*. **Mammary gland. Lactating Human. Paraffin section**. ×270. Observe the branching (*arrows*) of this alveolus, some of whose simple cuboidal **epithelial cells** (Ep) appear vacuolated (*arrowheads*). Note also that the **lumen** (L) contains a fatty secretory product (milk).

KEY					
Al	alveolus	**D**	duct	**L**	lumen
CT	connective tissue	**Ep**	epithelium	**Lo**	lobule

Selected Review of Histologic Images

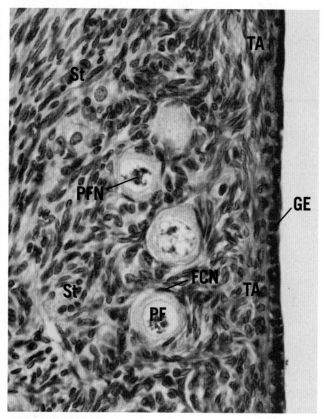

REVIEW FIGURE 18-1-1. Ovary cortex. Rabbit. Paraffin section. ×540.

This high-magnification photomicrograph of the ovarian cortex displays the **germinal epithelium** (GE) covering the **tunica albuginea** (TA) of the ovary. The highly cellular **stroma** (St) of the cortex houses the ovarian follicles. The small **primordial follicles** (PF), the **nuclei of the primary oocytes** (PFN), and the **nuclei of the flattened follicular cells** (FCN) are evident.

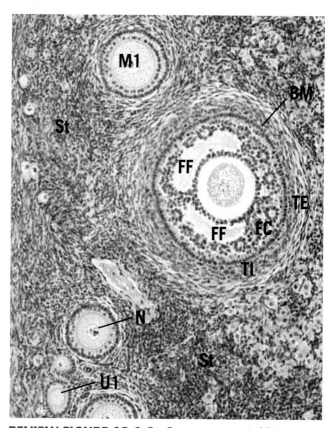

REVIEW FIGURE 18-1-2. Ovary cortex. Rabbit. Paraffin section. ×132.

The **stroma** (St) of the ovarian cortex envelops ovarian follicles in various stages of maturation. **Unilaminar primary follicles** (U1) are much smaller than the **multilaminar primary follicles** (M1). The **nuclei** (N) of the primary follicles are evident. The comparatively large secondary follicle is distinguishable by the **follicular fluid** (FF) accumulation among the **follicular cells** (FC). The **basement membrane** (BM) separates the follicular cells from the very cellular **theca interna** (TI), which is surrounded by the more fibrous **theca externa** (TE).

KEY					
BM	basement membrane	M1	multilaminar primary follicle	St	stroma
FC	follicular cell			TA	tunica albuginea
FCN	follicular cell	N	nucleus	TE	theca externa
FF	follicular fluid	PF	primordial follicle	TI	theca interna
GE	germinal epithelium	PFN	primary oocyte nucleus	U1	unilaminar primary follicle

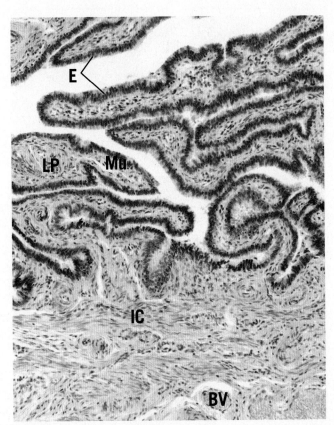

REVIEW FIGURE 18-1-3. Oviduct. Human. Paraffin section. ×132.

The oviduct is a muscular tube that extends from the vicinity of the ovary and ends in the lumen of the uterus. Its highly folded **mucosa** (Mu) is composed of a simple columnar **epithelium** (E) and a connective tissue **lamina propria** (LP) with a rich **vascular supply** (BV). The muscularis consists of two layers of smooth muscle, an **inner circular** (IC) and an outer longitudinal.

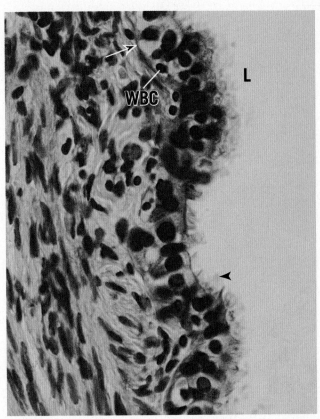

REVIEW FIGURE 18-1-4. Oviduct. Human. Paraffin section. ×540.

The mucosa of the oviduct has a connective tissue lamina propria and a simple columnar epithelium. The epithelium is composed of two cell types, a narrower peg cell and a wider ciliated cell whose **cilia** (*arrowhead*) project into the **lumen** (L) of the oviduct. The epithelium is separated from the lamina propria by a **basement membrane** (BM) (*arrow*). Frequently, **white blood cells** (WBC) penetrate the basement membrane as they migrate from the lamina propria into the lumen of the oviduct.

KEY					
BM	basement membrane	**IC**	inner circular layer	**Mu**	mucosa
BV	blood vessel (vascular supply)	**L**	lumen	**WBC**	white blood cell
E	simple columnar epithelium	**LP**	lamina propria		

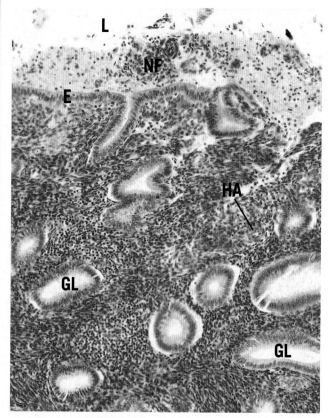

REVIEW FIGURE 18-2-1. Uterus. Menstrual phase. Human. Paraffin section. ×132.

During the menstrual phase of the uterus, the superficial layer of the endometrium is dislodged and is released into the **lumen** (L) of the uterus as **necrotic fragments** (NF). During the early menstrual phase, some of the **epithelium** (E) and some of the **uterine glands** (GL) are still intact as are the **helical arteries** (HA).

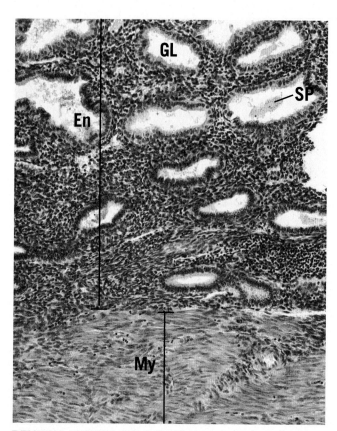

REVIEW FIGURE 18-2-2. Uterus. Late luteal (secretory) phase. Human. Paraffin section. ×132.

The **endometrium** (En) during the late luteal phase is characterized by intricate folding of the uterine **glands** (GL) and the presence of **secretory product** (SP) in their lumen. The **myometrium** (My) of the uterus is composed of three indistinct layers of smooth muscle cells.

KEY					
E	epithelium	**HA**	helical artery	**NF**	necrotic fragments
En	endometrium	**L**	lumen	**SP**	secretory product
GL	glands	**My**	myometrium		

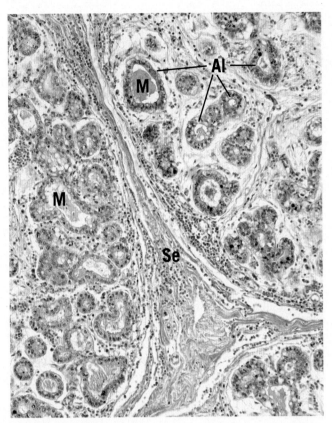

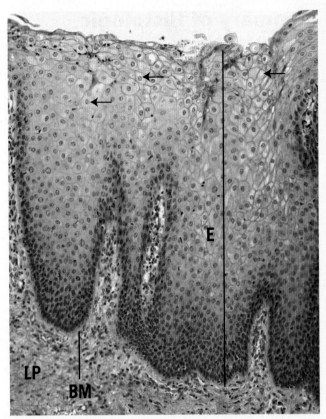

REVIEW FIGURE 18-2-3. Mammary gland. Lactating. Human. Paraffin section. ×132.

The lactating mammary gland is composed of many lobules separated from each other by connective tissue **septa** (Se). The lobes are composed of **alveoli** (Al) whose lumina contain **milk** (M) that is delivered into lactiferous ducts to be discharged into lactiferous sinuses at the base of the nipple.

REVIEW FIGURE 18-2-4. Vagina. Human. Paraffin section. ×132.

The human vagina is lined by a very thick stratified squamous nonkeratinized **epithelium** (E) whose surface cells are rich in lipids and glycogen. These are extracted during histologic preparation, leaving empty spaces (*arrows*) in the epithelial cells. The epithelium is separated from the **lamina propria** (LP) by a **basement membrane** (BM). Many of the small, round nuclei in the region of the lamina propria nearest the overlying epithelium belong to migrating white blood cells.

KEY					
Al	alveoli	**E**	epithelium	**M**	milk
BM	basement membrane	**LP**	lamina propria	**Se**	septa

Summary of Histologic Organization

I. Ovary

A. Cortex

The **cortex** of the **ovary** is covered by a modified mesothelium, the **germinal epithelium**. Deep to this simple cuboidal to simple squamous epithelium is the **tunica albuginea**, the fibrous connective tissue capsule of the ovary. The remainder of the ovarian connective tissue is more cellular and is referred to as the **stroma**. The cortex houses ovarian **follicles** in various stages of development.

1. Primordial Follicles

Primordial follicles consist of a **primary oocyte** surrounded by a single layer of flattened **follicular cells**.

2. Primary Follicles

a. *Unilaminar Primary Follicles*

Consist of a **primary oocyte** surrounded by a single layer of cuboidal **granulosa cells**.

b. *Multilaminar Primary Follicles*

Consist of a **primary oocyte** surrounded by several layers of **granulosa cells**. The **zona pellucida** is visible. The **theca interna** is begins to organize surrounding the granulosa cells.

3. Secondary (Vesicular) Follicle

The **secondary follicle** is distinguished from the primary multilaminar follicle by its larger size, by a well-established **theca interna** and **theca externa**, and especially by the presence of **follicular fluid** in small cavities formed from intercellular spaces of the **granulosa cells**. These fluid-filled cavities are known as **Call–Exner bodies**.

4. Graafian (Mature) Follicles

The **Graafian follicle** is very large; the Call–Exner bodies have coalesced into a single space, the **antrum**, filled with **follicular fluid**. The wall of the antrum is referred to as the **membrana granulosa**, and the region of the oocyte and granulosa cells jutting into the antrum is the **cumulus oophorus**. The layer of granulosa cells immediately surrounding the oocyte is the **corona radiata**. Long apical processes of these cells extend into the **zona pellucida**. The **theca interna** and **theca externa** are well developed; the former displays numerous cells and capillaries, whereas the latter is less cellular and more fibrous. The primary oocyte completes meiosis I and enters meiosis II to become the **secondary oocyte**, only to be arrested at metaphase just before or at ovulation.

5. Atretic Follicles

Atretic follicles are in a state of degeneration. Follicles in any stages of growth undergo atresia, but those in later stages are characterized by the presence of **fibroblasts** in the follicle and a degenerated oocyte.

B. Medulla

The **medulla** of the ovary is composed of a relatively loose fibroelastic connective tissue housing an extensive **vascular** supply, including spiral arteries and convoluted veins.

C. Corpus Luteum

Subsequent to the extrusion of the **secondary oocyte** with its attendant **granulosa cells**, the remnant of the **Graafian follicle** becomes partly filled with blood and is known as the **corpus hemorrhagicum**. Cells of the **membrana granulosa** are transformed into large **granulosa lutein cells**. Moreover, the cells of the **theca interna** also increase in size to become **theca lutein cells**, although they remain smaller than the **granulosa lutein cells**.

D. Corpus Albicans

The **corpus albicans** is a **corpus luteum** that is in the process of involution and hyalinization. It becomes fibrotic, with few **fibroblasts** among the intercellular materials. Eventually, the corpus albicans will become **scar tissues**.

II. Genital Ducts

A. Oviduct

1. Mucosa

The **mucosa** of the oviduct is highly folded in the **infundibulum** and **ampulla**. It is composed of a loose, cellular connective tissue, **lamina propria**, and a **ciliated simple columnar epithelial** lining. The epithelium is composed of **peg cells** and **ciliated cells**.

2. Muscularis

The **muscle coat** is composed of an **inner circular** and an **outer longitudinal smooth muscle layer**.

3. Serosa

The oviduct is invested by a **serosa**.

B. Uterus

1. Endometrium

The **endometrium** is subdivided into a **basal** and a **functional layer**. It is lined by a **nonciliated simple columnar epithelium**. The **lamina propria** varies with the phases of the menstrual cycle.

a. Proliferative Phase

The **glands** are straight and display mitotic figures, and the helical arteries grow into the functional layer.

b. Secretory Phase

Glands become tortuous, and the **helical arteries** become coiled. The **lumina** of the glands accumulate **secretory products**. **Fibroblasts** enlarge and accumulate glycogen.

c. Menstrual Phase

The **functional layer** is desquamated, and the lamina propria displays extravasated blood.

2. Myometrium

The **myometrium** is thick and consists of three poorly delineated **smooth muscle** layers: **inner longitudinal**, **middle circular**, and **outer longitudinal**. During pregnancy, the myometrium increases in size as a result of hypertrophy and hyperplasia of smooth muscle cells.

3. Serosa

Most of the uterus is covered by a **serosa**; the remainder is attached to surrounding tissues by an **adventitia**.

C. Placenta

1. Decidua Basalis

The **decidua basalis**, the maternally derived **endometrial layer**, is characterized by the presence of large, glycogen-rich **decidual cells**. **Coiled arteries** and straight **veins** open into the labyrinth-like **intervillous spaces**.

2. Chorionic Plate and Villi

The **chorionic plate** is a region of the **chorionic sac** of the fetus from which **chorionic villi** extend into the intervillous spaces of the **decidua basalis**. Each villus has a core of **fibromuscular connective tissue** surrounding **capillaries** (derived from the umbilical vessels). The villus is covered by **trophoblast cells**. During the first half of pregnancy, there are two layers of trophoblast cells, an inner cuboidal layer of **cytotrophoblasts**, and an outer layer of **syncytiotrophoblasts**. During the second half of pregnancy, only the **syncytiotrophoblasts** remain. However, at points where chorionic villi are anchored into the decidua basalis, **cytotrophoblasts** are present.

D. Vagina

1. Mucosa

The vagina is lined by a **stratified squamous nonkeratinized epithelium**. The **lamina propria**, composed of a **fibroelastic connective tissue**, possesses no glands. The **mucosa** is thrown into longitudinal folds known as **rugae**.

2. Submucosa

The **submucosa** is also composed of a fibroelastic type of connective tissue housing numerous blood vessels.

3. Muscularis

The **muscularis** is composed of interlacing bundles of **smooth muscle** fibers. Near its external orifice, the vagina is equipped with a **skeletal muscle sphincter**.

4. Adventitia

The vagina is connected to surrounding structures via its **adventitia**.

E. Mammary Glands

1. Inactive (Resting) Gland

The **inactive (resting) gland** is composed mainly of **dense irregular collagenous connective tissue** interspersed with lobules of **adipose tissue** and numerous **ducts**. Frequently, at the blind ends of ducts, **buds of alveoli** and attendant **myoepithelial cells** are present.

2. Active Gland

The **mammary gland** becomes active during pregnancy. The expanded **alveoli** that form numerous **lobules** are composed of **simple cuboidal cells**, resembling parotid glands or pancreas. However, larger sizes of the secretory units and their lumina along with the absence of striated ducts and pancreatic islets provide the histologic distinctions.

3. Lactating Gland

The **mammary gland** begins to lactate shortly after parturition. The numerous lobules may be comprised of different sizes of alveoli. The alveoli of the lactating lobules have dilated lumina and may resemble the large follicles of the thyroid gland. However, the presence of **ducts**, **myoepithelial cells**, and lobules in the resting state in the vicinity provides distinguishing characteristics. **Alveoli** and the **lumen** of the ducts may contain a fatty secretory product.

4. Areola and Nipple

The **areola** is composed of thin, **pigmented epidermis** displaying large **apocrine areolar glands**. Additionally, **sweat** and large **sebaceous glands** are present. The **dermis** presents numerous **smooth muscle fibers**. The **nipple** possesses several minute pores representing the distal ends of **lactiferous ducts**. These ducts arise from **lactiferous sinuses**, enlarged reservoirs at the base of the nipple. The **epidermis** covering the nipple is thin, and the dermis is richly supplied by **smooth muscle fibers** and **nerve endings**. Although the nipple possesses no hair follicles or sweat glands, it is richly endowed with **sebaceous glands**.

Chapter Review Questions

Questions 18-1 through 18-3 refer to the following clinical scenario.

A patient presents to an obstetrician for her first prenatal visit after testing positive for pregnancy. The patient reports that she is 8 weeks along in her first pregnancy and complains of severe morning sickness. Upon physical exam, the patient's body mass index is within normal range; however, her abdomen is noticeably round and is bigger than usual.

18-1. **Which clinical condition should be considered?**

    A. Endometriosis

    B. Hydatidiform mole

    C. Inflammatory pelvic disease

    D. Polycystic ovarian disease

18-2. **Ultrasonography of the patient would reveal which of the following?**

    A. Echogenic mass in the uterus without fetus

    B. Larger than normal fetus with minimal placenta

    C. Numerous cysts in the ovaries

    D. Placenta invading into the myometrium

18-3. **What is the most likely cause of this condition?**

    A. Cervical implantation

    B. Dispermy

    C. LH surge

    D. Spiral arterial spasm

18-4. **Which follicle contains the secondary oocyte?**

    A. Primordial follicle

    B. Unilaminar primary follicle

    C. Multilaminar primary follicle

    D. Secondary follicle

    E. Dominant Graafian follicle

18-5. **Endometrial biopsy reveals straight glands and intact lining epithelium. Which ovarian phase corresponds with the endometrial observation?**

    A. Follicular

    B. Luteal

    C. Menopausal

    D. Ovulation

MALE REPRODUCTIVE SYSTEM

CHAPTER OUTLINE

The male reproductive system, consisting of the two testes (the male gonads), a system of genital ducts, accessory glands, and the penis, functions in the formation of spermatozoa, the elaboration of male sex hormones, and the delivery of male gametes into the female reproductive tract. The penis also houses the urethra and, therefore, also functions in urination.

Testes

Each **testis** is an oval structure housed in its separate compartment within the scrotum. During embryonic development, the testes descend from the posterior abdominal wall into the scrotum and take the wall's covering with them. The **tunica vaginalis**, a peritoneal derivative, forms a serous sac over a part of the testes, providing a degree of movability for the testes within the scrotal sac. The **tunica albuginea**, the fibromuscular connective tissue capsule of the testis lined by a vascular connective tissue known as the **tunica vasculosa**, is thickened at the **mediastinum testis**, which give rise to septa that subdivide each testis into approximately 250 small, incomplete, pyramid-like compartments, known as the **lobuli testis** (Fig. 19-1).

- Each lobule houses one to four highly tortuous, **seminiferous tubules** lined by spermatozoa-producing **germinal (seminiferous) epithelium**. These tubules are surrounded by a richly vascularized connective tissue in which male hormone-forming **interstitial cells of Leydig** are embedded.

- Spermatozoa are formed only after puberty. They are produced in the seminiferous tubules and are conveyed via the short, straight **tubuli recti** into the labyrinth-like spaces, the **rete testis**, that occupy much of the mediastinum testis. The rete testis is drained of its spermatozoa by the approximately 20 short **ductuli efferentes** that lead into the **epididymis**.

The vascular supply of the testes is derived from the abdominal aorta as a **testicular artery**. A testicular artery and a **ductus deferens (vas deferens)** accompany each testis in its descent into the scrotum. The testicular artery is tortuous in the vicinity of the testis and is entwined by the **pampiniform plexus of veins**. These three structures, along with the accompanying plexus of nerves and lymph vessels form the **spermatic cord**, a relatively thick, cord-like structure (1 to 2 cm in diameter) that can be palpated through the skin of the scrotum in the live individual. Because the temperature of venous blood is cooler than that of arterial blood, the pampiniform plexus provides a countercurrent heat exchange, cooling the blood in the testicular artery by 2 to 3°C, permitting normal development of the spermatozoa.

Seminiferous Tubules

The walls of the **seminiferous tubules** are composed of collagenous connective tissue known as the **tunica propria** on the exterior, a **basement membrane**, and the thick **seminiferous (germinal) epithelium**. Four cell types constitute the basal-most layer of the seminiferous epithelium, and each cell type is in contact with the basement membrane (Figs. 19-2 and 19-3): **Sertoli cells**, and three types of **spermatogonia**, pale type A, dark type A, and type B (discussed in the section on Spermatogenesis).

Sertoli Cells

The tall, columnar-shaped **Sertoli cells** span the thickness of the germinal epithelium. These cells possess light, oval-shaped nuclei (see Fig. 19-2), as well as all the expected organelles, including numerous mitochondria, both rough and smooth endoplasmic reticula (ER), an abundant Golgi apparatus, well-developed endosomal compartments, many lysosomes, and a rich supply of cytoskeletal elements. The basal cell membrane of these cells possesses **follicle-stimulating hormone receptors**. Sertoli cells have numerous functions, including (Table 19-1):

- The formation of **occluding junctions** near their basal aspect that partition the lumen of the seminiferous tubule into two concentric compartments, the inner and broader **adluminal compartment** (that includes the center of the lumen) and the slimmer outer **basal compartment**. By doing so, they isolate the adluminal compartment from the connective tissue elements, establishing a **blood–testis barrier**, and thus protect the developing sperm cells (with recombined genetic content which the immune system has never encountered) from an autoimmune response. Of the developing germ cells, only the three types of spermatogonia occupy the basal compartment because as the primary spermatocyte forms and enters meiosis it migrates into the adluminal compartment and further spermatogenic development occurs in that compartment. Therefore, only Sertoli cells occupy both the basal and adluminal compartments.

- Secretion of **androgen-binding protein (ABP)**, in response to **follicle-stimulating hormone (FSH)** secreted by the anterior pituitary gland. ABP binds testosterone and dihydrotestosterone, forming a complex that enters the lumen of the seminiferous tubules, where it is maintained at a sufficiently high threshold level to permit spermatogenesis to occur.

- Secretion of the hormone **inhibin**, which blocks the release of FSH and **activin**, which enhances the release of FSH, both via a biofeedback mechanism.

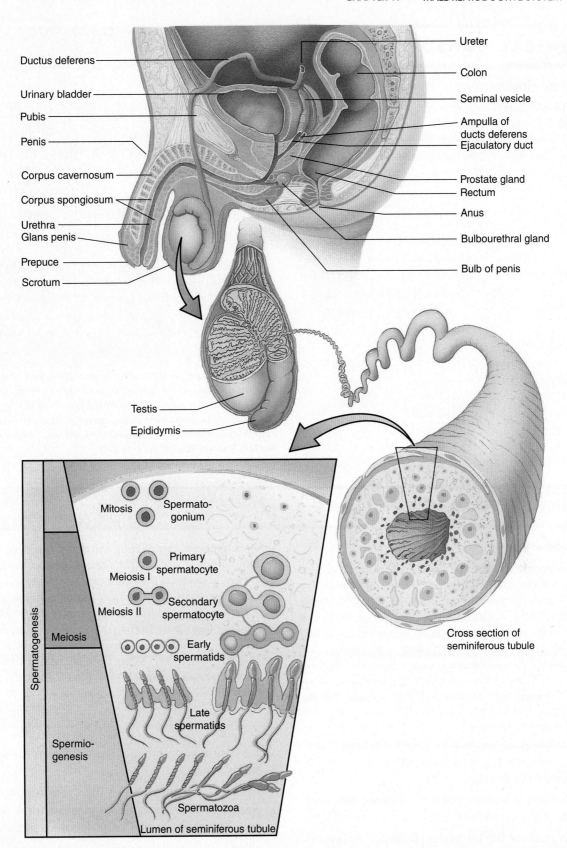

FIGURE 19-1. Schematic illustration of the male reproductive system, including the microscopic structure of the seminiferous tubule. Each testis is subdivided into ~250 lobules, lobuli testis, housing one to four highly convoluted **seminiferous tubules**. The wall of the seminiferous tubule is composed of slender connective tissue elements whose chief cellular components are **fibroblasts**. The **seminiferous (germinal) epithelium** is composed of spermatogenic cells and Sertoli cells. It is the **spermatogenic cells** that undergo **mitosis, meiosis**, and **spermiogenesis**. The **Sertoli cells** form zonulae occludentes with each other, thus separating the lumen of the seminiferous tubules into two concentric spaces.

CLINICAL CONSIDERATIONS 19-1

Cryptorchidism

Cryptorchidism is a developmental defect in which one or both testes fail to descend into the scrotum. When neither descends, it results in sterility because normal body temperature inhibits spermatogenesis. Usually, the condition can be surgically corrected; however, the patient's sperm may be abnormal.

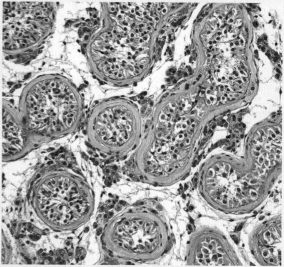

This figure is from the testis of a postpubertal patient demonstrating the absence of spermatogenesis in the seminiferous tubule as well as a very thick, hyalinized basement membrane. (Reprinted with permission from Strayer DS, et al., eds. *Rubin's Pathology: Mechanisms of Human Disease*, 8th ed. Philadelphia: Wolters Kluwer, 2020. Figure 23-27.)

CLINICAL CONSIDERATIONS 19-2

Scrotal Hyperthermia

The development of normal, healthy spermatozoa requires a lower intrascrotal temperature, about 35°C, than the normal body temperature of 36.5°C to 37.5°C. In order to maintain the appropriate testicular temperature, the dartos and the cremaster muscles move the testes farther away from or closer to the body wall. Additionally, the pampiniform plexus of veins cools the blood that the testicular arteries bring to the testes. In a "natural environment," the scrotum is not enclosed in clothing and the ambient temperature also cools the testes. However, men wearing jockey shorts bring the testes close to the body wall, thereby elevating the intrascrotal temperature. In the past 30 or so years, the advent of laptop computers has added an additional source that aggravates this problem. The heat generated by laptops sitting on the individual's lap for an hour or two can increase the intrascrotal temperature by almost 3°C. It has been suggested that this increase in temperature in the vicinity of the testicles may have deleterious effects on spermatogenesis.

- Formation of an apoprotein, called **testicular transferrin**, that transfers iron from serum transferrin to the developing gametes.

- Physical and nutritive support of spermatocytes, spermatids, and spermatozoa.

- Phagocytosis of the cytoplasm discarded by spermatids during spermiogenesis.

- Synthesis of a **transmission factor** that promotes the maintenance of stem cells responsible for gametogenesis.

- Manufacturing and releasing **Fas ligand**, a molecule, that drives cells, such as cytotoxic T lymphocytes, possessing **Fas receptors** into apoptosis, thereby preventing an immune response within the adluminal compartment.

- Secretion of a fructose-rich fluid that supports spermatozoa and provides a fluid medium for their transport through the seminiferous tubules and the genital ducts.

- Production, during embryonic development, of **antimüllerian hormone (müllerian-inhibiting factor)**, which triggers apoptosis of the müllerian ducts, thus ensuring the development of a male rather than a female genital tract. Additionally, the presence of dihydrotestosterone in the fetus encourages the

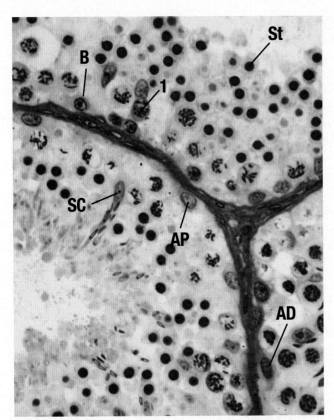

FIGURE 19-2. This high-magnification photomicrograph of three seminiferous tubule profiles display the three types of spermatogonia, **pale type A** (AP), **dark type A** (AD), and **type B** (B). Note the numerous **primary spermatocytes** (1), the **spermatids** (St), and the spermatozoa ensconced in the cytoplasmic processes of **Sertoli cells** (SC). Because secondary spermatocytes are short-lived, they are rarely seen in photomicrographs. The walls of seminiferous tubules are composed of slender connective tissue elements, known as the tunica propria, populated by fibroblasts and myoid cells. ×540.

development of male genitalia, whereas in its absence the female genitalia will develop even if the chromosomal complement calls for a male phenotype.

Spermatogenesis

Spermatogenesis, the process of producing haploid male gametes, has three phases (Table 19-2).

- **Spermatocytogenesis** is a process involving *mitosis* and maturation of diploid spermatogonia into diploid primary oocytes. **Pale type A spermatogonia** undergo mitosis to form two types of spermatogonia, more pale type A as well as **type B** spermatogonia, both of which are diploid. Type B spermatogonia divide via mitosis to form diploid **primary spermatocytes**. **Dark type A spermatogonia** represent a reserve population of cells that normally do not undergo cell division, but when they do, they form pale type A spermatogonia. All spermatogonia are located in the **basal compartment**, whereas primary spermatocytes migrate into the **adluminal compartment**.

- **Meiosis phase** starts when primary spermatocytes (**diploid cells, 2N**) undergo the first meiotic division, forming two **haploid (N) secondary spermatocytes**. Secondary spermatocytes immediately start the second meiotic division, in which chromatids separate, and each forms two **haploid (N) spermatids**.

- **Spermiogenesis** (see Fig. 19-3) is the process of cytodifferentiation of the spermatids into spermatozoa and involves no cell division. Instead, the spermatid loses much of its cytoplasm (the discarded cytoplasm is phagocytosed by Sertoli cells), forms an **acrosomal granule**, a long **cilium** known as a flagellum (plural **flagella**), associated **outer dense fibers**, and a **coarse**

Table 19-1	Selected Functions of Sertoli Cells
During Gestation	**After Puberty**
Synthesize and release antimüllerian hormone (müllerian-inhibiting factor) to suppress the formation of the female genital system and support the development of the male genital system	Physical and nutritional support of developing germ cells
	Synthesize and release ABP
	Establish blood–testis barrier
	Phagocytose cytoplasm shed during spermiogenesis
	Synthesize and release the hormone inhibin, which prevents the release of FSH by the adenohypophysis
	Synthesize and release the hormone activin, which prompts the release of FSH by the adenohypophysis
	Synthesize and release the apoprotein testicular transferrin that functions in transferring iron from serum transferrin to the developing gametes
	Secrete fructose-rich medium to provide nutrients for spermatozoa released into the male genital ducts

ABP, androgen-binding protein; FSH, follicle-stimulating hormone.

Table 19-2 Types of Spermatogenic Cells and Their Characteristics	
Spermatogonia	
Pale type A spermatogonia	possess a pale-staining nucleus, spherical mitochondria, a small Golgi complex, and abundant, free ribosomes. They are **mitotically active** (starting at puberty) and give rise either to more cells of the same type (to maintain the supply) or to type B spermatogonia.
Dark type A spermatogonia	represent mitotically **inactive** (reserve) cells (in the G_0 phase of the cell cycle) with dark nuclei; they have the potential to resume mitosis and produce pale type A cells.
Type B spermatogonia	undergo mitosis and give rise to primary spermatocytes.
Spermatocytes	
Primary spermatocytes	are large **diploid** cells with 4cDNA content. They undergo the **first meiotic division** (reductional division) to form secondary spermatocytes.
Secondary spermatocytes	are **haploid** cells with 2cDNA that quickly undergo the **second meiotic division** (equatorial division), without an intervening S phase, to form spermatids.
Spermatids	
Spermatids	are small **haploid** cells (containing only **1cDNA**) located near the lumen of the seminiferous tubule. Their nuclei often display regions of condensed chromatin. They possess a pair of centrioles, mitochondria, free ribosomes, SER, and a well-developed Golgi complex.

Reprinted with permission from Gartner LP. *BRS Cell Biology and Histology*, 8th ed. Philadelphia: Wolters Kluwer, 2019. p. 367.

fibrous sheath. The **spermatozoon** that is formed and released into the lumen of the seminiferous tubule is **nonmotile** and is incapable of fertilizing an ovum. The spermatozoa remain immotile until they leave the epididymis and become capable of fertilizing an ovum once they have been **capacitated** in the female reproductive system.

The process of spermatogenesis is dependent on several hormones, including **luteinizing hormone (LH)**, **prolactin**, and **FSH** from the adenohypophysis (see Fig. 19-3). Prolactin induces the interstitial cells of Leydig to express an increased number of **LH receptors**. Once LH binds to its receptors on the Leydig cells, these cells secrete **testosterone**, and, as noted above, FSH causes Sertoli cells to release **androgen-binding protein (ABP)**. ABP maintains a high enough concentration of testosterone in the seminiferous epithelium for spermatogenesis to occur.

Spermatogenesis occurs in a cyclic but asynchronous fashion along the length of the seminiferous tubule. These **cycles of the seminiferous epithelium** consist of repeated aggregates of cells undergoing spermatogenesis in varying stages of development. Each aggregate is composed of groups of spermatogenic cells that are connected to one another by **intercellular bridges**, forming a synchronized syncytium that migrates toward the lumen of the seminiferous tubule as a unit.

Interstitial Cells of Leydig

The loose, vascular connective tissue surrounding the seminiferous tubules houses, in addition to neural and vascular elements, small clusters of androgen-producing

CLINICAL CONSIDERATIONS 19-3

Control of Luteinizing Hormone and Follicle-Stimulating Hormone Release

Testosterone, manufactured by the interstitial cells of Leydig, acts as **negative feedback** for LH release; **inhibin**, produced by Sertoli cells, inhibits the release of **FSH**, whereas **activin**, also produced by Sertoli cells, enhances **FSH** release.

endocrine cells, the interstitial cells of Leydig (Fig. 19-4). These polygon-shaped cells usually possess a single nucleus with two or three dark nucleoli. As demonstrated by transmission electron microscopy, their **cytoplasm** houses an abundance of smooth ER, lipid deposits, and mitochondria with tubular cristae, all typical of endocrine cells that manufacture steroid hormones. These cells, at least in humans, also house crystalline inclusions, known as crystals of Reinke, whose function is not known. Beginning at puberty, interstitial cells of Leydig produce the male sex hormone testosterone (which makes spermatogenesis possible) and insulin-like factor 3 (INSL 3), which sustains spermatogenic cells by shielding them from entering apoptosis.

Genital Ducts

A system of **genital ducts** conveys the spermatozoa and the fluid component of the semen to the outside.

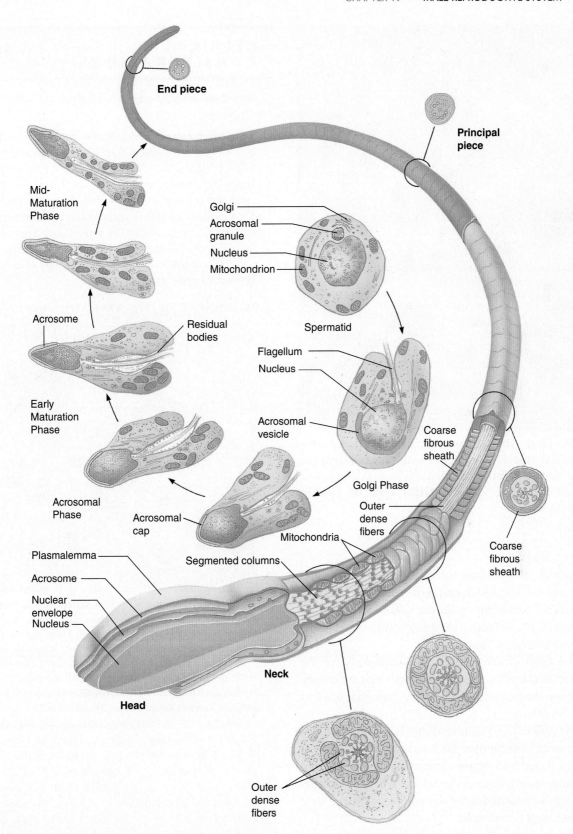

End piece

Principal piece

Mid-Maturation Phase

Golgi
Acrosomal granule
Nucleus
Mitochondrion

Acrosome
Residual bodies

Spermatid

Early Maturation Phase

Flagellum
Nucleus

Acrosomal vesicle

Coarse fibrous sheath

Acrosomal Phase

Acrosomal cap

Golgi Phase

Outer dense fibers

Coarse fibrous sheath

Mitochondria

Plasmalemma

Segmented columns

Acrosome

Nuclear envelope
Nucleus

Neck

Head

Outer dense fibers

FIGURE 19-3. Schematic diagram of a spermatid becoming transformed into a spermatozoon whose morphology is illustrated in three dimensions as well as in cross sections.

- The **seminiferous tubules** are connected by short straight tubules, the **tubuli recti**, to the **rete testis**, which is composed of labyrinthine spaces located within the **mediastinum testis**.

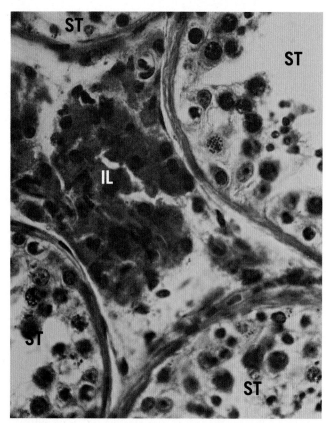

FIGURE 19-4. This high-magnification photomicrograph of the vascular connective tissue surrounding the **seminiferous tubules** (ST) displays a collection of testosterone-producing **interstitial cells of Leydig** (IL). ×540.

- From here, spermatozoa enter the first part of the **epididymis**, the 15 to 20 **ductuli efferentes** that lead into the second part of the epididymis, the **ductus epididymis** (Fig. 19-5). During their sojourn in the epididymis, spermatozoa mature.
  - The head of the epididymis is composed of the ductuli efferentes, whereas the body and tail consist of the ductus epididymis, a structure that is ~5 m in length.
  - The wall of the ductus epididymis is composed of a **smooth muscle coat** surrounding a loose connective tissue and a **pseudostratified stereociliated epithelium** that lines the lumen, where the epithelium is separated from the connective tissue by a basement membrane.
  - The epithelium is composed of short regenerative **basal cells** and tall **principal cells**.
  - These **principal cells** sport stereocilia (long, nonmotile microvilli) that phagocytose cytoplasmic remnants from spermiogenesis; phagocytose almost 90% of the fluid in the lumen; and synthesize and release the glycoprotein, **glycerophosphocholine**, which inhibits **capacitation** (the ability of the

CLINICAL CONSIDERATIONS 19-4

Testicular Cancer and Leydig Cell Tumors

Testicular cancer affects mostly men younger than age 40 years. It is discovered on palpation as a lump in the scrotum. If the lump is not associated with the testis it is usually benign, whereas if it is associated with the testis it is usually malignant; therefore, a lump noticed on the testis, whether or not it is painful, should be examined by a physician. Frequently, individuals with testicular cancer present with elevated blood α-**fetoprotein** and **human chorionic gonadotropin** levels.

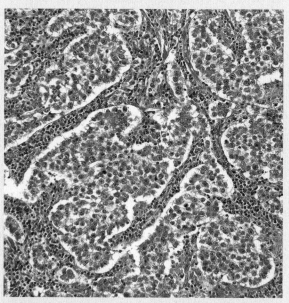

This figure is from the testis of a patient with a form of testicular cancer known as seminoma. Observe the clusters of tumor cells with large nuclei. These cells are enveloped by a connective tissue septa that appear quite cellular owing to the lymphocytic infiltration. (Reprinted with permission from Strayer DS, et al., eds. *Rubin's Pathology: Mechanisms of Human Disease*, 8th ed. Philadelphia: Wolters Kluwer, 2020. Figure 23-36B.)

Leydig cell tumors are unusual because they occur either in early childhood (age 5 to 10 years) or in middle-aged adults (age 30 to 60 years). They are usually encapsulated, can be as large as 10 cm in diameter, and usually present with a lobulated morphology. Histologically, the tumor cells resemble Leydig cells but are composed of many more cells, and their nuclei house a single, large, centrally located nucleolus. Approximately 30% of the cells possess Reinke crystals. Clinical signs in males include an enlarged and, frequently, tender testis; in young children, the production of a significant amount of testosterone may initiate early puberty. Fortunately, only 10% of the tumors are malignant; therefore, 90% of the tumors can be eliminated by orchiectomy.

spermatozoon to fertilize an ovum after it enters the female genital tract).

- Spermatozoa become **motile** near the end of the body of the epididymis.

- The head of spermatozoa picks up **glycerophosphocholine** from the fluid present in the lumen of the epididymis, which prevents them from being able to fertilize an ovum until that factor is removed from their plasma membrane in the female genital tract.

The **ductus deferens (vas deferens)** is the continuation of the tail of the epididymis (see Fig. 19-1). This thick, muscular structure passes through the inguinal canal, as a part of the spermatic cord, to gain access to the abdominal cavity. It is this structure that permits palpation of the spermatic cord through the wall of the scrotum.

- Just prior to reaching the prostate gland, the **seminal vesicle** empties its secretions into the ductus deferens, which terminates at this point.

- The continuation of the ductus deferens through the **prostate gland** is known as the **ejaculatory duct**. The prostate gland delivers its secretory product into the ejaculatory duct.
  - **The** right **and** left ejaculatory ducts **empty into the** prostatic urethra (**described below**), **which conveys both urine and semen to the outside.**

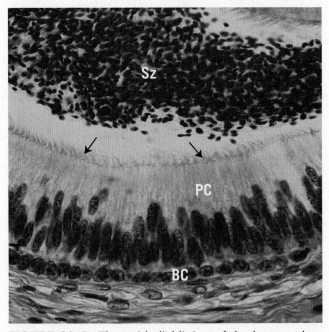

FIGURE 19-5. The epithelial lining of the human ductus epididymis is composed of short **basal cells** (BC) and tall, columnar **principal cells** (PC) whose stereocilia (*arrows*) protrude into the **spermatozoa** (Sz)-filled lumen. ×540.

Accessory Genital Glands

The **accessory glands** of the male reproductive system are the two **seminal vesicles** the **prostate gland** and the pair of small **bulbourethral glands**.

Seminal Vesicle

Each **seminal vesicle** is a 15-cm long, narrow gland that is highly folded on itself; they are located on the posterior aspect of the urinary bladder near its neck.

- The **pseudostratified columnar epithelium** that lines the lumen of the gland (Fig. 19-6) is composed of short regenerative **basal cells** and low columnar cells whose height is directly dependent on plasma testosterone levels. The columnar cells have short, stubby microvilli, a normal organelle content, lipid droplets, yellow, lipochrome pigment granules, as well as numerous secretory vesicles. The seminal vesicles produce a nutritive secretion rich in fructose, with a characteristic yellow color that constitutes ~70% of the ejaculate volume.

- The fibroelastic subepithelial connective tissue, known as the **lamina propria**, is surrounded by an inner circular and an outer longitudinal **smooth muscle coat** which is invested by a thin connective tissue **adventitia**.

- The **duct** of each seminal vesicle joins the ampulla of each ductus deferens forming the two **ejaculatory ducts** that penetrate the prostate gland to enter the urethra.

Prostate Gland

The **prostate gland** (Fig. 19-7) is composed of numerous individual **branched tubuloacinar glands** that surround, and whose ducts pierce, the wall of the prostatic urethra.

The gland possesses a fibroelastic capsule enriched with smooth muscle cells. Septa of the capsule infiltrate the substance of the gland, subdividing it into lobes.

- These glands are distributed into three concentric regions around the urethra and are named **mucosal**, **submucosal**, and **external (main) prostatic glands**.

- A **simple columnar** to **pseudostratified columnar epithelium** that lines the individual glands comprising the prostate is composed of two types of cells, short basal and low columnar. The former are regenerative cells whereas the latter manufacture and release the prostatic secretion.

  - The secretion of the prostate gland, regulated by testosterone, is a whitish, thin fluid containing **fibrinolysin**, **citric acid**, **serine protease (prostate-specific antigen, PSA)**, and **acid phosphatase**.

  - The secretions of the prostate gland are white in color and constitute ~30% of the ejaculate volume.

- **Prostatic concretions (corpora amylacea)**, whose function is not known, are frequently present in the lumina of the prostate gland. They increase in number with the age of the individual.

Bulbourethral Glands (Cowper's Glands)

The small, paired **bulbourethral glands (Cowper's glands)** are situated at the junction of the prostatic and membranous portions of the urethra. The fibroelastic connective tissue capsule of this gland contains some skeletal muscle fibers in addition to the fibroblasts and smooth muscle cells. Septa, derived from the capsule, subdivide this **compound tubuloacinar gland** into small lobules whose **simple cuboidal** to a **simple columnar** epithelial lining secretes a slippery fluid that is released into the membranous urethra, lubricating it just prior to the release of the ejaculate.

Urethra

The male **urethra** is ~20 cm long and extends from the urinary bladder to the tip of the penis, conveying urine from the bladder (and, during ejaculation, semen from the right and left ejaculatory ducts). It has three regions, named according to their locations:

- The 3- to 4-cm long **prostatic urethra** that pierces the substance of the prostate gland, whose lumen is lined by transitional epithelium.

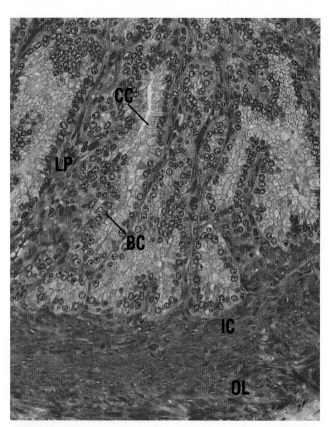

FIGURE 19-6. This medium-magnification photomicrograph of a monkey seminal vesicle displays the **short basal** (BC) and low **columnar** (CC) **cells** of the pseudostratified columnar epithelium, the **lamina propria** (LP), as well as its **inner circular** (IC) and **outer longitudinal** (OL) **smooth muscle layers**. ×270.

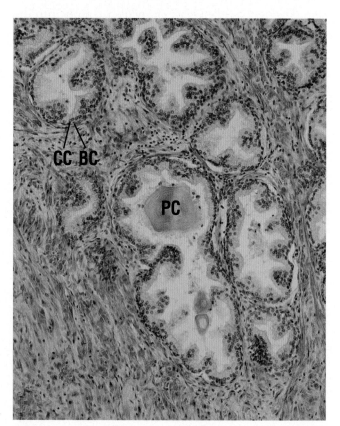

FIGURE 19-7. This low-magnification photomicrograph of the human prostate gland displays the smooth muscle cells, the two types of epithelial cells, short **basal cells** (BC) and the **columnar cells** (CC), as well as the **prostatic concretions** (PC) in the lumen. ×132.

CLINICAL CONSIDERATIONS 19-6

Benign Prostatic Hypertrophy and Adenocarcinoma of the Prostate

The prostate gland undergoes hypertrophy with age, resulting in **benign prostatic hypertrophy** (**BPH**), a condition that may constrict the urethral lumen, resulting in difficulty in urination. At age 50, about 40% of the male population is affected, and at age 80, about 95% of the male population is affected by this condition.

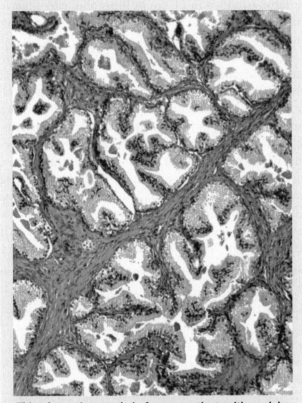

This photomicrograph is from a patient with nodular hyperplasia of the prostate. Observe that the gland is displaying cellular hypertrophy of the epithelium whose folding, in places, partially occludes its lumen. (Reprinted with permission from Strayer DS, et al., eds. *Rubin's Pathology: Mechanisms of Human Disease*, 8th ed. Philadelphia: Wolters Kluwer, 2020. Figure 23-45C.)

Adenocarcinoma of the prostate affects about 30% of the male population older than 75 years. Although this carcinoma is slow growing, it may metastasize to bone. Analysis of elevated levels of **prostate-specific antigen** (**PSA**) in the bloodstream is utilized as an early diagnostic test for prostatic cancer. Biopsy is required for accurate diagnosis.

- The 1- to 2-cm long **membranous urethra** that passes through the floor of the pelvis (perineum), whose lumen is lined by pseudostratified or stratified columnar epithelium.

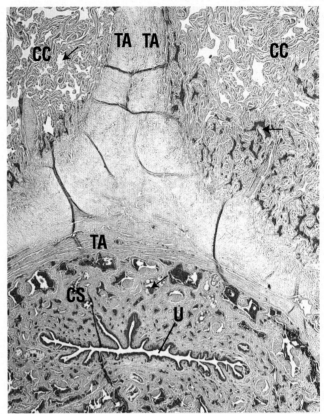

FIGURE 19-8. This very low-magnification cross section of a penis displays parts of the two **corpora cavernosa** (CC) and the single **corpus spongiosum** (CS). Observe the slit-like penile portion of the **urethra** (U), whose lumen is lined by a pseudostratified or stratified columnar epithelium. Note also the vascular spaces (*arrows*) within the erectile tissues of all three corpora as well as the **tunica albuginea** (TA) surrounding the three corpora. ×14.

- Skeletal muscle fibers from the perineum encircle the membranous urethra, forming the **external sphincter muscle** of the urethra, permitting voluntary control over the process of urination.

- The ~15-cm long **cavernous urethra** (**spongy urethra, penile urethra**) that passes through the length of the **penis** (Fig. 19-8), and its lumen is
  - lined by pseudostratified or stratified columnar epithelium.
  - The distal, expanded end of the cavernous urethra, located in the **glans penis**, called the **fossa navicularis**, is lined by a stratified squamous, nonkeratinized epithelium.

The richly vascularized fibroelastic connective tissue composing the **lamina propria** of all three regions of the urethra possesses mucous **glands of Littré**, whose secretion lubricates the lumen of the urethra. The entire urethra possesses an **inner longitudinal** and an **outer circular layer of smooth muscle** cells. The smooth muscle layers assist in moving the urine along the length of the urethra but do not contribute to the voluntary control of urination.

Penis

The **penis** transports urine to the outside and is also the male organ of copulation delivering semen into the female reproductive tract. It has three bodies composed of **erectile tissue**, the two dorsally positioned **corpora cavernosa** and a single, ventrally located **corpus spongiosum** (see Fig. 19-8). The distal end of the corpus spongiosum is expanded, forming the **glans penis** (head of the penis). Each of the three corpora possesses its own fibrous connective tissue capsule known as the **tunica albuginea**. The entire penis is invested by a thin skin that extends over the glans penis as a retractable wrapping, known as the **prepuce**.

Erection

Each erectile body, housing large endothelially lined **cavernous spaces**, is supplied by **helicine arteries** that are usually bypassed via arteriovenous shunts, maintaining the penis in a flaccid state. **Parasympathetic impulses** to these shunts cause vasoconstriction, directing blood into the helicine arteries whose smooth muscles become relaxed due to the local release of nitric oxide and thus blood flows into the cavernous spaces of the corpora cavernosa and corpus spongiosum. The erectile bodies (especially the two corpora cavernosa) become engorged with blood, and the fluid turgid pressure within the vascular spaces of the erectile tissues greatly enlarges the penis, causing it to become **erect** and **hard**. Subsequent to ejaculation or in the absence of continued stimulation, parasympathetic stimulation ceases; blood flow to the helicine arteries is diminished and blood slowly leaves the cavernous spaces. Detumescence follows, and the penis returns to its flaccid state.

Ejaculation

Ejaculation is the forceful expulsion of **semen** from the male reproductive tract. The force required for ejaculation is derived from rhythmic contraction of the thick smooth muscle layers of the **ductus (vas) deferens** and the rapid contraction of the **bulbospongiosus muscle** situated at and surrounding the proximal end of the corpus spongiosum.

Each ejaculate contains 200 to 400 million spermatozoa suspended in about 3 to 4 mL of **seminal fluid**. The accessory glands of the male reproductive system, the **prostate** and **bulbourethral glands**, as well as the **seminal vesicles** (and even the glands of Littré), contribute to the formation of the fluid portion of semen. Secretions of the bulbourethral glands lubricate the urethra, whereas secretions of the prostate assist the spermatozoa in achieving motility by neutralizing the acidic secretions of the ductus deferens and the female reproductive tract. Energy for the spermatozoa is provided by fructose-rich secretions of the seminal vesicles.

CLINICAL CONSIDERATIONS 19-7

Balanoposthitis and Phimosis

Accumulation of a thick, yellowish-white exudate underneath the foreskin of uncircumcised men can be a breeding ground for yeast and bacteria that, if not cleaned, may cause inflammation of the foreskin, known as **posthitis**, as well as inflammation of the glans penis, known as **balanitis**. When the two occur together, the condition is known as **balanoposthitis**. The condition may be accompanied by redness, pain, and itching as well as a swelling of the glans with a concomitant stricture of the urethra.

Phimosis, a tight foreskin that cannot easily be pulled over the glans penis, is a normal condition in uncircumcised infants, but in mature men the condition can be very painful and may result in interference with urination and sexual activity. As the penis becomes erect, the foreskin cannot expand to accommodate the increased girth and may result in balanoposthitis and urinary tract infections. Circumcision can usually alleviate this condition.

CLINICAL CONSIDERATIONS 19-8

Infertility

Approximately 7% of all men are **infertile**, that is, they are unable to father a child with a fertile woman. There are many possible reasons for infertility in males, such as chromosomal abnormalities; use of alcohol, tobacco, illicit drugs, and certain prescription medications; production of abnormal spermatozoa; having increased intrascrotal temperature. **Hypospermia**, a greatly reduced volume of ejaculate, is often associated with infertility containing less than 20 to 40 million spermatozoa per ejaculate. Interestingly, a study of more than 40,000 men from Europe, North America, New Zealand, and Australia indicated that there was a 50% decrease in sperm count in 2015 compared with sperm count in 1980 and the spermatozoa had reduced motility.

PLATE 19-1A   Testis

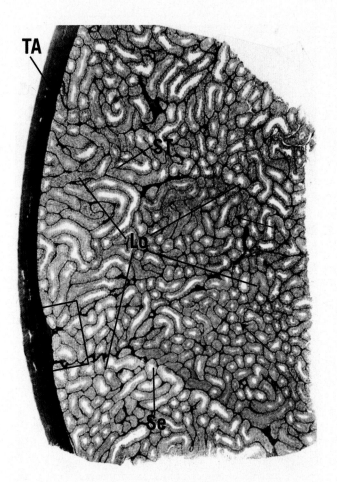

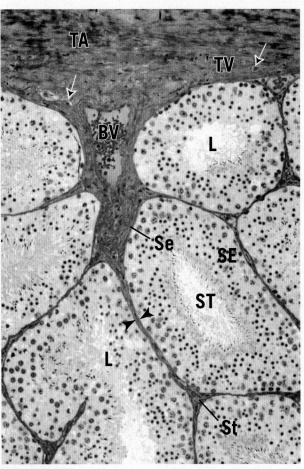

FIGURE 19-1-1. Testis. Monkey. Plastic section. ×14.

This low-magnification photomicrograph of the testis displays its thick **tunica albuginea** (TA), as well as the slender **septa** (Se) that attach to it. Observe that sections of **seminiferous tubules** (ST) present various geometric profiles, attesting to their highly convoluted form. Note that each **lobule** (Lo) is densely packed with seminiferous tubules, and the connective tissue stroma (*arrows*) occupies the remaining space. A region similar to the *boxed area* is presented at a higher magnification in Figure 19-1-2.

FIGURE 19-1-2. Testis. Seminiferous tubules. Monkey. Plastic section. ×132.

This photomicrograph is a higher magnification of a region similar to the *boxed area* of Figure 19-1-1. Observe that the **tunica vasculosa** (TV) of the **tunica albuginea** (TA) is a highly vascular region (*arrows*) and that **blood vessels** (BV) penetrate the lobuli testis in connective tissue **septa** (Se). The walls of the **seminiferous tubules** (ST) are closely apposed to each other (*arrowheads*), although in certain regions the cellular **stroma** (St) is evident. Observe that the **lumen** (L) of the seminiferous tubule is lined by a stratified **seminiferous epithelium** (SE).

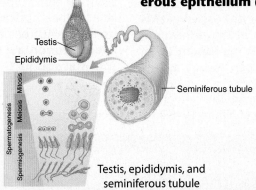

Testis, epididymis, and seminiferous tubule

KEY					
BV	blood vessel	**SE**	seminiferous epithelium	**St**	stroma
L	lumen	**Se**	septum	**TA**	tunica albuginea
Lo	lobule	**ST**	seminiferous tubules	**TV**	tunica vasculosa

PLATE 19-1B   Testis

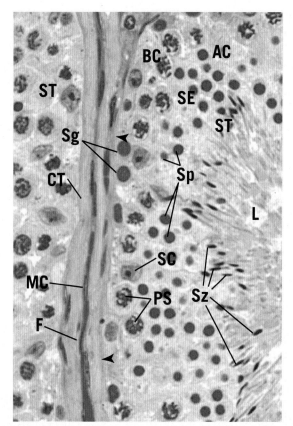

FIGURE 19-1-3. Testis. Seminiferous tubule. Monkey. Plastic section. ×540.

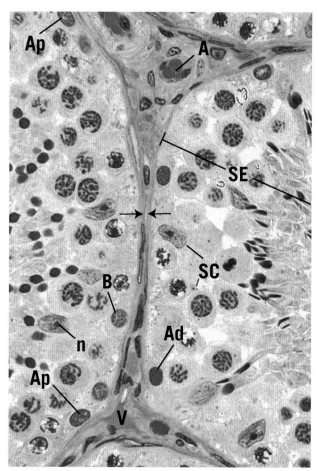

FIGURE 19-1-4. Testis. Seminiferous tubule. Monkey. Plastic section. ×540.

The adjacent walls of two **seminiferous tubules** (ST), in close proximity to each other, are composed of **myoid cells** (MC), **fibroblasts** (F), and fibromuscular **connective tissue** (CT). The stratified **seminiferous epithelium** (SE) is separated from the tubular wall by a basal membrane (*arrowheads*). **Spermatogonia** (Sg) lie on the basal membrane and are in the **basal compartment** (BC). The tall **Sertoli cells** (SC) span the thickness of the epithelium with their basal cell membranes in contact with the basement membrane and their apical cell membranes in contact with the lumen. The lateral membranes form tight junctions with neighboring Sertoli cells, partitioning the lumen into basal and adluminal compartments. **Primary spermatocytes** (PS), secondary spermatocytes, **spermatids** (Sp), and **spermatozoa** (Sz) are in the **adluminal compartment** (AC). Observe that the **lumen** (L) of the seminiferous tubule contains spermatozoa as well as cellular debris discarded during the transformation of spermatids into spermatozoa. Compare the cells of the seminiferous epithelium with those of Figure 19-1-4.

Observe that the fibromuscular walls of the two tubular cross sections are very close to each other (*arrows*); however, in regions, **arterioles** (A) and **venules** (V) are evident. The **Sertoli cells** (SC) may be recognized by their pale nuclei and dense **nucleoli** (n). In comparing the **seminiferous epithelia** (SE) of the tubules in the right and left halves of this photomicrograph, as well as those of Figure 19-1-3, it should be noted that their cellular compositions are different, indicative of the cyclic stages of the seminiferous epithelium. Note also that three types of spermatogonia are recognizable by their nuclear characteristics: **dark spermatogonia A** (Ad) possessing dark, flattened nuclei; **pale spermatogonia A** (Ap) with flattened pale nuclei; and **spermatogonia B** (B) with round nuclei.

KEY					
A	arterioles	**F**	fibroblast	**SE**	seminiferous epithelium
AC	adluminal compartment	**L**	lumen	**Sg**	spermatogonia
Ad	dark spermatogonia A	**MC**	myoid cell	**Sp**	spermatid
Ap	pale spermatogonia A	**n**	nucleoli	**ST**	seminiferous tubules
B	spermatogonia B	**PS**	primary spermatocyte	**Sz**	spermatozoa
BC	basal compartment	**SC**	Sertoli cell	**V**	venule
CT	connective tissue				

PLATE 19-2A   Testis

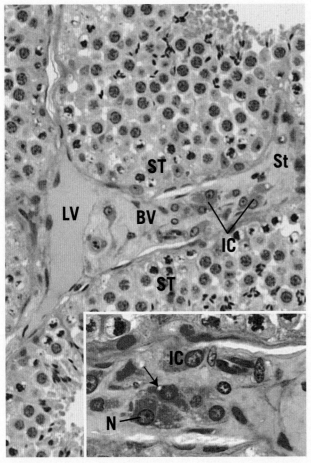

FIGURE 19-2-1. Interstitial cells. Testis. Monkey. Plastic section. ×270.

The **stroma** (St) surrounding **seminiferous tubules** (ST) possesses a rich **vascular supply** (BV) as well as extensive **lymphatic drainage** (LV). Much of the vascular elements are associated with the endocrine cells of the testis, the **interstitial cells of Leydig** (IC), which produce testosterone. *Inset*. **Interstitial cells**. **Testis**. **Monkey**. **Plastic section**. ×540. The **interstitial cells** (IC), located in small clumps, are recognizable by their round-to-oval **nuclei** (N) and the presence of lipid (*arrow*) within their cytoplasm.

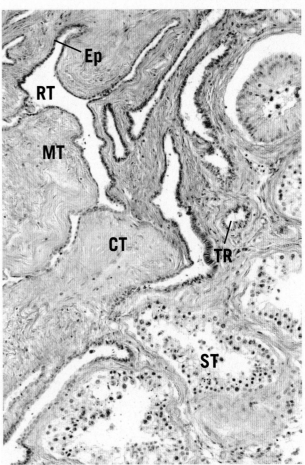

FIGURE 19-2-2. Rete testis. Human. Paraffin section. ×132.

The **rete testis** (RT), located in the **mediastinum testis** (MT), is composed of labyrinthine, anastomosing spaces lined by a simple cuboidal **epithelium** (Ep). The dense collagenous **connective tissue** (CT) of the mediastinum testis is evident, as are the profiles of **seminiferous tubules** (ST). Spermatozoa gain access to the rete testis via the short, straight **tubuli recti** (TR).

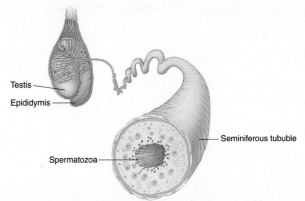

Testis, epididymis, and seminiferous tubule

KEY					
BV	blood vessel	**LV**	lymphatic vessels	**ST**	seminiferous tubules
CT	connective tissue	**MT**	mediastinum testis	**St**	stroma
Ep	epithelium	**N**	nuclei	**TR**	tubuli recti
IC	interstitial cells of Leydig	**RT**	rete testis		

PLATE 19-2B Epididymis

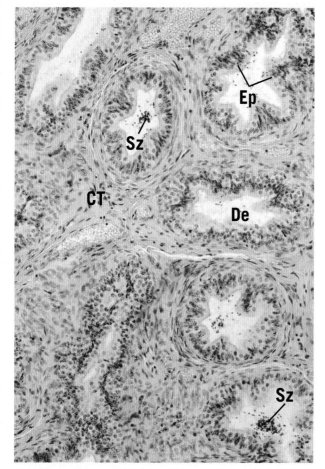

FIGURE 19-2-3. Ductuli efferentes. Human. Paraffin section. ×132.

The first part of the epididymis, the **ductuli efferentes** (De), receives **spermatozoa** (Sz) from the rete testis. The lumina of the ductuli are lined by a simple columnar **epithelium** (Ep), composed of tall and short cells, which are responsible for the characteristic fluted (uneven) appearance of these tubules. The thick fibroelastic **connective tissue** (CT) wall of the ductuli houses numerous smooth muscle cells (SM).

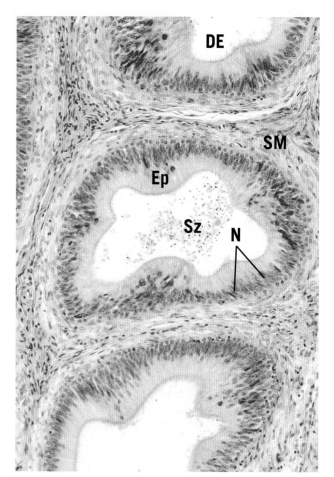

FIGURE 19-2-4. Ductus epididymis. Monkey. Plastic section. ×132.

The **ductus epididymis** (DE) may be distinguished from the ductuli efferentes with relative ease. Note that the **nuclei** (N) of the pseudostratified **epithelial lining** (Ep) are of two types, oval and round, whereas those of the ductuli are round. Observe that the lumen contains numerous **spermatozoa** (Sz) and that the epithelium sits on a basal lamina. The connective tissue wall of the ductus epididymis may be differentiated easily from its circularly arranged **smooth muscle coat** (SM).

KEY					
CT	connective tissue	Ep	epithelium	SM	smooth muscle
DE	ductus epididymis	N	nuclei	Sz	spermatozoa
De	ductuli efferentes				

PLATE 19-3A   Epididymis and Ductus Deferens

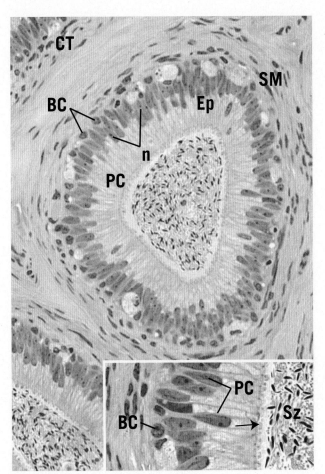

FIGURE 19-3-1. Ductus epididymis. Monkey. Plastic section. ×270.

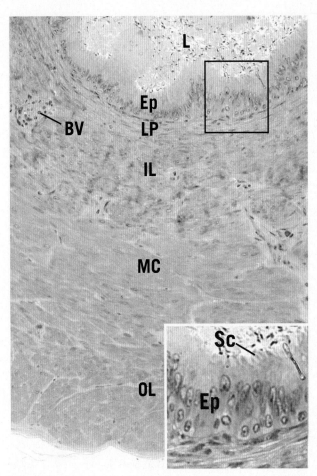

FIGURE 19-3-2. Ductus deferens. Monkey. Plastic section. ×132.

The pseudostratified stereociliated columnar **epithelium** (Ep) lining the lumen of the ductus epididymis is composed of two types of cells: short **basal cells** (BC), recognizable by their round nuclei, and tall columnar **principal cells** (PC), whose oval nuclei display one or more **nucleoli** (n). The **smooth muscle** (SM) cells, composing the wall of the epididymis, are circularly oriented and are surrounded by **connective tissue** (CT) elements. *Inset.* **Ductus epididymis. Monkey. Plastic section.** ×540. Observe the round nuclei of the **basal cells** (BC) and oval nuclei of the **principal cells** (PC). Clumped stereocilia (*arrows*) extend into the **spermatozoa** (Sz)-filled lumen.

Epididymis

The ductus deferens is a thick-walled, muscular tube that conveys spermatozoa from the ductus epididymis to the ejaculatory duct. The thick, muscular coat is composed of three layers of smooth muscle: **outer longitudinal** (OL), **middle circular** (MC), and **inner longitudinal** (IL). The fibroelastic **lamina propria** (LP) receives its **vascular supply** (BV) from vessels (*arrow*) that penetrate the three muscle layers. A pseudostratified columnar **epithelium** (Ep) lines the spermatozoa-filled **lumen** (L). The boxed area is presented at a higher magnification in the inset. *Inset.* **Ductus deferens. Monkey. Plastic section.** ×270. A higher magnification of the pseudostratified columnar **epithelium** (Ep) displays the presence of **stereocilia** (Sc).

KEY					
BC	basal cell	**L**	lumen	**OL**	outer longitudinal muscle layer
BV	blood vessel	**LP**	lamina propria		
CT	connective tissue	**MC**	middle circular muscle layer	**PC**	principal cell
Ep	epithelium			**Sc**	stereocilia
IL	inner longitudinal muscle layer	**n**	nucleoli	**SM**	smooth muscle
				Sz	spermatozoa

PLATE 19-3B Seminal Vesicle

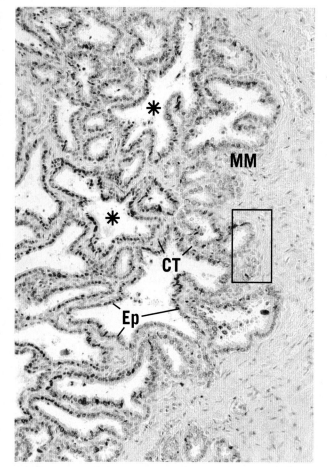

FIGURE 19-3-3. Seminal vesicle. Human. Paraffin section. ×132.

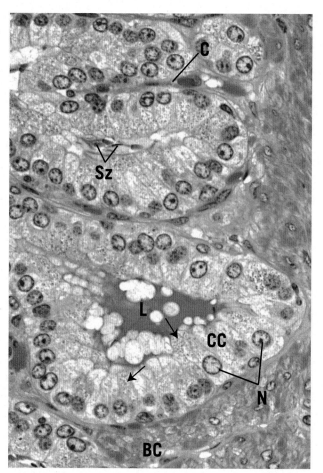

FIGURE 19-3-4. Seminal vesicle. Monkey. Plastic section. ×540.

The paired seminal vesicles are elongated tubular glands whose ducts join the ductus deferens just prior to the beginning of the ejaculatory ducts. The highly folded **mucous membrane** (MM) of the seminal vesicle is composed of pseudostratified **epithelium** (Ep) with a thin **connective tissue core** (CT). The folded membrane anastomoses with itself, partitioning off small spaces (*asterisks*) that, although continuous with the central lumen, appear to be discrete regions. A region similar to the *boxed area* is presented at a higher magnification in Figure 19-3-4.

This photomicrograph is a higher magnification of a region similar to the *boxed area* of Figure 19-3-3. Note that the tall **columnar cells** (CC) have basally located, round **nuclei** (N) and that their cytoplasm displays secretory granules (*arrows*). Short **basal cells** (BC) are occasionally present, which may function as regenerative cells for the epithelium. The secretory product is released into the **lumen** (L) as a thick fluid that coagulates in histologic sections. Observe the presence of numerous **capillaries** (C) in the connective tissue core deep to the epithelium. Although **spermatozoa** (Sz) are frequently noted in the lumen of the seminal vesicles, they are not stored in this structure.

KEY					
BC	basal cell	**CT**	connective tissue	**MM**	mucous membrane
C	capillaries	**Ep**	epithelium	**N**	nucleus
CC	columnar cell	**L**	lumen	**Sz**	spermatozoa

PLATE 19-4A Prostate

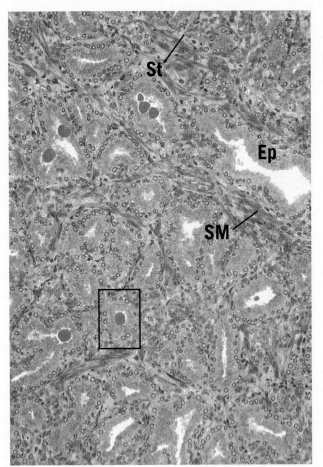

FIGURE 19-4-1. Prostate gland. Monkey. Plastic section. ×132.

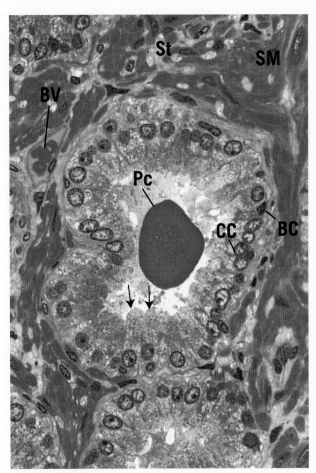

FIGURE 19-4-2. Prostate gland. Monkey. Plastic section. ×540.

The prostate gland, the largest of the male reproductive accessory glands, possesses a thick fibroelastic connective tissue capsule with which the connective tissue **stroma** (St) is continuous. Note that the stroma houses **smooth muscle** (SM) and blood vessels. The secretory portion of the prostate gland is composed of individual glands of varied shapes but consisting of a simple cuboidal-to-low columnar type of **epithelium** (Ep), although regions of pseudostratified columnar epithelia are readily apparent. A region similar to the *boxed area* is presented at a higher magnification in Figure 19-4-2.

This photomicrograph is a higher magnification of a region similar to the *boxed area* of Figure 19-4-1. Observe that the fibroelastic connective tissue **stroma** (St) presents numerous **blood vessels** (BV) and **smooth muscle cells** (SM). The parenchyma of the gland is composed of **columnar cells** (CC) as well as short **basal cells** (BC). Note that the dome-shaped apices (*arrows*) of some of the columnar cells appear to protrude into the lumen, which contains a **prostatic concretion** (Pc). The number of these concretions, which may calcify, increases with age.

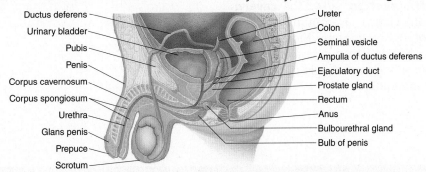

Male reproductive system

KEY					
BC	basal cell	**Ep**	epithelium	**SM**	smooth muscle
BV	blood vessel	**Pc**	prostatic concretion	**St**	stroma
CC	columnar cell				

PLATE 19-4B Penis and Urethra

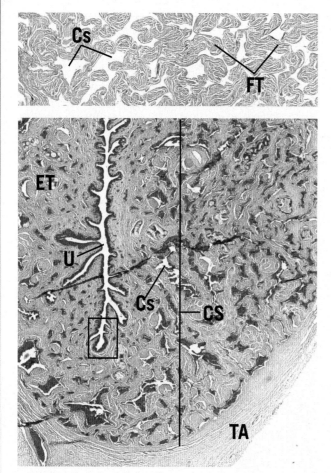

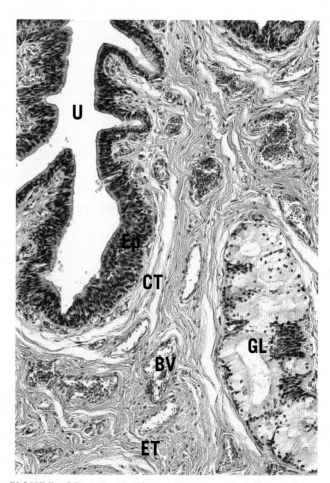

FIGURE 19-4-3. Penis. Human. x.s. Paraffin section. ×14.

FIGURE 19-4-4. Urethra. Human. Paraffin section. ×132.

The penis is composed of three erectile bodies: the two corpora cavernosa and the corpus spongiosum. The cross section of the **corpus spongiosum** (CS) displays the **urethra** (U), which is surrounded by **erectile tissue** (ET), whose irregular, endothelially lined **cavernous spaces** (Cs) contain blood. The spongy tissue is surrounded by the thick, fibrous **tunica albuginea** (TA). The three cavernous bodies are surrounded by a looser connective tissue sheath to which the skin (removed here) is attached. The *boxed area* is presented at a higher magnification in Figure 19-4-4. *Inset*. **Penis. Human. x.s. Paraffin section**. ×14. The **cavernous spaces** (Cs) of the corpus cavernosum are larger than those of the corpus spongiosum. Moreover, the **fibrous trabeculae** (FT) are thinner, resulting in the corpora cavernosa becoming more turgid during erection than the corpus spongiosum.

This photomicrograph is a higher magnification of the *boxed area* of Figure 19-4-3. Note that the spongy **urethra** (U) is lined by a pseudostratified columnar **epithelium** (Ep) surrounded by a loose **connective tissue sheath** (CT), housing a rich **vascular supply** (BV). The entire urethra is enveloped by the **erectile tissue** (ET) of the corpus spongiosum. Additionally, the mucous **glands of Littré** (GL) deliver their secretory product into the lumen of the urethra, lubricating its epithelial lining.

KEY					
BV	blood vessel	**Ep**	epithelium	**GL**	glands of Littré
CS	corpus spongiosum	**ET**	erectile tissue	**TA**	tunica albuginea
Cs	cavernous space	**FT**	fibrous trabeculae	**U**	urethra
CT	connective tissue				

PLATE 19-5 Epididymis, Electron Microscopy

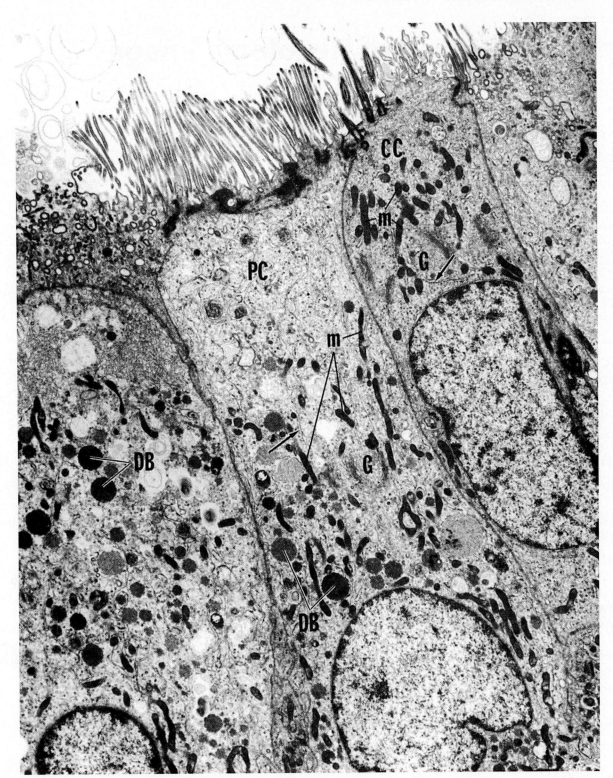

FIGURE 19-5-1. Epididymis. Rabbit. Electron microscopy. ×7,200.

The epithelial lining of the rabbit ductuli efferentes is composed of two types of tall columnar cells: **principal cells** (PC) and **ciliated cells** (CC). Note that both cell types possess numerous organelles, such as **Golgi** (G), **mitochondria** (m), and rough endoplasmic reticulum (*arrows*). Additionally, principal cells contain **dense bodies** (DB), probably a secretory material. (Courtesy of Dr. R. Jones.)

KEY					
CC	ciliated cell	**G**	Golgi apparatus	**PC**	principal cell
DB	dense bodies	**m**	mitochondrion		

Selected Review of Histologic Images

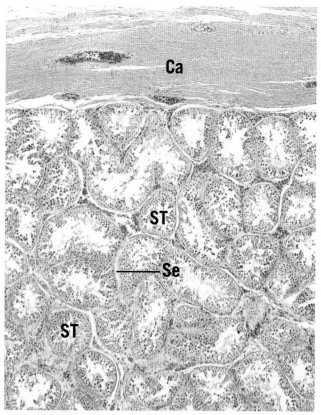

REVIEW FIGURE 19-1-1. Testis. Human. Paraffin section. ×56.

The testis has a connective tissue **capsule** (Ca) known as the tunica albuginea, which gives rise to slender **septa** (Se). Profiles of the highly convoluted **seminiferous tubules** (ST) are shown to be tightly packed.

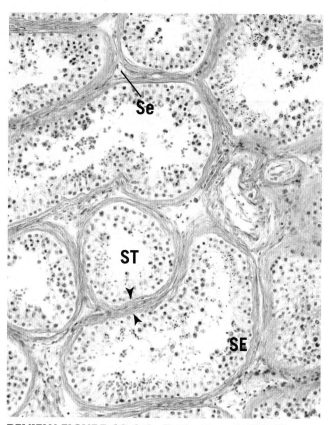

REVIEW FIGURE 19-1-2. Testis. Human. Paraffin section. ×132.

This is a higher magnification of an area similar to the one depicted in the previous figure. Note that the profiles of the **seminiferous tubules** (ST) are pressed against each other (*arrowheads*) so that the connective tissue **septa** (Se) appear to be quite slender. The seminiferous tubules are lined by **seminiferous epithelium** (SE) responsible for spermatogenesis.

KEY					
Ca	capsule	**SE**	seminiferous epithelium	**ST**	seminiferous tubule
Se	septa				

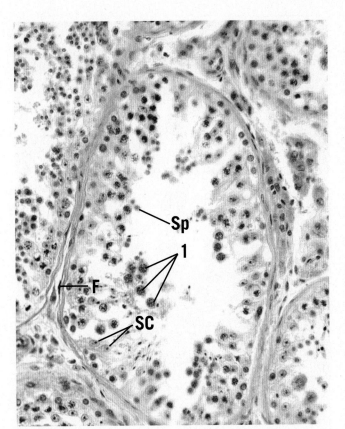

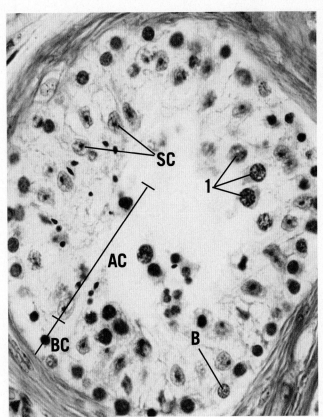

REVIEW FIGURE 19-1-3. Testis. Human. Paraffin section. ×270.

The profile of the seminiferous tubule depicted in this photomicrograph displays **fibroblasts** (F) that populate the connective tissue wall of the seminiferous tubule. Observe that some of the cell types of the seminiferous epithelium are labeled; namely **Sertoli cells** (SC), **primary spermatocytes** (1), and **spermatids** (Sp).

REVIEW FIGURE 19-1-4. Testis. Human. Paraffin section. ×540.

This high-magnification photomicrograph of a smaller profile of a seminiferous tubule approximates the **basal compartment** (BC) and the **adluminal compartment** (AC) created by the tight junctions formed by **Sertoli cells** (SC). **Spermatogonia B** (B) and **primary spermatocytes** (1) are labeled.

KEY					
1	primary spermatocyte	**BC**	basal compartment	**SC**	Sertoli cell
AC	adluminal compartment	**F**	fibroblast	**Sp**	spermatid
B	spermatogonia B				

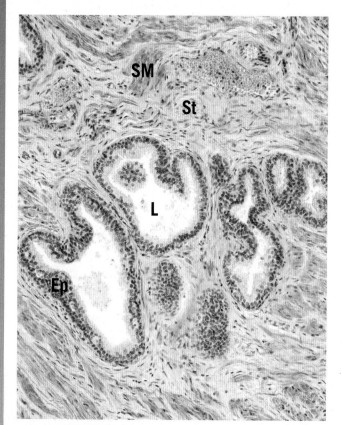

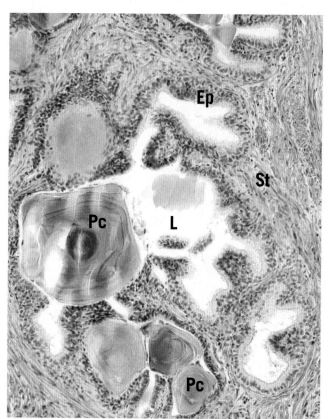

REVIEW FIGURE 19-2-1. Prostate gland young. Human. Paraffin section. ×132.

The prostate gland of a young man displays its fibro-elastic connective tissue **stroma** (St) which also has **smooth muscle** (SM) fibers scattered throughout. The **epithelium** (Ep) of the gland is simple columnar to stratified columnar and surrounds its **lumen** (L).

REVIEW FIGURE 19-2-2. Prostate gland old. Human. Paraffin section. ×132.

The prostate gland of an older individual displays the accumulation of **prostatic concretions** (PC) in its **lumen** (L). Otherwise, the **epithelium** (Ep) and the **stroma** (St) of the gland resemble that of a younger individual.

KEY					
Ep	epithelium	**Pc**	prostatic concretions	**St**	stroma
L	lumen	**SM**	smooth muscle		

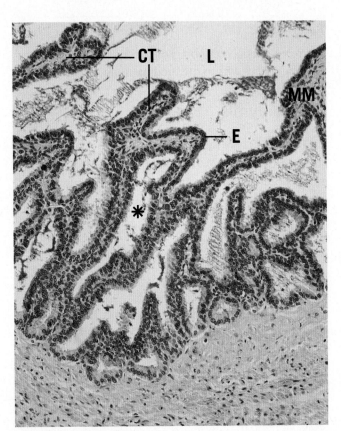

REVIEW FIGURE 19-2-3. Seminal vesicle. Human. Paraffin section. ×132.

The tubular-shaped seminal vesicles have a highly convoluted **mucous membrane** (MM) that anastomoses with itself and forms enclosed regions (*asterisk*) of the **lumen** (L). The **pseudostratified columnar epithelium** (E) overlies a slender **connective tissue** (CT) core.

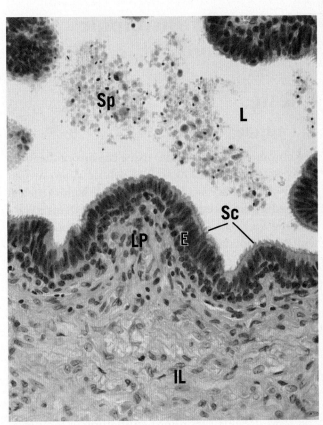

REVIEW FIGURE 19-2-4. Ductus deferens. Human. Paraffin section. ×270.

The ductus deferens, also known as the vas deferens, is a very muscular tube that conducts spermatozoa from the epididymis to the ejaculatory duct. The **lumen** (L) contains, in addition to **spermatozoa** (Sp), cell remnants shed by the spermatids and not phagocytosed by Sertoli cells along the way. The **pseudostratified epithelium** (E) lining the lumen is separated from the fibroelastic **lamina propria** (LP) by a basement membrane. The thick muscular coat is composed of three layers of smooth muscle cells: **inner longitudinal** (IL), middle circular, and an outer longitudinal.

KEY					
CT	connective tissue	**IL**	inner longitudinal layer	**Sc**	stereocilia
E	pseudostratified columnar epithelium	**L**	lumen	**Sp**	spermatozoa
		LP	lamina propria		

Summary of Histologic Organization

I. Testes

A. Capsule

The fibromuscular connective tissue **capsule** of the testes is known as the **tunica albuginea**, whose inner vascular layer is the **tunica vasculosa**. The capsule is thickened at the **mediastinum testis** from which **septa** emanate, subdividing the testis into ~250 incomplete **lobuli testis**, with each containing one to four **seminiferous tubules** embedded in a connective tissue **stroma**.

B. Seminiferous Tubules

Each highly convoluted **seminiferous tubule** is composed of a fibromuscular **tunica propria**, which is separated from the **seminiferous epithelium** by a **basal membrane**.

1. Seminiferous Epithelium

The **seminiferous (germinal) epithelium** is composed of sustentacular **Sertoli cells** and a stratified layer of developing **male gametes**. Sertoli cells establish a blood–testis barrier by forming occluding junctions with each other, thus subdividing the seminiferous tubule into **adluminal** and **basal compartments**. The basal compartment houses **spermatogonia A** (both **light** and **dark**), **spermatogonia B**, and the basal aspects of Sertoli cells. The adluminal compartment contains the apical portions of Sertoli cells, **primary spermatocytes**, **secondary spermatocytes**, **spermatids**, and **spermatozoa**.

2. Tunica Propria

The **tunica propria** consists of loose collagenous connective tissue, **fibroblasts**, and **myoid cells**.

C. Stroma

The loose vascular connective tissue **stroma** surrounding seminiferous tubules houses small clusters of large, vacuolated-appearing endocrine cells, the **interstitial cells (of Leydig)**.

II. Genital Ducts

A. Tubuli Recti

Short, straight tubes, the **tubuli recti**, lined by **Sertoli-like cells** initially and **simple cuboidal epithelium** later, connect the seminiferous tubules to the **rete testis**.

B. Rete Testis

The **rete testis** is composed of cuboidal cell–lined labyrinthine spaces within the **mediastinum testis**.

C. Epididymis

1. Ductuli Efferentes

The **ductuli efferentes** compose the **head of the epididymis**, whose lumina are lined by **simple columnar** (tall ciliated and low nonciliated) **epithelium**. The walls of the ductules consist of fibroelastic connective tissue and **smooth muscle cells**.

2. Ductus Epididymis

The **ductus epididymis** comprises the **body** and **tail** of the epididymis. Its lumen is lined by a **pseudostratified** type of **epithelium** composed of short **basal** and tall **principal cells** bearing **stereocilia** (long microvilli). The epithelium is separated by a **basal membrane** from the connective tissue wall that houses **smooth muscle cells**.

D. Ductus (Vas) Deferens

The enlarged continuation of the ductus epididymis, the **ductus deferens**, is a highly muscular structure. The **mucosal lining** of its small **lumen** is composed of **pseudostratified stereociliated epithelium** lying on a thin fibroelastic **lamina propria**. Its thick, muscular coat is composed of three layers of **smooth muscle**: an **inner** and **outer longitudinal** and a **middle circular** layer. A loose, fibroelastic **adventitia** surrounds the outer longitudinal muscle layer.

III. Accessory Glands

A. Seminal Vesicles

As the **seminal vesicles**, two highly convoluted tubular structures, secrete their products into the dilated ampullae of ductus deferens, they continue as the paired **ejaculatory ducts**, traversing the prostate gland. The highly folded **mucous membrane** of the seminal vesicle is composed of a **pseudostratified epithelium**, whose columnar cells are interspersed with short **basal cells**, sitting on a fibroelastic **lamina propria**. The muscular coat is composed of **inner circular** and **outer longitudinal** layers of **smooth muscle** and is invested by a fibrous **adventitia**.

B. Prostate Gland

The ejaculatory ducts join the urethra as these three structures traverse the substance of the **prostate gland**, whose **capsule** is composed of fibroelastic connective tissue and **smooth muscle cells**. The dense **stroma** of the gland is continuous with the capsule. The **parenchyma** of the prostate is composed of numerous individual glands disposed in three layers: **mucosal**, **submucosal**, and **external (main)**. The **lumina** of these three groups drain into three systems of **ducts** that lead into the expanded **urethral sinus**. The folded mucosa of the glands is composed of **simple cuboidal**-to-**columnar** (with regions of pseudostratified columnar) **epithelia** supported by fibroelastic vascular **stroma** displaying **smooth muscle cells**. Frequently, the lumina of the glands of older men possess round-to-ovoid **prostatic concretions** that are often lamellated and may become calcified.

C. Bulbourethral Glands

Each small **bulbourethral (Cowper's) gland** possesses a thin connective tissue **capsule** whose septa subdivide the gland into **lobules**. The **cuboidal-to-columnar cells** lining the lumen of the gland possess flattened, basally located **nuclei**. The main **duct** of each gland delivers its mucous secretory product into the **cavernous (spongy) urethra**.

IV. Penis

The **penis**, ensheathed in **skin**, possesses a thick, collagenous capsule, the **tunica albuginea**, that encloses the three cylindrical bodies of **erectile tissue**. The two dorsally positioned **corpora cavernosa** are incompletely separated from each other by **septa** derived from the tunica albuginea. The **corpus cavernosum urethrae (corpus spongiosum)** contains the spongy portion of the urethra. The vascular spaces of the erectile tissues are lined by **endothelium**.

V. Urethra

The male **urethra** is subdivided into three regions: **prostatic**, **membranous**, and **spongy (penile)** urethra.

A. Epithelium

The **prostatic portion** is lined by **transitional epithelium**, whereas the **membranous** and **spongy portions** are lined by **pseudostratified-to-stratified columnar epithelium**. The **spongy urethra** frequently displays regions of **stratified squamous epithelium**. Goblet cells and **intraepithelial glands** are also present.

B. Lamina Propria

The **lamina propria** is composed of a type of **loose connective tissue** housing **elastic fibers** and **glands of Littré**. **Smooth muscle**, oriented longitudinally and circularly, is also evident.

Chapter Review Questions

19-1. Which of the following is the path that spermatozoa follow?

A. Seminiferous tubules, tubuli recti, ductus epididymis, ductuli efferentes, vas deferens

B. Seminiferous tubules, ductus epididymis,
ductuli efferentes, tubuli recti, vas deferens

C. Seminiferous tubules, tubuli recti, rete testis, ductuli efferentes, ductus epididymis, vas
deferens

D. Seminiferous tubules, tubuli recti, ductuli efferentes, ductus epididymis, vas deferens

E. Seminiferous tubules, rete testis, tubuli recti,
ductus epididymis, ductuli efferentes, vas
deferens

19-2. Which cells in the male reproductive system secrete steroid hormones in response to LH?

A. Dark A spermatogonia A

B. Primary spermatocytes

C. Interstitial cells of Leydig

D. Sertoli cells

E. Spermatids

19-3. Which cells secrete antimüllerian hormone?

A. Sertoli cells

B. Interstitial cells of Leydig

C. Spermatogonia B

D. Pale A spermatogonia

E. Dark A spermatogonia

19-4. What clinical diagnosis should be considered
for a patient with elevated levels of blood
α-fetoprotein?

A. Testicular cancer

B. Adenocarcinoma of the prostate

C. Benign prostatic hypertrophy

D. Cryptorchidism

E. Phimosis

19-5. Which of the following cells participates in
spermiogenesis?

A. Pale type spermatogonia A

B. Type B spermatogonia

C. Primary spermatocyte

D. Secondary spermatocyte

E. Spermatid

SPECIAL SENSES

CHAPTER

20

CHAPTER OUTLINE

The organs of special senses include the gustatory, olfactory, somatosensory, visual, auditory, and vestibular systems. The gustatory apparatus, consisting of taste buds, is discussed in Chapter 14, Digestive System I, and the olfactory epithelium is presented in Chapter 13, Respiratory System. Sensory endings are located at the peripheral termini of dendrites. These specialized receptors (Table 20-1) are members of the general somatic or general visceral afferent pathways. Some are specialized to respond to stimuli, such as pressure, touch, temperature, as well as pain and itch, on the external surface of the body (**exteroceptors**, discussed in Chapter 12); others are designed to collect sensory information from internal body organs monitoring the activity of these organs as components of the general visceral afferent pathways (**interoceptors**). Additionally, specialized receptors are incorporated into muscles and tendons to perceive the localization of the body in three-dimensional space (**proprioceptors**, discussed in Chapter 7).

This chapter details the microscopic morphology of the eye, involved with visual sensations, and the ear, involved with auditory and vestibular sensations.

Eye

The eye is a special sensory organ conveying rays of light originating in the external environment and focusing them onto photosensitive cells of the retina. The intensity, location, and wavelengths of the transmitted light are partially processed by the retina, and the information is transmitted as three-dimensional color images of the external milieu for further processing and interpretation by the visual cortex of the brain.

- The two eyes are set apart by a certain distance resulting in overlapping visual fields, which make such three-dimensional imaging possible.

- Each eyeball sits within the bony orbit and is cushioned by periorbital fat. A group of **extrinsic skeletal muscles** inserts into the fibrous outer tunic of the eye to move it to direct the pupil to the object of interest.

- The anterior surface of the eye is protected by the eyelid and is bathed in **tears**, a fluid medium with a complex mixture of proteins, the antibacterial enzyme **lysozyme**, salts, peptides, secreted by the **lacrimal gland**.

Table 20-1	Specialized Receptors, Their Function and Location	
Receptor	**Type**	**Function and Location**
Peritrichial nerve endings	Nonencapsulated	Are nonmyelinated and have no associated Schwann cells. Most are coupled with hair follicles and react to the hair's motion. The sensation is interpreted as touch or being tickled.
Merkel's disks	Nonencapsulated	Mechanoreceptors located in the stratum basale of the epidermis
Meissner's corpuscles	Encapsulated	Located in the dermal papillae of the dermis and respond to touch sensations
Pacinian corpuscles	Encapsulated	Resemble an onion because epithelioid cells form concentric layers around a naked nerve ending. These corpuscles, located in the hypodermis, mesocolon, and mesentery respond to vibration, pressure, and deep touch.
Ruffini's endings	Encapsulated	Are composed of highly branched nerve termini surrounded by fibroblast-like cells. They respond to pressure and stretch and are located in nail beds, periodontal ligament, dermis of the skin, and capsules of joints.
Krause's end bulbs	Encapsulated	These spherical capsules containing a naked nerve ending are located in the connective tissues just deep to the epithelium, capsules of joints, peritoneum, and in the dermis of the skin. Their function is not known.
Muscle spindles	Encapsulated	Described in the chapter on Muscle. They respond to alteration in the length and rate of change in muscle and thus function in proprioception.
Golgi tendon organs	Encapsulated	Described in the chapter on Muscle. Respond to changes in the tension and the rate of tension change around a joint, thus function in proprioception.
Thermoreceptors	Nonencapsulated	They are assumed to be naked nerve endings located in the epidermis that respond to temperature. Their morphology is not known.
Nociceptors	Nonencapsulated	Branched naked nerve endings located in the epidermis. They are stimulated by extremes in temperature, by damage to the epidermis and underlying structures as well as to certain chemicals as pain sensation.

- The interior of the eyeball is subdivided into three chambers (Fig. 20-1):
  - **Anterior chamber** is a narrow space between the **cornea** and the anterior aspect of the **iris**. This space is filled with a watery fluid called the **aqueous humor**.
  - **Posterior chamber** is a narrow space between the posterior aspect of the **iris** and the anterior surface of the **lens**, filled with **aqueous humor**. The anterior and posterior chambers are continuous with each other via the **pupil** of the iris. The aqueous humor provides nutrients to the avascular cornea and the lens.
  - **Vitreous chamber** is the largest space, positioned posterior to the lens, and is filled with a translucent gelatinous substance called the **vitreous humor (body)**. The vitreous chamber and the posterior chamber are continuous via the periphery of the lens; thus, the aqueous humor produced by the **ciliary processes** enters the vitreous chamber and hydrates the vitreous body. The aqueous humor and the vitreous body provide adequate intraocular pressure to maintain the shape of the eye.

Three coats constitute the wall of the eyeball: the outer fibrous tunic (corneoscleral layer), the middle vascular tunic (uvea), and the inner neural (retinal) tunic.

Fibrous Tunic

The **fibrous tunic (corneoscleral layer)** is composed of the opaque, white **sclera** that covers the posterior aspect of the eyeball, the transparent **cornea** that covers the anterior one-sixth of the eye, and the junction between the two known as the **corneoscleral junction** or **limbus** (Fig. 20-2).

The transparent cornea is highly convex and is responsible for most of the refraction of the incoming light. It is supplied with a rich network of free nerve endings providing somatosensory perceptions; however, it is avascular and thus relies on the diffusion of nutrients from the aqueous humor in the anterior chamber. The cornea is composed of six layers (Figs. 20-2 and 20-3):

- The external-most **corneal epithelium** is comprised of several layers of cells forming a nonkeratinized stratified squamous lining.

- **Bowman's membrane**, a thin fibrillar lamina, composed mostly of type I collagen fibers, supports the corneal epithelium.

- The transparent **stroma** is the thickest constituent of the cornea composed of ~250 lamellae of type I collagen fibers that are parallel to each other within each lamella but not to those in the adjacent lamellae. Associated with these lamellae are slender elastic fibers, glycosaminoglycans, and fibroblasts.

- **Pre-Descemet layer (Dua layer)** deep to the stroma is a more recently recognized layer composed of tough type I collagen fibers contributing structural support to the cornea.

- **Descemet's membrane** is a thick basement membrane for the innermost layer of the cornea.

- The innermost simple squamous **corneal endothelium** is in contact with the aqueous humor of the anterior chamber and maintains the cornea in a mildly dehydrated condition, which contributes to its transparency.

The **corneoscleral junction (limbus)** is where the cornea transitions to the opaque sclera (Fig. 20-4). Here, the corneal epithelium becomes continuous with the stratified columnar epithelium of the **conjunctiva**, the mucosa for the exposed anterior aspects of the sclera, and the inner surfaces of the eyelid. A **trabecular meshwork** comprising of seemingly unorganized collagenous networks forms between the Descemet's membrane and the stroma (Fig. 20-5). The spaces between the trabecular meshwork eventually become continuous with an endothelium-lined **canal of Schlemm**, which drains aqueous humor from the anterior chamber of the eye to enter the venous network. The stroma of the cornea continues as the substance of the **sclera**. The type I collagen fibers in the sclera are not as precisely aligned, contributing to the opacity of the structure.

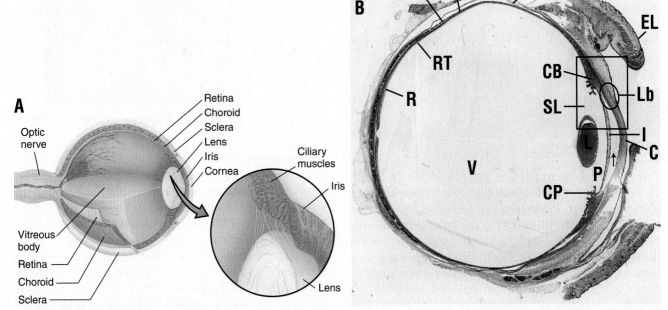

FIGURE 20-1. Anatomy of the eye. **A.** Illustration of eye anatomy. The eye is a hollow spherical globe comprised of three layers of tissues: the fibrous, vascular, and retinal tunics. The space within the eye is subdivided into the aqueous humor-filled anterior and posterior chambers, and the vitreous humor-filled posterior chamber. The iris is an extension of the vascular and retinal tunics, which function as a diaphragm that regulates the diameter of the pupil to adjust the amount of light entering the eye. The lens, positioned posterior to the iris, is held in place and its convexity is regulated by the actions of the ciliary body and the suspensory ligaments.

B. Human. Paraffin section. ×4.

This human eyeball is not sectioned at the equatorial plane; therefore, the pupil is not in the plane of section; instead, causing the iris to appear as if it were a continuous sheet of tissue. The **vitreous** (V), **posterior** (P), and **anterior** (arrow) chambers are apparent although the vitreous body and aqueous humor that occupy them are removed during tissue processing. Observe the three layers of the eye: The **fibrous tunic** (FT) has three subdivisions: the **cornea** (C), **limbus** (Lb), and **sclera** (S); the **vascular tunic** (VT) is composed of the **iris** (I), **ciliary body** (CB), and the **uvea** (U); the **retinal tunic** (RT) consists of the **retina** (R) and its nonsensory extension lining the interior of the iris and the ciliary body. The **lens** (L) does not belong to any of the tunics and is held in place by the **suspensory ligaments** (SL) extending from the ciliary body. Actions of the **ciliary muscle** of the ciliary body can exert tension on the peripheral rim of the lens via suspensory ligament, thus its convexity. The **ciliary processes** (CP) that produce aqueous humor are the infoldings of the vascular tunic covered with an extension of the retinal tunic. Note the **eyelid** (EL) protecting the exposed portion of the eye. Higher magnification of the *boxed area* is presented in Figure 20-2.

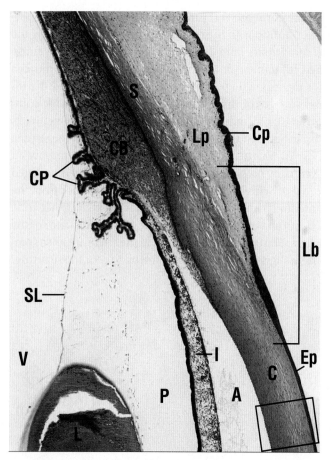

FIGURE 20-2. Human. Paraffin section. ×25.

This is a photomicrograph of the *boxed area* in Figure 20-1B. Observe the **limbus** (Lb), where the **cornea** (C) transitions to the **sclera** (S). Note the transition of the corneal **epithelium** (Ep) to the **conjunctival epithelium** (Cp) at the limbus, which is supported by the **lamina propria** (Lp). Higher magnification of the area similar to the *boxed region* of the cornea is presented in Figure 20-3. Observe in this image, the **anterior** (A) and the **posterior** (P) chambers separated by the **iris** (I), and the **vitreous** (V) chamber posterior to the **lens** (L). The **ciliary body** (CB), **ciliary processes** (CP), and the **suspensory ligaments** (SL) are also apparent.

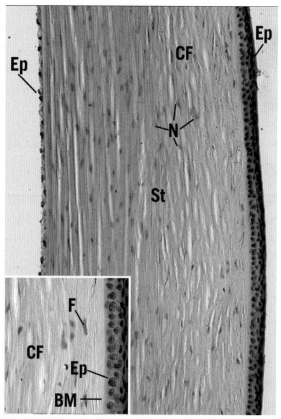

FIGURE 20-3. Cornea. Monkey. Paraffin section. ×132.

The cornea is a multilayered, transparent structure. Its anterior surface is covered by a stratified squamous nonkeratinized **epithelium** (Ep) on the right-hand side of the image, deep to which is a thin, acellular Bowman's membrane. The bulk of the cornea, the **stroma** (St), is composed of regularly arranged **collagen fibers** (CF) and intervening fibroblasts, whose **nuclei** (N) are evident. The posterior surface of the cornea is lined by a simple squamous-to-cuboidal **epithelium** (Ep) on the left-hand side of the image. A thin, acellular Descemet's membrane lies between the simple epithelium and the Dua layer. *Inset.* **Cornea. Monkey. Paraffin section.** ×270. A higher magnification of the anterior surface displays the stratified squamous **epithelium** (Ep) as well as the acellular **Bowman's membrane** (BM). Note the regularly arranged bundles of **collagen fibers** (CF) and intervening **fibroblasts** (F), whose nucleus is labeled by the lead line.

CLINICAL CONSIDERATIONS 20-1

Glaucoma

Glaucoma is a condition of high intraocular pressure caused by an obstruction that prevents the aqueous humor from exiting the anterior chamber of the eye. If left untreated, the pressure can reduce the blood flow through the vessels in the uvea and cause damages to the optic nerve and the retina to such an extent that blindness may result. Occasionally, pigment cells that line the posterior aspect of the iris become detached and enter the aqueous humor of the anterior chamber. As these pigment cells accumulate, a condition known as pigment dispersion syndrome, they become trapped in the trabecular network thwarting the normal outflow of the aqueous humor through the canal of Schlemm, thereby causing a special type of glaucoma known as pigmentary glaucoma.

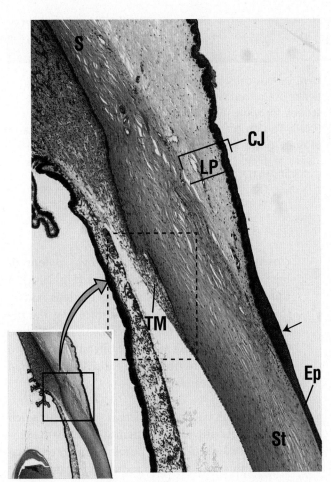

FIGURE 20-4. Corneoscleral junction. Human. Paraffin section. ×42.

The corneal **epithelium** (Ep) becomes slightly thickened (*arrow*) and then transitions to the stratified columnar epithelium of the **conjunctiva** (CJ) with the underlying **lamina propria** (LP). The **stroma** (St) of the cornea loses its precise organization and continues as the substance of the **sclera** (S). Deep to Descemet's membrane, the **trabecular meshwork** (TM) appears in the limbus, channeling the aqueous humor toward the **canal of Schlemm** (CS). A higher magnification of the *boxed area* is presented in Figure 20-5.

Vascular Tunic

The **vascular tunic (uvea)** consists of several regions: the anteriorly positioned **iris** and **ciliary body** and the largest posterior aspect the **choroid** which is highly vascular and pigmented (see Fig. 20-1). **Melanocytes** are disseminated throughout this layer and synthesize melanin, but unlike the melanocytes in the skin, the pigment is retained in their cytoplasm.

- **Iris** is the anterior-most aspect of the vascular tunic with a central aperture known as the **pupil**. Iris functions to regulate the size of the pupil and in turn, the amount of light that enters the eye. The melanin in

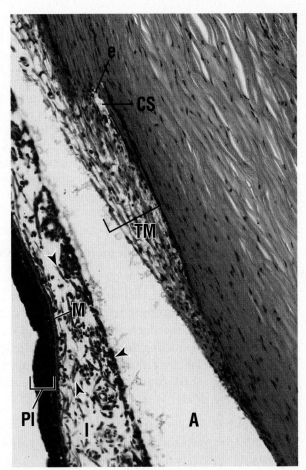

FIGURE 20-5. Canal of Schlemm. Human. Paraffin section. ×132.

This is a photomicrograph of the *boxed area* in Figure 20-4, highlighting the **trabecular meshwork** (TM) of the limbus. The aqueous humor in the **anterior chamber** (A) travels through the trabecular meshwork and eventually drains into the **endothelium** (e)-lined **canal of Schlemm** (CS). Note the higher magnification of the **iris** (I) with melanocytes (*arrowheads*) identifiable by the brown melanin in the cytoplasm. The anterior surface of the iris has no epithelial lining and is in contact with the aqueous humor in the anterior chamber. The posterior surface however has a darkly pigmented epithelial lining derived from the retinal tunic, called the **pars iridica** (PI). Just anterior to the pars iridica, observe a thin strip of **smooth muscles** (M). These are the radially oriented dilator pupillae.

the melanocytes prevents light from passing through the iris except at the pupil (Fig. 20-6; also see Fig. 20-5). Additionally, the abundance of melanin produced by the melanocytes in the iris confers different eye colors, in that a large amount of melanin imparts dark color to the eyes, whereas less melanin renders the eyes light in color. Iris is covered on its posterior side by an extension of the modified retinal tunic (called **pars iridica**), but its anterior surface has no epithelial lining; thus, its stroma baths in the aqueous humor (see Fig. 20-5).

CLINICAL CONSIDERATIONS 20-2

Floppy Iris Syndrome

Occasionally, removal of the lens during cataract surgery results in the displacement of the pupillary rim of the iris toward the space previously occupied by the lens. This condition, known as **floppy iris syndrome** (intraoperative floppy iris syndrome), is caused by a reduction in the normal turgidity of the iris. Although this condition may have various causes, the most common reason is the patient's use of certain α-blockers, such as tamsulosin, prescribed for some men with benign prostatic hypertrophy (BPH). This drug acts to relax the smooth muscles of the prostate gland and urinary bladder; however, it also relaxes the dilator muscle of the iris, causing the iris to be somewhat flaccid.

Two intrinsic muscles within the iris regulate the pupil size.

- **Sphincter pupillae** are circular muscles surrounding the pupil, contracting in response to a parasympathetic signal that reduces the pupil size and the amount of light entering the eye (see Fig. 20-6).
- **Dilator pupillae** are radially oriented and, upon sympathetic signal, contract to increase the pupil size (see Fig. 20-5).

- **Ciliary body** is a thickened, circular region of the vascular tunic between the iris and the choroid, which appears wedge-shaped in a cross-sectional image (Fig. 20-2; also see Fig. 20-7). The thickening of the ciliary body is largely owing to the circular **ciliary muscle**, the third intrinsic muscle of the eye. The innermost aspect of the ciliary body has numerous projections of connective tissue stroma, collectively known as **ciliary processes**, covered by the modified region of the retinal tunic (**pars ciliaris**). Ciliary processes produce aqueous humor and anchor **suspensory (zonule) ligaments**, which attach to the peripheral rim of the lens, holding it in place. In addition, the ciliary muscles and suspensory ligaments participate in lens **accommodation**.

  - Contraction of the circular ciliary muscle reduces the tension on the suspensory ligament, which allows the lens to relax and become rounded. The rounded lens refracts incoming light more to focus on the near objects.
  - Relaxation of the ciliary muscle increases the tension on the suspensory ligament which pulls on the lens flat. The flatter lens refracts incoming light less to focus on the far objects.

- Lens is a crystalline structure suspended in place by the suspensory ligaments. Although this structure does not belong to the vascular tunic, its function of refracting the incoming light just the right amount is regulated by the actions of the ciliary muscles. Histologically, the lens is composed of closely packed, elongated cells known as **lens fibers** arranged parallel to each other (Fig. 20-8). A thin layer of cuboidal cells forms the lens epithelium that covers the anterior surface and the peripheral rim, but not the posterior surface. The lens epithelial cells divide at the peripheral rim and give rise to the new lens fibers. The entire lens is covered by an acellular capsule.

- Choroid is a thin layer of connective tissue with a rich vascular supply providing nutrient support to the retinal tunic (see Fig. 20-2). The heavily pigmented melanocytes in this structure also reduce the scattering of the light entering through the pupil.

Retinal Tunic

The innermost **retinal tunic** derives directly from the outpocketing of the developing brain as a spherical **optic vesicle**. The distal end of each optic vesicle folds inward transforming it into an **optic cup**, comprised of the **outer and inner retinal epithelium** separated by a narrow space, known as the **intraretinal space**. The outer retinal epithelium gives rise to a single layer of pigmented cells that form the **retinal pigment epithelium**, whereas the inner retinal epithelium gives rise to rods, cones, and a variety of neural and glial cells. As development continues, the intraretinal space eventually disappears; because these two layers are not tightly held together by cell–cell junctions, this space can potentially reopen resulting in a condition described as a detached retina. The retinal tunic has three regions: **pars iridica**, **pars ciliaris**, and **pars optica**.

- **Pars iridica**, the anterior-most aspect of the retinal tunic, lines the posterior surface of the iris and is comprised of two layers of heavily pigmented cuboidal cells (see Fig. 20-6). This region does not perform a sensory function.

- **Pars ciliaris** does not perform a sensory function. Positioned between pars iridica and pars optica, it lines the inner surface of the ciliary body and forms

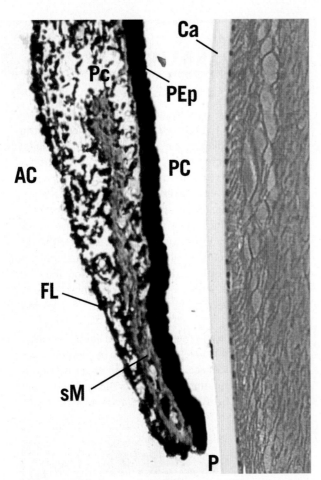

FIGURE 20-6. Iris. Monkey. Paraffin section. ×132.

The iris is a pigmented diaphragm that delineates the **pupil** (P) of the eye. It separates the **anterior chamber** (AC) from the **posterior chamber** (PC). The iris is composed of three layers: an outer discontinuous layer of melanocytes and fibroblasts; the intermediate **fibrous layer** (FL), housing **pigment cells** (Pc) and fibroblasts; and the posterior double-layered **pigmented epithelium** (PEp). The **sphincter** (sM) and dilatator muscles are composed of smooth muscle and smooth muscle–like myoepithelial cells, respectively. Observe the lens positioned posterior to the iris and surrounded by a thick capsule (Ca).

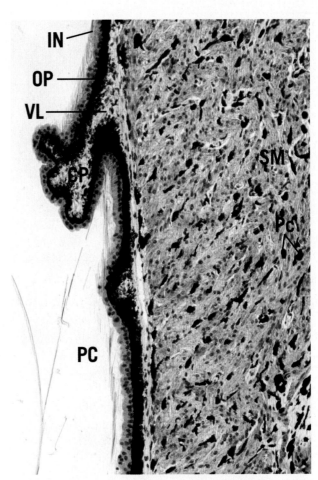

FIGURE 20-7. Ciliary body. Monkey. Paraffin section. ×132.

The ciliary body is composed of **ciliary processes** (CP) projecting into the **posterior chamber** (PC), from which suspensory ligaments (zonular fibers) extend to the lens. The bulk of the ciliary body is composed of **smooth muscle** (SM) disposed more or less in three layers, not evident in this photomicrograph. Numerous **pigment cells** (Pc) are present in this region. Note that the epithelium of the ciliary body is the pars ciliaris of the retinal tunic, composed of two layers: an **outer pigmented** (OP) and an **inner nonpigmented** (IN) epithelium. The narrow **vascular layer** (VL) intervenes between the epithelium and ciliary muscles. The base, or root, of the iris is anchored to the ciliary body.

CLINICAL CONSIDERATIONS 20-3

Blue Eye Color

Until approximately 6,000 to 10,000 years ago, every human being had brown eyes; then, a small mutation in the switch that turned off the *OCA2* gene resulted in the inability of that individual to manufacture P protein in the iris. Protein P is involved in melanin formation; therefore, the person with this particular mutation was able to synthesize melanin normally except in the iris, and, instead of having brown eyes, that person's eyes were blue. Thus, it is believed that all blue-eyed individuals are descendants of that one person born in the 6th to 8th millennium BCE.

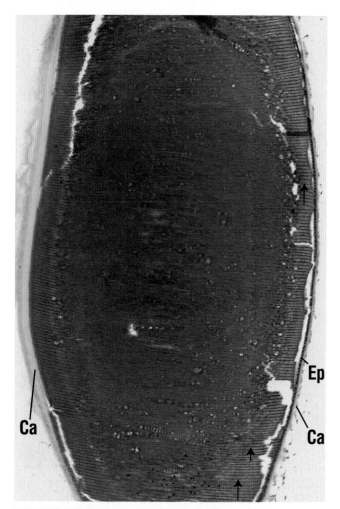

FIGURE 20-8. Lens. Human. Paraffin section. ×52.

The lens is a biconvex, flexible, transparent disc covered by a homogenous **capsule** (Ca). The lens **epithelium** (Ep), comprising of a single layer of cuboidal cells, covers the anterior and lateral surfaces but not the posterior surface. The lens fibers (*arrows*), constituting the bulk of the lens, are composed of closely packed, hexagon-shaped cells.

the epithelial component of the ciliary processes. It is composed of two layers of cuboidal cells: the pigmented external layer and the nonpigmented internal layer (see Fig. 20-7). The boundary between the thicker retina and the thinner pars ciliaris of the retinal tunic is known as the **ora serrata**.

- **Pars optica (retina)** makes up the posterior two-thirds of the retinal tunic. It is thicker and performs the special sensory function in registering and relaying visual information. The two photoreceptor cells of the retina are **rhodopsin-synthesizing rods** and **iodopsin-forming cones**. When stimulated by light, the impulses generated by the rods and cones are transmitted through a chain of interneurons and eventually to the brain via the optic nerve. The rods, cones, interneurons, and their synapses in the retina are supported

CLINICAL CONSIDERATIONS 20-4

Age-Related Eye Disorders

Presbyopia is age-related farsightedness. With increasing age, the lens elasticity diminishes and the reduced rounding of the lens, even when the ciliary muscle is fully contracted, causes the inability to focus on near objects, requiring convex (reading) glasses.

In **myopia** and **hyperopia**, as an individual ages, the longitudinal axis of the eye changes, as may the curvature of the cornea, and the lens, instead of focusing the image on the retina, focuses it either in front of the retina (**myopic vision**) or behind the retina (**hyperopic vision**). The condition may be corrected with lenses (eyeglasses or contact lenses) or by refractive surgery, assisting the lens in focusing on the retina.

Cataract, a common condition of aging, is caused by excessive ultraviolet radiation and by pigments and other substances accumulating in the lens, making it opaque and thus impairing vision. This condition may be corrected by excising the lens and replacing it with a plastic lens.

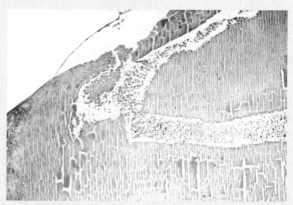

This photomicrograph is from the lens of a patient who presented with age-related cataract. Observe the presence of cortical extracellular clefts and globules. (Reprinted with permission from Mills SE, et al., eds. *Sternberg's Diagnostic Surgical Pathology*, 6th ed. Philadelphia: Wolters Kluwer, 2015. p. 1081, Figure 24-25.)

by numerous glial cells. The precise organization and alignment of these cells and their cellular regions impart 10 histologically distinct layers to the retina (Table 20-2 and Fig. 20-9). The thickness of the inner nine layers varies (thinner anteriorly and thicker posteriorly) and are modified even further in two discrete regions, the **optic disc** and the **fovea centralis**. The optic disc is where all the axons from the retina converge and exit the eye, thus the 10-layer organization is absent. The fovea centralis is positioned directly in line with the pupil and contains tightly packed cones that disrupt the 10 layers into the thinner, depressed region in the retina, while providing the greatest visual acuity of the entire retina (Fig. 20-10; also see Fig. 20-2).

The 10 layers of the retina from external to internal are as follows (see Fig. 20-9 and Table 20-2).

Layer 1: Retinal pigment epithelium consists of a single layer of pigmented cuboidal cells with microvilli on its internal aspect (adjacent to the layer 2). This layer functions in **esterifying vitamin A** and transporting it to the rods and cones, **phagocytosing** the shed tips of rods and cones, and **synthesizing melanin**, which absorbs light after rods and cones have been stimulated. The tight junctions between the neighboring pigment cells contribute to the **blood–retinal barrier** regulating the movement of ion, protein, and water into and out of the retina.

Layer 2: Receptors of **rods and cones** are the photosensitive regions of these cells, shaped like rods and cones, respectively (Figs. 20-11 and 20-12). The receptors are embedded within the microvilli of the retinal pigment epithelial cells but there are no cell–cell junctions tightly holding the two layers together. In the detached retina, the separation occurs between this layer and the retinal pigment epithelium.

- **Rods** are sensitive to low light intensity and possess many flattened discs containing **rhodopsin** (an integral membrane protein, **opsin**, bound to **retinal**, the aldehyde form of **vitamin A**) in their outer receptor segment. When light is absorbed by rhodopsin, it dissociates into **retinal** and **opsin** (bleaching), permitting diffusion of bound Ca^{2+} into the outer segment. Excess levels of Ca^{2+} hyperpolarize the cell by closing Na^+ channels, thus preventing the entry of Na^+ into the cell. The electrical potential thus generated is relayed to other rods via gap junctions and then along the pathway to the optic nerve. Dissociated retinal and opsin reassemble, and the Ca^{2+} ions are recaptured, establishing a normal resting potential.

- **Cones**, sensitive to light of high intensity, producing **greater visual acuity**, are much more numerous than rods, and they produce **iodopsin**, the photopigment responsible for distinguishing color. Three different moieties of opsin are sensitive to red, green, or blue light. The mechanism of transducing photon energy into electrical energy for transmission to the brain via the optic nerve is similar to that described in the rods.

Layer 3: External limiting membrane is not a true membrane; instead, it is a thin histologically distinct layer composed of cell–cell junctions made among the supporting Müller cells with each other and with rods and cones. The Müller cells are tall cells extending through all 9 inner layers of the retina. They form a cellular medium providing structural, metabolic, and nutrient support to rods, cones, and interneurons.

Layer 4: Outer nuclear layer is the region in which nuclei of rods and cones are concentrated.

Layer 5: Outer plexiform layer is where the axons of the rods and cones synapse with dendrites of the bipolar and horizontal cells.

Layer 6: Inner nuclear layer is formed by aggregates of nuclei that belong to glial cells and bipolar cells.

Layer 7: Inner plexiform layer is where synapses occur between axons of the bipolar cells and dendrites of the ganglion cells.

Table 20-2	Layers of the Retina
Layer	**Description**
Pigment epithelium	Synthesizes melanin that absorbs light that activates rods and cones, phagocytoses the shed tips of rods and cones, and esterifies vitamin A
Receptors of rods and cones	Photosensitivity; rods are sensitive to low light intensity, and cones are sensitive to bright light and perceive color
External limiting membrane	Zonulae adherentes formed between the photoreceptor cells and Müller cells (therefore, it is not a membrane)
Outer nuclear layer	Houses the nuclear regions of rods and cones
Outer plexiform layer	Region of synapse between axons, photoreceptor cells, and dendrites of horizontal and bipolar cells
Inner nuclear layer	Houses the nuclear regions of Müller, bipolar, amacrine, and horizontal cells
Inner plexiform layer	Region where synapses occur among axons and dendrites of amacrine, bipolar, and ganglion cells
Ganglion cell layer	Region of the cell bodies of multipolar neurons as well as of neuroglial cells
Optic nerve fiber layer	Region where the unmyelinated axons of ganglion cells join to form the optic nerve. Once the fibers pierce the sclera, they become myelinated
Inner limiting membrane	Composed of the expanded terminal processes of Müller cells and their basal lamina

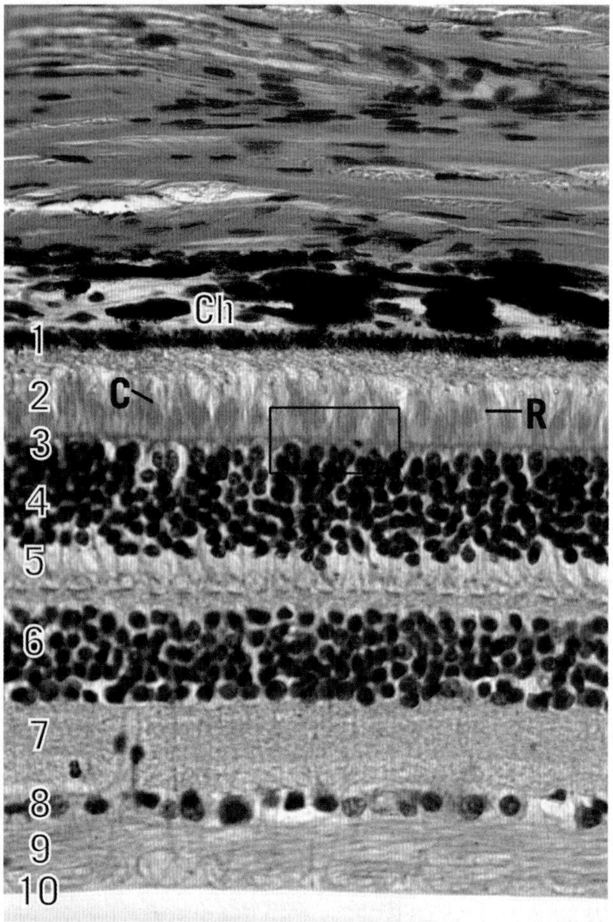

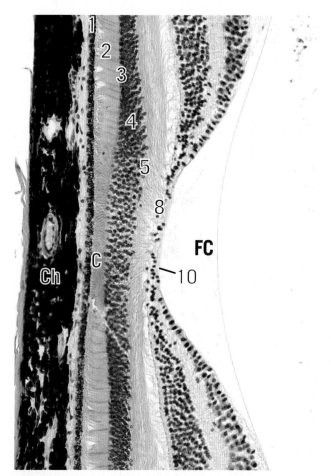

FIGURE 20-9. Retina. Pars optica. Monkey. Paraffin section. ×270.

The pars optica of the retina is composed of 10 distinct layers. The pigment **epithelium** (1), the outermost layer, is closely apposed to the vascular and pigmented **choroid** (Ch). Various regions of the **rods** (R) and **cones** (C) characterize the next four layers. These are the **receptors of rods and cones** (2), **external limiting membrane** (3), **outer nuclear layer** (4), and **outer plexiform layer** (5). The **inner nuclear layer** (6) houses the nuclear regions of the horizontal, amacrine, bipolar, and Müller cells. The **inner plexiform layer** (7) is a region of synapse formation, whereas the **ganglion cell layer** (8) houses the cell bodies of multipolar neurons and associated neuroglia. The centrally directed (toward the central nervous system) fibers of these ganglion cells form the **optic nerve fiber layer** (9), whereas the **inner limiting membrane** (10) is composed of the expanded processes of Müller cells along the inner surface of the eye. A region similar to the *boxed area* is presented in Figure 20-12, a scanning electron micrograph of the rods and cones.

Layer 8: Ganglion cell layer is the region housing nuclei that belong to ganglion cells and glial cells. A minor subpopulation of ganglion cells possesses the light-sensitive pigment melanopsin that responds to

FIGURE 20-10. Fovea centralis. Monkey. Paraffin section. ×132.

The retina is greatly reduced in thickness at the **fovea centralis** (FC) of the macula lutea. This is the region of greatest visual acuity, and **cones** (C) are the only photoreceptor cells in this area. Note that the retinal layers present are the pigmented **epithelium** (1), **receptors of cones** (2), **external limiting membrane** (3), **outer nuclear layer** (4), **outer plexiform layer** (5), **ganglion cell layers** (8), and **inner limiting membrane** (10). Because of the presence of numerous melanocytes, the vascular **choroid** (Ch) appears dark.

blue light even in individuals who are blind. The axons of these ganglion cells project to the suprachiasmatic nucleus, the region of the brain responsible for the regulation of circadian rhythm.

Layer 9: Optic nerve fiber layer is formed by axons emanating from the ganglion cells which converge at the optic disc and exit the eye as the optic nerve.

Layer 10: Inner limiting membrane is not a true membrane; instead, it consists of the innermost aspects of the Müller cells.

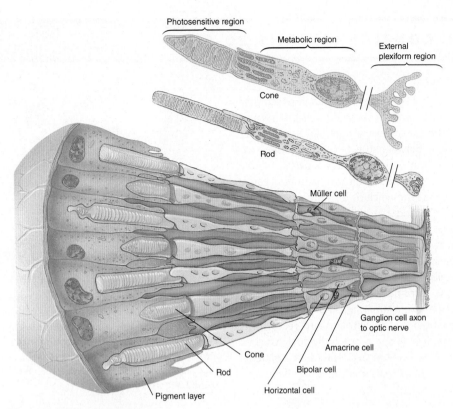

FIGURE 20-11. Illustration of the retina.

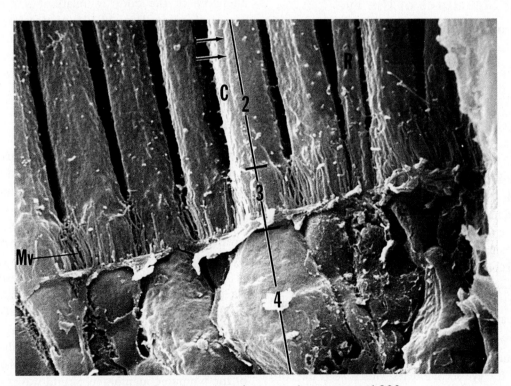

FIGURE 20-12. Rods and cones. Monkey. Scanning electron microscopy. ×6,300.

This scanning electron micrograph of the monkey retina displays regions of several **cones** (C) that display their thicker morphology and wider nuclear zone and of a few **rods** (R) whose diameter is narrower, with a thinner nuclear zone. The inner segments of the **lamina of rods and cones** (2), **external limiting membrane** (3), and **outer nuclear layer** (4) are clearly recognizable. The **microvilli** (Mv) noted in the vicinity of the external limiting membrane belong to the Müller cells, which were removed during specimen preparation. Observe the longitudinal ridges (*arrows*) along the surface of the inner segments. (From Borwein B, et al. The ultrastructure of monkey foveal photoreceptors, with special reference to the structure, shape, size, and spacing of the foveal cones. *Am J Anat* 1980;159(2):125–146. Copyright © 1980 Wiley-Liss, Inc. Reprinted by permission of John Wiley & Sons, Inc.)

CLINICAL CONSIDERATIONS 20-5

Retinal Disorders

Detached retina may result from a trauma in which the neural and pigmented layers of the retina become separated, reopening the embryonic intraretinal space. The prolonged separation between the two layers results in ischemic damage to the neurons, causing partial blindness, but it may be corrected by surgical intervention. Early symptoms of detached retina include a sudden increase in floaters, flashes of light, and a reduction in the visual field sometimes described as a curtain blocking a field of vision. **Retinoblastoma** is a malignancy of a very young child, usually detected at about age 2 years, although at the time of diagnosis the child may be 5 or 6 years old. Approximately a third of the cases have familial components, but at least 60% occur without a familial incidence. The tumor appears white with regions of calcification and yellow foci of necrosis. The tumor may spread by individual cells invading the optic nerve as well as the choroid. The patient has to lose the eyeball to prevent metastasis.

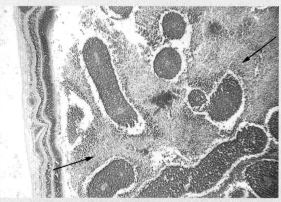

This photomicrograph is from the eyeball of a child with retinoblastoma. Observe the relatively normal retina on the left-hand side of the image. The *arrows* indicate regions of necrosis in a field of perivascular tumor cells. (Reprinted with permission from Mills SE, et al., eds. *Sternberg's Diagnostic Surgical Pathology*, 6th ed. Philadelphia: Wolters Kluwer, 2015. p. 1082, Figure 24-29.)

Accessory Structures of the Eye

Accessory structures of the eye include the conjunctiva, eyelids, and lacrimal gland.

- The **conjunctiva** is a transparent mucous membrane that lines the inside of the eyelids and reflects onto the anterior surface of the sclera. It is comprised of stratified columnar epithelium supported by the loose connective tissue, lamina propria. The conjunctival epithelium becomes continuous with the corneal epithelium at the corneoscleral junction.

- The **eyelids** covered by skin anteriorly and conjunctiva posteriorly have an ill-defined dense irregular connective tissue core known as the **tarsal plate**, providing structural support (Fig. 20-13). They also contain modified sebaceous glands, known as the **meibomian glands**, whose lipid-rich secretions are responsible for altering the surface tension of the watery tears and slowing evaporation. Orbicularis oculi, a circular skeletal muscle, is also within the substance of the eyelid.

- The **lacrimal glands** positioned on the anterolateral aspects of the eye secrete **tears**, which keep the conjunctiva and cornea moist and have antimicrobial effect attributable to the **lysozyme**, an antibacterial enzyme (Fig. 20-14).

Ear

The **ear** functions in the reception of sound as well as in the perception of the orientation of the head and therefore of the body in relation to the directional forces of gravity (Fig. 20-15). Anatomically, the ear is subdivided into the external, middle, and inner ears. Although the sense of hearing requires all three components, the sense of balance is perceived by parts of the inner ear only.

External and Middle Ear

The **external ear** is composed of the **auricle (pinna)**, a semicircular skin-covered protrusion whose shape is maintained by an elastic cartilage core, functioning to gather sound and direct it to the **external auditory meatus** (see Fig. 20-15). This tube is supported by elastic cartilage externally and bone internally and is separated from the middle ear by the thin **tympanic membrane**.

The **tympanic cavity** of the **middle ear** houses the three **auditory ossicles**: the outermost **malleus** (hammer), the middle **incus** (anvil), and the innermost **stapes** (stirrup). This cavity is connected to the **nasopharynx** via the cartilaginous **auditory (eustachian) tube**, which permits equalization of atmospheric pressures on either side of the tympanic membrane. Sound waves are funneled by the auricle to the tympanic membrane, whose vibrations are amplified and transmitted by the movements of the ossicles to the **oval window** of the inner ear's **cochlea**.

Inner Ear

The inner ear, functioning in both hearing and balance, is housed within the petrous region of the temporal bone

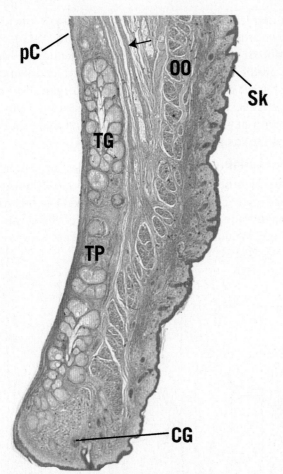

FIGURE 20-13. Eyelid. Paraffin section. ×14.

The external aspect of the eyelid is covered by thin **skin** (Sk). The deep surface of the eyelid is lined by a stratified columnar epithelium, the **palpebral conjunctiva** (pC). The substance of the eyelid is formed by the thick connective tissue **tarsal plate** (TP) and **tarsal glands** (TG). Two skeletal muscles are associated with the upper eyelid: the circularly disposed **orbicularis oculi** (OO) and the longitudinally oriented levator palpebrae superioris. Although the latter muscle is not present in this photomicrograph, its connective tissue aponeurosis is evident (*arrow*). Eyelashes and the sebaceous **ciliary glands** (CG) are present at the free end of the lid.

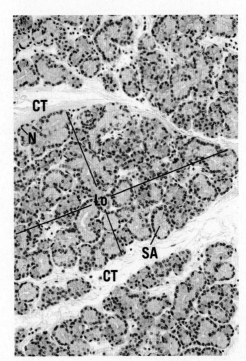

FIGURE 20-14. Lacrimal gland. Monkey. Paraffin section. ×132.

Lacrimal glands are compound tubuloacinar glands, separated into lobes and **lobules** (Lo) by **connective tissue** (CT) elements. Because these glands produce a lysozyme-rich, watery secretion, they are composed of numerous **serous acini** (SA), as evidenced by the round, basally located **nuclei** (N) of the secretory cells.

and is comprised of the **bony labyrinth** on the exterior and the **membranous labyrinth** in the interior. The space between the bony and membranous labyrinth is filled with **perilymph**, which is similar to cerebrospinal fluid in composition. The membranous labyrinth, a continuous tubular network lined with a delicate layer of cells, is filled with **endolymph** whose components are similar to the intracellular fluid. The **bony labyrinth** is subdivided into **semicircular canals**, **vestibule**, and **cochlea** (see Fig. 20-15). The portions of the membranous labyrinth in these three subdivisions of the bony labyrinth house special sensory structures responsible for sensing sound and equilibrium.

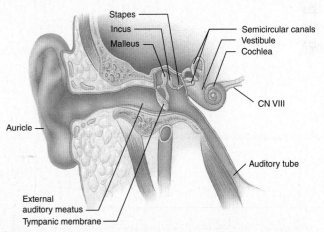

FIGURE 20-15. Illustration of ear anatomy. The external ear, the auricle, and the external auditory meatus gather sound and channel it to the tympanic membrane that vibrates and transmits the mechanical energy to the three ossicles of the middle ear cavity, the malleus, incus, and stapes. The inner ear composed of the bony labyrinth houses the membranous labyrinth within its perilymph-filled space. The membranous labyrinth is filled with endolymph and houses sensory structures responsible for sensing the sound and the sense of balance, equilibrium, and movement. This sensory information is conducted to the brain through the vestibulocochlear nerve (cranial nerve VIII).

Cochlea and Cochlear Duct

Cochlea, the snail shell-shaped region of the bony labyrinth, is situated closest to the middle ear and houses the segment of the membranous labyrinth known as the **cochlear duct** (Fig. 20-16). The endolymph-filled cochlear duct, also known as **scala media**, is coiled within the spiral of the cochlea and compartmentalizes the perilymph-filled space between it and the bony labyrinth into **scala vestibuli** (located superiorly) and the **scala tympani** (positioned inferiorly). The superior and inferior boundaries of the cochlear duct are named the **vestibular membrane** and the **basilar membrane**, respectively. At the apex of the cochlea where the cochlear duct ends, the scala vestibuli and scala tympani communicate with each other via a small opening known as the **helicotrema** (Figs. 20-16 and 20-17). The **vestibular membrane** functions to maintain the **high ion gradient** between the perilymph and endolymph. The basilar membrane hosts the **spiral organ of Corti**, responsible for transducing sound (reaching them in the form of pressure waves) into electrical signals transmitted to the brain.

- The **spiral organ of Corti** is comprised of neuroepithelial **inner** and **outer hair cells** whose kinocilia and stereocilia are embedded in the gel-like **tectorial membrane**. Additional components of the organ of Corti include various supporting and accessory cells (Fig. 20-18).

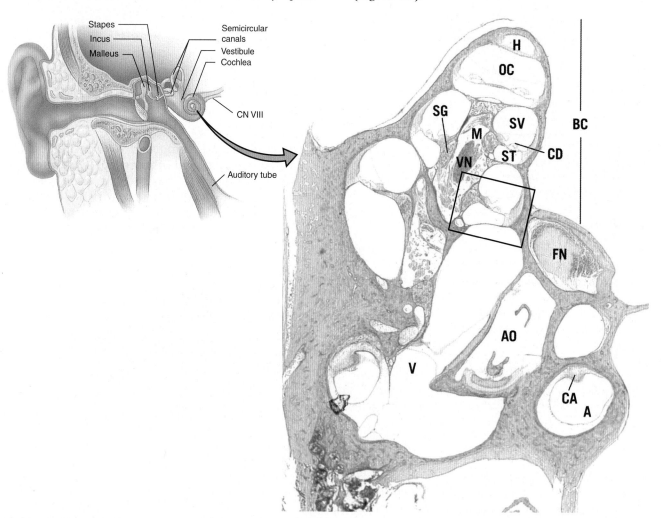

FIGURE 20-16. Inner ear. Paraffin section. ×21.

This photomicrograph is a survey section of the petrous portion of the temporal bone displaying the various components of the inner ear. Note that the spirally disposed **bony cochlea** (BC) encases the endolymph-filled **cochlear duct** (CD) and the perilymph-filled **scala tympani** (ST) and **scala vestibuli** (SV). The apex of the cochlea displays the **helicotrema** (H), the point of communication between the scala tympani and the scala vestibuli. Innervation to the spiral **organ of Corti** (OC), located within the cochlear duct, is derived from the **spiral ganglion** (SG), housed in the **modiolus** (M). Two cranial nerves, **vestibulocochlear** (VN) and **facial** (FN), are evident in this photomicrograph. The **vestibule** (V), as well as sections of the **ampullae** (A) of the semicircular canals containing the **crista ampullaris** (CA), is clearly recognizable. Finally, note one of the **auditory ossicles** (AO) of the middle ear. An area similar to the *boxed area* is presented at higher magnification in Figure 20-17.

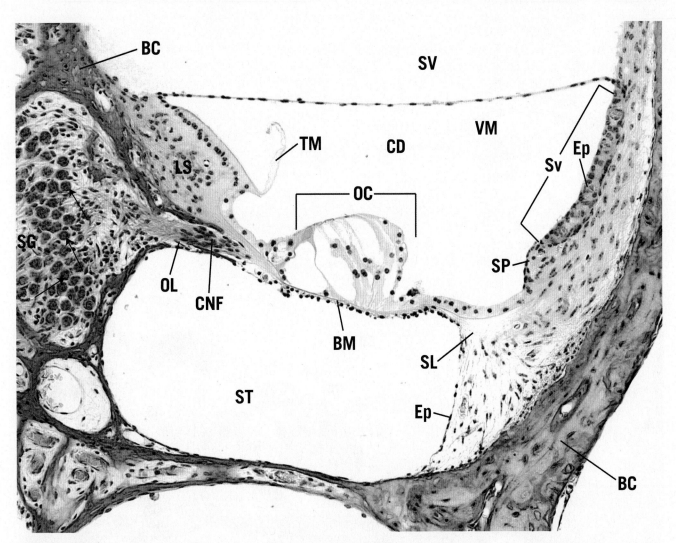

FIGURE 20-17. Cochlea. Paraffin section. ×211.

This photomicrograph is a higher magnification of a region similar to the *boxed area* in Figure 20-16, one of the turns of the cochlea. Observe that the **scala vestibuli** (SV) and **scala tympani** (ST), enclosed in the **bony cochlea** (BC), are **epithelium** (Ep)-lined spaces, filled with perilymph. The **cochlear duct** (CD), filled with endolymph, is separated from the scala vestibuli by the thin **vestibular membrane** (VM) and from the scala tympani by the **basilar membrane** (BM). Within the bony casing lies the **spiral ganglion** (SG), containing the large cell bodies (*arrows*) of primary sensory neurons. **Cochlear nerve fibers** (CNF) from the spiral ganglion traverse bony tunnels of the **osseous spiral lamina** (OL) to reach the hair cells of the spiral **organ of Corti** (OC). This structure, responsible for the sense of hearing, is an extremely complex entity. It rests on the basilar membrane, a taut, collagenous sheet extending from the **spiral ligament** (SL) to the **limbus spiralis** (LS). Attached to the limbus spiralis is the **tectorial membrane** (TM) (whose elevation in this photomicrograph is an artifact of fixation), which overlies the spiral organ of Corti. Observe the presence of the **stria vascularis** (Sv), which extends from the vestibular membrane to the **spiral prominence** (SP). The stria vascularis possesses a pseudostratified **epithelium** (Ep) composed of basal, dark, and light cells, which are intimately associated with a rich capillary network. It is believed that endolymph is elaborated by some or all of these cells. The morphology of the spiral organ of Corti is presented at higher magnification in Figure 20-18.

- Vibration of the **basilar membrane**, induced by disturbances in the perilymph, results in bending of the kinocilia and stereocilia, causing the hair cells to release their neurotransmitter substances to excite the bipolar cells of the spiral ganglion and eventually, the transmission of the impulse to the brain via the **cochlear branch** of the **vestibulocochlear nerve** (**cranial nerve VIII**).

- Although the basilar membrane vibrates at many frequencies, certain regions vibrate optimally at specific frequencies. Low-frequency sound waves are detected farther away from the oval window.

- Cell bodies of bipolar neurons are aggregated within the modiolus, the bony center of the cochlea. It is the dendrites of these neurons that synapse with the hair cells of the spiral organ of Corti and, if excited,

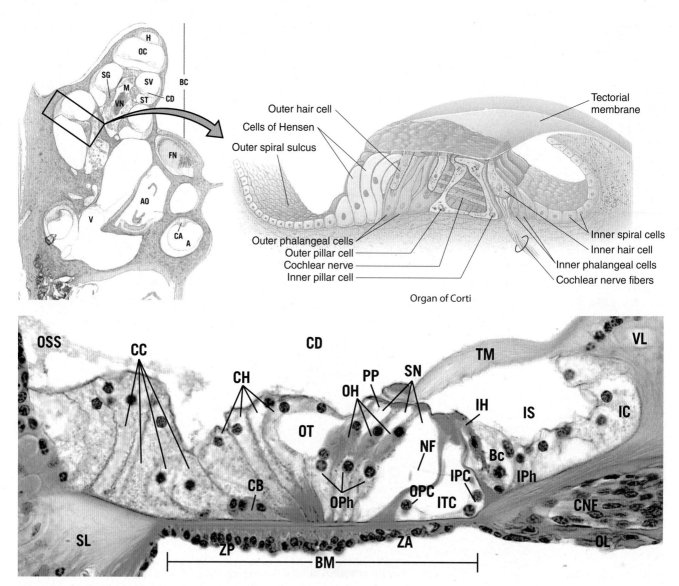

FIGURE 20-18. Illustration and spiral organ of Corti (montage). Paraffin section. ×540.

The spiral organ of Corti lies on the **basilar membrane** (BM), whose two regions, the **zona pectinata** (ZP) and the **zona arcuata** (ZA), are delineated by the base of the **outer pillar cells** (OPC). The basilar membrane extends from the **spiral ligament** (SL) to the **tympanic lip** (TL) of the limbus spiralis. The **tectorial membrane** (TM) is anchored to the **vestibular lip** (VL) of the limbus spiralis. The tectorial membrane forms a roof over the **internal spiral sulcus** (IS). Observe the **cochlear nerve fibers** (CNF) traversing the tunnels of the **osseous spiral lamina** (OL). The lateral wall of the internal spiral sulcus is formed by the single row of **inner hair cells** (IH), flanked by the **inner phalangeal cells** (IPh) and **border cells** (Bc). The floor of the internal spiral sulcus is formed by **inner sulcus cells** (IC). Proceeding laterally, the **inner pillar cell** (IPC) and **outer pillar cell** (OPC) form the **inner tunnel of Corti** (ITC). The **spaces of Nuel** (SN) separate the three rows of **outer hair cells** (OH) from each other and from the outer pillar cells. Fine **nerve fibers** (NF) and **phalangeal processes** (PP) traverse these spaces. The outer hair cells are supported by **outer phalangeal cells** (OPh). The space between the **cells of Hensen** (CH) and the outermost row of outer phalangeal cells is the **outer tunnel** (OT). Lateral to the cells of Hensen are the darker-staining, deeper positioned **cells of Boettcher** (CB) and the lighter staining, larger **cells of Claudius** (CC), which enclose the **outer spiral sulcus** (OSS). Note that the space above the spiral organ of Corti is the **cochlear duct** (CD), whereas the space below the basilar membrane is the scala tympani.

transmit the impulses along their axons. The collection of these axons form the cochlear branch of the vestibulocochlear nerve.

- Oscillations set in motion at the **oval window** are dissipated at the secondary tympanic membrane covering the **round window** of the cochlea.

Utricle and Saccule in the Vestibule

The **vestibule** of the bony labyrinth contains the endolymph-filled dilations of the membranous labyrinths, **utricle**, and **saccule**. Both the utricle and the saccule host special sensory structures known as the **maculae** arranged perpendicular to each other. Each macula is comprised of **neuroepithelial hair cells** whose stereocilia and **kinocilia** (nonmotile cilia) project into the **otolithic membrane**, a proteinaceous substance containing calcium carbonate crystals called **otoliths** (Fig. 20-19). Linear acceleration in the horizontal or vertical plane causes the kinocilia and stereocilia of the hair cells to bend, causing the macula of the utricle or saccule to generate impulse, transmitting it to the brain via the **vestibular branch** of the **vestibulocochlear (CN VIII) nerve**.

Semicircular Canals and Ducts

The semicircular canals of the bony labyrinth each house the endolymph-filled semicircular ducts that are arranged at right angles to each other. At the base of the semicircular canal, near the vestibule, the semicircular ducts converge into three swellings called the ampullae, each hosting a collection of hair cells known as the **crista ampullaris** (Fig. 20-20). The stereocilia and kinocilia of these neuroepithelial cells project into a proteinaceous material known as the **cupula**. Crista ampullaris detect angular acceleration along any of the three axes which are registered and interpreted as a vector in three dimensions.

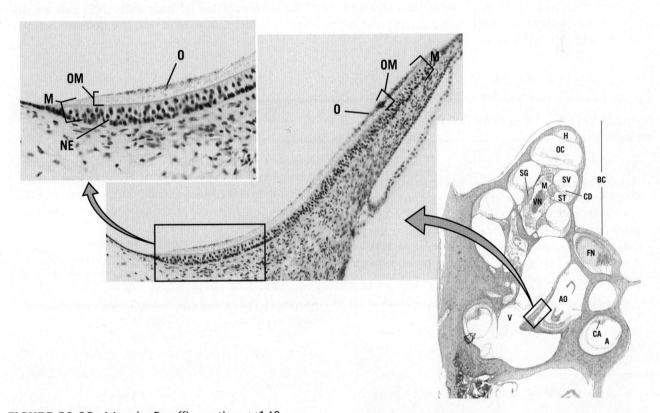

FIGURE 20-19. Macula. Paraffin section. ×140.

This is a higher magnification of the region similar to the *boxed area* in the survey inner ear photomicrograph. The endolymph-filled utricle and saccule within the vestibule house the special sensory structures, **maculae** (M) comprised of **neuroepithelial hair cells** (NE) whose kinocilia and stereocilia are embedded in the **otolithic membrane** (OM). *Inset* (**Macula**. Paraffin section. ×**400**.) is a higher magnification of the boxed area detailing the **neuroepithelial cells** (NE) and their hair embedded in the **otolithic membrane** (OM) with the small, crystalline **otoliths** (O).

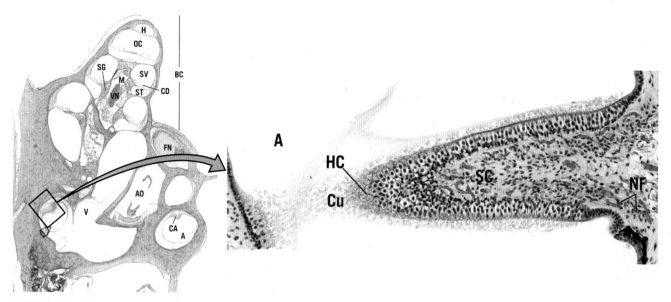

FIGURE 20-20. Crista ampullaris. Paraffin section. ×132.

The **crista ampullaris** (CA) is housed within the expanded **ampulla** (A) of each semicircular duct. **Nerve fibers** (NF) enter the connective tissue core of the crista and reach the **neuroepithelial hair cells** (HC) that are supported by **sustentacular cells** (SC). Kinocilia and stereocilia of the hair cells extend into the gelatinous cupula (Cu) associated with the crista.

CLINICAL CONSIDERATIONS 20-6

Ear Disorders

Conductive hearing loss may arise from a middle ear infection (otitis media), an obstruction, or otosclerosis of the middle ear.

Nerve deafness results from a lesion in the cochlear portion of the vestibulocochlear nerve (cranial nerve VIII). This condition may be the result of disease, prolonged exposure to loud sounds, and/or drugs.

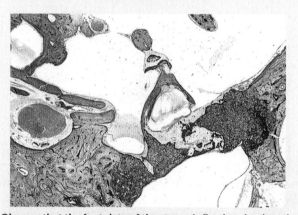

Observe that the footplate of the stapes is fixed to the densely sclerotic bone forming the perimeter of the oval window. (Reprinted with permission from Mills SE, et al., eds. *Sternberg's Diagnostic Surgical Pathology*, 6th ed. Philadelphia: Wolters Kluwer, 2015. p. 1037, Figure 23-22.)

Ménière's disease is an inner ear disorder characterized by symptoms such as hearing loss owing to excess fluid accumulation in the endolymphatic duct, vertigo, tinnitus, nausea, and vomiting. In severe cases, surgical treatment may be required.

The condition known as **acoustic neuroma** is a benign tumor whose cells of origin are Schwann's cells of the vestibulocochlear nerve (cranial nerve VIII). It is manifested by loss of hearing, loss of balance, vertigo, and tinnitus. If the tumor is not treated early enough, it may involve other cranial nerves in its vicinity. Recent studies suggest the possibility that long-term exposures to the electromagnetic radiation emitted by cell phones may be a causative factor in the development of acoustic neuroma in susceptible individuals.

Selected Review of Histologic Images

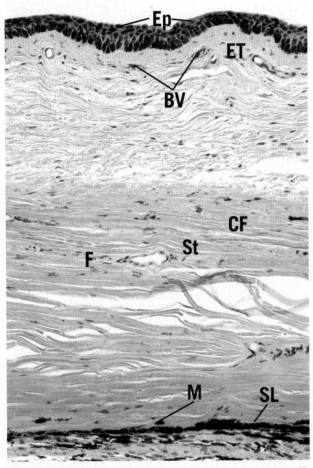

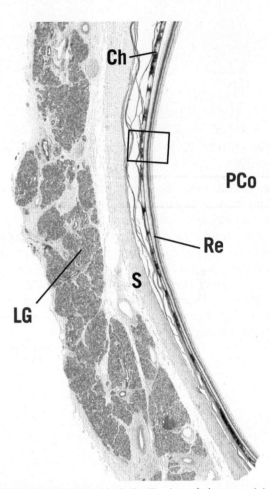

REVIEW FIGURE 20-1-1. Sclera. Monkey. Paraffin section. ×132.

The sclera is similar to and continuous with the cornea, but it is not transparent. Note that the **epithelium (Ep)** of the conjunctiva covers the anterior surface of the sclera. Deep to the epithelium is the loose **episcleral tissue** (ET), whose small **blood vessels** (BV) are evident. The **stroma** (St) is composed of thick **collagen fiber** (CF) bundles, between which numerous **fibroblasts** (F) can be seen. The deepest layer of the sclera is the **suprachoroid lamina** (SL), whose **melanocytes** (M) containing dark melanin pigment characterize this layer.

REVIEW FIGURE 20-1-2. Tunics of the eye. Monkey. Paraffin section. ×14.

This survey photomicrograph is of an anterolateral section of the globe of the eye, as evidenced by the presence of the **lacrimal gland** (LG). Note that the three layers of the globe of the eye are extremely thin in relation to its diameter. The **sclera** (S) is the outermost layer. The pigment **choroid** (Ch) and multilayered **retina** (Re) are easily distinguishable even at this low magnification. The **posterior compartment** (PCo) lies behind the lens and houses the vitreous body. Higher magnification of the boxed area is shown in Review Plate 20-2A

KEY						
BV	blood vessel	**F**	fibroblasts	**Re**	retina
CF	collagen fibers	**LG**	lacrimal gland	**S**	sclera
Ch	choroid	**M**	melanocytes	**SL**	suprachoroid lamina
Ep	epithelium	**PCo**	posterior compartment	**St**	stroma
ET	episcleral tissue				

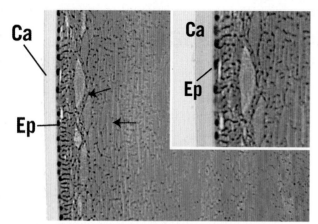

REVIEW FIGURE 20-1-3. Lens. Monkey. Paraffin section. ×132.

The lens is a biconvex, flexible, transparent disc covered by a homogenous **capsule** (Ca), deep to which lies the simple cuboidal lens **epithelium** (Ep). The fibers (*arrows*), constituting the bulk of the lens, are composed of closely packed, hexagon-shaped cells whose longitudinal axes are oriented parallel to the surface. The lens is avascular, hence the absence of blood vessels. *Inset.* **Lens. Monkey. Paraffin section.** ×270. Note the presence of the homogeneous **capsule** (Ca) overlying the simple cuboidal lens **epithelium** (Ep).

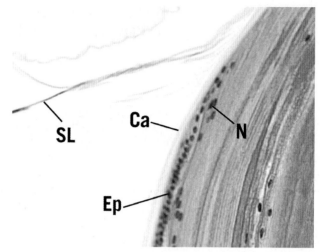

REVIEW FIGURE 20-1-4. Lens. Monkey. Paraffin section. ×132.

The equator of the lens displays the presence of younger cells that still possess their **nuclei** (N) and organelles but lose them as these cells mature. Note the **suspensory ligaments** (SL), **capsule** (Ca), and the lens **epithelium** (Ep).

KEY

Ca	Capsule	**N**	nucleus	**SL**	suspensory ligaments
Ep	epithelium				

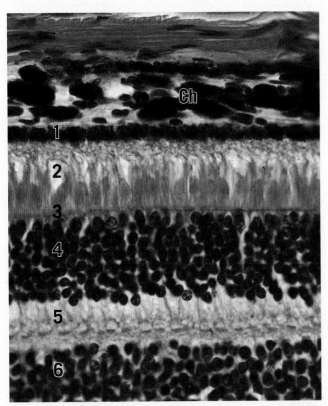

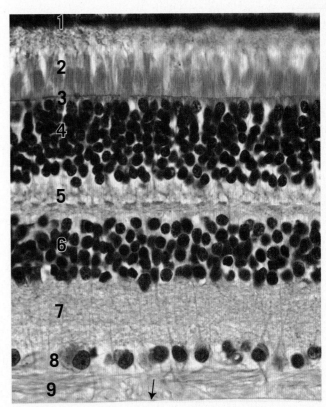

REVIEW FIGURE 20-2-1. Retina. Monkey. Paraffin section. ×540.

REVIEW FIGURE 20-2-2. Retina. Monkey. Paraffin section. ×540.

The **choroid layer** (Ch) of the eyeball is sandwiched between the sclera and the outermost layer, the **pigment epithelium** (1) of the retina. The **lamina of rods and cones** (2), the **external limiting membrane** (3), the **outer nuclear layer** (4), and the **outer plexiform layer** (5) compose the various layers of the rods and cones. The **inner nuclear layer** (6) houses the nuclear regions of the horizontal, amacrine, bipolar, and Müller cells.

This photomicrograph is similar to Review Figure 20-2-1, but it includes the entire thickness of the retina. The **pigment epithelium** (1) abuts the **lamina of rods and cones** (2). **The external limiting membrane** (3), the **outer nuclear layer** (4), and the **outer plexiform layer** (5), as well as the **lamina of rods and cones** (2), compose the various layers of the rods and cones. The **inner nuclear layer** (6) houses the nuclear regions of the horizontal, amacrine, bipolar, and Müller cells. Synapses among the axons and dendrites of amacrine, ganglion, and bipolar cells occur in the **inner plexiform layer** (7). Observe the **ganglion cells layer** (8), the **optic nerve fiber layer** (9), and the **inner limiting membrane** (*arrow*) that constitute the innermost three layers of the retina.

KEY							
1	pigment epithelium	4	outer nuclear layer	8	ganglion cell layer
2	lamina of rods and cones	5	outer plexiform layer	9	optic nerve fiber layer
3	external limiting membrane	6	inner nuclear layer	Ch	choroid layer
		7	inner plexiform layer		

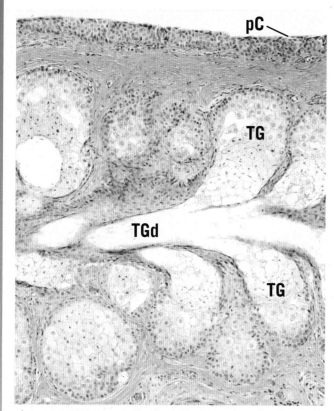

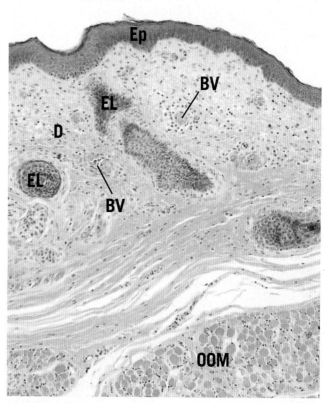

REVIEW FIGURE 20-2-3. Eyelid. Human. Paraffin section. ×132.

This photomicrograph is a higher magnification of the region of the tarsal gland near the free edge (margin) of the eyelid. The duct of the **tarsal gland** (TGd) receives meibum, the lipid-rich secretion, from the lobes of the **tarsal gland** (TG), also known as meibomian glands, and delivers it to the free edge of the eyelids. The **palpebral conjunctiva** (pC) is a stratified columnar to low columnar epithelium interspersed with goblet cells.

REVIEW FIGURE 20-2-4. Eyelid. Human. Paraffin section. ×132.

This photomicrograph is a higher magnification of the skin aspect near the margin of the eyelid. Note that the interface of the **epidermis** (Ep) and **dermis** (D) is relatively smooth, displaying a virtual absence of a rete apparatus. Observe that the dermis is well supplied by **blood vessels** (BV), and the presence of **eyelashes** (EL) is also evident. The **orbicularis oculi muscle** (OOM) of the eyelid is composed of skeletal muscle.

KEY					
BV	blood vessel	**Ep**	epidermis	**TG**	tarsal gland
D	dermis	**OOM**	orbicularis oculi muscle	**TGd**	duct of the tarsal gland
EL	eyelash	**pC**	palpebral conjunctiva		

Summary of Histologic Organization

I. Eye

A. Fibrous Tunic

1. Cornea

The **cornea** is composed of six layers. From superficial to deep, they are

a. *Stratified Squamous Nonkeratinized Epithelium*

b. *Bowman's Membrane*

The outer, homogeneous layer of the stroma.

c. *Stroma*

A transparent, dense, regular, collagenous connective tissue housing **fibroblasts** and occasional **lymphoid cells**, constituting the bulk of the cornea.

d. *Dua Layer*

A thin, collagenous membrane that provides protection for the cornea.

e. *Descemet's Membrane*

A thick, basal lamina.

f. *Corneal Endothelium*

Not a true endothelium, a simple **squamous-to-cuboidal epithelium**.

2. Corneoscleral junction (Limbus)

Trabecular meshwork and endothelium-lined canal of Schlemm conduct and drain aqueous humor from the anterior chamber.

3. Sclera

The **sclera**, the white of the eye, is composed of three layers: the outer **episcleral tissue** housing blood vessels; the middle **stroma**, composed of dense, regular, collagenous connective tissue; and the **suprachoroid lamina**, a loose connective tissue housing **fibroblasts** and **melanocytes**.

B. Vascular Tunic

The **vascular tunic (uvea)** is a pigmented, vascular layer housing smooth muscles. It is composed of the **choroid**, the **ciliary body**, and the **iris**.

1. Choroid

The **choroid** is composed of four layers. The **suprachoroid layer** is shared with the sclera and houses **fibroblasts** and **melanocytes**. The **vascular** and **choriocapillary layers** house larger vessels and capillaries, respectively. The **glassy membrane (of Bruch)**, interposed between the choroid and the retina, is composed of basal lamina, collagen, and elastic fibers.

2. Ciliary Body

The **ciliary body** is the region of the vascular tunic located between the **ora serrata** and the iris. The ciliary body is composed of the numerous, radially arranged, **aqueous humor–forming ciliary processes** that together compose the **ciliary crown** from which **suspensory ligaments** extend to the lens. Three layers of **smooth muscle**, oriented more or less meridianally, radially, and circularly, function in visual accommodation. The **vascular layer** and **glassy membrane** of the choroid continue into the ciliary body. The inner aspect of the ciliary body is covered by the inner nonpigmented and outer pigmented layers of the **retina (pars ciliaris)** forming the **ciliary epithelium**.

3. Iris

The **iris**, separating the **anterior** from the **posterior chamber**, is attached to the ciliary body along its outer circumference. The free edge of the iris forms the boundary of the **pupil** of the eye. The iris is composed of three layers: the outer (frequently incomplete) **simple squamous epithelial layer**, a continuation of the corneal epithelium; the intermediate **fibrous layer**, composed of the nonvascular **anterior stromal** and vascular **general stromal layers** that house numerous **melanocytes** and **fibroblasts**; and the posterior **pigmented epithelium (pars iridica** of the **retina)**. The **sphincter** and **dilator muscles** of the pupil are composed of myoepithelial cells.

C. Retinal Tunic

The **retinal tunic**, the deepest of the three layers, consists of the **pars iridica**, **pars ciliaris**, and **pars optica**. The last of these is the only region of the retina that is sensitive to light, extending as far anteriorly as the **ora serrata**, where it is continuous with the pars ciliaris.

1. Pars Optica

The **pars optica** is composed of 10 layers. From the exterior to the interior, they are:

a. *Pigment Epithelium*

The **pigment epithelium** is attached to the choroid membrane.

b. *Lamina of Rods and Cones*

The **outer** and **inner segments** of the photoreceptor cells; the rest of the cell parts of the rods and cones constitutes the next three layers.

c. External Limiting Membrane

The **external limiting membrane** is not a true membrane. It is merely a junctional specialization between the photoreceptor cells and processes of **Müller** (supportive) **cells**.

d. Outer Nuclear Layer

The **outer nuclear layer** houses the cell bodies (and nuclei) of the photoreceptor cells. At the **fovea centralis**, only cones are present.

e. Outer Plexiform Layer

The **outer plexiform layer** is the region of synapse formation between the **axons** of photoreceptor cells and the processes of **bipolar** and **horizontal cells**.

f. Inner Nuclear Layer

The **inner nuclear layer** houses the **cell bodies of Müller**, **amacrine** (associative), **bipolar**, and **horizontal cells**.

g. Inner Plexiform Layer

The **inner plexiform layer** is the region of synapses between **dendrites** of **ganglia cells** and **axons** of **bipolar cells**. Moreover, processes of **Müller** and **amacrine cells** are also present in this layer.

h. Ganglion Cell Layer

The **ganglion cell layer** houses the **cell bodies of multipolar neurons**, which are the final link in the neuronal chain of the retina, and their **axons** form the optic nerve. Additionally, **neuroglia** are located in this layer.

i. Optic Nerve Fiber Layer

The **optic nerve fiber layer** is composed of the **unmyelinated axons** of the **ganglion cells**, which converge at the optic disc and leave the eye as the optic nerve.

j. Inner Limiting Membrane

The **inner limiting membrane** is composed of the expanded terminal processes of **Müller cells**.

2. Pars Ciliaris and Pars Iridica Retinae

At the **pars ciliaris** and **pars iridica retinae**, the retinal layer has been reduced to a thin epithelial layer consisting of a columnar and a pigmented layer lining the ciliary body and iris.

D. Lens

The **lens** is a biconvex, flexible, transparent disc that focuses the incident rays of light on the retina. It is composed of three layers, an elastic **capsule** (basement membrane), an anteriorly placed **simple cuboidal epithelium**, and **lens fibers**, modified epithelial cells derived from the **equator** of the lens.

E. Lacrimal Gland

The **lacrimal gland** is external to the eye, located in the superolateral aspect of the orbit. It is a **compound tubuloacinar gland**, producing a lysozyme-rich serous fluid with a slightly alkaline pH.

F. Eyelid

The **eyelid** is covered by **thin skin** on its external aspect and by **conjunctiva**, a mucous membrane, on its inner aspect. A thick, dense, fibrous connective tissue **tarsal plate** maintains and reinforces the eyelid. Associated with the tarsal plate are the **tarsal glands**, secreting an oily sebum that is delivered to the margin of the eyelid. Muscles controlling the eyelid are located within its substance. Associated with the eyelashes are **sebaceous glands**. Ciliary glands are located between eyelashes.

II. Ear

A. External Ear

1. Auricle

The **auricle** is covered by thin skin and is supported by a highly flexible **elastic cartilage plate**.

2. External Auditory Meatus

The **external auditory meatus** is a **cartilaginous tube** lined by skin, containing **ceruminous glands** and some fine **hair**. The skin of the external meatus is continuous with the external covering of the tympanic membrane. In the medial aspect of the meatus, the cartilage is replaced by **bone**.

3. Tympanic Membrane

The **tympanic membrane** is a thin, taut membrane separating the external from the middle ear. It is lined by **stratified squamous keratinized epithelium** externally and low **cuboidal epithelium** internally and possesses a core of **collagen fibers** disposed in two layers.

B. Middle Ear

The **middle ear** is composed of the **simple cuboidal epithelium**–lined **tympanic cavity** containing the three **ossicles** (**malleus, incus**, and **stapes**). The tympanic cavity communicates with the nasopharynx via the cartilaginous and bony **auditory tube**. The medial wall of the middle ear communicates with the inner ear via the **oval (vestibular)** and **round (cochlear) windows**.

C. Inner Ear

The inner ear is a complex three-dimensional structure comprised of the bony labyrinth forming the outer shell for the delicate membranous labyrinth within. The membranous labyrinth is a complex system of a continuous tube with dilations, filled with endolymph, and houses special sensory structures. The spaces between the bony and the membranous labyrinth are filled with perilymph.

1. Cochlea and Cochlear Duct

The **bony cochlea** houses the endolymph-filled **cochlear duct (scala media)** that subdivides the perilymph-filled cochlea into the superiorly positioned **scala vestibuli** and the inferiorly located **scala tympani**. The **cochlear duct** houses the **spiral organ of Corti** that lies on the **basilar membrane**. The spiral organ of Corti is composed of **inner hair cells** and **outer hair cells** whose kinocilia and stereocilia are embedded into the overlying **tectorial membrane**. Additional components of the organ of Corti include various supporting and accessory cells. Bipolar neurons whose cell bodies (and their nuclei) are positioned within the modiolus, forming the **spiral ganglion**, receive impulses from the hair cells and transmit them through their axons that emerge as the **cochlear branch** of the **cranial nerve VIII (CNVIII,** **vestibulocochlear nerve)**. The **stria vascularis**, which synthesizes and maintains endolymph, constitutes the outer wall of the cochlear duct.

2. Vestibule, Utricle, and Saccule

The bony vestibule houses the two dilations of the membranous labyrinth, the **utricle** and **saccule**, both filled with **endolymph** and house **maculae**. Each **macula** is composed of simple **columnar epithelium** composed of two cell types, neuroepithelial **hair cells** and **supporting cells**. The free surface of the macula displays the **otolithic membrane**, housing small particles called **otoliths**.

3. Semicircular Canals, Semicircular Ducts, and Ampullae

The three bony **semicircular canals** are oriented perpendicular to each other. Within each canal is the endolymph-filled semicircular duct, the extensions of the membranous labyrinth. The base of each semicircular duct dilates as the **ampulla** which houses a **crista**, the sensory structure composed of neuroepithelial **hair cells** and **supporting cells**. A gelatinous **cupula** is located at the free surface of the crista, but it contains no otoliths.

Chapter Review Questions

Questions 20-1 to 20-3 refer to the following clinical scenario. A mixed martial art fighter presents to her doctor immediately after losing the bout because of a knockout kick to the left temple. The patient complains of ringing in her left ear and flashes of light in her left eye. During the MRI imaging session, the patient complains that she is unable to hear well from the left ear and reports altered vision in her left eye as though a dark curtain is blocking part of her visual field.

20-1. Which histologic alteration may explain the patient's vision changes?

   A. Hematoma pressing on the sympathetic nerve fibers

   B. Loosened suspensory ligament

   C. Narrowed diameter of the canal Schlemm

   D. Reopening of the intraretinal space

20-2. The MRI reveals fluid in the middle ear. Based on this imaging outcome, what is the likely cause of the hearing deficit?

   A. Endolymph buildup in the cochlear duct

   B. Dampened movements of ossicles

   C. Hematoma in the modiolus

   D. Inappropriate stimulation of maculae

20-3. Four weeks after the match, the hearing test reveals the return of most of her hearing except for the deficit in registering low-frequency sound. Which region of the ear may have acquired permanent damage?

   A. Cochlear duct near helicotrema

   B. Cochlear duct near the oval window

   C. Interface between the stapes and the oval window

   D. The round window

20-4. When a photon enters the eye, which layer of the retina does it encounter first?

   A. Inner limiting membrane

   B. Outer plexiform layer

   C. Photoreceptor layer

   D. Retinal pigment epithelium

20-5. Which sensory structure registers the angular motion of the head?

   A. Cristae ampullaris

   B. Helicotrema

   C. Maculae

   D. Organ of Corti

   E. Otolith

Appendix A

TISSUES THAT RESEMBLE EACH OTHER

Tissue are comprised of cells and extracellular matrix (ECM), and, depending on the proportions of different cell types and ECM components, distinct characteristics emerge in histologic images. Just as we can easily distinguish individuals, such as friends and family members, at first glance, a competent histology student has pattern recognition skills to do the same when looking at histologic images through the microscope, on digital devices, on papers, or in any other medium. However, just as with people, some tissues or organs resemble each other to such an extent that, at first glance, and sometimes even on closer observation, it is not so easy to tell them apart. Additionally, color differences between tissues, unless specifically designed to characterize particular tissue components, should be disregarded because the intensity of the dyes used may vary depending on tissue preparation procedures. Instead, features such as cellular morphologies, ECM distributions, and tissue architectural features should be examined to recognize the provenance of a particular sample. This Appendix is designed to illustrate tissues that closely resemble each other and specify how they may be distinguished from each other.

Each page of the Appendix has two to three images of histological look-alikes presented one above the other. The table next to each image identifies the tissue and highlights the differences in bullet points.

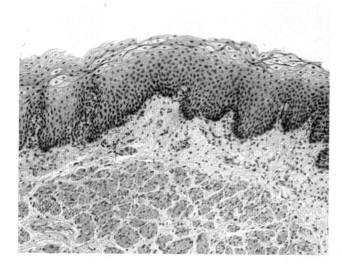

FIGURE A-1. Stratified nonkeratinized squamous epithelium.
- Several layers of epithelial cells
- Cells in the deeper layer are cuboidal
- The apical cells are flat with small, condensed nuclei

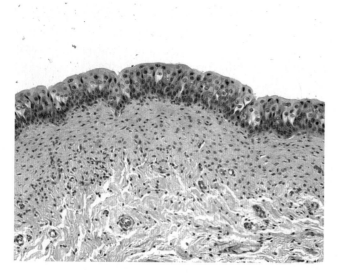

FIGURE A-2. Transitional epithelium.
- Fewer layers of epithelial cells than Figure A-1
- The apical layers have plump to dome-shaped cells
- Some of the apical cells are binucleate

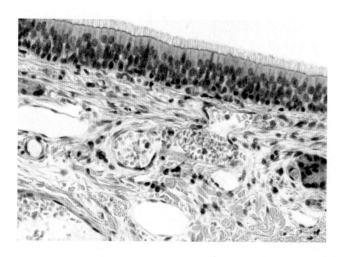

FIGURE A-3. Pseudostratified columnar epithelium.
- Single layer of diverse epithelial cell types all in contact with the basement membrane
- The nuclei are crowded and staggered, giving the stratified impression but they do not form even rows
- Apical compartments of the cells and the epithelia are often devoid of nuclei
- If present, cilia are a distinguishing feature

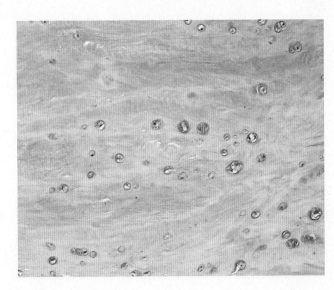

FIGURE A-4. Fibrocartilage.
- Round chondrocytes in lacunae arranged in more or less linear fashion
- Parallel arrays of type I collagen fibers separating rows of chondrocytes
- Occasional groups of chondrocytes in a lacuna may be present

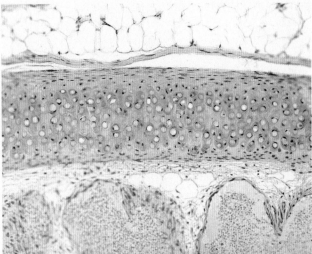

FIGURE A-5. Hyaline cartilage.
- Chondrocytes in lacunae are round in the middle and flatter in the periphery of the cartilage
- Homogeneous matrix but areas surrounding lacunae may stain darker
- Isogenous groups of chondrocytes in a lacuna may be observed more frequently than in Figure A-4

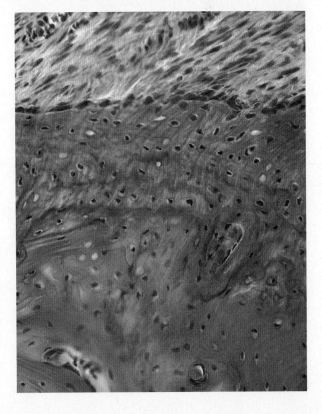

FIGURE A-6. Woven/primary/immature bone.
- Osteocytes in lacunae are not as rounded nor as pale staining
- Canaliculi connecting neighboring lacunae maybe observed
- Matrix is more eosinophilic with abundant type I collagen fibers, some organized into layers, some in haphazard arrangements
- Flat to cuboidal osteoblasts on the surface of the bone tissue maybe observed

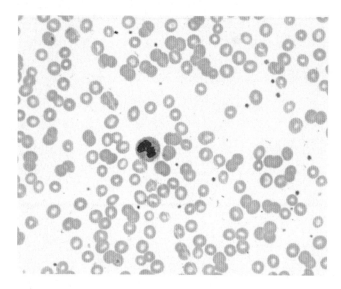

FIGURE A-7. Monocyte.
- Large cell
- Kidney-shaped nucleus
- Generally more euchromatic nucleus compared to Figure A-8
- Relatively large amount of cytoplasm

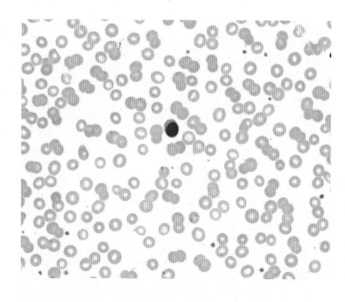

FIGURE A-8. Lymphocyte.
- Smaller cell than in Figure A-7
- Round, small, heterochromatic nucleus
- Scant cytoplasm
- Perinuclear clearing (Golgi apparatus) maybe observed

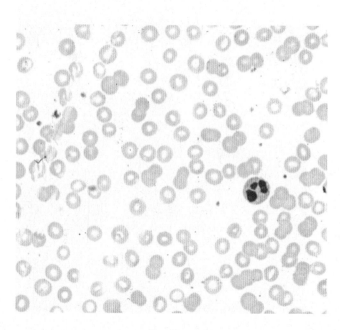

FIGURE A-9. Neutrophil.
- Size is in between monocyte and lymphocyte
- Three- to four-lobed, heterochromatic nuclei
- Good amount of cytoplasm
- Small granules maybe observed in the cytoplasm

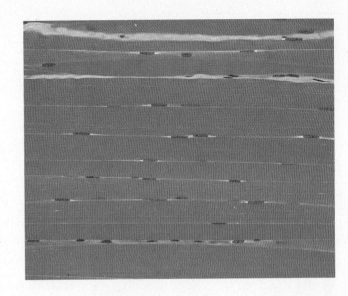

FIGURE A-10. Skeletal muscle (longitudinal section).
- Long, cylindrical, multinucleated cells arranged parallel to each other
- Nuclei are aligned at the periphery of the cell

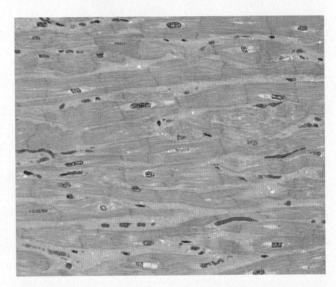

FIGURE A-11. Cardiac muscle (longitudinal section).
- Elongated, striated, branching cells that are not as long as those in Figure A-10
- Single or sometimes two nuclei positioned in the center
- Intercalated discs between cells
- Tissue as a whole is more vascular
- Pale-staining regions owing to glycogen storage observed in the cytoplasm
- Lipofuscin in cytoplasm maybe observed

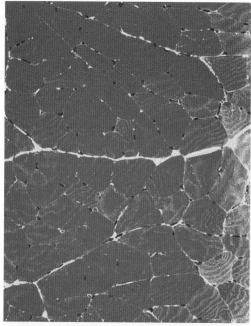

FIGURE A-12. Skeletal muscle (cross section).
- Large polygonal outline of skeletal muscle cells
- Flattened nuclei in the periphery
- Cytoplasm is densely filled with myofibrils

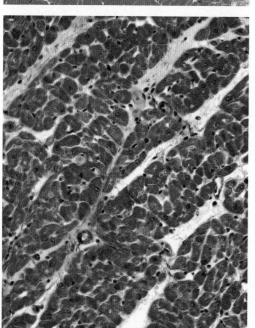

FIGURE A-13. Cardiac muscle (cross section).
- Irregularly shaped, heterogenous outline of cardiac muscle cells
- More vascularity
- Ovoid, more euchromatic nuclei toward the center of the cell
- Pale-staining regions owing to glycogen storage may be observed
- Lipofuscin inclusions may be observed

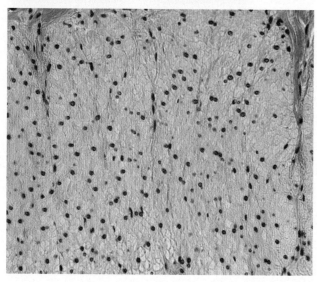

FIGURE A-14. Smooth muscle (cross section).
- Circular outlines of smooth muscle cells in different sizes are closely packed together
- Small, circular, condensed nuclei are in the center of some but not in every cross section

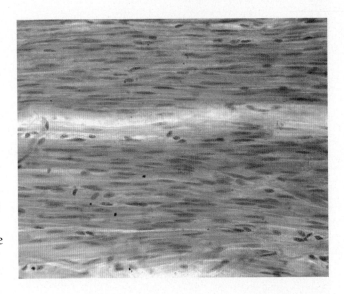

FIGURE A-15. Smooth muscle (longitudinal section).
- Spindle-shaped cells with spindle-shaped nuclei inside the cell boundary
- Usually do not exhibit wavy appearance as a whole

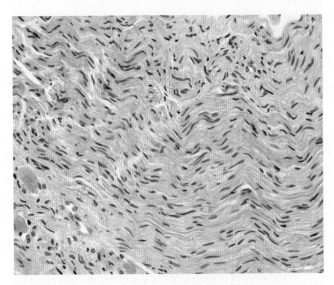

FIGURE A-16. Peripheral nerve (longitudinal section).
- Alternating darker- and pale-staining patterns owing to axons surrounded by myelin sheaths
- Flattened nuclei of varying size are in the periphery of the pale-staining myelin sheath
- May exhibit waviness
- Nodes of Ranvier may be observed

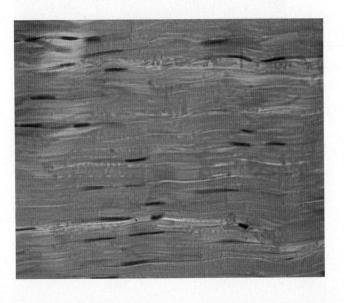

FIGURE A-17. Dense regular connective tissue (longitudinal section).
- Dense, noncellular, eosinophilic collagen fibers are arranged in parallel
- Flattened, dense nuclei of fibrocytes are positioned in between the fibers
- Not as cellular or vascular as those in Figures A-15 and A-16

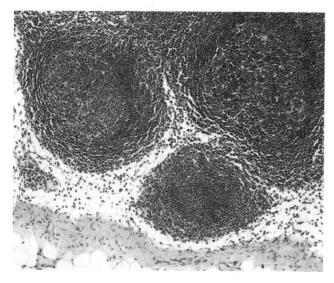

FIGURE A-18. Lymph node.
- Organized into cortex and medulla
- Subcapsular sinus is observed just deep to the dense connective tissue capsule
- Cortex is organized into outer cortex with lymphoid nodules and inner cortex without lymphoid nodules
- Medulla is organized into medullary cords and sinuses

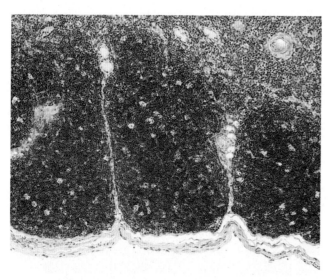

FIGURE A-19. Thymus.
- Organized into incomplete lobes, each with cortex and medulla
- Cortex stains dark owing to densely packed, small thymocytes, with sporadic pale-staining spots because of epithelial reticular cells and macrophages
- There are no lymphoid nodules
- Medulla stains lighter and houses thymic (Hassall's) corpuscles

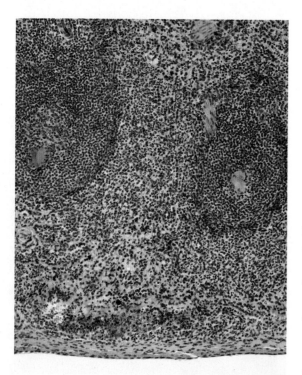

FIGURE A-20. Spleen.
- Organized into red and white pulps instead of cortex and medulla
- White pulp is comprised of lymphoid nodules with or without germinal centers
- Each lymphoid nodule (white pulp) has an associated central artery surrounded by periarterial lymphoid sheath
- Red pulp is organized into splenic cords and sinusoids

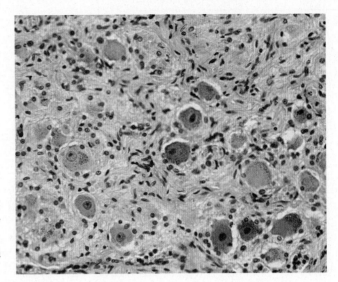

FIGURE A-21. Dorsal root (spinal) ganglion.
- Displays round, unipolar neuron cell bodies with centrally positioned nuclei
- Cuboidal to round satellite cells surround the neuron cell bodies

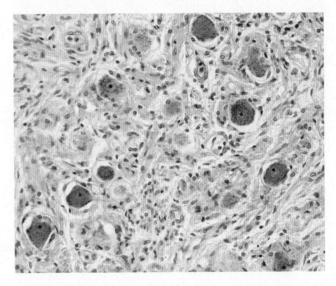

FIGURE A-22. Sympathetic ganglion.
- Displays slightly more angular cell bodies of the multipolar neurons with eccentrically positioned nuclei
- The supporting cells surrounding the neuron cell bodies are flattened

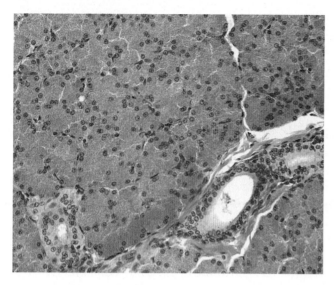

FIGURE A-23. Parotid gland.
- Compound acinar exocrine gland composed of serous acini
- Serous acini outnumber the cross-sectional profiles of ducts

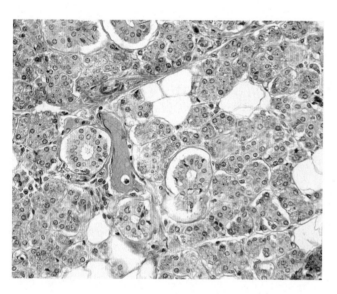

FIGURE A-24. Submandibular gland.
- Compound tubuloacinar exocrine gland
- Secretory units are mostly serous acini with minor mucous tubules and serous demilunes
- There are more cross-sectional profiles of ducts than in Figure A-23

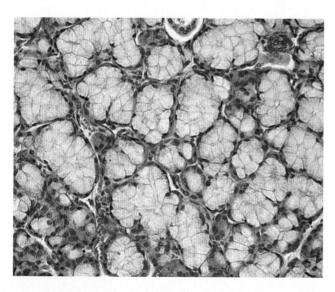

FIGURE A-25. Sublingual gland.
- Compound tubuloacinar exocrine gland
- Secretory units are mostly mucous tubules with minor serous acini and serous demilunes
- There are more cross-sectional profiles of ducts than in Figure A-23

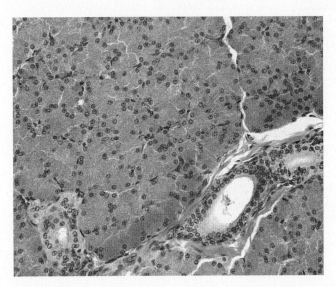

FIGURE A-26. Parotid gland.
- Compound acinar exocrine gland composed of serous acini
- Serous acini outnumber the cross-sectional profiles of ducts

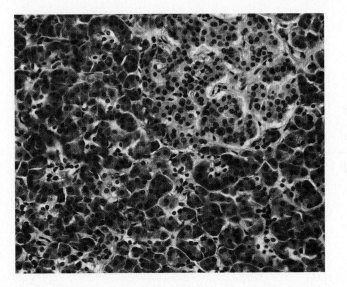

FIGURE A-27. Pancreas.
- Both exocrine and endocrine gland
- Exocrine component is compound acinar exocrine gland
- There are centroacinar cells with dense nuclei and clear cytoplasm
- There are no striated ducts
- Pancreatic islets (of Langerhans) are vascular, have no ducts, and are surrounded by a thin capsule

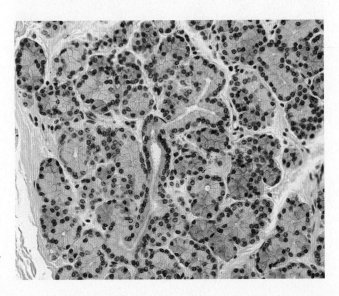

FIGURE A-28. Lacrimal gland.
- Compound tubuloacinar exocrine gland
- Secretory units are mostly serous acini with larger lumina than those of the parotid gland

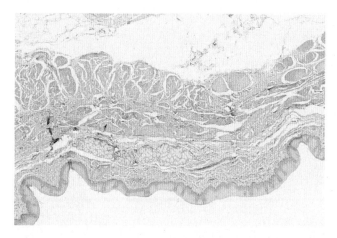

FIGURE A-29. Esophagus.

- Lined by a nonkeratinized stratified squamous epithelium, which is thinner than that in Figures A-30 and A-31
- Displays a proper four-layer organization
- Houses esophageal glands in the submucosa

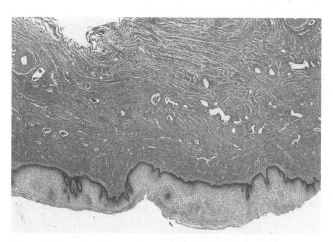

FIGURE A-30. Vagina.

- Lined by a nonkeratinized stratified squamous epithelium, which is thicker than that in Figure A-29
- Epithelial cells appear plumper and vacuolated owing to lipids and glycogen storage, which are extracted during tissue preparation
- The tissue layers are not as distinctive but instead are comprised of a mixture of collagen, elastic, and smooth muscle fibers
- There are no glands
- Lamina propria is richly endowed with lymphoid cells

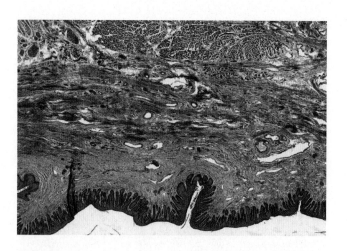

FIGURE A-31. Anal canal.

- Lined by a nonkeratinized stratified squamous epithelium, which is thicker than in Figure A-29
- Organized into four layers, but it is not as distinct as in Figure A-29
- There are no submucosal glands
- In the vicinity, rectal mucosa and keratinized stratified squamous epithelium of the anus may be observed

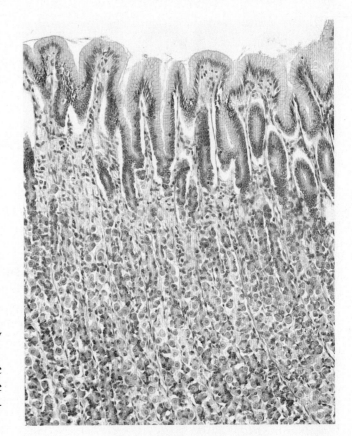

FIGURE A-32. Fundus of the stomach.

- Displays long, parallel gastric glands and relatively shallow gastric pits
- Gastric glands possess chief cells (concentrated in the base) and parietal cells (concentrated in the middle portion), diffuse neuroendocrine system cells, mucous neck cells, and stem cells

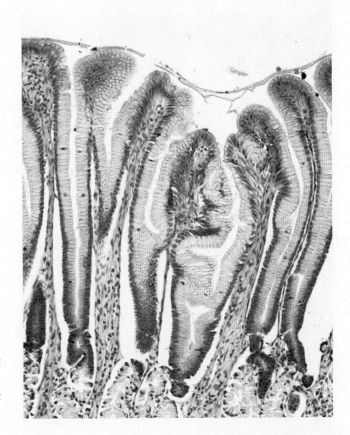

FIGURE A-33. Pylorus of the stomach.

- Displays much deeper and somewhat coiled gastric pits and coiled gastric glands
- The glands manufacture a mucous substance and have no chief cells and only a few parietal cells

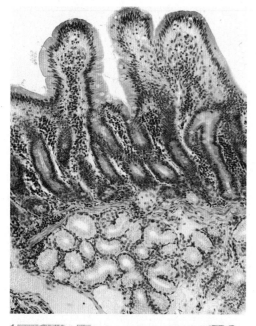

FIGURE A-34. Duodenum.
- Displays blunt villi
- Houses compound tubular exocrine glands known as the duodenal (Brunner's) glands in the submucosa

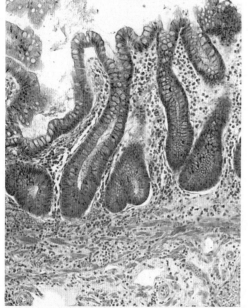

FIGURE A-35. Jejunum.
- Displays tall, well-developed villi
- Epithelial cells are mostly enterocytes proximally, but the goblet cells increase distally
- Possesses the most well-developed plicae circularis
- Has neither submucosal glands nor prominent lymphoid nodules

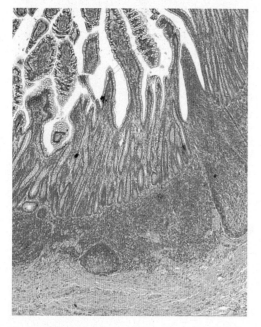

FIGURE A-36. Ileum.
- Displays long, narrower villi
- Goblet cells increase in the epithelial lining
- Possesses large and abundant lymphoid nodules, Peyer's patches, in the lamina propria that may extend into the submucosa

FIGURE A-37. Colon.

- Has a large diameter and much larger lumen compared to the small intestine or the appendix (same magnification as Figure A-38)
- Its mucosa and submucosa maybe thrown into folds, but these are not permanent structures
- There are no villi
- There are abundant simple tubular exocrine glands in the lamina propria
- Outer longitudinal layer of muscularis externa forms taeniae coli

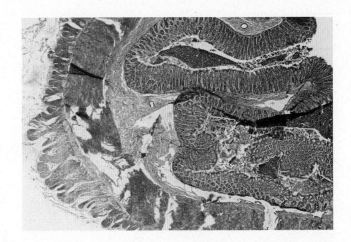

FIGURE A-38. Appendix.

- Much smaller tube with a narrow lumen (same magnification as Figure A-37)
- Mucosa resembles the colonic mucosa, but there are far fewer glands
- Displays numerous lymphoid nodules in the lamina propria that may extend into the submucosa
- The outer longitudinal layer of muscularis externa does not form taeniae coli but, instead, is uniform in thickness

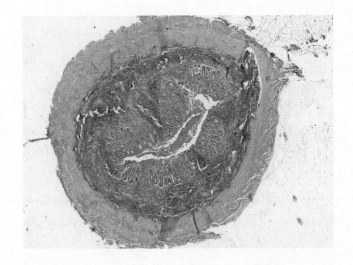

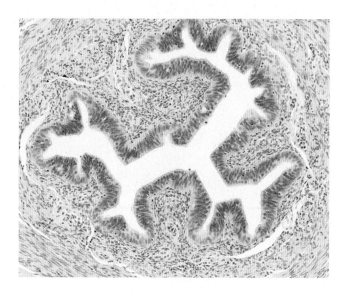

FIGURE A-39. Uterine tube.

- Lined by ciliated simple columnar epithelium composed of peg cells and ciliated cells

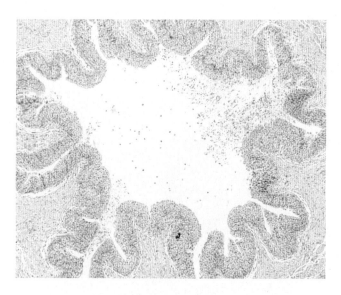

FIGURE A-40. Ureter.

- Lined by transitional epithelium

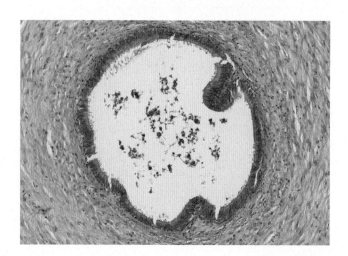

FIGURE A-41. Vas deferens.

- Lined by pseudostratified columnar epithelium with cells that possess stereocilia

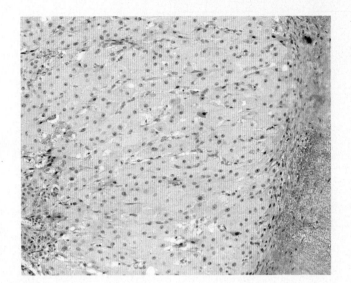

FIGURE A-42. Corpus luteum.

- Has two types of parenchymal cells surrounded by ovarian stroma
- The larger and more abundant granulosa lutein cells are arranged in cords
- The smaller, spindle-shaped theca lutein cells are wedged in between the cords and in the periphery

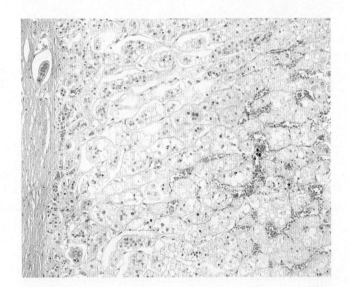

FIGURE A-43. Adrenal cortex.

- Organized into three regions, from superficial to deep: zona glomerulosa, zona fasciculata, and zona reticularis (not shown in this figure)
- Cells of the zona fasciculata, the spongiocytes, are arranged in parallel columns

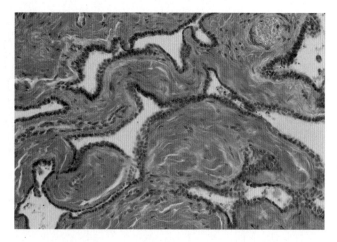

FIGURE A-44. Rete testis.

- Irregular channels lined by a mixture of epithelial lining of simple cuboidal, pseudostratified columnar, and stratified columnar type
- Surrounded by dense irregular connective tissue of the mediastina testis

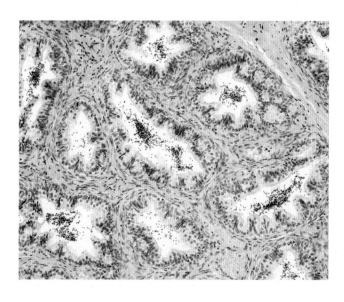

FIGURE A-45. Ductuli efferentes.

- Displays a fluted (uneven) lumen owing to the epithelial lining composed of patches of tall cells alternating with patches of short cells

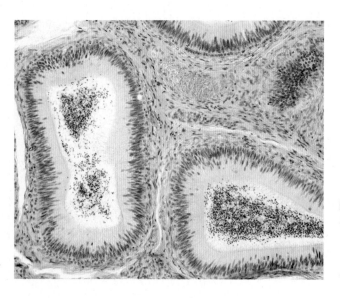

FIGURE A-46. Ductus epididymis.

- Displays regular lumina lined by pseudostratified columnar epithelium whose principal cells are uniform in size
- Stereocilia are prominent and characteristic

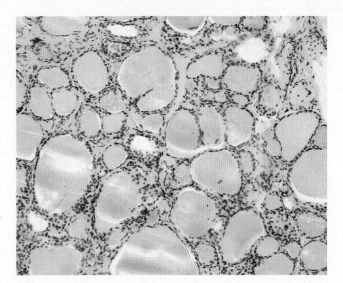

FIGURE A-47. Thyroid gland.
- Composed of colloid-filled follicles
- Thyroid lacks ducts and lobular organization
- Lining epithelium may vary between simple cuboidal to simple columnar epithelia depending on the activity level of the thyroid
- Pale parafollicular cells may be intermixed in the follicular lining and in between the follicles

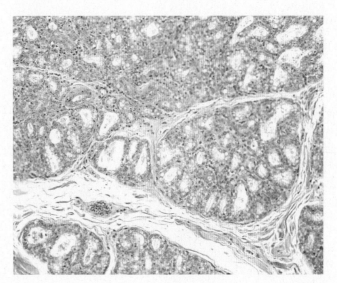

FIGURE A-48. Lactating mammary gland.
- Compound tubuloalveolar exocrine gland organized into lobules and lobes
- Alveoli display branching and may contain milk, not colloid
- System of ducts are present
- Simple cuboidal epithelium comprises the secretory units
- Myoepithelial cells are associated with secretory units and the ducts

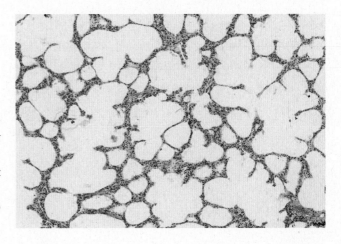

FIGURE A-49. Lung.
- Spherical alveoli are lined by simple squamous epithelium and filled with air, not colloid or secretory products
- Several alveoli opening into the common alveolar sac or alveolar duct may be observed
- Connective tissue stroma and vasculature are limited to the thin alveolar septa

Appendix B
ANSWERS TO CHAPTER REVIEW QUESTIONS

Chapter 2

2-1. D
2-2. A
2-3. B
2-4. C
2-5. D

Chapter 3

3-1. D
3-2. B
3-3. A
3-4. A
3-5. A

Chapter 4

4-1. C
4-2. A
4-3. C
4-4. B
4-5. C

Chapter 5

5-1. D
5-2. C
5-3. A
5-4. C
5-5. A

Chapter 6

6-1. B
6-2. C
6-3. E
6-4. D
6-5. D

Chapter 7

7-1. B
7-2. C
7-3. E
7-4. C
7-5. B

Chapter 8

8-1. E
8-2. B
8-3. A
8-4. B
8-5. E

Chapter 9

9-1. C
9-2. A
9-3. E
9-4. C
9-5. C

Chapter 10

10-1. B
10-2. D
10-3. E
10-4. A
10-5. D

Chapter 11

11-1. B
11-2. E
11-3. A
11-4. B
11-5. C

Chapter 12
12-1. B
12-2. C
12-3. C
12-4. D
12-5. C

Chapter 13
13-1. B
13-2. C
13-3. C
13-4. D
13-5. C

Chapter 14
14-1. C
14-2. D
14-3. A
14-4. D
14-5. A

Chapter 15
15-1. A
15-2. C
15-3. B
15-4. B
15-5. D

Chapter 16
16-1. B
16-2. B
16-3. C
16-4. E
16-5. D

Chapter 17
17-1. D
17-2. A
17-3. B
17-4. A
17-5. C

Chapter 18
18-1. B
18-2. A
18-3. B
18-4. E
18-5. A

Chapter 19
19-1. C
19-2. D
19-3. A
19-4. A
19-5. E

Chapter 20
20-1. D
20-2. B
20-3. A
20-4. A
20-5. A

Index

(*Note*: Page numbers in *italics* denote figures; those followed by "t" denote tables)